Pregnancy and Childbirth

'for my children; in binding me to the earth, they freed me to fly'
Suzanne Yates

For Elsevier

Publisher: Sarena Wolfaard
Development Editor: Helen Leng
Project Manager: Nayagi Athmanathan / Anne Dickie
Designer/Design Direction: Charles Gray
Illustration Manager: Bruce Hogarth
Illustrator: Diane Mercer

Pregnancy and Childbirth

A holistic approach to massage and bodywork

Suzanne Yates BA(Hons) DipHSEC MRSS(T) APNT PGCE(PCET)
Shiatsu and massage therapist, and childbirth educator
Director of Well Mother-Education for Maternity Care, Bristol, UK

Foreword by
Michele Kolakowski BA RMT CD(DONA) CIMI
Registered Massage Therapist, Certified Birth Doula (DONA), Certified Infant Massage Instructor
Supervisor, Health Center of Integrated Therapies, Longmont United Hospital
Co-Developer & Faculty, Cortiva Institute Maternity and Infant Massage Program
Colorado, USA

Penny Bussell Stansfield BA (Hons) LMT CD(DONA) CCE
Licensed Massage Therapist, Certified Birth Doula and Doula Trainer (DONA), Certified Childbirth Educator
Co-Developer & Faculty, Cortiva Institute Maternity and Infant Massage Program
New Jersey, USA

Photographers Sherrie Keuhlein and Amanda Hartman

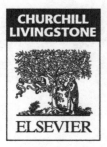

CHURCHILL LIVINGSTONE

ELSEVIER

Edinburgh London New York Oxford Philadelphia St Louis Sydney Toronto 2010

CHURCHILL
LIVINGSTONE
ELSEVIER

First published 2010, © Elsevier Limited. All rights reserved.

ISBN 978-0-7020-3055-0

British Library Cataloguing in Publication Data
A catalogue record for this book is available from the British Library

Library of Congress Cataloging in Publication Data
A catalog record for this book is available from the Library of Congress

Notice
Neither the publisher nor the author assumes any responsibility for any loss or injury and/or damage to persons or property arising out of or related to any use of the material contained in this book. It is the responsibility of the treating practitioner, relying on independent expertise and knowledge of the patient, to determine the best treatment and method of application for the patient.

The Publisher

ELSEVIER   your source for books,
journals and multimedia
in the health sciences
www.elsevierhealth.com

Working together to grow
libraries in developing countries

www.elsevier.com | www.bookaid.org | www.sabre.org

ELSEVIER   BOOK AID
International   Sabre Foundation

The Publisher's policy is to use paper manufactured from sustainable forests

Printed in China

Contents

Foreword

In 2006, we collaborated with teachers across the United States to create a comprehensive curriculum in pregnancy, labor, postpartum massage and bodywork. At the time, it was challenging to find one reference book that provided everything we needed-rich multicultural perspectives on the most common of miracles; the requisite depth and detail on the complex maternal transformations and the accompanying embryological/fetal development; possible deviations from healthy changes with complications, high risk conditions and unexpected outcomes; a treasure trove of massage therapy and bodywork techniques; professional issues to prepare practitioners to work effectively in a variety of venues; and most importantly, the wisdom of holistic care for childbearing women. Suzanne Yates has achieved this and taken massage and bodywork to a new level with her new book, 'Pregnancy and Childbirth – A Holistic Approach to Massage and Bodywork.'

Readers will benefit from an impressive compilation of Suzanne's twenty years of study and experience, plus additional contributions from maternity care specialists around the world. Suzanne brilliantly combines Eastern and Western theories and techniques in one book that offers maternity care specialists an unsurpassed spectrum of treatment options to meet each woman's unique needs throughout her pregnancy, childbirth and postpartum time. 'Pregnancy and Childbirth – A Holistic Approach to Massage and Bodywork' has the essential information that massage therapists, bodyworkers and other maternity care providers need to inform, guide and expand their practices. Experienced maternity care veterans will also benefit from the profound depth and detail that makes this book an indispensable reference guide.

In Section 1, Suzanne thoroughly details both Eastern and Western theories of the fascinating maternal changes as well as embryological/fetal development. This provides a solid foundation of knowledge and understanding for the reader to build upon. Section 2 contains a thorough overview of the practical application of massage therapy and bodywork with case studies, open dialogues on controversial topics such as leg and abdominal massage, guidelines for working with higher risk maternity clients, personal patient stories and insightful professional issues. We are thrilled to see breast massage, perineum care and scar tissue recovery included, as they are also important aspects of holistic maternity care. Readers will further benefit from each chapter's reflective questions, summary of implications, excellent references and further recommended reading to engage their critical thinking skills and further their studies.

'Pregnancy and Childbirth – A Holistic Approach to Massage and Bodywork' is certainly one of the 'bibles' for maternity care specialists, and we are delighted to have it as an essential book in our professional libraries, at the hospitals and clinics where we work and in the maternity massage classroom. Thank you Suzanne for elevating maternity massage and bodywork to a higher level. It brings us great joy to think of all the maternity care providers, the women and babies around the world who will benefit from the caring, skilled touch so beautifully shared in this exquisite book!

Michele Kolakowski & Penny Bussell Stansfield

Acknowledgements

This book has truly been a collaborative effort: from the early ideas for the project, to the writing and the editing and final stages of production. In addition to those listed as contributors and to the wonderful team at Elsevier who have given me fantastic support and advice from the conception of this book, many other people have also been involved. I would especially like to thank the models for the photographs: Clare Sandham and baby Donny, Tanya Meyers, Cynthia Grundmann, Caroline Martin, Pamela Hammond, Natalie Zinman and Robyn Sanford. Also my thanks to those clients and bodyworkers who contributed their testimonials of the value of bodywork.

Some other people not listed as contributors have also made some contributions to the text: Jan Carusone (of massage suppliers Know Your Body Best, Toronto), Fi Mazurka (medical herbalist and massage therapist), Alice Lyon (midwife) and Chris Andrews (midwife/chiropractor). Debra Betts (acupuncturist) was helpful in discussing many of the ideas and in suggesting contributors. Nicola Endicott, Anne Badger and Heidi Armstrong, my co-teachers, made invaluable comments from a reader's point of view, as did my administrator Becky Matthews.

And in the background were many others who have helped with the development of this text:

My other co-teachers who in recent years have helped me expand and develop my work.

Becky Matthews who did my admin so I had time to write the book.

Sponsors of my courses, especially those who had faith in my work during the early days. In particular: Gill Tree of Essentials for Health, London who helped me develop the Pregnancy Massage Diploma for her school and where I continue to teach introductory days; Marina Morton of the Shambahla Shiatsu School in Vienna who brought my work to an Austrian audience, translating both my course handouts and my teaching and Birgit Fromm-Leichtfried who has also helped with the translations; Gina Debrito and Laure Huret who brought my work to France, Gina for organising the courses and Laure for translation of the course materials; Patricia Carusone of the sadly now defunct Boston School and Jenny Dorrington, director of the Australian Shiatsu College, Jane Brennan of the Wellington School of Massage Therapy and all the other people who have organised courses for me over the years.

My massage teachers, from my early informal teaching in the early 1980s to the Maitri Foundation near Stroud where I did my diploma. My shiatsu teachers, especially Sonia Moriceau who encouraged me to teach shiatsu and more recently Kazunori Sasaki Sensei who helped me contact more directly the work of Masunaga and Kawada Yuichi Sensei who validated much of my work with the Extraordinary Vessels. Elizabeth Noble, with whom I trained in Boston in 1989 who set me on the path of integrating exercise into my bodywork; she was an early source of inspiration in setting up Well Mother.

My children, Rosa and Bram, who for years put up with my sitting up in the attic writing; they brought me into this work and I hope they have not suffered too much from my dedication to it!

All of my students, without whom I would never have developed my work. Firstly the pregnant women to whom I taught weekly ante- and postnatal classes in Bristol from 1990 to 2002 and later my professional (midwives, massage and shiatsu therapy) students, from 1998. And last, but by certainly no means least, the many hundreds of pregnant women with whom I have had the honour to work individually during their pregnancies, sometimes attending their births, and supporting them in their new lives with their partners and babies. They make it all worthwhile.

Picture credits

The following images have been redrawn with permission.

Chapter 1

Figures 1.1, 1.2, 1.3, 1.5A and B, 1.6, 1.7, 1.8, 1.9 Henderson, C., Macdonald, S., 2004. Mayes' Midwifery: A Textbook for Midwives, thirteenth ed. Baillère Tindall, Edinburgh. **Figures 1.10, 1.12, 1.14** Coad, J., Dunstall, M., 2001. Anatomy and Physiology for Midwives. Mosby, Edinburgh. **Figures 1.13** Moore, K.L., Persaud, T.V.N., 2008. Before We Are Born, seventh edn. Saunders, Philadelphia.

Chapter 2

Figures 2.1, 2.4 Coad, J., Dunstall, M., 2001. Anatomy and Physiology for Midwives, Mosby, Edinburgh. **Figures 2.3A-C, 2.5A and B, 2.6, 2.8, 2.9, 2.10A and B, 2.11, 2.12, 2.13, 2.14** Henderson, C., Macdonald, S., 2004. Mayes' Midwifery: A Textbook for Midwives, thirteenth ed. Baillère Tindall, Edinburgh.

Chapter 3

Figures 3.1A and B Coad, J., Dunstall, M., 2001. Anatomy and Physiology for Midwives. Mosby, Edinburgh.

Chapter 4

Figures 4.1, 4.3, 4.4, 4.5, 4.6 Maciocia, G., 2006. The Channels of Acupuncture. Churchill Livingstone, Edinburgh. **Figure 4.2** Yates, S., 2003. Shiatsu for Midwives. Books for Midwives, Oxford.

Chapter 9

Figures 9.23, 9.33 Yates, S., 2003. Shiatsu for Midwives. Books for Midwives, Oxford.

Chapter 10

Figures 10.2, 10.3, 10.4, 10.5, 10.6, 10.7, 10.8, 10.9, 10.10, 10.11A, 10.11B, 10.12, 10.13, 10.14 Yates, S., 2003. Shiatsu for Midwives. Books for Midwives, Oxford.

Chapter 12

Figure 12.2 Yates, S., 2003. Shiatsu for Midwives. Books for Midwives, Oxford.

Chapter 14

Figure 14.1 Henderson, C., Macdonald, S., 2004. Mayes' Midwifery: A Textbook for Midwives, thirteenth ed. Baillère Tindall, Edinburgh.

Preface

When I first had the vision for this text, which was even before writing *Shiatsu for Midwives*, I wanted it to be a 'Bible' for bodyworkers. It would be the bodywork equivalent of *Mayes Midwifery*. It would include everything that a bodyworker could possibly need to inform their practice! After 6 years of writing, however, I now realise how ambitious a plan that was. *Mayes Midwifery* is in its thirteenth edition and has been enriched over many years by the contributions and experience of numerous practitioners. This is only the first edition of this text, but none the less I have endeavoured to enrich it through the contributions of several workers and experts in the field. I offer it humbly as a textbook on bodywork which has more depth than any texts published on this subject so far, but which I am sure can be developed and improved.

I regret that for reasons of space I had to omit some of my passions, such as preconceptual care and work with the newborn. Although others have made their contributions to this text, for which I am eternally grateful, the ultimate responsibility for any unintended inaccuracies or misrepresentations is entirely mine as the main writer.

I hope that this text helps the process of bodyworkers taking their place in the provision of maternity care in the 21st century. In order to do that we need to be able to demonstrate that we have not only sound knowledge of the suitability of techniques but also a detailed knowledge of anatomy and physiology and of the medical approach. If we are working with eastern approaches, we need to have a detailed grasp of that theory. We are not going to be taken seriously, either by primary care providers or by women themselves, if we cannot demonstrate the soundness of our knowledge.

For too long we have accepted texts and courses of inadequate quality. How ridiculous it is to assume that anyone can learn about pregnancy in a 1- or 2-day course, when midwives train for 3 years or more. The need for more rigorous training courses is gradually being acknowledged by the industry. This text is not intended to be a substitute for training, but rather to complement courses: to enable therapists to identify appropriate courses and then provide information to support them in their training. Ultimately this text cannot stand alone and needs to be supported by relevant changes in training and in ongoing professional development and research. There are still areas where more research and understanding needs to be developed, areas for discussion and ongoing collaboration and continued learning from different practices of bodywork in different cultures worldwide.

When I think back to my early work in the field I can see that on some levels I did not really know what I was doing. I had an open heart, a desire to learn and connect with the women I was working with, a passion and enthusiasm for the work and a desire to make a difference. However, I wish I knew then what I know now, 20 years later. This is why I have written this book: to share the knowledge which I have built up from many different sources, courses, reading, study and most of all the hundreds of mothers I have worked with, the hundreds of therapists and the thousands of women they jointly have worked with.

As we move on through this new century, I see a great future for the use of bodywork in maternity care. One day I hope that bodywork will be part of mainstream care, as indeed, it once was in many traditional cultures. As more midwives begin to integrate different therapies into their practice, so more research will emerge about their effectiveness. In our infatuation with modern technological medicine, we have moved away from the original forms of touch-based healing, seeing them as primitive and ineffective. It is true that not all aspects of traditional healing should be kept and that many aspects of modern medicine are fundamental to the care we expect. This is not a time to return to the past, nor a time for 'either, or', but a time to move forward and to integrate the best aspects of both approaches.

My principal aim remains simple: to enable women to connect with their bodies and their babies at this fundamental time in their lives. Ultimately this connection makes a difference to us all.

'For the first time since I've been pregnant, I felt totally OK to be me, supported and even happy to be going through all the issues I am dealing with at the moment ... thank you for all the work and inspiration you give in this field; it's a good way to influence our world'
(Pregnant shiatsu student)

Suzanne Yates, Bristol

Contributors

Primary contributor

Cindy McNeely MT
Registered Massage Therapist
Ontario, Canada
Trimesters: Massage Therapy Education
Ontario, Canada
Collaborated with the overall planning of the book and advised on all practical sections.
2 Western approach to labour.
14 Working with higher-risk maternity clients

Contributors

Yosef (Jon) Barrett MBBCh MD FRCSC FRCOG
Obstetrician
Chief Maternal Fetal Medicine and Program
Research Director
Sunnybrook Health Sciences Center
Toronto, Canada
2 Western approach to labour

Jacky Bloemraad-de Boer LicAc CertReflex OrthoNut DiplBWM Doula Cert
Obstetric Acupuncture Practice in Association with
Amsterdam Midwifery Centre
Amsterdam
The Netherlands
2 Western approach to labour
6 Eastern approach to labour

Jane Coad BSc PhD PGCEA
Associate Professor of Human Nutrition,
Massey University
Institute of Food, Nutrition & Human Health
Palmerston North New Zealand
1 Western approach to pregnancy

Michael Dooley MMs FRCOG FFFP MBBS
Obstetrician
The Poundbury Clinic
Dorchester, UK
3 Western approach to the postpartum

Rhiannon Harris
Clinical Aromatherapist
Co-director of Essential Oil Resource Consultants
Editor of the International Journal of Clinical
Aromatherapy
La Martre, Provence, France
8.8 Section on the primary role of aromatherapy in maternity care

Sandra Hill MA(Fine Art), BAc(ICOM)
Acupuncturist and Shiatsu Therapist
Visiting Lecturer Westminster University,
School of Integrated Health;
Postgraduate Teaching College of Integrated
Chinese Medicine;
MSc Program College of Traditional Acupuncture
London, UK
5 Eastern approach to pregnancy

Caroline Martin RMT DipMT DipSIM
Registered Massage Therapist
Part-time Massage Therapy Instructor,
Centennial College
Owner and Operator of Martin Therapy Services Ltd
Ontario, Canada
Practical bodywork in pregnancy, labour, the postpartum
8.2 Orthopaedic assessment and the maternity client

Averille Morgan MSc BAppSc(Osteo)
Osteopath
Lecturer in obstetric osteopathy for postgraduate
pathways in London and Paris
Masters programmes in Munich and Barcelona
Section 1 Theory Advisor on some sections
Section 2 Practical bodywork Advisor on some sections

Lea Papworth MTCM DiplAcu DiplCHM RM
Acupuncturist, Chinese herbalist and registered
midwife
Hawthorn
South Australia
2 Western approach to labour
6 Eastern approach to labour
7 Eastern approach to the postpartum

Glossary

Western terms

amenorrhoea absence of periods/menstruation

anabolic building up of cells

angiogenesis growth

aponeurosis layers of flat connective tissue (fascia) between muscles

asynclitic when the fetal head is angled going into the pelvis so that only one parietal bone presents in the pelvis

autolysis breaking down of muscle fibres

blastocyst early cells from fertilised egg

Braxton Hicks contractions painless contractions measurable from first trimester

CAPs contraction-associated proteins

catabolic breaking down of cells

cephalo pelvic disproportion (CPD) when the fetal head (cephalo) is too big for the woman (pelvic)

chloasma gravidarum darker patches of skin over forehead and arm

cholelithiasis gallstones

cornus top of the uterus

decidua part of uterine lining, endometrium which forms part of the placenta

diatasis separation

diuresis increased urination

dystocia dysfunctional labour. Shoulder dystocia – when the shoulders of the baby gets stuck at delivery

embryoblast early cells which will develop into the embryo

endometrium the inner lining of the uterus in pregnancy

fetal heart rates/tones (FHR/FHT)

follicle the group of cells containing the egg

galactopoiesis maintenance of breastfeeding

gap junction proteins

haemangioma benign tumours which will disappear, formed from endothelial cells (i.e. cells lining blood vessels) so red in appearance

haemolysis breaking open of red blood cells

hyperaemia lack of blood

hyperaemic blood congestion

hypervolaemia fluid overload

hypocapnia reduced CO_2 in blood

hypotonia lack of muscle tone

intrapartum the period during labour

involution return of organs to pre pregnant state

ischaemia constrictions of blood flow

Kraamverzorgester the name of the helper in Holland who comes for the first week to 10 days postpartum to help the mother

lactogenesis initiation of breastfeeding

leucorrhoea thick whitish vaginal discharge

linea nigra dark line of skin pigmentation in the centre of the abdomen

lithotomy supine position in labour in stirrups

LUS lower uterine segment

macrocosmia large fetus

meconium fetal faecal excretion

morula early cells from fertilised egg

mucorrhoea clear mucous discharge

multipara woman with a second or subsequent pregnancy

myometrium middle layer of the uterus

natriuresis excretion of sodium

nocturia waking in the night due to need to urinate

oocyte the egg

operculum plug of mucus covering cervix

partogram chart to measure progress in labour

perimetrium also outer layer and forms broad ligament

perinatal the period around labour, before, during and the immediate postpartum

peritoneum outer layer of the uterus

polycythaemia more red blood cells in the blood

primapara woman with her first pregnancy

ptaylism increased salivation

retraction when the uterine muscle lengthens again after a contraction but not back to its original length prior to the contraction, i.e. it retains some of the shortened length

salpingitus inflammation of the fallopian tube

stenosis narrowing, e.g. of blood vessel

trophoblast early cells which will develop into the placenta

UUS upper uterine segment

vascularisation blood flow

vasoconstriction constriction of blood flow

zygote early cluster of cells from fertilised egg

Eastern terms

Blood nutritive energy; blood flows in blood vessels but also in meridians and vessels.

cun Chinese measurement of one thumb width to measure point location

Extraordinary Vessels core meridians which regulate Jing and Qi.

fundus top portion of uterus

hyperemesis extreme vomiting

Jing/Essence fluid-like substance which is the source of life. The most dense material manifestation of Qi.

Meridians energy pathways in the body which circulate Qi and organ energy.

olighydramnio insufficient amnitotic fluid

polyhydramnios excessive amniotic fluid

pruritis localised itching

Qi invisible energy in the body, creative principle, life's animating force.

Shen the spirit of a person.

Tao the whole.

Tsubos points along the meridians.

Yin and Yang the two main forces in the universe:
Yin – earth, night, more inward moving, resting/forming, contraction
Yang – heaven, day, more outward moving, active/transforming, expansion.

Abbreviations

ARM artificial rupture of the membranes
ASIS anterior superior iliac spine
BP blood pressure
CPD cephalo pelvic disproportion
CTG cardiotocograph
CTS carpal tunnel syndrome
CVsystem Cardiovascular system
dBP sBP diastolic or systolic blood pressure
DIC disseminated intravascular coagulation
DVT deep vein thrombosis
FBS fetal blood sampling
FSH follicle stimulating hormone
GA general anaesthesia
GDM gestational diabetes mellitus
GI gastrointestinal
hcG human chorionic gonadrotrophin
HELLP haemolysis, elevated liver enzymes and low platelet count
IVF in vitro fertilisation
L Lumbar
LH lutenizing hormone
LOA ROA left or right occiput anterior
LOP LOP left or right occiput posterior
LOT ROT left or right occiput transverse
LSCS lower section caesarean section
LUS lower uterine section
MET muscle energy technique
NMT neuro muscular technique
OC obstetric cholestasis
PCOS polycystic ovary syndrome
PE pulmonary embolism
PET pre eclampsia/toxaemia
PGI pelvic girdle instability
PIH pregnancy induced hypertension
PUPPS pruritic urticarial papules and plaques of pregnancy

RLS restless leg syndrome
ROM range of motion
SGA or LGA small or large for gestational age
SHS supine hypotensive syndrome
SIJ sacro iliac joint
SPL symphysis pubis laxity
T thoracic
TED thrombo emobolitic disease
TFL tensor fascia lata
TMJ temporo mandibular joint
TOS thoracic outlet syndrome
UTI urinary tract infection
VBAC vaginal birth after caesarean

Meridians
BL Bladder
GB Gall Bladder
HP Heart Protector
HT Heart
KD Kidney
LI Large Intestine
LU Lung
LV Liver
SI Small Intestine
SP Spleen
ST Stomach
TH Triple Heater

Extraordinary vessels
CV Conception Vessel
GDV Girdle Vessel
GV Governing Vessel
PV Penetrating Vessel

Introduction

Working with pregnant women is not simply about adapting normal bodywork techniques as there is a particular 'energetics' of pregnancy. This is why we have described the eastern and western theoretical views of pregnancy in so much detail. Together, they offer a way of looking at the body which can lead to a better understanding of the most appropriate practical approach for each client.

The book is divided into two sections: a theoretical section and a practical section. The two sections are designed to be read separately but the reader can cross-refer from one to the other, as relevant. The theoretical section is itself divided into two, describing western and eastern approaches. The practical section draws together eastern and western approaches by integrating them into ideas on how to work with the different areas of the body.

The theory is separated into eastern and western approaches because this reflects the fact that the theories have evolved separately, but we hope that at some point in the future they may blend together to become an holistic way of looking at the body. Indeed this is already happening. Quantum physics and biology are moving towards some aspects of traditional Chinese medicine such as the idea of a unified energy field, which is essentially the Tao. As this happens then we hope that eastern and western healing traditions can merge to provide integrated medical care.

The eastern theory described is based on traditional Chinese theory, partly because this is the theory with which the authors are most familiar and partly because it is a traditional medical system which has survived to the present day intact and uninterrupted. However, there are other traditional medicines worldwide which have contained and contain similar themes. For example, the role of the healer in many societies has been primarily to support health in order to prevent disease. The theory was usually based on observing patterns in nature and applying them to the body. We hope that whatever discipline therapists work with, they will find relevant and useful ideas in this book.

We have sometimes made reference to the differences between traditional cultures and modern cultures. We are aware that a whole book can be written on this huge subject, but rather than individually note the many thousands of examples of different traditional practices worldwide, we are talking in general terms about traditional cultures being based more on people living closer to the cycles and rhythms of nature. Of course, there are many variations in these types of cultures and this is expressed in both positive and negative aspects. We do not want to unduly glorify traditional culture per se, as there may be aspects which are not beneficial; however, we feel that some practices are worth noting and it is valuable to reflect on how those aspects may be integrated into modern cultures.

We have tried to cite as much published evidence as possible. There are fewer references available for eastern bodywork and in general there is not a great deal of research on massage or on shiatsu and bodywork. This does not mean, however, that these practices are of less value than modern medicine which is more research based. Furthermore it can be argued that bodywork does not have the potentially negative implications of many aspects of modern medicine. To begin to validate the role of bodywork we have drawn on studies which have been done on the role of stress and the presence of support people in labour, which can give indications as to the potential benefits. There is a need for more research in the field of bodywork but it can be difficult to have access to funding. Nevertheless, where possible, we encourage bodyworkers to collaborate with local researchers and hospitals and try to get their work recorded so that its effects can be investigated and analysed.

We would have liked to include more information on aftercare but realised that this could indeed be a whole other book. Instead, we give some basic information on the main themes of aftercare.

Each section is clearly indexed so that the reader can move between the sections.

Further reading

Western theory

Baker, P.N., 2006. Obstetrics by Ten Teachers. Hodder Arnold, London.

Balaskas, J., 2004. The Water Birth Book. Thorsons, London.

Blackburn, S., 2007. Maternal, Fetal and Neonatal Physiology: A Clinical Perspective, third ed. Saunders, St Louis.

Brizendine, L., 2007. The Female Brain: Hormonal Changes through a Woman's Life. Bantam, London.

Buckley, S.J., 2006. Gentle Birth Gentle Mothering. One Moon Press, Anstead, Australia.

Calais-Germain, B., 2000. Le périnée féminin et accouchement. Editions DésIris, Meolans-Revel, France.

Coad, J., Dunstall, M., 2005. Anatomy and Physiology for Midwives, second ed. Churchill Livingstone, Edinburgh.

Cooper, C., 2004. Twins and Multiple Births: The Essential Parenting Guide from Birth to Adulthood. Vermilio, London.

Davis, E., 2004. Heart and Hands: A Midwife's Guide to Pregnancy and Birth, fourth ed. Celestial Arts, Berkeley, CA.

De Gasquet, B., 2004. Abdominauz: arrêtez le massacre. Robert Jauze, Paris.

Dick-Read, G., 2007. Childbirth Without Fear. Pinter and Martin, London.

Fraser, D.M., Cooper, M.A., 2003. Myles Textbook for Midwives. Churchill Livingstone, Edinburgh.

Gaskin, I.M., 2003. Ina May's Guide to Childbirth. Bantam, London.

Glenville, M., 2000. Natural Solutions to Infertility: How to Increase your Chances of Conceiving and Preventing Miscarriage. Piatkus Books, London.

Goer, H., Wheeler, R., 1999. The Thinking Woman's Guide to a Better Birth. Perigee Trade, New York.

Henderson, C., MacDonald, S., 2004. Mayes' Midwifery: A Textbook for Midwives. Baillière Tindall, Edinburgh.

Karlton Terry & Team, 2006. Pre and perinatal healing to relieve the shock of trauma to both mother and newborn. Institute for Pre- and Perinatal Education, Denver, CO.

Kitzinger, S., 1991. Homebirth: The Essential Guide to Giving Birth Outside of the Hospital. Dorling Kindersley, London.

Kitzinger, S., 2008. New Pregnancy and Childbirth. Dorling Kindersley, London.

Moberg, K.U., 2003. The Oxytocin Factor: Tapping the Hormone of Calm, Love and Healing. Da Capo Press, Cambridge, MA.

Motha, G., 2008. The Gentle Birth Method. Thorsons, London.

Northrup, C., 2006. Women's Bodies Women's Wisdom: Creating Physical and Emotional Health and Healing. Bantam, London.

Odent, M., 1999. The Scientification of Love. Free Association Books, London.

Odent, M., 2004. The Caesarean Birth. Free Association Books, London.

Odent, M., 2005. Birth Reborn. Souvenir Press, London.

Odent, M., 2007. Birth and Breastfeeding. Clairview Books, Forest Row, East Sussex.

Sadler, T., 2003. Langman's Medical Embryology, nineth ed. Lippincott Williams & Wilkins, Philadelphia.

Simkin, P., Ancheta, R., 2005. The Labor Progress Handbook, second ed. Blackwell, Oxford.

Verny, T., Kelly, J., 1982. Secret Life of the Unborn Child. Sphere, London.

Wagner, M., 1994. Pursuing the Birth Machine: The Search for Appropriate Birth Technology. Ace Graphics, Camperdown Australia.

Water birth

There are a number of specific books on water birth. Please read as many as you can. Recommended are books on the subject by Janet Balaskas and sections on water birth in the books by Sheila Kitzinger (see list above).

DVDs

Harper, Barbara, 2005. Gentle Birth Choices. Quantum Leap.

Lake, Ricky with Michel Odenet, Abby Epstein et al., 2007. The business of being born. New Line Home Video.

Pascali-Bonaro, Debra, 2009. Orgasmic birth. ESI Distribution.

Tonetti-Vladimirova, Elena, 2008. Birth as we know it. Birth into Being.

Eastern theory

Beresford Cooke, C., 2003. Shiatsu Theory and Practice: A Comprehensive Text for the Student and Professional, second ed. Churchill Livingstone, Edinburgh.

Deadman, P., Al-Khafaji, M., Baker, K., 1998. A manual of acupuncture. J. Chin. Med. (Hove).

Flaws, B., 2005. Chinese Medical Obstetrics. Blue Poppy Press, Boulder, CO.

Fu Ke Xin Fa Yao Jue, 2005. A Heart Approach to Gynecology: Essentials in Verse (S. Yu, Trans.). Paradigm Publications, Taos, NM.

Fu, Q.-Z., 1995. Fu Qing-zhu's Gynecology (S.-Z. Yang, D.-W. Liu, Trans.), second ed. Blue Poppy Press, Boulder, CO.

Low, R.H., 1984. The Secondary Vessels of Acupuncture: A Detailed Account of their Energies, Meridians and Control Points. Thorsons, Wellingborough.

Maciocia, G., 1998. Obstetrics and Gynecology in Chinese Medicine. Churchill Livingstone, Edinburgh.

Maciocia, G., 2006. The Channels of Acupuncture: Clinical Use of the Secondary Channels and Eight Extraordinary Vessels. Elsevier, Churchill Livingstone, Edinburgh.

Rochat de la Vallée, E., 2007. Pregnancy and Gestation in Chinese Classical Texts. Monkey Press, Cambridge.

Zhao, X., 2006. Traditional Chinese Medicine for Women: Reflections of the Moon on Water. Virago Press, London.

Jin, Y., 1998. Handbook of Obstetrics and Gynecology in Chinese Medicine: An Integrated Approach (C. Hakim, Trans.). Eastland Press, Seattle.

Yuen, J.C., 2005. Channel Systems of Chinese Medicine: The Eight Extraordinary Vessels: 12–13 April 2003. New England School of Acupuncture Continuing Education Department.

Section 1

Theory: western and eastern approaches

CONTENTS

CHAPTER **1** | Western approach to pregnancy

Chapter contents

See eastern theory chapters (p. 131–178)

For more information on:

Emotional response to pregnancy

See practical pregnancy section (chapter 9 p. 225)

For more information on:

How to translate the implications in practical adaptations of work

See high-risk chapter (p. 367)

For more information on:

For complications

Learning outcomes

- The changes in the maternal systems during pregnancy
- The process of fetal and placental development
- Different tests to assess fetal and maternal well-being
- Issues relating to miscarriage

Definition of pregnancy and overview of changes

The duration of pregnancy averages 266 days (38 weeks) after ovulation or 280 days (40 weeks) from the first day of the last menstrual period. This equals approximately 10 lunar months (which are 28 days) or just over 9 calendar months. During these months the uterus develops from a small thick-walled lumen (cavity) into a large thin-walled organ. For the woman, pregnancy is defined as starting from the date of the last period. This means that for the first 2 weeks (average in a 28-day cycle) of the pregnancy she is not actually pregnant. Fetal development is usually measured from conception and lasts 38 weeks. This means there may be apparent discrepancies between measurements, for example 2 weeks' fetal development is the fourth week of pregnancy for the mother.

The woman

All the physiological systems in the body are affected in some way. Most of the changes are progressive and can be attributed to either hormonal response or physical alterations due to fetal size. The maternal neuroendocrine system is the ultimate regulator, controlling both the length and integrity of gestation. Some women find their bodies accommodate the changes relatively easily and experience pregnancy as a healthy time in their life, with some adaptations to their normal lifestyle patterns by the end. Other women find that some of their systems do not adapt as well and they may experience discomfort or even ill health. It is important to understand possible complications within systems as well as the potential benefits of pregnancy. Complications within systems and pre-existing health issues complicating pregnancy are discussed in the 'higher risk' chapter (p. 367).

It is necessary to be aware of the increased demands caused by pregnancy on women who may not be in the best of health at the time of conception, such as obese women or women with pre-existing health issues. Some systems, especially the renal and circulatory systems, are more prone to complications. Further, there may be issues facing women who have needed medical help to begin the pregnancy: they may begin by doubting their body's ability to cope with the pregnancy. Bodywork may be partly about helping these women to learn to work with their bodies.

The fetus

For the fetus, most of the physiological systems are developed during the first trimester and this explains the high rate of miscarriage. Severe abnormalities in fetal growth often lead to fetal death and the end of pregnancy. However, there can be problems at any stage of the pregnancy. Sadly, fetuses sometimes die during the last trimester and even during the birth process itself. The chances of this happening, however, go down significantly after 9 weeks of fetal development, when the main organ systems are formed.

Detailed discussions of the development of the different fetal systems is less relevant to the therapist, but it is important, especially if the therapist wants to include an awareness of the fetus in their work, to understand the general pattern of development, particularly the development of the senses.

Supporting the development of the fetus are the placenta, the fetal membranes (amnion and chorion) and the amniotic fluid. These protect and nourish the fetus and are essential structures.

Maternal well-being and the growth of the fetus: a case for bodywork

The allopathic medical view used to be that the fetus would be able to take what it needed while in utero regardless of the health state of the mother, except in more extreme cases. This is to some extent validated by the fact that babies can be carried to term by cocaine users, albeit with health issues. However, this idea is being challenged to come more in line with some traditional cultural views (compare, for example, Japanese views in eastern theory chapter) that the fetal environment profoundly affects fetal development. This is a complex area to explore and it is difficult to isolate the most important factors. The reality is probably that many factors add up to determine the fetal environment and thus the health of the future adult. These factors include genetics, nutrition, stress and environmental factors. Teratogens are examples of extreme negative influences, such as exposure to alcohol, drugs (e.g. thalidomide) and disease. Fetal environment is determined by the development of the placenta and amniotic sac which are largely genetically determined. Fetal development is affected by genes and the environment but limited by nutrient and oxygen supply, for example the fetus adapts to under-nutrition by altering metabolism and blood flow to protect the brain, at the expense of other organs (Barker 1998). Much of this work is still in its early stages and is controversial, but we feel it is interesting to refer to as it may help validate the importance of the bodywork space in providing strategies for helping to reduce stress, supporting good nutrition and being aware of maternal emotions and environment.

Nathanielsz goes as far as to say 'the quality of life in the womb, our temporary home before we were born, programmes our susceptibility to coronary artery disease, stroke, diabetes, obesity and a multitude of other conditions in later life' (Nathanielsz 1999). And 'that programming of a lifetime health by the conditions in the womb is equally, if not more important than our genes in determining how we perform mentally and physically during our life'. He draws upon research by Bateson (2004). A range of adult-related chronic disorders including osteoporosis, mood disorders and psychoses have been intimately related to pre- and perinatal developmental influences (Gluckman & Hanson 2004).

Recent research on nutrition in pregnancy suggests that good nutrition in pregnancy will affect the long-term health of the unborn child (Stein et al 1995). Research is being carried out in the area of nutrition and its implications by an EU-funded project, EARNEST ('Early nutrition programming – long-term follow-up of efficacy and safety trials and integrated epidemiological, genetic, animal, consumer and economic research'; Press Release 07). Bodyworkers, if appropriately qualified, may advise on nutrition and at least highlight its importance for their clients.

Stress and emotional support is an area in which bodywork may play a role. Exactly how stress affects the unborn child and the implications for the future adult are unclear; however, early studies indicate the potential negative implications of long-term stress on both short- and long-term maternal and fetal health. If the mother is chronically stressed the fetus will absorb excess cortisol and other 'fight or flight' hormones. These will affect the fetus in the same way as the mother and shunt blood flow from the viscera and organs and suppress forebrain function (Christensen 2000; Gitau et al 1998, 2005; Lesage et al 2004; Leutwyler 1998; O'Connor et al 2002, 2003, 2005; Sandman et al 1994; Sapolsky 1997; Teixeira et al 1999; van den Bergh et al 2005).

1.1 Changes for the pregnant woman

The 40 weeks of pregnancy are divided into three trimesters. Weeks 0–13 are trimester 1; weeks 14–26 are trimester 2 and weeks 27–40 are trimester 3.

Changes in maternal systems by trimester of pregnancy: summary

Trimester 1

- Neuroendocrine system changes underpin changes in all systems.
- Initial changes in cardiovascular system: cardiac volume and output begin to increase contributing to increased renal plasma flow and glomerular filtration.
- Blood pressure decreases slightly.
- Changes in musculoskeletal system minimal – maternal weight gain usually small and the woman may even lose weight.
- Effects of stress, nutrition, drug, alcohol abuse and other teratogenic influences are at their most marked in terms of fetal development.
- Uterus is still a pelvic organ. Fundus of the uterus can be palpated at the pubic border at around 12 weeks.

First signs and symptoms

- Cessation of menses, although brief or scant bleeding may occur, especially around time of implantation.
- Breast tenderness and tingling around 4–6 weeks. Increased vascularity and colostrum leakage may occur around 3 months. Enlargement of sebaceous glands around the nipple (Montgomery's glands) may be apparent.
- Nausea or vomiting may be experienced. This usually begins about 6 weeks after last period and continues for 6–12 weeks.
- Increase in urination which subsides around 12 weeks.
- Fatigue.
- Headaches, migraines, may be experienced due to tension or endocrine changes.
- Goodell's sign (softening of cervix and vagina with increased leukorrheal discharge).
- Hegar sign (softening and increased compressibility of the lower uterine segment (LUS).
- Jacquemier-Chadwick's sign (bluish purple discoloration of the vaginal mucosa, cervix and vulva by 8 weeks).
- 8–10 weeks fetal heart tones can be auscultated by Doppler ultrasonography.

Trimester 2

- Continuing of changes in cardiovascular (CV) system: maternal blood volume rises significantly and haematocrit and haemoglobin levels fall. Blood pressure decreases slightly and heart rate increases by 10–20 beats per minute.
- Beginning of major changes in musculoskeletal system primarily due to increasing weight.
- Gastrointestinal (GI) system changes more evident. Decreased motility of GI tract may lead to heartburn and constipation.
- Uterus moves into abdominal cavity and movements of the fetus can be felt from 16–20 weeks.

Other changes

- Uterus now ovoid in shape as length increases over width. Uterus moves into abdominal cavity and begins to displace the intestines. Tension and stretching of broad ligament may lead to low, sharp, painful sensations. Normally contractions in the second trimester are irregular and painless.
- Increasing vascularity of the vagina and pelvic viscera may result in increased sensitivity and heightened arousal and sexual interest. Mucorrhea (clear mucous discharge) is not uncommon as a result of the hyperactivity of the vaginal glandular tissues and this may increase sexual sensitivity. Spontaneous orgasm may occur.
- Leukorrhea (thick whitish vaginal discharge) often occurs.
- Perineal structures enlarge.
- Breasts become more nodular, nipples larger and more deeply pigmented.
- Increased skin pigmentation, especially along abdominal midline (linea nigra) and darkening of skin over forehead and cheeks (chloasma gravidarum).
- Spider nevi and capillary haemangiomas (benign tumour) may appear. Breakdown of underlying connective tissue may result in stretch marks.
- Increased oestrogen may result in hyperaemic (blood congested) soft swollen gums that bleed easily and increased salivation (ptalyism) may occur.
- Glomerular filtration rates increase. Bladder and ureter tone decrease and ureters become more tortuous.
- Fluid retention.
- Protein and carbohydrate requirements increase, contributing to weight gain.

Trimester 3

- The CV system continues to have to make adaptations in order to support increased demands for oxygen. The heart is displaced slightly to the left, blood pressure rises slightly and cardiac output remains unchanged. Blood volume peaks at 30–34 weeks. Oedema occurs as blood return from the lower extremities is decreased. Incidence of varicose veins increases.
- The renal system continues to adapt.
- There are continuing effects on the GI system as the growing uterus displaces stomach and intestines. The upper portion of the stomach may become herniated.
- Increased changes in the musculoskeletal system: increased elasticity of connective and collagen tissue leads to increased mobility of pelvic joints, especially symphysis pubis and sacroiliac joint. Stress on ligaments and muscles of lower back. This is combined with increasing weight gain.

- At the end of this trimester there is an initiation of hormonal changes to stimulate labour.

Other changes
- There is additional weight and pressure from the enlarged uterus.
- The fetus can be palpated through the uterine wall and begins to settle into position for birth.
- Broad ligament pain can become more intense.

- Thoracic breathing predominates.
- Fatigue, dyspnoea (shortness of breath) and increased urination may be experienced.
- There can be varicosities of the perineum and rectum due to increasing pelvic congestion caused by pressure from the growing fetus and relaxation of smooth muscle in the veins.
- Bladder pulled up, urethra stretched and increase in UTIs (urinary tract infections).

Systems overview

Changes with most implication for bodyworkers: summary

- Effects of progesterone and relaxin relaxing connective tissue, smooth muscle and ligaments, especially in the pelvis (see neuroendocrine effects).
- Increased blood flow and changes in composition of blood (see cardiovascular effects).
- Increasing size of the fetus and weight gain (see musculoskeletal effects).

1.2 Reproductive system

The most obvious changes in the body occur in this system. There are substantial changes in the uterus. It grows from a pelvic organ to fill the whole abdominal cavity to provide the space for the developing fetus to grow. Within the uterus a new organ is developed to support these changes, namely the placenta.

These changes are regulated by hormones. From an eastern perspective this is related to the Extraordinary Vessel energies. Cessation of menstruation and breast tenderness are among the first physical changes.

The menstrual cycle and conception
Proliferative (10 days or more)
Between 5 and 15 primordial follicles begin to grow under the influence of FSH (follicle stimulating hormone). Under normal conditions, in each cycle only one of these follicles reaches full maturity. Most follicles degenerate without reaching full maturity. The mature follicle secretes oestrogen. As oestrogen levels increase then LH (luteinising hormone, produced by the pituitary) is secreted, which causes the maturing of a follicle and its ovum. Cells of the endometrium (lining of the uterus) begin to proliferate under the influence of oestrogen. This phase has most variation in time. It is longer in women who have longer cycles and shorter in women with shorter cycles.

Ovulation
On about day 12 of a 28 day cycle, there is a surge of oestrogen which stimulates LH levels to rise which leads to ovulation. The woman's temperature rises and her mucus becomes more sticky.

At ovulation a single mature egg (occasionally more than one) rises to the surface of the protective follicle and is released into the adjacent fallopian tube. The egg (oocyte) is 100 times bigger than a sperm. If more than one egg matures and is fertilised, non-identical twins will be conceived.

The corpus luteum is formed by the remaining follicular cells and takes up cholesterol from the bloodstream, which colours it yellow. It produces oestrogen and progesterone and the lining of the uterus thickens. The cells of the endometrium reach a thickness of 2–3 mm and glands and arterioles grow longer and more coiled.

If conception occurs it is within 12–24 hours after ovulation.

Secretory or luteal phase (14 days)
The corpus luteum grows and secretes progesterone and oestrogen. These hormones influence the glands to become more tortuous and produce secretions. The endometrium continues to thicken, reaching a maximum of 4–6 mm; some of this is swelling caused by fluid retention. Endometrial glands secrete their nutrient fluid. This phase always lasts on average 14 days (range 12–16 days) and precedes menstruation. It needs to be at least 10 days long to support conception.

Progesterone acts to slightly increase the woman's temperature.

If there is no conception, then the corpus luteum disintegrates about 10 days after ovulation. If conception occurs then the corpus luteum remains in the ovary, secreting more oestrogen and progesterone under the influence of hCG (human chorionic gonadotropin). The fertilised egg undergoes a process of rapid cell division and after around 10 days implants on the wall of the uterus (these changes are described in fetal development, p. 44–54). No menstruation will occur, although sometimes around the time of implantation there can be a small blood loss known as 'implantation bleeding'.

Changes in the ovaries, uterus and breasts

The uterus

A non-pregnant uterus weighs approx 50 g with a cavity of approximately 10 ml. It is composed of three layers:

- Inner layer – *endometrium*.
- Middle layer – smooth muscle – *myometrium*. This is composed of three muscle layers which are not very distinctive in the non-pregnant state.
- Outer layer – *peritoneum* which drapes over the uterus anteriorly to form a fold between the uterus and the bladder and over the uterine tubes to cover the myometrium. This is the *perimetrium* – it forms the *broad ligament* and maintains the anatomical position of the uterus.

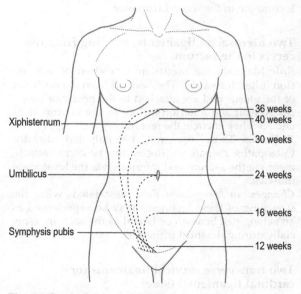

Fig. 1.1 Fundal height and changing size of uterus in pregnancy.

Xiphisternum

Umbilicus

Symphysis pubis

36 weeks
40 weeks
30 weeks
24 weeks
16 weeks
12 weeks

The uterus grows from a lime-sized organ in the pelvis to reach the xiphoid process by the eighth month of pregnancy (Fig. 1.1 and Table 1.1).

The *endometrium* thickens into the *decidua*. The three layers of the *myometrium* become defined as the uterine muscles develop new fibres. As pregnancy progresses there is great increase in the length and thickness of existing muscle fibres (hypertrophy) in the upper uterine segment (UUS). In early pregnancy the *uterine isthmus* (the constricted part of the uterus between the uterine neck (the cervix) and the uterine body) increases from about 7 to 25 mm. From 32 to 34 weeks the isthmus forms the lower uterine segment (LUS). As effacement of the cervix commences (at approximately 36 weeks) the external os (outmost part of the cervix) is incorporated into the LUS. The LUS and the cervix are not rich in muscle fibres.

The blastocyst usually implants in the fundus of the uterus, partly because the muscle fibres are richer. By 12 weeks the fetus fills the uterine cavity and the fundus can just be palpated at the pelvic brim. As the uterus expands during pregnancy it loses its anteverted and anteflexed configuration and becomes erect, tilting and then rotating to the right under the pressure of the descending colon.

Many people do not realise that the uterus is never completely quiescent and exhibits low-frequency activity throughout pregnancy. *Braxton Hicks contractions* are painless contractions which are measurable from the first trimester. They do not dilate the cervix but assist in the circulation of blood to the placenta. They are usually irregular and weak, unsynchronised and multifocal in origin.

Clinical implications/observations for the bodyworker

We have observed that if the mother overexerts herself, especially towards the end of the second trimester when she has possibly had many weeks of feeling well, she may experience more intense and even slightly painful Braxton Hicks, as the uterus needs to send more blood to the placenta as blood is being shunted to other muscles in her body. These are a sign that she needs to slow her physical pace down once more.

However, if there is blood loss, pain or stronger contractions these may be a sign of premature labour

Table 1.1 Changes in size of uterus (after Resnik 1999)				
	Weight	**Length × weight × depth**	**Capacity**	**Total uterine volume**
Pre-pregnancy	50–70 g	7.5 × 5×3.5 cm	10 ml	<300 cm^3 (early pregnancy)
Term	800–1200 g	30 × 25 × 22.5	5000 ml	4500 cm^3

or miscarriage or other complications and the woman needs to refer to her primary care provider.

Uterine ligaments (reviewed by Averille Morgan, personal correspondence)

The growth of the uterus affects the ligaments which support the uterus in the pelvis (Fig. 1.2). These ligaments are formed from external uterine connective tissue. They soften and thicken under the influence of progesterone and relaxin which increase the mobility and capacity of the pelvis. As they soften, pain may be caused in the pelvic area at the site of their attachment. The cervical ligaments give support to the uterus and work reciprocally with the pelvic floor muscles (PFM). Osteopathic or chiropractic, soft tissue techniques may ease the uterus or ligament strain.

Broad ligaments (two; the side ligaments)

Role It is the main supporting ligament of the mesenteries and GIT and gives some support to the uterus. The round ligament is part of the broad ligament (as is the ovarian ligament). It is formed from a loose double fold of the perimetrium, which extends from the lateral borders of the uterus to the side walls of the pelvis.

Palpation It can be palpated with the hand over the lower area of abdomen, i.e. holding over the lower abdominal fascia and cupping the bowel mesenteries in the palm of the hand.

Changes in pregnancy In the first trimester as these stretch they may cause low, sharp pain in the lower abdomen. During the second trimester the pain is usually less but increases by the third trimester and may be referred to the sides, back and buttocks, especially from 6–7 months.

Two round ligaments: the front ligaments

Role Maintain the uterus in a position of anteversion (tilted forwards). They are part of the broad ligament. They arise at the *cornua* (one of the two horns of the uterus, a bluntly rounded superior lateral extremity of the uterine body that marks the site of the entrance of the fallopian tube) of the uterus and descend through the broad ligament and inguinal canals to the labia majora, attaching into the connective tissue of the pubic mons.

Palpation They can be found one third of the way down an imaginary line drawn between the umbilicus and the ASIS (anterior superior iliac spine).

Changes in pregnancy Usually during pregnancy they feel tender. As they stretch, pain may be felt from the top of the uterus to the groin, sometimes extending to the vulvar and upper thigh fascia. Pain is usually one-sided, depending on fetal position, and is common in the second trimester.

Two uterosacral ligaments: running from the cervix to the sacrum

Role Maintain the uterus in a position of anteversion (tilted forwards). They extend from the posterior of the uterus and are attached to the posterior pelvic cavity wall and anterior surface of the sacrum at S2 and S3. They encircle the rectum.

Palpation These can not be palpated directly. Osteopaths palpate indirectly the posterior attachment via the sacrum and inferiorly via the levator ani muscles.

Changes in pregnancy Pain associated with the stretching of these ligaments may be experienced as an aching just beneath or lateral to the sacrum, especially during the third trimester.

Two transverse cervical ligaments (or cardinal ligaments) (side)

Role They give an important support to the uterus and, if they become overstretched, can cause the uterus to prolapse. They extend from the cervix laterally to the side walls of the pelvis. They aid the PFM to guide the fetal descent and rotation at the lower pelvic cavity.

Palpation Cannot be palpated directly but osteopaths palpate via the attachment to the ilia laterally.

Changes in pregnancy Pain which can be referred to the side of the groin.

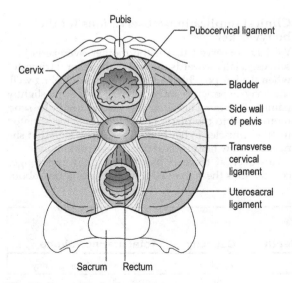

Fig. 1.2 The uterine ligaments.

Pubocervical – cervix to pubis
Role Aid in the lift of the urethra and vagina while the PFM are contracted. They support the anterior position of the fetus and posterior presentation of the cervix. They are strong ligaments.

Blood supply to the uterus
The vasculature of the uterus undergoes a number of changes during pregnancy. Uterine blood flow increases, vessel diameter increases and vascular resistance falls. These changes accommodate the increased blood flow to the placenta which is maintained under conditions of low blood pressure.

Nerves to the uterus
- *Parasympathetic* – rising from second, third and fourth sacral segments.
- *Sympathetic* – via presacral nerve (branching from the aortic plexus) and branches from the lumbar sympathetic chain.

This has sometimes led bodyworkers to be cautious of working over the sacral area, especially in the first trimester, for the fear it may cause miscarriage or early labour. There is no evidence that work over the sacrum overstimulates these nerves. Indeed, our sedentary lifestyle is likely to cause compressions of the nerves which can be released through bodywork. Furthermore nerve stimulation is not the mechanism by which contractions begin; contractions are hormonally regulated.

The cervix
This increases in width in pregnancy. Oestrogen increases the blood supply to the cervix resulting in a local coloration and softer tissue texture. Cervical mucosa proliferates and glands become more complex and secrete thickened mucus which forms a plug or *operculum* protecting the cervix from ascending infection. The plug is held laterally by projections of thickened mucus in the mouths of the mucus-secreting glands. It is this plug that is released as 'the show' at the onset of labour when the cervix starts to be drawn up to form the lower uterine segment.

There can be issues with the cervix dilating too early in the pregnancy; cervical incompetence (see 'higher risk', p. 367–390).

Vagina
Blood flow increases to the vagina resulting in softer, more distensible vaginal tissue. The purplish coloration of the vagina and cervix was traditionally recognised as an indicator of pregnancy (Jacquemier-Chadwick's sign). The increased blood flow means that the pulsating of the uterine arteries can be felt through the lateral fornices. Increased vaginal discharge has low pH and is white with an inoffensive odour. The cells acquire a boat-shaped appearance. Bodyworkers can reassure their clients that this increased discharge is normal.

The placenta
For further information see p. 45–47 (fetal development) and (complications, p. 378–379) (higher risk).

The placenta is essentially the fetus's support system and any problems with it may endanger its life and well-being. It transfers nutrients and gases from the mother to the fetus and removes waste products from the fetus. Further, because by the end of pregnancy it is a large, well-vasculated organ, problems with it may lead to haemorrhage and so can be life-threatening to the woman as well as to the fetus.

The placenta has a role in regulating the hormones of pregnancy. Early placental tissue produces hCG as well as progesterone, and the developed placenta produces progesterone and oestrogen.

Breasts
The breasts are essentially modified exocrine glands consisting of epithelial glandular tissue with an extensive system of branching ducts surrounded by adipose tissue and separated from the pectoralis major muscle of the chest and the ribs by connective tissue (Fig. 1.3). They are highly innervated with rich vascular and lymphatic systems. The basic glandular unit is the alveolus. There is a system of branching ducts from the alveolus which merge into the larger lactiferous or mammary ducts. At the base of the nipple the ducts dilate forming ampullae. These are surrounded by fibro-muscular tissue and provide an area of milk storage. The breast consists of 15–20 lobes arranged in spokes around the nipple and separated from each other by connective tissue. The areolar area around the nipple contains small sebaceous glands (tubercules of Mongomery) which provide nipple lubrication and antisepsis. Washing the nipple with soap can remove these protective secretions and lead to drying and cracking of the nipples, thus increasing the risk of infection.

In pregnancy, vascularisation increases, resulting in a marbled appearance of skin owing to the dilation of superficial veins. The breasts may feel sensitive and tingle from around 4 to 6 weeks because of the engorgement of blood. Increased vascularity and colostrum (pre-milk) leakage may occur from around 3 months. By the second trimester the breasts become more nodular, the nipples larger and more deeply pigmented.

Clinical implications for the bodyworker of the changes in the reproductive organs: summary

- Eastern approaches see the uterus and the breasts as being influenced by the Extraordinary Vessels, especially the Penetrating Vessel. Blood flow to the uterus is regulated by the Penetrating Vessel but Spleen, Liver and Kidney are all important for regulating energy flows to the uterus.
- Need to be able to identify possible causes of abdominal pain to know whether it is safe to proceed with bodywork and how (or whether) to refer urgently. Some of these are discussed in more detail in the high risk section.

Possible causes of abdominal pain
Stretching of uterine ligaments
- Broad: low sharp abdominal pain especially in first trimester.
- Round: from top of uterus to groin.
- Work can proceed in accordance with the comfort of the client.

Placental abruption
- Immediate referral required.

Retroverted uterus at around week 14–15
- This is accompanied by inability to urinate.
- Immediate referral required.

Fibroids and cysts
- Work can proceed in accordance with the comfort of the client but if suspect undiagnosed fibroids and cysts refer back to primary care giver for further diagnosis and monitoring.

Uterine bleeding
- Any case of active uterine bleeding needs immediate medical attention.
- Otherwise health history needs to be established to determine work.

Possible causes of bleeding
First trimester
- Implantation bleeding in first trimester: if mild not necessarily an issue.
- Miscarriage. If it is known that it is a 'miscarriage' and the woman knows that the fetus has died and there is no medical treatment apart from dilatation and curettage, it is the woman's choice to proceed with work.
- Ectopic pregnancy or hydatiform mole: immediate referral if active bleeding.

Second and third trimesters
- Placenta praevia: may be from mild to severe.
- Placental abruption: may present with mild bleeding, but is a medical emergency. Other signs are shock and a hard uterus.

Size of uterus
- Need to be aware of the physical location and size of the uterus for the safety and effectiveness of abdominal work and in order to establish the most effective connection with the fetus. Appropriate pressure, applied on the woman's out breath, over the uterus will not increase intrauterine pressure. If there is a lot of amniotic fluid (polyhydramnios, see higher risk section), avoid pressure.

Structural abnormality of the uterus
- This may be a cause of miscarriage or pre-term labour.
- Malpresentation of fetus may be due to abnormalities of the uterus.
- Pain or urinary tract infections may be due to the shape of the uterus, and malformations of the uterus, although rare, are possible.
- Refer if there is a suspected urinary tract infection. It is an emergency if accompanied by severe abdominal pain.

Ligament pain
- Need to be aware of the symptoms of stretching of the uterine ligaments during the different trimesters and pain sites.
- Broad: low sharp abdominal pain in the first trimester in front and side, second and third trimester sides of abdomen, back and buttocks.
- Round: top of uterus to groin sometimes in vulva and upper thigh.
- Uterosacral: sacral pain.

Breasts
- There is tenderness of breast tissue from early pregnancy.

Contractions
- Painful Braxton Hicks contractions may indicate that the woman is over-exerting herself or may be an indication of premature labour. Questioning is required as to activity level and to establish cause. If suspect premature labour then immediate referral required.

Female genital circumcision (see also higher risk section)
Be aware of and sensitive to the issues raised by this procedure:

- Increased likelihood of urinary tract infections.

- Discomfort during sex and possible marital tension.
- Possible history of infection, endometriosis and pain.
- Emotional and cultural issues, particularly if the woman is not living in her own society.

Referral issues
Immediate referral with no bodywork
- Undiagnosed vaginal bleeding.
- Abdominal pain if severe and especially if accompanied by inability to pass urine.

- Suspected ectopic pregnancy.
- Severe vaginal pain.
- Inability to pass urine.
- Suspected premature labour.
- Strong contractions before due date.

Referral but bodywork may proceed
- Suspected mild urinary tract infection (UTI) with no other complications (such as ectopic, molar, uterine issues).
- Suspected fibroids or cysts.

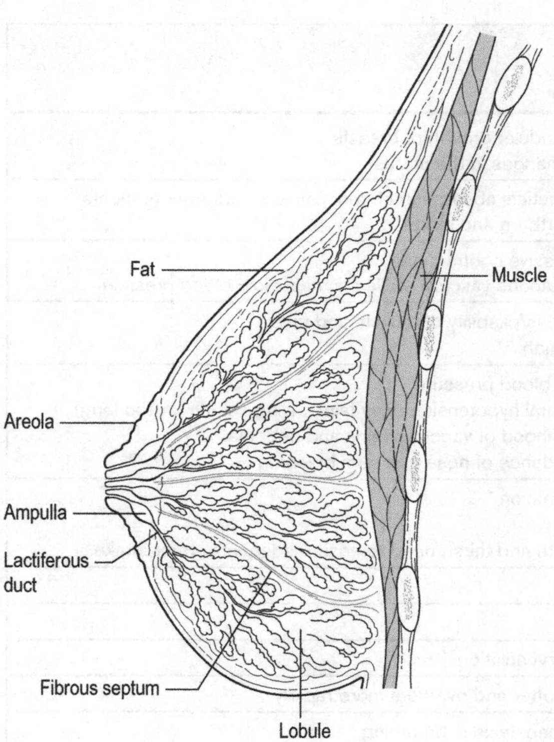

Fig. 1.3 The breast.

1.3 Neuroendocrine system

Major hormonal changes underpin the changes of the first trimester in preparing the woman's body to support the fetus throughout the rest of the pregnancy. Hormonal levels become more stable during mid-pregnancy with more changes at the end of pregnancy, during birth and the early postnatal period. They affect all of the physiological systems in the woman's body, including her emotions, as well as the growth and development of the fetus. Bodywork may have a role in supporting the body to regulate and adapt to the hormonal changes by inducing relaxation and reducing cortisol levels in the woman's body which may in turn affect the fetus. Eastern approaches may include work with the Extraordinary Vessels which are closely linked with the neuroendocrine system.

Due to advances in neuroendocrinology, hormones are now seen as part of a complex system encompassing local hormonal changes, changes in the endocrine glands, the brain and the nervous system, the digestive system, the limbic system and neuropeptides.

Prolonged stress is understood to affect this delicate hormonal balance partly through the link with the nervous system and the fact that some hormones are also neurotransmitters.

Five hormones which are also neurotransmitters have a fairly direct link with moods:

- Serotonin – emotional calmness
- Adrenaline/noradrenaline (epinephrine/norepinephrine) – controls stress
- Dopamine – pleasure
- Acetylcholine – indigestion
- GABA (gamma-aminobutyric acid) – relaxation.

The release of adrenaline and the fear fight reflex is regulated by a neuronal pathway. Adrenaline is the body's short-term response to stress and cortisol is its long-term response.

The main hormones of pregnancy are oestrogens, progesterone, relaxin and human placental lactogen (hPL).

Hormonal changes

The physiological adaptation to pregnancy is mediated by the increase of secretion of the steroid hormones progesterone, oestrogens, hPL and relaxin. Steroid hormones are initially produced from the corpus luteum under the influence of hCG as well as by placental tissue. The placenta synthesises a range of hormones and releasing factors similar to those originating from the hypothalamus and other maternal endocrine organs. Placental products reach both maternal and fetal circulation, regulating maternal physiology and fetal development.

The maternal endocrine system is affected by this increase in steroid hormones as other hormones augment the effects of oestrogen and progesterone. For example the secretion of melancocyte stimulating hormone (MSH) and cortisol increase in pregnancy, affecting skin pigmentation and improving some pathological conditions such as eczema.

The overall regulators of this system are the pituitary and the hypothalamus.

Steroid hormones

Progesterone Progesterone levels increase gradually at first. By 5–6 weeks placental production of progesterone is adequate to support the pregnancy. There is little change between weeks 5 and 10 but it increases more markedly after week 10 (Tulchinsky & Hobel 1973). By the end of the first trimester, progesterone levels are 50% higher than luteal levels and by term they are threefold. For effects of progesterone see Table 1.2.

Table 1.2 The effects of progesterone

Effect	Implication
Prepares the uterus for pregnancy, maintains pregnancy	Stimulates glandular growth of breasts Enables the changes in the uterus
Relaxes smooth muscle: – digestive tract linings	Maximises intestinal absorption of iron, calcium and other nutrients Increased heartburn and reflux
Relaxes smooth muscle: – uterus	Prevents excessive contractions Relaxation of uterine vascular walls maintains low blood pressure
Relaxes smooth muscle	Relative softness/pliability of muscle and fascia Nasal congestion
Vasodilation of vascular smooth muscle Decreased peripheral resistance	Maintains low blood pressure Possible postural hypotension (may faint if lying supine for too long) Increased likelihood of varicose veins and oedema Increased incidence of nose and gum bleeding
Affects sodium and water secretion	Increase in urination Oedema Affects appetite and thirst; need to ensure adequate water intake
Is mildly catabolic (breaks down cells)	
Affects metabolic rate	
Increases sensitivity to carbon dioxide	Possible hyperventilation
Increases basal body temperature	Women feel hotter and overheat more rapidly
Increases respiratory efficiency in line with increased cardiac output	Maintains homeostasis in breathing
Inhibits prolactin secretion	
Helps suppress maternal immunological responses to fetal antigens	Helps prevent rejection of fetus
Emotional effects: helps balance cortisol effects	Calming, slowing down, brain less focused, natural protector against stress Sleepiness Some mothers may resist this slowing down and it may explain some of the weepiness, clinginess and crankiness

Oestrogens The primary oestrogen of pregnancy is oestriol. Early in pregnancy oestrone and oestradiol levels increase. Oestriol levels do not begin to rise until the 9th week when fetal adrenal glands begin to synthesize the precursor dehydroepiandrosterone sulphate (DHEAS) for placental production of oestriol. Oestriol is an indicator of fetal well-being and decreased oestriol may indicate fetal distress. Oestriol measurement is part of the Bart's triple test for Down's syndrome. Oestrone and oestradiol levels increase about 100 times and oestriol levels about 1000 times during the course of pregnancy (Heinrichs & Gibbons 1989).

See Table 1.3 for the effects of oestrogens.

Human chorionic gonadotropin (hCG) This is maximal at 60–90 days and falls to a low level which is maintained through pregnancy. Persistently low levels of hCG are associated with abnormal placental development or ectopic pregnancy. It has a similar structure to LH and acts on LH receptors, prolonging the life of the corpus luteum.

Effects
- Luteotrophic (stimulatory) effect on corpus luteum maintaining synthesis and secretion of oestrogen and progesterone.
- Stimulates placental progesterone production.
- May be responsible for nausea and vomiting.
- Stimulates maternal thyroid gland; increases appetite and fat deposition.
- Increases sensitivity to glucose.
- Decreases osmotic threshold for thirst and release of ADH.
- Suppresses maternal lymphocyte activity.
- Promotes myometrial growth (uterus).
- Inhibits myometrial contractility (uterus).
- Modulates trophoblastic invasions (early placental development).

Table 1.3 The effects of oestrogens (after Blackburn 2003, Cunningham & Whitridge 1997, Garnica & Chan Wy 1996, Sichel & Driscoll 1999)

Effect	Implication
Stimulate growth (angiogenesis)	Prepare the uterus for ovulation and fertilisation Support the uterus to increase in size and vascularisation (increased blood flow), markedly promoting the growth of the endometrium Promote growth effects in the breasts Lustrous hair growth Skin changes Tumours, including fibroids and cysts, may grow larger
Stimulate fluid retention and increase the ability of connective tissue to retain water	Sinus congestion and oedema
Increase metabolic efficiency of use of sugar and carbohydrate and balance salt, water and insulin levels	
Suppress spontaneous uterine contractions	
Affect distribution of collagen in the tunica media of the large vessel walls	Increase venous distensibility Increased incidence of varicose veins Affect skin and contribute to the smoothing out of wrinkles
Prime endometrium for progesterone action	
Mildly anabolic (building up organs and tissues)	
Increase calcification of bones	
Stimulate the rise of oxytocin	Oxytocin (Uvnas-Moberg & Francis 2003) is a 'feel good' hormone (promotes labour contractions and stimulates let-down reflex in breastfeeding mothers; for further information see labour and postnatal sections)
Emotionally, the 'feminine' hormones	Support female secondary sex characteristics 'Feel good' hormones; promote mood stability even sense of euphoria May be associated with increased sexual behaviour

- Affects fetal nervous tissue development.
- Affects male sexual differentiation and stimulates fetal testes to produce testosterone.
- Stimulates fetal adrenal glands to increase production of corticosteroids.

Human placental lactogen (hPL) As hCG levels fall there is an increased secretion of hPL. hPL increases in parallel with the size of the placenta and correlates well with fetal and placental weight. It has properties similar to growth hormone and prolactin, being lactogenic and stimulating growth of maternal and fetal tissues. It appears to protect the fetus from rejection and low levels of hPL are associated with pregnancy failure and spontaneous abortion. hPL is antagonistic to insulin, resulting in raised plasma glucose levels. This diabetogenic effect of pregnancy adjusts glucose and fat metabolism to the advantage of the fetus.

Relaxin Less has been researched about this hormone, but along with progesterone it is responsible for supporting many of the changes in the ligaments of the pelvis. It is an insulin-like hormone secreted by the corpus luteum and later by the myometrium, decidua and placenta. Its levels are high in the first trimester, decrease in the second trimester and increase again so that by the end of pregnancy they have increased tenfold. They are greatly reduced by 6 weeks postnatally but can stay for up to 5 months postnatally (Burrows et al 1996, Buster & Sauer 1989).

Effects
- Appears to inhibit uterine activity early in pregnancy.
- Softens and helps lengthen the cervix and has been used clinically in cervical ripening during induction of labour.
- Appears to act with progesterone in softening and relaxing the cartilage and connective tissue of the sacroiliac joints, the symphysis pubis, the pelvic ligaments and connective tissue to allow mobilisation and growth of the uterus into the abdomen and in preparation for the movement of the pelvis during birth.
- Cuts collagen production and increases collagen breakdown which also help to soften the connective tissue.

Adrenal and pituitary hormones

The adrenal gland increases in both size and activity in pregnancy. The adrenal cortex (composed of regular endocrine tissue) produces, synthesises and secretes corticosteroids, the most important being cortisol and aldosterone. The adrenal medulla (composed of neurosecretory tissue) is the source of adrenaline and noradrenaline. Both cortisol and adrenaline are involved in the stress response. The short-term stress response (fight and flight) which activates the sympathetic nervous system involves the release of adrenaline directly into the blood. The longer-term stress response (linked with how often the short-term stress response is activated) involves the release of cortisol.

Cortisol Oestrogen stimulates adrenal cortisol production by inhibiting the metabolism of cortisol and increasing the synthesis of cortisol-binding protein (transcortin). Progesterone increases tissue resistance to cortisol by competing at the receptor level and binding to the cortisol-binding protein. During pregnancy there is an increase in cortisol production:

- Cortisol levels increase in response to the increased cardiac output and decreased fasting glucose levels in the second trimester.
- Cortisol increases greatly in the third trimester and may contribute to depression.
- High levels of cortisol are linked with premature labour.

Effects of cortisol This increase in cortisol serves to aid:

- Glucose metabolism.
- Regulation of blood pressure.
- Insulin release.
- Immune and inflammatory response.

It has a positive effect on certain conditions such as rheumatoid arthritis and eczema.

Excessive cortisol production, however, will negatively affect cognitive performance, the thyroid gland, blood sugar levels, decrease bone density and muscle tissue, raise blood pressure and immune response.

Emotionally, the more 'wired' 'stressed' effects of cortisol are balanced by the more calming effects of progesterone and oestrogen. The impact of cortisol is to make the woman more alert and vigilant about her safety, nutrition and surroundings.

Aldosterone Maintains sodium homeostasis in the blood by increasing sodium reabsorption in the kidneys in exchange for potassium and hydrogen ions. It therefore influences potassium and pH levels in the blood. It causes increased water retention which increases volume of blood, raising blood pressure, and therefore plays a role in the regulation of blood pressure. It is controlled mainly by the renin–angiotensin mechanism (RAS) in the kidneys and this is why water retention may be an indication of kidney issues.

Pituitary gland This increases in size in pregnancy. It has a key role in regulating hormonal changes of pregnancy and was once referred to as the 'master gland'. It actually consists of the anterior and posterior glands. The anterior gland is responsible for producing many hormones. Growth hormone (GH), lutenising hormone (LH) and follicle stimulating hormone (FSH) are all suppressed in pregnancy. Thyroid stimulating hormone (TSH) is unchanged. There is a small rise in adrenocorticotropic hormone (ACTH) and melanocyte stimulating hormone (MSH).

The posterior pituitary serves as a storage and release site for two hormones: antidiuretic hormone (ADH) and oyxtocin. Oxytocin is increased by the end of pregnancy.

MSH Its synthesis increases so pigment dispersal is increased in melanocytes, resulting in deeper pigmentation (Ances & Pomerantz 1974). Pregnant women frequently tan more deeply or develop irregular pigmented patches. Increased MSH is responsible for the skin coloration of the linea nigra.

Prolactin Levels of prolactin increase progressively through pregnancy to values 20 × higher than prepregnant levels. This is the hormone responsible for milk production and has been linked with irritability and anger (Sichel & Driscoll 1999).

ACTH This may be linked with changes in the placenta. It is linked in with cortisol balance and rises rapidly in labour.

Oxytocin It plays an important role in labour. Levels vary considerably. There is an increase in the production of oxytocin from the second half of pregnancy. Oestrogen stimulates oxytocin receptors and stimulates the production of oxytocin.

Effects Oxytocin used to be understood as the birth and breastfeeding hormone but is now understood to be present at other times.

Thyroid hormones

These increase. Pregnancy mimics hyperthyroidism in a number of respects – increasing body temperature, stimulating appetite and feelings of fatigue. In 70% of pregnant women the thyroid gland enlarges because thyroid activity increases and renal iodine loss is increased. Ancient Egyptians used the observation of pregnancy-induced goitre as confirmation of pregnancy (Glinoer & Lemone 1992). Now with better diets, unless women are at the threshold of iodine deficiency goitre is rare in pregnancy. Basal metabolic rate increases by 20–25% from the 4th month of pregnancy but much of the increase is related to the increased surface area of the woman and the increased work she has to do to maintain maternal and fetal tissue requirements. Nausea and vomiting have been linked not only to changes in hCG but also directly to a rise in free T4. Studies have been done which show the women who have higher levels of both hCG and T4 and TSH have more severe vomiting (Mori et al 1988).

About 50–70% of pregnant women experience morning sickness and it has been reported to have a positive effect on pregnancy outcome, associated with decreased risk of miscarriage, preterm birth, low birth weight (LBW) and maternal death. It is suggested that morning sickness, resulting from secretion of hCG and thyroxine, reduces maternal energy intake and stimulates early placental growth. Evidence also suggests there may be a positive relationship between morning sickness and preconceptional body mass index (BMI), so that women who are underweight will experience less severe symptoms of morning sickness compared with women with normal preconceptional BMIs (Huxley 2000).

Clinical implications for the bodyworker of the changes in the neuroendocrine system: summary

The Extraordinary Vessels regulate reproductive hormones. Work to balance energy flow in these meridians is important.

The effects of the different hormones

- The many and complex effects of the hormone changes and their interplay with the nervous system underpin many of the maternal changes in pregnancy such as: sickness, increased blood sugar, increased sensitivity of skin, diabetes, sinus congestion, cardiovascular effects, including blood pressure effects, metabolic effects especially glucose and gestational diabetes.
- Learn the effects of the different hormones (Tables 1.2 and 1.3).
- The effects on the cardiovascular and musculoskeletal systems in particular will affect bodywork. There is relative pelvic joint instability and softness of connective tissue. As the tissue is softer, jerky movements and excessive tapotement need to be avoided. Care needs to be taken with stretches and it needs to be recognised that tissue will respond relatively more quickly to the effects of bodywork.
- The changing hormones levels have many emotional effects.

Relaxation

- Emphasise relaxation: bodywork may help the body adapt to the hormonal changes and reduce the effects of stress.

Referral issues

- There are not really the same urgent referral issues as for other systems although these changes may be underlying some of the other referral issues.

1.4 Haematological, haemostatic and cardiovascular systems

Many changes occur in these systems due to the increased circulating maternal blood mass, fetal nutritional requirements and placental circulatory systems. Maternal blood volume increases by up to 30–40% and the composition and circulation of the blood also alters. Increases in cardiac output, stroke volume and heart rate support increased oxygen distribution. There is a slightly increased risk of clotting disorders but for a low-risk woman the risk of serious disease is low and the major issue is usually varicose veins. However, when superimposed upon an existing disease state, the changes may create dangerous issues for the woman.

Haematological and haemostatic changes

Many changes happen within the blood which have a protective role for maternal homeostasis and are important for fetal development. They also enable the mother to tolerate blood loss and placental separation at delivery. Although they increase the risk for complications such as *iron deficiency anaemia, thromboembolisms and coagulopathies*, the risk is still low and, for most women, homeostatic imbalance is maintained.

Blood volume, blood and plasma changes

These result in the *'hypervolemia* of pregnancy' – an increase in blood volume and blood plasma.

Circulating maternal blood volume increases by about 30% and sometimes more (up to 40% primipara, 60% multipara). This represents an increase of approximately 1.5 L (Chesley 1972). The increased blood volume is due to an increase in plasma volume, with a lesser increase in total red blood cell (RBC) count. Blood volume changes begin at 6–8 weeks, peak at 30–34 weeks, then reach a plateau towards term.

Plasma volume change begins at 6–8 weeks, increases rapidly in the second trimester, followed by a slower but progressive increase which reaches its maximum around 28–32 weeks. At its peak it is about 50% greater than pre-pregnancy levels. The enlarged plasma volume is accommodated by changes in vascularisation of the uterus, breast, muscles, kidneys and skin. Increased blood flow to the uterus accounts for about $\frac{1}{6}$ of the increase. Uterine blood flow increases by about 150%. Renal blood flow is the next most significant. Plasma proteins (albumin) are also diluted.

Plasma volume, placental mass and birth weight are closely associated and fetal growth correlates more to plasma changes than increases in RBC. The exact aetiology is poorly understood but is influenced by hormonal influences on the vasculature of the circulatory system which lead to decreased venous tone, increased capacity of the veins and muscles and decreased vascular resistance. The vascular system expands as progesterone stimulates the vasodilation of the vascular smooth muscle and oestrogen stimulates angiogenesis (formation of new blood vessels and vascular beds) and increased blood flow.

Both progesterone and oestrogen, along with aldosterone, affect the renin–angiotensin system (RAS; hormone system regulating long-term blood pressure and volume). RAS responds to the under-filled vascular system by increasing sodium and water retention; thus blood volume increases by about 40%.

White blood cells

Total white blood cell (WBC) count increases slightly during early pregnancy, beginning in the second month, and levels off during the second and third trimesters. Total lymphocyte count is unchanged.

Red blood cells
Haemodilution

The increase in plasma volume leads to a state of *haemodilution* as red blood cell mass does not increase as much as plasma volume. Red blood cell mass increases by about 18–20% in women who take no iron supplements. It begins to expand in the second trimester and peaks in the third trimester. Levels of Hb are at their lowest between 16 and 22 weeks. Lack of haemodilution or plasma volume expansion is associated with a poor pregnancy prognosis. This physiological response indicates that a degree of haemodilution is a normal part of pregnancy adaptations and it is no longer considered desirable to try to retain a pre-pregnancy level of Hb. Routine iron supplementation has been questioned and iron tends only to be prescribed when anaemia is diagnosed. Haemodilution does not seem to affect iron stores.

Iron

Women can become anaemic in pregnancy because of the increased demands for oxygen. It is estimated that approximately 56% of women in developing countries and 18% of women in developed countries have anaemia in pregnancy (Jacobs et al 1972). The most common cause is poor iron stores at the beginning of pregnancy, poor dietary intake of iron, folic acid deficiency and loss of blood. Loss of blood could be through placental issues, haemorrhoids or bowel issues. When anaemia is diagnosed in the second trimester it is associated with poor outcome such as an increase in pre-term delivery and low-birth-weight babies. If it is diagnosed in the third trimester it is usually associated with haemodilution and less with poor outcome.

The most accurate and appropriate method of determining iron status and therefore anaemia seems to be measurement of serum ferritin levels (Jacobs et al 1972). Serum ferritin, the major iron storage protein, becomes depleted before clinical indicators reveal anaemia. It is stable and not affected by recent ingestion of iron. It is, however, greatly affected by infection or inflammation and so C-reactive protein (CRP) is usually also tested. The most common anaemias in pregnancy are iron deficiency anaemia, megaloblastic anaemia of pregnancy (folic acid deficiency), sickle cell disorders and thalassaemia (Garn et al 1981, Goldenberg et al 1998, Klebanoff et al 1991, Lu et al 1991, Scholl & Schroeder 1999).

Haemostasis: changes in clotting factors and risk of deep vein thrombosis (DVT)

Pregnancy has been called an acquired hypercoagulable state: there is an increased risk of inappropriate or excessive thrombosis (blood clot) formation. There are two main factors which lead to this increased risk: clotting factor changes and stasis of blood flow. However, the risk for a healthy pregnant woman developing a serious disorder is low as these changes are balanced by other changes such as plasminogen elevation. The risk is six times greater than in a non-pregnant woman but is still low (0.6–3 per 1000 pregnant women), especially as these women include women with medical conditions (De Swiet 1985). However, the therapist needs to be alert to the signs of potential thrombosis as thromboembolic disease (TED) is the greatest single cause of maternal mortality in developed countries (Gates 2000).

Clotting factors

The net effect of changes in haemostasis is increased activity of most coagulation factors and a lowering of factors that inhibit coagulation. There is a moderate rise in all coagulation factors except factors XIII and XI and a dramatic rise in fibrinogen and factors III, X and VIII. This state promotes clot formation, extension and stability (Hathaway & Bonnar 1987).

This is balanced by changes in plasminogen which is elevated while tissue plasmin inhibitors are decreased. This helps retain the dynamic equilibrium between clotting and clot lysis (breaking down of clots) and thus overall haemostatic balance during pregnancy (Hathaway & Bonnar 1987, Comeglio et al 1996).

The number of platelets decreases slightly towards term but generally remains within the non-pregnant range. Bleeding time decreases by about 30%.

The change in clotting factors particularly in late pregnancy seems to be compensatory in preparation for labour. This state is further magnified during the intra-partum period which protects the woman from haemorrhage and excessive blood loss by providing for rapid haemostasis following delivery of the placenta.

Stasis of blood flow

During pregnancy there are various factors which affect blood flow:

- The effects of progesterone on venous muscle tone increases stasis especially in lower extremities.
- There is restriction of blood flow caused by the enlarged gravid uterus which includes flow to the legs and compression of the inferior vena cava. This is more noticeable in supine and semi-reclining positions but less so in lateral positions, especially left, and forward leaning.
- Increased venous capacitance leads to increased distensibility, decreased flow in the lower extremities and venous stasis. By late pregnancy the velocity of venous blood flow in the lower extremities has been reduced by half and venous pressure has risen an average of 10 mmHg. There is compression of the left iliac vein by the right iliac and ovarian veins which means that the diameter of the major leg veins increases more on the left than on the right. During pregnancy 85% of deep vein thromboses occur on the left (versus 55% in non-pregnant woman) (Arafeh 1997).

Problems which can be caused by the hypercoaguable state

There are three main types of problems: coagulopathies, thrombosis and varicose veins, in order of seriousness. Varicose veins are fairly common and present few cautions. Coagulopathies and thrombosis are discussed in the higher risk section.

Varicose veins

The changes in pregnancy aggravate the incidence of varicose veins in the legs, vulva and anus (haemorrhoids). There are several factors at play:

Increased femoral venous pressure

Hormone changes The effects of progesterone relaxing vascular tone and increased coagulants in blood slow the flow of the blood through the veins.

Impediments to venous return: weight of fetus and lack of movement The weight of the fetus may compress the pelvic veins (inferior vena cava, iliac and femoral), especially if the mother is sitting down or standing for long periods of time without regular movement, and create stasis in the veins of the legs.

Valvular insufficiency The primary site may be with the saphenofemoral junction (where the superficial saphenous vein empties into the deep femoral vein), or with the valves of the other superficial lower extremity veins becoming unable to work properly. This causes back flow and other valvular incompetence, creating the development of varicosities.

Weakness of the venous walls: primary idiopathic dilation This may be supported by familial history and lead to venous expansion and varicosities.

Oedema

Lymphostatic oedema

This type of oedema often accompanies varicose veins. It is largely due to changes in the RAS system and the dilution of plasma proteins, but also to the effects of progesterone relaxing vascular tone, impeded venous return and an increase in femoral venous pressure. The net reduction in plasma albumin reduces plasma colloid osmotic pressure interfering with the return of fluid. There is an increase in interstitial fluid, mostly due to alterations in capillary permeability and changes in interstitial ground substance (Theunissen & Parer 1994).

It is seen in up to 70% of pregnant women, is more common as pregnancy progresses and in obese women. It is associated with large babies (Davison 1997).

Treatment of lymphostatic oedema
- Avoid supine position.
- Avoid upright position for extended periods.
- Rest in left lateral with legs slightly elevated.
- Elevate legs and feet regularly.
- Use water immersion.
- Use support hose.
- Avoid wearing tight clothing on lower extremities.
- Engage in regular exercise.
- Restrict the intake of foods and beverages high in salt.
- Responds to manual lymphatic drainage.

Circulatory: the cardiovascular response

Changes are especially marked in this system to meet the increased demands of maternal and fetal tissues. These changes are mediated both indirectly by hormones (especially circulating oestrogens, progesterone and prostaglandins (PG)) and directly by mechanical effects.

Anatomical changes such as the upward displacement of the diaphragm by the gravid uterus shift the heart upward and laterally and rotate it forward.

There is a slight cardiac enlargement and the left border is straightened. The size and positioning of the uterus, the strength of the abdominal muscles and the configuration of the abdomen and thorax determine the extent of these changes (Cunningham & Whitridge 1997).

There are changes in blood volume, cardiac output, heart rate, systemic blood pressure, vascular resistance and distribution of blood flow. Stroke volume, heart rate and cardiac output increase significantly, whereas systemic vascular resistance, pulmonary and vascular resistance (PVR) and colloid osmotic pressure decrease (Clark et al 1989).

All these changes enable homeostasis to be maintained.

Cardiac disease and pregnancy

Heart disease affects less than 1% of pregnancies and causes 10 deaths per million in England and Wales (Caulin-Glaser & Setaro 1999).

However, symptoms of heart disease (breathlessness, palpitation, fainting and oedema) are present in over 90% of pregnant women (De Swiet & Fidler 1981).

Superimposed on a pre-existing cardiac disease state, pregnancy can be dangerous and even potentially fatal. However, other diseases may benefit from the increase in cardiac output, decrease in systemic vascular resistance and increased heart rate.

Heart and blood vessel remodelling

Heart

The heart increases in size by about 12% and is accompanied by some remodelling. The changes are like the ventricular hypertrophy of an athlete's heart in continuous training. In fact formerly Eastern Bloc countries would coerce female athletes to bear one child to improve their fitness! Over a third of the female medal winners in the 1956 Russian Olympics were pregnant and the cardiovascular changes were partly responsible for their performance (De Swiet 1998).

Stroke volume

Stroke volume increases by 8 weeks.

Cardiac output

Cardiac output (heart rate × stroke volume) is one of the most significant haemodynamic changes. It is generally agreed that it increases by about 40% through pregnancy but uncertainty remains about the exact timing and pattern of the component changes (Duvekot & Peters 1998).

Recent data tend to suggest that cardiac output rises significantly during the first trimester, initially as a result of increased heart rate which is subsequently followed by increased stroke volume. By 8 weeks it is already 22% higher than pre-pregnancy (Capeless &

Clapp 1989). It rises more slowly until the third trimester when values, measured in the left lateral recumbent position, are 30–50% higher than in nonpregnant women. It peaks at 32 weeks with no significant changes thereafter. As pregnancy advances, the heart rate increases by about 10–20 beats per minute. It varies according to position, especially in the third trimester. A change from the left lateral recumbent to supine can lead to a 25–30% decrease in cardiac output. The compression of the inferior vena cava by the uterus results in a decrease in venous return and cardiac output (20–30%).

The increase in cardiac output is not related to the metabolic requirements of the mother and fetus but most likely due to the development of placental circulation. Myocontractility (i.e. more contractility of heart muscles) is increased throughout pregnancy which stimulates a degree of ventricular hypertrophy (enlargement of heart chambers) (Benedetti 1990, Capeless & Clapp 1989, Clark et al 1989, Mabie et al 1994, Manga 1999, Morton 1991).

Heart rate guidelines for exercise

Most guidelines advocate a maximal heart rate of 60–70% for women who were sedentary prior to pregnancy and the upper range of 60–90% of maximal heart rate for women wishing to maintain fitness during pregnancy (Table 1.4).

Blood pressure

This remains fairly stable unless there are complications, although it can change with position. Venous pressures do not change much. There is little change in systolic pressure. Diastolic blood pressure decreases in early pregnancy reaching a minimum mid-pregnancy and then returns close to pre-pregnant values towards term (Manga 1999).

Supine hypotensive syndrome (SHS)

Blood pressure may be affected dramatically by posture from the second trimester as the fetus increases in size. If a woman is lying supine, the increased

weight of the uterus may impede venous return from the inferior vena cava resulting in an apparent decrease in cardiac output. This is known as supine hypotensive syndrome, i.e. a drop in blood pressure.

About 90% of pregnant women experience obstruction of the inferior vena cava in supine but only 8% of women experience a significant decreasing heart rate and blood pressure leading to symptoms of weakness, light-headedness, nausea, dizziness or syncope (temporary loss of consciousness) (Kerr 1965; Manga 1999).

Causes
- Progesterone relaxing vascular smooth muscle.
- Oestrogen induced myocardial hypertrophy (changes in cardiac muscles).
- Changes in utero-placental circulation causing a vascular shunt, i.e. causing blood to be shunted from the heart.
- Pressure of the fetal head on the iliac veins.

Implications The concern is that the drop in blood pressure may affect uterine circulation. However, no one knows to what extent. Different texts vary in their suggestions. Henderson and Macdonald (2004) suggest that the supine position should be avoided throughout the entirety of the second and third trimesters. Myles (Fraser & Cooper 2003), however, suggests avoidance of the supine position only late in the second trimester. Some women are comfortable lying on their backs, even doing gentle exercise, for a significant part of the pregnancy. Others are not comfortable lying fully supine after 4–5 months. It is obviously related to the weight as well as the position of the fetus, and therefore may be more of a problem for women with big babies and women with twins or triplets. Guidelines given to limit supine positioning are more exercise guidelines (RCOG 2006).

Given the difficulties in establishing safe times for bodywork, the potential limitations of the fully supine position can be readily addressed by replacing it with a semi-reclining position.

If the woman wants to lie supine and shows any symptoms of SHS then it can be corrected by immediately repositioning to left lateral to release the pressure from the inferior vena cava which is more on the right side.

Distribution of blood flow

- The increase in blood flow of up to 40% correlates with birth weight and, as it begins early in pregnancy, is thought to be hormonally driven.
- Much of the increased cardiac output is distributed to the placenta. Uterine blood flow increases by about 150% so that at term it is receiving 10–20% of cardiac output.

Table 1.4 Modified heart rate target zones for aerobic exercise in pregnancy (from RCOG 2006)

Maternal age (years)	Heart rate target zone (beats/minute)
<20	140–155
20–29	135–150
30–39	130–145
>40	125–140

Clinical implications for bodyworkers of changes in haemostasis and the cardiovascular system: summary

Energy work includes focus with Heart, Heart Protector, Spleen, Liver, Penetrating Vessel.

PET/HELLP
- Learn the risk factors and signs of PET and HELLP (pre-eclampsia toxaemia; haemolytic anaemia, elevated liver enzymes and low platelet count; see high risk section):
  - High blood pressure, protein in the urine, generalised, firmer oedema which does not alter with elevation, rest or exercise.
- Learn how to identify if it is developing into eclampsia.

TED
Assess risk factors (p. 27) for possible risk of TED; refer as appropriate.
- Consult re bodywork treatment for clients with TED.
- Be aware of benefits of mobilisations and bodywork in preventing TED and varicose veins.
- Learn the signs of DIC: i.e. shock.

Signs of suspected thrombosis
1. One-sided oedema.
2. Pain or tenderness in the calf.
3. Swelling or redness in the calf.
4. Fever or raised temperature.
5. Positive Homans sign (dorsal flexion of the foot).

Anaemia
- Understand the symptoms of anaemia and iron deficiency, which are:
  - Tiredness, breathless and paleness.

- Assess that the mother is taking in adequate dietary iron and folic acid and is not losing blood.
- Be aware that healthy pregnant women may suffer from breathlessness, palpitation and fainting but that if she rests and allows the symptoms to subside, then there are no adverse effects. The woman needs to be encouraged to listen to her body and not overexert.

Supine hypotensive syndrome
- Learn how to identify supine hypotension (SHS):
  - Feelings of faintness, nausea, sweatiness.
- Correct with immediate left lateral positioning.

Exercise
- Be aware of current exercise guidelines when advising re exercise.

Referral issues
Urgent referral with no bodywork
- Concerns re possible thrombosis.
- Current undiagnosed vaginal blood loss.
- Eclampsia see box 8.3 p185.

Referral as aftercare but bodywork can proceed
- Concerns re oedema and blood pressure; signs which are milder pre-eclampsia.
- Refer the mother to her primary care-giver for appropriate treatment if there is any concern re anaemia.

- Renal blood flow increases to 35–60% by end of first trimester.
- Pulmonary blood flow increases by 50%.
- Mammary blood flow is increased.
- Venous return is diminished. This increases the likelihood of varicosities.
- Distribution of blood to the skin is increased which stimulates growth of nails and hair.
- Increased flow to mucous membranes can result in increased congestion of mucosa, which is demonstrated by increased incidence of sinusitis, nosebleeds and snoring in pregnancy (Manga 1999).

1.5 Musculoskeletal system

This is one of the prime systems addressed through bodywork. Changes in individual muscles become increasingly marked as the pregnancy progresses and give the characteristic gait of the pregnant mother (Fig. 1.4).

Postural effects

Postural alterations are due largely to changes in the pelvis resulting from:

- Increasing weight of the fetus, which shifts the mother's centre of gravity and brings about changes in the abdominal wall.
- Softening of the pelvic joints, ligaments and muscles.
- Changes in breast size also affect posture.

As the weight of the uterus increases, the centre of gravity moves forward. This may lead to problems with balance, increasing the risk of falls. If there is inadequate muscular support from the lower back and abdomen then the pelvis can tip forward, resulting in poor posture (Heckman & Sassard 1994).

Backache occurs in up to 70% of women, mostly from the fifth month of pregnancy onwards. This can be caused by postural change or due to muscle spasm caused by pressure on nerve roots (Fast et al 1990). There may be an increase in intravertebral disc disorders due to possible increase in mechanical stress.

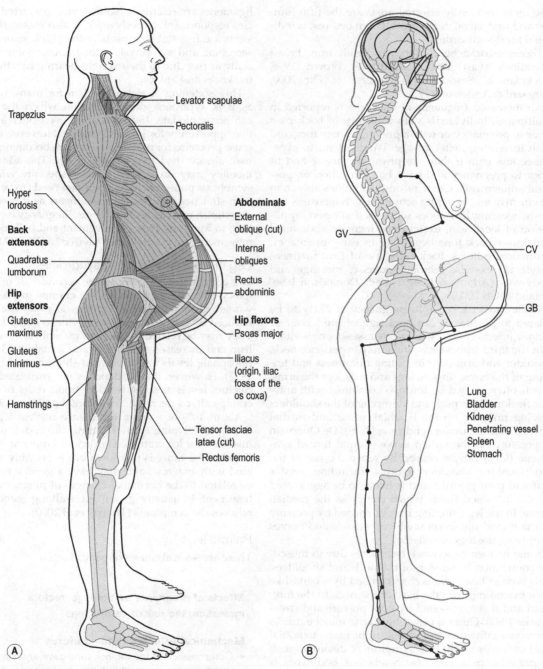

Fig. 1.4A and B Postural patterning.

The most frequently affected areas are the fifth lumbar and first sacral nerve roots. Often bed rest is indicated for disc disorders.

Thoracic backache earlier may result from breast alterations (Fast 1990, Gilleard & Brown 1996, Heckman & Sassard 1994, Ireland & Ott 2000, Ostgaard & Anderson 1991).

An increased frequency of backache is reported in multiparas, individuals with a history of back pain prior to pregnancy or with a previous pregnancy, and with increasing maternal age. Women tend to experience less pain if they are physically active and fit prior to pregnancy and have had education on postural adjustments. Other recommendations shown to be effective are: avoiding activity which increases lordosis, wearing low shoes with good support, application of local heat, exercises to increase abdominal and lower back tone beginning in early pregnancy, abdominal pillows, back rubs, use of firm mattress, pelvic tilt exercise, aerobic exercise, massage and bodywork (Adams & Keegan 1998, Donaldson 1998, Ireland & Ott 2000).

While most backache in pregnancy is likely to be related to posture, it can be a sign of pre-labour or kidney infections and so accurate assessment is vital.

In the third trimester women may experience neck, shoulder and arm pain including numbness and tingling of the arms, fingers, legs and toes. For the arms, this is often caused by lordosis combined with anterior flexion of the neck and slumping of the shoulders placing pressure on the brachial, ulnar and medial nerves: thoracic outlet syndrome (TOS). De Quervain is pressure on the radian nerve. Carpal tunnel syndrome (CTS) can be caused by repetitive use of the wrist and/or shoulder injuries, including rotator cuff and poor posture, and is likely to be aggravated by the increased fluids which compress the median nerve. In the legs, tingling may be caused by pressure of the gravid uterus on the blood vessels and nerves supplying the legs or oedema.

Some women experience headaches due to muscular contraction or tension of the neck and shoulders. This type of headache is characterised by a band-like pain extending from the base of the neck to the forehead and it is aggravated by poor posture and stress (Burke 1993). Other types of headache may be due to hormonal influences but care must be taken to note if the headaches might be a symptom of disorders such as pre-eclampsia. For most headaches, bodywork is likely to be effective.

Hormonal effects

Progesterone and relaxin relax smooth muscles, soften connective tissue, cartilage, joints and ligaments of the pelvis. This means that the fascia, muscles and ligaments are relatively 'softer' and contracted muscles respond well to bodywork. It also means that all joints are less stable, especially the pelvic joints (hip, sacroiliac and symphysis pubis). Other joints especially at risk due to their weight-bearing function are the knees and ankles.

This 'softening' is not a problem for many women as it is a physiological adaptation which the body can accommodate. Indeed it may even offer a positive opportunity for postural change. However, it may cause problems for mothers who before becoming pregnant already had hypermobile joints. The additional mobility may cause joint issues, especially with the symphysis pubis. For all women care needs to be taken with stretches and resisted movements as it is easy to overstretch muscles and ligaments. Pregnancy is not the time to force any type of movement and ballistic-type movements are generally not advised (ACOG 2006).

Leg cramps/restless leg syndrome

Leg cramps are common in the second half of pregnancy. The specific basis for leg cramps in pregnant women remains unclear. Cramps at night are often reduced by gentle leg exercises prior to going to bed. They may be related to calcium/phosphorus metabolism and increased neuromuscular irritability. Raised phosphate levels are implicated (Blackburn & Loper 1992). However, the incidence is not correlated with calcium levels as some women report relief from leg cramps after a decrease in milk intake (Pitkin 1985).

About 10% of women experience restless leg syndrome 10–20 minutes after getting into bed. It is often mistaken for leg cramps. The legs feel more and more fidgety. The cause is unknown but is possibly associated with anaemia, and may have a genetic basis or be related to the hormonal changes of pregnancy. No treatment is usually given but walking sometimes relieves the symptoms (Thorpy et al 2000).

Painful legs

There are several causes of painful legs.

Effects of pregnancy on the legs: factors increasing the risk of painful legs

Mechanical effects of gravid uterus
- Compression of the inferior vena cava and iliac veins, especially when supine.
- Altered gait and posture.

Systemic effects of pregnancy
- Relaxation of cartilage and collagen; reduced pelvic girdle stability; altered gait and posture.

- Reduced concentration of serum albumin causing increased colloid osmotic pressure and dependent oedema.
- Increased concentrations of clotting factors VII, VIII, IX and X.
- Diminished activity of anti-thrombin III.
- Alterations in endocrine milieu.

(above three increase risk of TEDs and care needs to be taken with assessment to ensure no DVT)

- Alteration in calcium and phosphorus metabolism and diet.

Iatrogenic effects of pregnancy
- Lithotomy position with pressure problems secondary to stirrups.
- Operative delivery.

(From Lee et al 1990: 290.)

Chorea gravidarum

This is rapid, brief, non-rhythmical, involuntary, jerky movements of the limbs and non-patterned facial grimacing. There is an incidence of 1 in 139 000 women (Nyman et al 1997). The cause is unknown but it is related to streptococcal infections and is most common in women with a history of rheumatic fever or heart disease (Aminoff 1999).

Calcium metabolism

There is an increased turnover of calcium in early pregnancy with increased bone resorption and decreased bone volume. The maternal skeleton is conserved if dietary calcium is adequate (Coad & Dunstall 2001: 245). There is no marked change in maternal skeletal mass or bone density and clinical deficiency of calcium is rarely observed.

The pelvis: structure and muscles

The pelvis is where the main connective tissue changes occur to accommodate the increasing size of the uterus and fetus. A woman with healthy musculature who does not put on excessive weight adapts to these changes. However, for some women the changes here may cause problems: the main issue is pelvic girdle instability.

The bony structure

The pelvis is a basin-like structure comprising the:

- Sacrum.
- Coccyx.
- Two innominate bones, with three regions: the ilium, the ischium and the pubis.

It is divided into the:

- False or major pelvis, which consists of the ala (blades) of the iliac bones and forms part of the posterior abdominal wall.
- True or minor pelvis which consists of the bones below the pelvic brim. The pelvic brim is formed in continuity by the pubic crest, pectineal line of pubis, the arcuate line of the ilium, the ala and the promontory of the sacrum.

True pelvis
- Houses the pelvic contents.
- Provides exit for the fetus.
- Allows weight transference from the trunk to the lower limb.

Divided into three regions:

- Upper pelvic aperture or pelvic inlet.
- Pelvic cavity.
- Lower pelvic aperture or pelvic outlet.

The structure of the joints and ligaments of the pelvis

Ligaments of the pelvis (Fig. 1.5):

- Sacrospinous.
- Sacrotuberous.
- Iliolumbar.

Sacroiliac (SI) joint

Functions to transmit weight from the body above to the hipbone. It comprises two joints:

- Synovial joint – between the auricular surfaces of the ilium and the sacrum.
- A fibrous joint – between the iliac tuberosity and the sacral tuberosity.

Ligaments The sacroiliac joint is connected by the most comprehensive ligamentous complex in the body. It is the main joint where there are likely to be issues in pregnancy due to relative instability and increased weight-bearing function.

The tendency due to its function in weight-bearing (exaggerated in pregnancy) is for the sacrum to move forward and downward and its inferior end to rotate upward. The ligaments prevent this movement.

Posterior sacroiliac ligaments
- Interosseous sacroiliac ligaments.
- Anterior sacroiliac ligament.

They are big and strong and do not loosen or tighten easily, but if they do then there can be problems such as sacroiliac pain and pelvic girdle instability. There is a gradual stretch to increase the pelvic diameters for

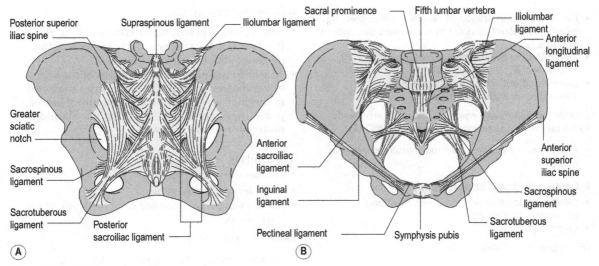

Fig. 1.5A and B Ligaments of the pelvis.

fetal descent (Fig. 1.6). The more supple and tensile the ligaments are, the more effective the coordinated spread. The SI ligaments have a direct anatomical connection with the lumbar and abdominal fascias which both aid the pelvis in softening and stability (Morgan 2008, personal communication).

If the pelvis is out of alignment prior to pregnancy then the problems could either improve or deteriorate.

Pubic symphysis

This is a fibro-cartilaginous joint which consists of two bones with cartilage-covered articular surfaces united by fibrous material.

In every pregnancy there is a natural increase in the width of the symphysis pubis due to the laxity of connective tissue under hormonal (relaxin and progesterone) influence as well as the increasing weight of the uterus. However, there can be excessive movement of the joint. It has also been noted that severe dysfunction and pain may occur irrespective of clinical evidence of joint disruption. This is known as SPI (symphysis pubis instability). As it is often linked with a general instability in the pelvis and combined with sacroiliac instability, it tends to be referred to as part of a pattern of 'pelvic girdle instability' (PGI).

Pelvic girdle instability (PGI): symphysis pubis instability/diastasis (SPI/SPD/DSP)

This is a condition which has now become acknowledged (Albert et al 2002, Larsen et al 1999, Ostgaard

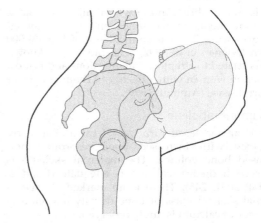

Fig. 1.6 Fetus putting pressure on the pelvic bones.

et al 1994) but is still poorly defined and understood. Previously it was often confused with other types of pelvic discomfort and even attributed to bowel pain. It is usually diagnosed when there is pain in the pubic bone itself which causes limitations in movement. It is due to the pubic bones becoming overly unstable and 'grinding' together. In its early stages, the pain may not necessarily be experienced at the moment of placing strain on the joint (through standing/walking/movement of the joint) but several hours later. This can make it hard to know what is happening. Later, it may be painful all the time and worse while actually doing the movements which aggravate it.

The true incidence is not known, although it has been estimated to be 1 in 36 (Owens et al 2002). In clinical practice bodyworkers are finding as many as 1 in 6 women suffering some kind of symphysis pubis discomfort, even if it is mild.

If it is diagnosed and treated early on, through appropriate lifestyle and bodywork, it need not develop into a major problem. It may cause some discomfort in pregnancy but provided care is taken in labour then it usually resolves quickly in the postnatal period. If untreated, however, it can lead to the woman being confined to bed in the later stages of pregnancy, being unable to walk or lift and being in considerable pain. If it is aggravated during labour, it may remain an issue in the postnatal period for months or even years. It potentially has an immense impact on the woman's emotional well-being. If she is in pain it may lead to feelings of isolation and depression and affect bonding, breastfeeding and family relationships (Shepherd & Fry 1996).

Symptoms

The pain may be insidious or sudden. As well as being felt in the pubis, pain may be felt in the groin and medial aspect of thighs, either unilaterally or bilaterally. It may be similar to pain in the groin areas experienced due to pressure of the fetus's head coming down and engaging at the end of pregnancy, or the fetus's body pushing against the woman and causing feelings of being bruised, or simply heavy feelings of muscle fatigue. It is not always easy to differentiate, although symphysis pubis pain is usually more sharp, even 'burning' and felt more specifically in the joint. It eases when care is taken to keep the legs adducted and is aggravated with leg abduction movements.

This pain can be mild to severe and is exacerbated by walking and all weight-bearing activities, particularly those which include lifting one leg, such as going up the stairs, parting the legs, or by movement in bed. It is also aggravated by any position which abducts the legs. There is a characteristic waddling gait. It is not to be confused with urinary tract infection which would be diagnosed by a more internal feeling of burning.

It is frequently accompanied by low back or sacroiliac pain and suprapubic pain. Symphysial 'clicking' or grinding may be audible and can be felt by the woman.

It can come on gradually in pregnancy, during labour (if the woman labours in positions with the legs abducted, especially with weight-bearing, and especially in the lithotomy position, i.e. lying on the back with legs apart) or following delivery:

- If it is caused by trauma in labour, it is likely to recur more severely and earlier on in subsequent pregnancies if it is not dealt with.

- If it is caused in the first pregnancy by softening of the tissue it is likely to occur during the third trimester.
- If it is during a second pregnancy it is likely to occur earlier.

Assessment

There is a condition known as symphysis pubis diastasis which is when the pubic bone is 10 mm apart (Lindsey et al 1988). However, this 'diagnosis' is controversial as many women suffer pain without the joint being apart. This is why assessment is usually based on pain and limitation of movement and the condition is referred to as dysfunction or instability.

The signs are groin pain when:

- Walking.
- Turning over in bed at night.
- Getting in and out of the car.
- After doing stretches or during doing stretches which involve abduction.
- Weight-bearing.
- Lifting.

In the early stages pain may not be felt while undertaking the aggravating movements but a few hours after. Eventually when it gets worse, pain will be experienced during the activities which aggravate it, or even constantly.

If the assessment is uncertain then it is acceptable to suggest protocols for symphysis pubis pain because they will not do harm and if they make no difference then it is probably related to another issue.

Risk factors

- Women who tend to hyper flexibility when they are not pregnant: the additional flexibility caused by the hormonal changes of pregnancy can be a problem (Gamble et al 1986, Kristiansson et al 1996).
- Women who have overstretched the joint prior to pregnancy; this could be through lots of ballet or gymnastics as a child.
- Women with pre-existing pelvic injuries which place uneven strain on the symphysis pubis. Previous injury (e.g. fall or skiing accident) may have put the pelvic bones out of alignment which can mean that there is uneven pulling on each side.
- Strain injuries which occur during pregnancy, such as sudden twisting and moving, pulling the softening musculature.
- Weak abdominal and/or pelvic floor muscles.
- Previous forceps delivery or lithotomy position in a previous labour which may have forced the bones apart excessively.

Some therapists have noticed an emotional component. It seems to occur in women when they are in need of emotional and physical support. The body generates symptoms which mean that the woman cannot lift and has to accept support.

Treatment

Professional uncertainty still remains as to the best approach and the European COST Commission recommended the need for consistent terminology and evidence-based treatment (ECC 2004). The use of stabilising exercises in the postpartum (Stuge et al 2004) and acupuncture (Elden et al 2005) indicate promising approaches. Yvonne Coldron suggested that a combination of treatment approaches should be considered (Coldron 2005). Christine Andrews, chiropractor and midwife, is currently completing her PhD thesis on the issue (Andrews 2008).

In our clinical experience, the main guidance is addressing lifestyle issues which aggravate the problem. During pregnancy the simplest advice is to imagine that the legs are tied together or that one is wearing a tight miniskirt for a week. This means keeping the legs adducted as much as possible, especially when changing position. It also means avoiding, where possible, lifting and weight-bearing activities.

Exercises to strengthen the supporting musculature, particularly abdominal and pelvic floor and lower back, tend to be beneficial. Good posture is also essential as hyperlordotic patterning tends to aggravate the issue.

Postnatally symptoms may continue for sometime, especially if they are aggravated through delivery, and often there is a recurrence around menstruation due to the hormonal changes.

There is a lot that can be done to address this issue through appropriate bodywork. The main aim of treatment is first to avoid excessive strain on the joint and secondly to strengthen abdominal and pelvic floor muscles along with relevant muscle groups and address ligament weakness. Energy-based approaches can also be successful.

There is no medical treatment in pregnancy. A support belt can be prescribed by a physiotherapist for use both antenatally and postnatally. It is usually important that the mother does not wear this all the time, as while it may give support it will also tend to weaken the supporting musculature which needs to be strengthened. Some women find simply wearing more supportive underwear is sufficient.

If the bone remains severely disrupted, as in diastasis, then post-pregnancy an operation can be carried out to insert a metal plate across the joint, but this has questionable outcomes. It would be considered only as a last resort when all other approaches had failed and is not commonly used.

Muscles supporting the pelvis

There are many muscles which support the pelvis. Here we specifically discuss the pelvic floor and abdominal muscle changes in pregnancy as many therapists do not have as much knowledge of these important muscle groups.

The pelvic floor muscles (PFM) and the perineum

The pelvic floor is key to female health due to its support of the pelvis and pelvic organs, although 50% of Caucasian women suffer from some form of dysfunction.

Perineal muscles

Complex muscles (Fig. 1.7):

- Superficial level: pelvic floor.
- Deeper level forming a hammock.

Pelvic floor

The outer layer of the pelvic floor is the floor to the bony basin of the pelvis. It consists of a muscle sheet which forms a figure of eight swung in loops around the urethra and vagina at the front and the anus at the back. It is suspended mainly between the bony points of the pubis and the coccyx. Another part, the transverse, is attached between the two ischions. At the junction where these two parts cross it is called the central tendon. They include the:

- Bulbocavernosus muscles.
- Ischiocarvernous muscles.
- Transverse perineal muscles.

The deeper layer of the pelvic floor is known as the levator ani and is approximately 3–5 cm in depth. When the levator ani muscles are contracted the pelvic floor and perineum are lifted upwards. They include the:

- Pubococcygeus muscles.
- Iliococcygeus muscles.
- Ischiococcygeus muscles.

Functions

The pelvic floor is important for support, elimination and sexuality:

1. It acts as a base of support for the pelvic organs (the bladder, uterus and bowel) and their

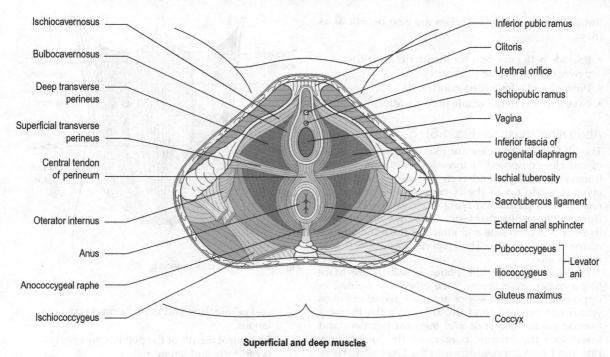

Superficial and deep muscles

Fig. 1.7 The perineal muscles.

contents. In pregnancy it has to provide a lot more support to all these organs due to the changes and increased weight.

2. It has to withstand increases in pressure in the abdominal and pelvic cavity. When laughing, coughing or sneezing, there is increased pressure on the pelvic floor muscles. Pregnancy, because of the increasing weight of the uterus, places a constant and increasing pressure on the muscles. Pressure is also exerted on them during the pushing of the second stage of labour.

3. It provides sphincter control of the perineal openings (urethra, vagina and anus) – important during elimination and sex.

Problems with a weak pelvic floor

Since the muscles are supported like a hammock, if they are not strong enough, they start to provide insufficient support to the pelvic organs. The uterus can prolapse and eventually herniate through the vaginal wall. The onset of any problems in the weakness of these muscles may be slow. Often it may start as vague aches or fatigue in the area. Escape of urine when laughing or coughing may also be a sign. Sometimes urinary stress incontinence only occurs during pregnancy and appears to clear up afterwards. However, the fact that it has occurred indicates a weakness. Exercise can alleviate incontinence, along with special weights or use of ultrasound, but if the condition is allowed to progress too far then surgery may be needed.

As the pelvic floor and abdominals give support to the pelvis and its contents as well as both having attachments at the pubic bone, weak pelvic floor and weak abdominals are often interlinked.

Exercise of the pelvic floor

Exercise of the pelvic floor involves contracting the muscles (strength), holding (endurance), releasing (relaxation). Work needs to be done to work with both slow twitch and fast twitch fibres.

These muscles are not exercised during any form of sport, yoga, movement, etc. but specific exercises to improve the muscle tone and strength were developed by Professor Kegel, professor of obstetrics and gynaecology at the University of California. He realised that a great deal of female surgery on the pelvic floor was unnecessary and could be corrected through exercise. The exercises are also beneficial as they:

- Provide better support for the uterus and other pelvic organs during pregnancy.
- Prevent and alleviate haemorrhoids.
- Give support to the whole pelvic girdle.

Abdominal muscles (Fig. 1.8)

The abdominal muscles are like an elaborate corset of muscles composed of three layers of muscles: the transverse, oblique and recti muscles. The deepest layer is made up of the transverse muscles, acting rather like a girdle and lying horizontally. They run from the thoracolumbar fasica, iliac crest and inguinal ligaments at each side and attach to the inner surface of the lower six ribs. Their aponeurosis inserts into the linea alba.

The next layer are the obliques, which are more like a corset, overlapping each other and pulling in opposite directions. Deeper are the internal obliques which run upwards and inwards from the thoraco-lumbar fascia, iliac crest and inguinal ligament and insert into the inferior borders of the lower three ribs and by an aponeurosis into the linea alba. There may be discomfort under the ribs as the fetus grows and exerts pressure on these muscles. The external obliques are superficial and run at right angles to the internal obliques. They insert into the anterior half of the iliac crest, pubic crest and by an aponeurosis into the linea alba and their origin is the outer surface of the lower eight ribs. The inguinal ligament is formed from the lower border of each external oblique.

The most superficial layer is formed by the recti muscles which go in a vertical panel composed of two vertical lines like braces. They all join up in the mid-line which is made up of connective tissue. They are enclosed in the aponeuroses formed by the other abdominal muscles. They attach superiorly to the cartilages of ribs 5, 6 and 7 and to the xiphisternum and inferiorly to the crest of the pubis.

In pregnancy, they all stretch out from the mid-line.

Role of abdominal muscles

They act along with the pelvic floor to give pelvic stability:

1. To maintain proper positions of the abdominal and pelvic organs (including the uterus in pregnancy).
2. To assist in deliberate breathing, singing, shouting, coughing, sneezing, etc., straining

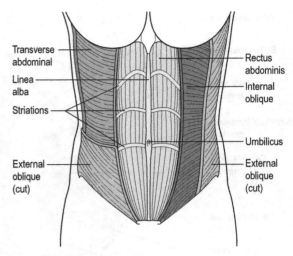

Fig. 1.8 The abdominal muscles.

and elimination and in the second stage of labour.

3. To control the tilt of the pelvis – anteriorly/posteriorly and laterally.
4. To flex the trunk sideways laterally, raise up from lying and rotation.
5. To stabilise the lower back. The transverse is particularly important in this regard.

(After Richardson & Jull 1995.)

Weakness of abdominal muscles is a common cause of backache. When, as a human race, our position changed from four-legged creatures to adopt the erect position, the role of the abdominal muscles changed and they do less work. Abdominal muscles tend to be underexercised due to our sedentary lifestyle. Weak abdominal muscles are not able to give adequate support to the pelvis and lumbar spine. They may also contribute to pelvic girdle instability and symphysis pubis instability.

The centre seam of muscles: the recti muscles (Fig. 1.9)

These muscles in particular have to do a lot of stretching and can pull apart. Some degree of separation of these muscles is to be expected, but excessive separation, of more than two to three fingers, means that the abdominal wall has become significantly weakened and care needs to be taken in the type of exercise done (e.g. no sitting up from lying down, no sit-ups) and lifting must also be avoided. The entire abdominal corset needs to be toned during pregnancy to help

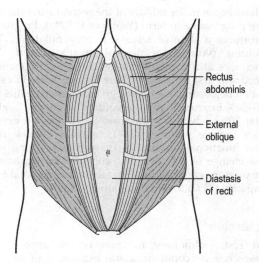

Rectus abdominis

External oblique

Diastasis of recti

Fig. 1.9 Rectus abdominis muscles.

minimise this separation and so that during labour the muscles are able to work effectively in the bearing down phase of labour.

Some people argue that abdominal exercises should not be done because the abdominal wall needs to stretch. It is true that some degree of stretching is natural and inevitable; however, due to the modern sedentary lifestyle, for most women the abdominal muscles are not used enough in day-to-day activity and work to keep them toned is important, provided they realise that the aim is not to have a 'flat tummy' and they do the exercises correctly.

The most important is to emphasise first respiratory exercise i.e. synchronising the abdominal and pelvic floor muscles during respiration to align the cavities from within and secondary skeletal muscle action to support the natural progression of postural and visceral position changes.

(Averille Morgan, personal communication, 2008)

There is also a myth that strong abdominal muscles inhibit labour. In fact the reverse is true: they help, particularly with second stage. It is true that tension in the abdomen will not aid in labour and primiparae in particular may need to be encouraged to relax the obliques, multifidus, hip rotators and PFM.

All fours is an effective position in which to exercise abdominal muscles in pregnancy, especially as many women will be uncomfortable in the supine position.

Clinical implications for bodyworkers of changes in the muscoloskeletal system

- The connective tissue is relatively softer than pre-pregnancy and this needs to be taken into account in assessing muscle responsiveness. Care needs to be taken when performing stretches or mobilisations as it is much easier to overextend muscles and ligaments.
- There is also relative instability of joints, especially in the pelvis.
- Be aware of increased blood supply to tissue.
- Be aware of changes in the abdominal wall, what degree of change is normal and what causes problems: recti muscle separation less than three fingers width is considered physiological.
- Be aware of how to differentiate types of back pain, e.g. backache, round ligament pain, or other discomforts, and how they might differ from the type of backache associated with pre-term labour or kidney issues.
  - Pre-term labour: other symptoms such as contractions.
  - Kidney pain at level of kidneys, changes in urination patterns (Kidney pain).
- Be able to differentiate between causes of painful legs or arms as being muscoloskeletal or due to cardiovascular changes including possible thrombosis.
- Be able to differentiate between different types of headaches: e.g. musculoskeletal, hormonal, PET.
- Eastern terms: MS system relates to Spleen (Muscle), Liver (joints and ligaments), Kidney (bones).

Immediate referral issues
- Suspect DVT.
- Premature labour.
- Eclampsia.

1.6 Respiratory system

Respiration has to increase to meet the increased metabolic demands for both mother and baby. Changes are mediated by hormonal and biochemical changes as well as by the enlarging uterus. The muscles and cartilage in the thoracic region relax, the chest broadens, and tidal volume (VT) is improved with a conversion from abdominal to thoracic breathing. This leads to a 50% increase in air volume per minute. These changes result in a mild respiratory alkalosis (excess base (alkali) in the body fluids). For the fetus this mild alkalosis is essential for the exchange of gases across the placenta (Wilkening & Meschia 1983).

The stress put on the maternal respiratory system is small compared with the demands put on the cardiovascular system. This means that women who have pre-existing respiratory disease are much less likely to deteriorate in pregnancy than those with cardiac disease (Coad & Dunstall 2001: 236).

Mechanical changes: enlarging uterus

Early in pregnancy, and therefore not because of the enlarging uterus, the diaphragm is displaced upwards by 4 cm (De Swiet 1998 in Coad & Dunstall 2001: 236). Near the end of pregnancy, the enlarging uterus displaces the diaphragm upward as there is increased flaring of the lower ribs. This is known as 'rib flare' and many women feel slightly bruised and constricted. These anatomical changes do not completely reverse post-pregnancy, hence changes in body shape, and it is said that this increased flaring is beneficial to opera singers!

Diaphragmatic movement, however, actually increases and the major work of breathing is accomplished by the diaphragm rather than the costal muscles (Bolt et al 2001, Wilkening & Meschia 1983). Hyperventilation is common due to compression of lower parts of the lungs by the uterus. There are also changes in ventilation due to decreased CO_2 (hypocapnia).

Hormonal factors

Higher progesterone levels are thought to be a major factor in the changes as progesterone is a respiratory stimulant. The respiratory centre is more sensitive to CO_2 as progesterone lowers the sensibility of the peripheral and central chemoreceptors for carbon dioxide (Skatrud et al 1978). This may mean that if pregnant women do not breathe well, they can suffer from dizziness or visual disturbances more readily than non-pregnant women. It is a factor to consider when exercising.

As progesterone increases in pregnancy the increased responsiveness to PCO_2 results in an increased tidal volume and minute volume (Miller et al 2002, Wise et al 2006). Progesterone may also play a role in decreasing airway resistance, reducing the work of breathing and facilitating a greater air-flow in pregnancy.

Hormonal influences cause the muscles and cartilage in the thoracic region to relax so the chest broadens. Relaxation of the ligamentous rib attachments increases rib cage elasticity – this is similar to changes in the pelvis and mediated by similar factors, especially relaxin (Sherwood et al 1993).

Changes in lung function and volumes

These begin in the middle of the second trimester and are progressive to term (Wolfe et al 1998). Pregnancy produces a state of relative hyperventilation. Tidal volume (volume of normal breath at rest, VT) increases at a constant rate of 25–40% (75% increase occurs in first trimester). There is an increase in ventilation beginning in early pregnancy which results in a 40–50% increase in minute volume (resting 50%, alveolar 70%). There is a progressive decrease in expiratory reserve volume (ERV), residual volume (RV) and functional residual capacity (FRC). Along with the change in VT there is a concomitant increase in inspiratory capacity (IC), thereby allowing total lung capacity (TLC) to remain relatively stable.

Exercise

At rest, pulmonary function is not impaired as there is a concomitant lateral expansion of rib cage and increased tidal volume. During mild activity expected increases in oxygen consumption occur. In high-intensity exercise the increase is less than expected, suggesting that pregnant women are unable to maintain high levels of aerobic activity. This is why moderate exercise is recommended as being more beneficial than intense activity in pregnancy.

Dyspnoea

Many pregnant women experience dyspnoea (shortness of breath) in early pregnancy, before there are changes in intra-abdominal pressures. About 60–70% of women experience this, beginning in the first or second trimester with a maximal incidence between 28 and 31 weeks (De Swiet 1991).

The cause is thought to be due to increased respiratory drive and load, changes in oxygenation or a combination of the two. This may cause discomfort and anxiety. It can be quite uncomfortable and anxiety-provoking and may cause women to decrease usual activity levels. It can occur at rest or with mild exertion (Wise et al 2006).

Respiratory effects

Capillaries in the upper respiratory tract become engorged, which can create difficulties in breathing via the nose and aggravate respiratory infections. Laryngeal changes and oedema of the vocal cords caused by vascular dilation can promote hoarseness and deepening of the voice and a persistent cough.

The altered cell-mediated immunity may place the woman at risk for upper respiratory infections.

Nose

There is a heightened sense of smell. There is also a greater likelihood of nasal congestion. Nasal mucosa becomes hyperaemic (gorged with blood) and congested due to the changes in oestrogen.

Asthma

It affects about 0.4–1.3% of pregnant women. Women who had asthma prior to pregnancy may find that it can either improve, worsen or remain unchanged.

Smoking

In addition to affecting fertility, risks of smoking in pregnancy include: a spontaneous abortion rate two times greater than in the non-smoking population, an increased risk of abruption, placenta praevia, early or late bleeding, premature rupture of membranes and prolonged rupture of the membranes, and pre-term labour, low birth weight and intra-cuterine growth restrictions (Abel 1983, Andres 1999, Heffner et al 1993, Malloy et al 1992, Weinberger & Weiss 1999).

Clinical implications for the bodyworker regarding changes in the respiratory system

- The eastern view is to support the Lung.
- There are physiological changes in the rib cage and diaphragm which mean that they are more sensitive to pressure in bodywork techniques.
- Women are likely to suffer from blocked sinuses, nasal congestions, blocked throat.
- This system is important to promote deep breathing as without good breathing there may be issues such as shortness of breath, dizziness and so on.
- When teaching breathing, be aware of the role of the diaphragm; teach both abdominal and diaphragmatic breathing.
- Be aware of exercise implications: moderate exercise is considered advisable due to the state of relative hyperventilation.
- Positioning considerations: if the woman has sinus congestion or is finding it hard to breathe, side or semi-recumbent may be preferable to forward leaning.

Referral issues

- There are not really any emergency situations which arise in this system.

1.7 Renal system

Kidneys

The kidneys are fundamental organs in the regulation of homeostasis, and underlying disease or problems in the renal system can potentially cause severe implications for the pregnancy.

Pregnancy is characterised by sodium retention and increased maternal intravascular and extracellular volume which must be mediated by the kidneys. They also have to serve as the primary excretory organ for fetal waste.

Kidneys:

- Regulate water and electrolyte balance.
- Excrete metabolic waste products and foreign substances.
- Regulate vitamin D activity and erythrocyte (red blood cell) production (via erythropoietin which is a naturally occurring hormone, produced by the kidneys) and gluconeogenesis (generation of glucose) (Vander et al 2000).

They also play an important role in the control of arterial blood pressure through the renin–angiotensin system (RAS) and regulation of sodium balance.

Hormonal effects, particularly the influence of progesterone on smooth muscle, pressure from the enlarging uterus, effects of position and activity and alterations in the cardiovascular system, all affect the kidneys. There is a close relationship between changes in the cardiovascular system and changes in the renal system which affect cardiac output, increased blood and plasma volume, and alterations in the venous system and plasma proteins.

During pregnancy the renal system goes through a variety of structural and functional changes with many of the structural changes continuing into the postpartum period.

Functional changes

Kidneys increase their tubular reabsorption rate of sodium to achieve increased circulating blood volume and haemodilution. There is an increased glomerular filtration rate (GFR) from early pregnancy, by 40–50%. The changes begin soon after conception, peak at 9–16 weeks and remain relatively stable around 36 weeks (Davison 1987, Duvekot et al 1993).

This results in more sodium, glucose and amino acids in the filtrate. However, the pregnant woman remains in sodium balance and responds normally to changes in sodium and water balance as most sodium is reabsorbed.

The increased GFR also reduces serum BUN, plasma urea, uric acid and creatinine by the end of the first trimester. GFR is measured by insulin or creatinine clearance. For women with impaired kidney function, changes in creatinine and insulin can give an indication of how the kidneys are functioning in pregnancy.

Glycosuria: insulin resistance and proteinuria

The tendency to become insulin-resistant in the latter part of pregnancy results in increased blood glucose. Glucose excretion may be up to 10 times greater than the non-pregnant levels. This does not necessarily indicate diabetes, as few women with glycosuria have abnormal glucose tolerance test results. However, some women do develop gestational diabetes and this will need to be checked. Mild proteinuria is also relatively common and does not necessarily indicate PET.

Effects of position on renal function

As pregnancy progresses there is pooling of the blood in the pelvis and lower extremities while sitting, lying supine or standing. This leads to a relative hypovolaemia and decreased cardiac output. These effects are magnified with women with PET. Renal plasma flow is maximal in the left lateral position (Manga 1999).

Structural changes

Kidneys enlarge due to the increased renal blood flow and vascular volume. There is a dilatation of the renal pelvis and ureters.

Recent ultrasound studies have demonstrated dilatation of the urinary tract in 50% of women in the second and third trimesters due to the effect of progesterone relaxing smooth muscle (Faúndes et al 1998).

As pregnancy progresses the ureters are displaced by the growing uterus. In most women the right ureter is dilated more than the left (Faúndes et al 1998, Hertzberg et al 1993).

The calyces of kidneys and the ureters appear to be distended as due to hormonal changes they lose some of their peristaltic activity in pregnancy. The ureters elongate and become tortuous so they can accommodate an increased volume of urine. This is associated with an increased risk of infection. Women with urinary tract infections are at increased risk of going into premature labour or miscarriage (Culpepper & Jack 1990, Davison & Linheimer 1999).

Urine output increases. Renal volume increases by 30% due to increase in blood flow (Christensen et al 1989).

Changes in blood flow

Renal blood flow increases by 35–60% by the end of the first trimester and then decreases from the second trimester to term. This change is accompanied by increased glomerular filtration rate (GFR), decreased renal vascular resistance (RVR) and activation of the renin–angiotensin–aldosterone system. These changes begin before significant expansion of plasma volume and are thought to be related to the decrease in systemic vascular restrictions (SVR).

Bladder

Bladder tone decreases due to the effects of progesterone on smooth muscle. This means that capacity increases and may be up to 1 L by term. These two factors (changes in tone and function) mean that the vesico-ureteral sphincters are compromised and reflux of urine may go from the bladder into the ureters, increasing the chance of urinary infection. This is of particular importance when advising regarding pelvic floor exercises. The old advice was to tell women to stop and start the urine flow. Now it is recognised that this is not wise and women should empty their bladder before doing pelvic floor exercises.

Problems caused by changes in the renal system

Urinary tract infections

Due to the structural changes there is an increased incidence of UTIs. In the first trimester, these may be a cause of miscarriage and in the second and third with premature labour. Early detection is therefore important. The signs of UTI can be abdominal bladder pain, burning pain, increased urination, pain on urination.

Prevention is important. It is important to encourage the woman to be aware of good perineal hygiene and to ensure adequate water intake.

Urinary frequency, incontinence and nocturia

Urinary frequency (more than seven daytime voidings) is common in about 60% of women (Mikhail & Anyaegbunam 1995). It is often stated that urinary frequency is most common in the first and third trimesters due to the compression of the bladder by the uterus, but there is little research to support this belief. Thorp notes that urinary frequency is progressive and maximum at term. It is mostly due to the effects of hormonal changes, hypervolaemia (fluid overload) and increased renal blood flow (RBF) and GFR. The pressure of the uterus probably influences it during the last weeks of pregnancy only (Thorp et al 1999).

Urinary stress incontinence is experienced by about 30–50% of pregnant women (versus about 8% of non-pregnant women).

Nocturia

Nocturia (waking in the night to urinate) is due to patterns of sodium excretion. It is thought that during the day, water and sodium are trapped in the lower extremities because of venous stasis and pressure of the uterus on the iliac vein and inferior vena cava. At night this pressure is reduced as the mother lies down, promoting increased venous return, cardiac output, renal blood flow and glomerular filtration.

Treatment There is no medical treatment for nocturia. Advice usually given is:

- Restriction of fluids in the evening.
- Ensure adequate intake over 24 hours of fluids.
- Encourage voiding.
- Limit intake of diuretics (e.g. coffee, tea, cola with caffeine).
- Teach the woman the signs of UTI.
- Use the left lateral recumbent position to promote diuresis.

Proteinuria

Mild proteinuria is common in pregnancy and usually benign, although with coexisting hypertension it can indicate complications of pre-eclampsia.

High-risk issues
Lymphostatic oedema

Oedema can be related to failure of the kidneys and the heart (lymphodynamic oedema). This is more serious and can be linked with PET.

Kidneys and pre-eclampsia

Due to the links between the renal and cardiovascular system, the kidneys are affected by pre-eclampsia along with the heart.

Hypertension

The kidneys play a critical role in regulation of blood pressure through the renin–angiotensin system and regulation of sodium balance. Pre-eclampsia is associated with a suppression of the renin–angiotensin–aldosterone system.

Implications of changes in renal system for bodyworkers

- Energy approaches are about supporting the Kidneys and Jing.
- The renal system is fundamental in supporting pregnancy and issues within it tend to be potentially serious. Clients with pre-existing kidney problems are 'higher risk'.

- Study the links between the renal and cardiovascular systems and learn the issues related to oedema, varicose veins and TEDs, pre-eclampsia, raised blood pressure.
- Recognise the signs of UTIs: abdominal bladder pain, burning and increased urination, pain on urination.
- Many women suffer from managing urinary frequency, oedema and nocturia. Note the appropriate self-care for these clients.
- Understand the different types of oedema, their causes, appropriate treatment and aftercare.

Immediate referral issues

- Issues with this system are potentially serious and often need immediate referral.
- PET.
- Lymphodynamic oedema.
- Severe UTI, especially in first trimester and if accompanied by signs of premature labour.

Referral after bodywork session

- Suspect UTI with no other issues.

1.8 Gastrointestinal system

Maternal nutrition is one of the most important factors affecting pregnancy outcome. This system must digest and absorb nutrients needed for fetal and placental growth and development and meet the altered maternal metabolic demands as well as eliminate unneeded by-products and waste materials.

The changes are due to the pressure of the growing uterus and hormonal influences of progesterone on smooth muscle and the effects of oestrogen on liver function.

Disturbances here are the most common cause of complaint by pregnant women. Over 50% experience an increased appetite and thirst due to the effects of progesterone. These changes in appetite do not necessarily reflect changes in fetal growth or maternal metabolism as appetite tends to increase from mid-pregnancy but declines in later pregnancy due to increasing pressure from the uterus. While most of the complaints are irritating, such as constipation, heartburn and so on, they are not potentially dangerous. However, some conditions are serious and do warrant immediate referal, for example cholestasis, gallstones or biliary colic.

Nutritional requirements of the mother

An additional 300 metric calories per day are needed in the second and third trimesters to meet energy and growth demands of the mother and fetus and to conserve protein for cell growth. It is vital that the woman takes in proper amounts of protein, fat and vitamins and minerals. The risk of dehydration is increased. There is a requirement for long-chain fatty acids which are present in oily fish, nuts and seeds (Hughes 1998, Odent 2002). Reducing consumption of tea, coffee and fizzy drinks is usually recommended, and eating a varied diet. Guidance varies, so refer to current guidelines in the relevant country.

Both excessive weight gain and insufficient weight gain can be problematic. The fetus adapts to maternal undernutrition by slowing growth and reducing energy expenditure and a number of adult-onset diseases are associated with impaired fetal nutrition (Barker 1998). Maternal obesity is associated with an increased incidence of congenital malformations (Prentice & Goldberg 1996) and difficulties in pregnancy and delivery.

Many vitamin allowances are increased by 20–100% and it is important the mother has the correct amounts to support the development of the fetus.

Important vitamins in pregnancy

- **Vitamin E:** tissue growth and integrity of cell tissue. **Source:** vegetable oils, grains, milk, eggs, fish, meat.
- **Vitamin C:** increases iron absorption and needed for collagen formation and tissue formation and integrity. **Source:** citrus fruit, tomatoes, other fruits and vegetables.
- **Thiamin (B$_1$)** – riboflavins, niacin, vitamins B$_6$ and B$_{12}$ – serve as coenzymes for protein and energy metabolism. **Source:** pork, wheatgerm and yeast.
- **Zinc:** supplementation has been reported to increase birth weight in those who are deficient. **Source:** oysters, steak, crab meat, red meat, milk products.
- **Iron:** transfer of O$_2$ in haemoglobin molecule. Oxidation processes electron transfer chain. **Source:** meat, vegetables, pumpkin seeds, beetroot, parsley, nuts, sesame seeds, dried beans.

Excessive vitamin supplementation or marked deficiency may both have an effect on the baby and the practice of routine supplementation is controversial. Vitamin A in particular may present a teratogenic risk (Rosa et al 1986). Folic acid (vitamin B$_9$) consumed at higher levels than from diet alone periconceptually is linked with reduction in neural tube defects (NTD) (Smithells et al 1981) and is recommended in many countries. The Institute of Medicine recommends that pregnant women with balanced diets do not need routine supplementation except for iron if they are anaemic (Institute of Medicine 1990).

Food cravings

Many women experience food cravings and aversions, often beginning in the first trimester, but also later. These cravings do not usually indicate mineral/vitamin deficiencies but may be a response to hormonal changes. Common cravings include fruit, pickles, kippers and cheese. 'Pica' is the term used to describe an extreme craving for a non-nutritious substance. Women may experience this type of craving for coal, soap, dirt, disinfectant, toothpaste, mothballs and ice.

Aversion to foods is particularly marked in the first trimester and is often towards less beneficial foods such as tea, coffee, fried food and eggs, alcohol and smoking. It is often a response to nausea and vomiting.

While the sense of taste may be dulled in pregnancy, the sense of smell may be enhanced.

Mouth

Gums may become hyperaemic, oedematous and spongy because of the effects of oestrogen on blood flow and connective tissue consistency. Gums bleed more easily and are sensitive to vigorous tooth brushing. Gingivitis and periodontal disease occur in a large proportion of pregnant women and are more extreme with increased maternal age and parity and when there are pre-existing dental problems.

Contrary to folk belief that a tooth is lost for every baby, there is no evidence of demineralisation of dentine as fetal calcium stores are drawn from maternal body stores (the skeleton) and not from maternal teeth (Blackburn & Loper 1992).

There is a more acidic pH of saliva, but volume does not usually change. Rarely there is excessive production of saliva, ptyalism or ptyalorrhoea. This may occur with hyperemesis gravidarum (extreme nausea and vomiting, see p. 40).

Oesophagus

The lower oesophageal sphincter tone decreases because of the effects of progesterone on smooth muscle which is linked with an increased incidence of acid reflux. There is also an increase of hiatus hernia in later pregnancy due to increasing pressure from the gravid uterus.

Heartburn

Heartburn affects about 30–70% of women. It is worse with multiple pregnancies, polyhydramnios (excess amniotic fluid), obesity and with excessive bending. Often simply eating sitting upright, as opposed to slouching, can make a difference. Alcohol, coffee and chocolate all exacerbate heartburn by reducing muscle tone. Gastric reflux can be reduced by advising more frequent intake of smaller meals and avoidance of seasoned food. Many women take antacid preparations but these can have side-effects such as:

- Aluminium salts – diarrhoea.
- Magnesium salts – constipation.
- Phosphorus may affect calcium/phosphorus balance and exacerbate cramp.
- Sodium may affect water balance.
- Long-term use of antacids is associated with malabsorption, particularly of drugs and dietary minerals.

Stomach

There are some inconclusive studies which suggest that acid secretion tends to decrease, which may explain why the remission of symptoms of peptic ulcers is not uncommon. GI motility is decreased.

In late pregnancy the stomach drapes loosely over the uterine fundus so gastric emptying is delayed and this may increase the likelihood of heartburn and nausea.

Intestine and colon

Due to the progesterone-induced relaxation of smooth muscle, gut tone and motility are increased and transit time in the gut increases. This has potentially beneficial effects on absorption (Parry et al 1970). Improved absorption of several nutrients such as iron and calcium has been measured (Hytten 1991). The increased absorption of iron in late pregnancy coincides with raised placental uptake and decreased maternal stores. However, progesterone may inhibit transport mechanisms of other nutrients such as B vitamins.

Pancreas

The oestrogen receptors in the pancreas may increase the risk of pancreatitis in pregnancy. It is usually caused by cholelithiasis (gallstones blocking pancreatic duct) or due to the increased amount of lipids (hypertriglycerides). This can be serious. The symptoms are nausea, vomiting and abdominal pain which could be confused with other issues in pregnancy, most notably hyperemesis gravidarum and premature labour. There are also changes in the islet cells associated with increased production and secretion of insulin.

Nausea and vomiting

Between 50% and 90% of women experience some degree of nausea during the first trimester although some women (less than 10%) experience nausea throughout the entire gestation. It is more common in westernised, urban populations and is affected by ethnicity, occupational status and age. It generally begins between 4 and 6 weeks, tends to peak at around 8–12 weeks, and usually resolves by 3–4 months. About 50% of women experience it more in the morning, others after or before eating, in the evening or at other times throughout the day (Flaxman & Sherman 2000, Maxwell & Niebyl 1982, Rubin & Janovitz 1991).

Hyperemesis gravidarum

About 2% of women (Maxwell & Niebyl 1982, Meetze et al 1992) experience a more extreme form of sickness known as hyperemesis gravidarum. This is characterised by intractable nausea and vomiting causing extreme dehydration, electrolyte imbalances, metabolic disturbances and nutritional deficiencies. These women may need to be hospitalised to have intravenous fluids.

Theories about the causes of nausea and vomiting in pregnancy

There are various theories about the causes which include: mechanical, endocrinological, allergic, metabolic, genetic and psychosomatic factors but there is no substantial research to back them up. The major schools of thought consider that it is hormonally caused.

The hormonal theories postulate that the rapidly increasing and high levels of oestrogen, human chorionic gonadotropin (hCG) and possibly thyroxine are involved. Serum hCG peaks in the first trimester (released by syncytiotrophoblast cells). Nausea has been associated with good pregnancy outcomes and this is why it is often considered a favourable sign.

The effects of progesterone on gastric smooth muscle tone, especially on the lower oesophageal sphincter and delayed gastric emptying, suggest how the steroid hormones may be involved.

Another theory is that it may have an adaptive function to protect the embryo from potentially toxic substances in foods such as animal products, caffeinated beverages and alcohol, which may also help explain why it is less common in non-industrialised countries (Flaxman & Sherman 2000, Huxley 2000).

Treatment

- Some suggest small, frequent, high-carbohydrate, low-fat meals although others suggest high-protein meals.
- Avoid strong odours, fatty or spicy foods and cold liquids.
- Consume dry crackers and toast or oatcakes before rising and through the day.
- Consume ginger (soda, tea, cookies, etc.).
- Suck on hard candy or umeboshi plums.
- Use sea bands or stimulate HC6 (De Aloysio & Penacchioni 1992, Jewell & Young 2000).
- Lie down when first experiencing symptoms.
- Relaxation skills.

Constipation

About 10–30% of women experience constipation and it tends to be worse in the first and third trimesters (Bonapace & Fisher 1998, Steinlauf & Traube 1999). It probably arises primarily from alterations in water transport and reabsorption in the large intestine. Decreased intestinal motility and prolonged transit time increase electrolyte and water absorption. There is also some compression of the rectosigmoid area by the enlarging uterus and changes in diet and activity.

Treatment

- Drink fluids.
- Eat high-fibre foods such as fruits and raw vegetables, bran and wheat.
- Light exercise.
- Avoid using mineral oil as it absorbs fat-soluble vitamins including vitamin K.
- Be aware of possible side-effects of laxatives (e.g. fluid accumulation, sodium retention and oedema and cramping).

Haemorrhoids

Constipation may aggravate haemorrhoids. These vein walls are relaxed due to the effects of progesterone and bear increased pressure due to the expanding uterus. Further, increased venous pressure in the pelvic veins leads to venous congestion and engorgement and enlargement of the haemorrhoidal veins.

Treatment

- Prevent constipation and straining.
- Use topical creams.
- Do pelvic floor exercises.

Liver and gallbladder

Gallbladder

Progesterone affects the smooth muscle tone of the gallbladder resulting in flaccidity, increased bile volume storage and decreased emptying rate. Water reabsorption by gallbladder epithelium cells is decreased and so bile is more dilute and contains less cholesterol. There is a tendency to retain bile salts and this can lead to the formation of cholesterol-based gallstones in pregnancy.

Liver

The liver is the organ which is most affected by the displacement of the uterus, being displaced superiorly, posteriorly and anteriorly. The liver edge may be palpable by late in the third trimester although its size does not increase. Hepatic blood flow is not significantly altered despite the blood changes. This means that the proportion of blood flow to the liver is decreased by one third. Liver production of plasma proteins, bilirubin, serum enzymes and serum lipids are altered with a fall in albumin, an increase in fibrinogen and an increase in cholesterol synthesis. These changes arise from the effects of oestrogen and to some extent haemodilution.

Higher risk: pre-eclampsia and the HELLP syndrome

Both of these conditions involve the liver.

Clinical implications for bodyworkers of changes in the gastrointestinal system

- Energy approaches include: Stomach, Spleen, Liver, Gall Bladder, Large Intestine, Small Intestine.
- Recognise the possible causes of itching and know how to recognise obstetric cholestasis (OC): itching in hands and feet (see higher risk section).
- Good aftercare advice is important when dealing with GI issues such as constipation, heartburn and so on.
- Be able to identify if abdominal pain could be related to (cholelithiasis) gallstones. This is serious (see abdominal pain chart, p. 254, box 9.2).
- Be aware of differences between nausea and hyperemesis.
- Extreme vomiting may also be linked with other situations, e.g., hydatiform mole, infection or potential miscarriage, and needs referral.

Immediate referral issues with no bodywork
- Severe continuous unexplained abdominal pain: could be liver issues, gallstones, cholestasis, or biliary colic.
- Extreme vomiting.
- Hyperemesis; client may need fluids.

Referral after bodywork
- Milder abdominal pain, as medical diagnosis may be needed to ascertain cause.
- Skin itching and suspected OC.
- Milder vomiting.

1.9 Immune, sensory, nervous, metabolic and integumentary systems

Immune system response and host defence system

There are many changes in the mother's immune system affecting both innate (includes inflammatory response and phagocytosis) and adaptive (specific immune responses such as cell- and antibody-mediated response) immunity. These changes involve a balancing act between helping the mother's host defence system tolerate the fetus without overly increasing the risk of maternal infections and influencing the course of chronic disorders such as autoimmune disease.

Innate and adaptive immunity responses

The number of white blood cells increases and cells respond more readily to changes. High levels of oestrogen and progesterone decrease the number of helper T-cells and increase the number of suppressor cells. Yeast infections increase in pregnancy, possibly because of the effect of oestrogen on the flora of the reproductive tract (Priddy 1997).

Local concentrations of corticosteroids around the fetus and placenta suppress phagocytic activity, especially in response to Gram-negative bacteria. This means there is less ability to respond to Gram-negative infections of the reproductive tract such as gonococcal infection.

Susceptibility to infection

Due to changes in maternal immune responses, women may have increased susceptibility to viral infection. Women appear to have increased immunological responses to bacterial infection. Some immunological conditions improve in pregnancy, others worsen. Historically, pregnant women were observed to contract smallpox and poliomyelitis more readily. Today viral hepatitis infections pose a major threat to pregnant women.

Women who lack immunity to primary cytomegalovirus (CMV) have increased susceptibility to infections in pregnancy; this is associated with fetal congenital abnormalities. Pregnant women have increased susceptibility to listeriosis, influenza, varicella, herpes, rubella, hepatitis and human papillomavirus.

The pregnancy-induced suppression of helper T-cell numbers may be permanent so pregnancy can cause a progression of HIV-related disease.

Both acute and chronic maternal infections are associated with pre-term labour. There has also been increasing evidence of the role of vaginal and cervical organisms and chorioamnionitis in the initiation of pre-term labour and premature rupture of the membranes (Lockwood & Kuczynski 1999).

Pregnant women with autoimmune disease

This is variable as some women experience improvement, while others experience exacerbation or no changes, depending on the disorder.

Transplacental passage of maternal antibodies

Both protective and potentially damaging antibodies cross the placenta. Maternal IgC antibodies are the only ones to cross in significant amounts. This provides passive immunity against many disorders through the passage of antibodies acquired by the mother from previous infection or immunisation. Depending on maternal antibody complement, passive immunity may be acquired by the fetus against tetanus, diphtheria, polio, measles, mumps, group B streptococcus (GBS), *Escherichia coli*, hepatitis B, salmonella and other disorders.

However, potentially damaging antibodies, such as in Rhesus incompatibility, also cross the placenta. Some examples of these include Graves disease which can lead to transient neonatal hyperthyroidism in a few infants (about 1%), myasthenia gravis which results in transient myasthenia, fetal thrombocytopenia and systemic lupus erythematosus (SLE).

Clinical implications of changes in immune system

If the bodyworker has any concerns about risk of or active infection then it is important to refer to the primary caregiver for diagnosis and appropriate treatment.

Sensory system changes

Eyes

The pregnant woman develops a mild corneal oedema, especially during the third trimester, as well as corneal hyposensitivity, probably because of the increased thickness and fluid retention. There is also a progressive decrease in blood flow to the conjunctiva which is sensitive to oestrogen. Subconjunctival haemorrhages may occur during pregnancy.

Ears, nose and larynx

Changes here are related to modifications in fluid dynamics, vascular permeability, increased protein syntheses, vasomotor alterations of the nervous system along with hormonal (especially oestrogen) influences.

Rhinitis is seen in up to 30% of all pregnant women, especially those who smoke. There may be ear stuffiness or blocked ears due to oestrogen-induced changes in the mucous membranes of the eustachian tube, oedema of the nasophayrnx and alterations in fluid dynamics and pressures of the middle ear.

There can be oedema of the vocal chords and women may note hoarseness, deepening or cracking of the voice, or a persistent cough. Snoring is more common during pregnancy and an increase in hypertension, pre-eclampsia and intrauterine growth restriction (IUGR) has been reported in snorers.

Sleep

Sleep patterns change. There is an increased desire for sleep in the first trimester. By the second half of gestation pregnant women have less overall sleep time and more night awaking than non-pregnant women.

Progesterone may affect neuronal activity in the brain, reducing the level of excitatory neurotransmitters.

REM sleep increases from 25 weeks, peaking at 33–36 weeks. Stage 4 non-REM sleep decreases – it is this type that appears important for tissue repair and recovery from fatigue.

During the second half of pregnancy women tend to sleep less as they are disturbed by nocturia, dyspnoea, heartburn, nasal congestion, muscle aches, stress and anxiety and fetal activity.

Metabolic factors

These include: carbohydrate, protein and fat metabolism, calcium and phosphorus metabolism, bilirubin metabolism and thermoregulation – basal metabolic rate.

Major changes in metabolism occur in pregnancy. These are essential so that the mother can provide adequate nutrients to support fetal growth and development. They are linked closely with the endocrine system. These changes also alter the course of pregnancy in women with chronic disorders such as diabetes mellitus.

The changes are directed towards:

1. Ensuring satisfactory growth and development of the fetus.
2. Providing the fetus with adequate stores of energy and substrate for the transition to extrauterine life.
3. Meeting maternal needs to cope with the increased physiological demands of pregnancy.
4. Providing energy and substrate stores for the demands of pregnancy, labour and lactation.

The first two demands compete with the second two.

Pregnancy is primarily an anabolic state in which food intake and appetite are increased, activity is decreased, approximately 3.5 kg of fat is deposited, energy reserves of approximately 30 000 kcal are established, and 900 g of new protein is synthesised (by mother, fetus and placenta). The overall energy cost of pregnancy is estimated at 75 000 to 85 000 kcal (Baird 1986, King 2000). Anabolic aspects are most prominent during the first half to two-thirds of pregnancy when accumulation of maternal fat and increase blood volume lead to maternal weight gain. Insulin increases in response to glucose with a normal or slight increase in peripheral insulin sensitivity and serum glucose levels. There is a resulting uptake in nutrients and maternal fat accumulated. During the second half to final third of pregnancy the woman's metabolic status becomes more catabolic as stored fat is used; counter-insulin hormones increase leading to insulin resistance. During this phase weigh gain is primarily due to the growing fetus and placenta: 90% of the growth of the fetus is in the last half of pregnancy.

Basal metabolic rate (BMR)

Increases during pregnancy by as much as 15–30%.

Carbohydrate metabolism

Pregnancy is primarily anabolic: food intake and appetite increase and activity decreases. Pregnancy has been described as a 'state of accelerated starvation' (because there is an increased tendency to become ketotic) (Frienkel et al 1972).

Insulin and pregnancy as a diabetogenic state

This is due to elevated blood glucose levels in association with increasing insulin resistance. For most women this does not present an issue but regular tests are carried out to test glucose tolerance. HPL is antagonistic to insulin, resulting in raised plasma glucose levels. This diabetogenic effect of pregnancy adjusts glucose and fat metabolism to the advantage of the fetus.

Calcium and phosphorous

There is an increase in the amount and efficiency of intestinal calcium absorption.

Temperature control

Maternal temperature usually increases by 0.5°C (0.3°F). Both core and skin temperature increase. Core temperature peaks by mid-pregnancy and then decreases by late pregnancy. The amount of heat generated increases by 30–35% and many pregnant women become more sensitive to hot weather conditions.

Fetal temperature is linked to maternal temperature and there has been concern about the effects of elevated maternal temperature on the fetus. Research has focused on effects of raised temperature due to fever secondary to illness, exercise and use of hot tubs but has been inconclusive. There is a link between raised temperature secondary to fever around the time of neural tube closure (22–28 days) and central nervous system disorders in the fetus (Graham et al 1998) but this may be due to the underlying effects of the illness. Prolonged exercises in heat or high humidity may result in a higher maternal temperature than exercise in a cool, dry or water environment.

Milunksy et al (1992) found that hot tub exposure posed a greater risk than sauna use with no risk from electric blanket use. Prospective studies from Finland of sauna use in pregnancy have not shown an increased risk. However, the maximal temperature in these studies was 38.1°C (100.6°F) that is to say below the value of 38.9°C (102°F) thought to be critical (McMurray et al 1993).

It seems sensible to advise pregnant women to monitor their temperature and comfort levels during pregnancy and not to elevate levels unduly through extreme exercise in hot weather. Hot packs would be better used on the extremities rather than over the pelvic area.

Fat

Women lay down 1–4 kg fat. Body fat drops by 15–33 weeks after pregnancy depending on extent of lactation.

Implications for bodyworkers of changes in metabolic system

- There are many changes in the sense organs which are not usually serious but may affect the woman's well-being, e.g. blocked noses, throat congestion, coughing, snoring, sleeplessness.

- Be alert to signs of possible onset of diabetes, which are: increased thirst and urination. Refer if concerns.
- Mild proteinuria is common in pregnancy and usually benign, although with coexisting hypertension it can indicate complications of pre-eclampsia.
- Core body temperature is higher so the woman is likely to feel the effects of heat more readily. Monitor her comfort levels during bodywork and exercise.
- Good nutrition is fundamental to support pregnancy. If the therapist is appropriately trained then relevant nutritional guidance may be suggested. Otherwise advise eating a sensible diet, referring to the current diet guidelines in the country of practice.

Referral issues
Refer after bodywork
- Refer if suspected diabetes. Remind the woman that this may impact on blood sugar levels.

Integumentary system

Skin

The skin undergoes changes which are thought to be primarily hormonal due to the increase in MSH. There are alterations in skin pigmentation such as the linea nigra (pigmentation of the linea alba). Melasma (chloasma) or 'mask' of pregnancy occurs in 50–70% of pregnant women. It is characterised by irregular blotchy areas of pigmentation on the face. Freckles and scars may deepen. Some conditions such as eczema may improve. However, eczema may also worsen.

Types of skin itching in pregnancy

As the skin can be sensitive, women can feel a little more sensitivity to heat. There can be itching due to skin conditions such as chickenpox or eczema. However, additionally, three types of skin itching have been noted:

1. *Pruritis* in pregnancy: localised itching usually of the abdomen, occurs in about 20% women in the third trimester (Coad & Dunstall 2001: 244).
2. *PUPPPS*: PUPPS, or pruritic urticarial papules and plaques of pregnancy, also called PEOP, polymorphic eruption of pregnancy. Usually PUPPPS is red and there is itching and inflammation, especially near/around stretch marks low on the abdomen. It can be quite uncomfortable.

3. *Cholestasis.* This is potentially serious. It is characterised by extreme itching of hands and feet and is described in the higher risk section.

The first two conditions, while uncomfortable, are due to hormonal changes and do not have serious health implications. The woman may, however, scratch them obsessively so that they become open wounds and then there is a potential risk of infection. They often respond well to certain kinds of topical creams and in particular to oat baths.

Changes in connective tissue

Stretch marks (striae gravidarum) are linear tears in dermal collagen and commonly noted. They are most prominent by 6–7 months. They appear initially over the abdomen and then on the breasts, thighs and inguinal area. Some women complain of stretching feelings in the skin. They are more frequently seen in younger women with a large total weight gain and in Caucasian women (90%). They are less frequently in Asian and African-American women. These differences are due to the fact that the way skin stretches is genetically determined. The marks usually fade after pregnancy but never completely disappear, remaining as depressed, irregular silvery-white bands. The cause is unclear but believed to arise from hormonal alterations combined with stretching.

Vascular changes

Women may experience the development of vascular spiders.

Implications for bodyworkers in changes in the integumentary system

- There are many issues related to the increased stretching of the skin, such as increased sensitivity to touch, to stretching and to oils and lotions. Relief may be afforded by some oils.
- Normal cautions for working with areas of inflammation apply. If the woman has scratched the skin and there are open sores then the therapist must work with gloves or through the clothes due to the increased risk of infection.

Referral issues after bodywork

- Refer skin itching if it seems to be caused by potential cholestasis.

1.10 Embryonic development, fetal growth

Including the development of the placenta and the amniotic sac.

Conception

An egg (oocyte) is fertilised by a sperm (spermatozoa). Once the oocyte enters the uterine tube it has an estimated lifespan of 6–24 hours while spermatozoa have been estimated to remain in a viable state for 30–80 hours following their arrival in the vaginal cavity. Only one of the 2–4 million spermatozoa released during ejaculation fuses with the oocyte.

When the sperm enter the genital tract, over 99% of them are lost by leakage from the vagina. The remainder undergo a series of changes before they are ready for fertilisation. The first of these is called *capacitation*. In this process the cell membrane modifies itself. Then the sperm bind with the zona pellucida, the outer layer of the oocyte. Once the sperm and egg fuse, changes occur in the oocyte cytoplasm so that no further sperm can penetrate.

Fertilisation occurs when one sperm penetrates the tough outer membrane of the egg and arrives to its nucleus, fusing to form one cell – the *zygote*. The zygote immediately divides into two cells, which divide again and continue to divide. This cluster of cells is called the *morula*.

The baby's DNA is created within minutes of the egg and sperm fusing.

Twins

If two eggs are produced at the same time and fertilised by separate sperm, non-identical twins are conceived. The propensity to release two eggs simultaneously is genetic and is more common in women over 35.

Identical twins are produced from a single sperm and egg which during early divisions form two separate embryos with the same DNA – this is thought to be completely random.

Week 1 after conception (Fig. 1.10)

There is a rapid division of cells into germ layers from which all organs and tissues develop. It takes about 4 days for the morula to reach the uterus, by which time it contains around 100 cells grouped around a fluid-filled centre. It is now known as a *blastocyst* and is ready for implantation in the uterine wall.

It takes about 10 days from fertilisation for the blastocyst to become implanted in the lining of the uterus. During this time no nutrients from the mother are available. The rapid cell division occurs with no significant increase in total mass compared to the zygote. The ovum has a large amount of nutrients which help support this development until implantation occurs.

Even at this early stage of fetal development, problems may occur. The blastocyst may embed in a fallopian tube rather than in the uterus. This is an *ectopic*

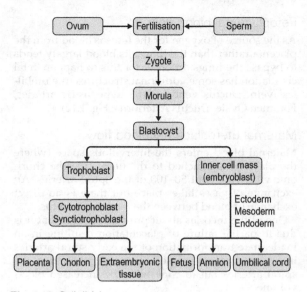

Fig. 1.10 Cell division.

pregnancy and potentially dangerous, if the cells continue to grow. It is also possible for the fertilised egg to arrive in the uterus and then not to be able to implant. This is often for reasons to do with the uterine wall, such as excessive scarring. This causes an early miscarriage.

The blastocyst divides into two main cell masses, the *trophoblast* and the *embryoblast*. The trophoblast cells will form the placenta and the embryoblast cells will form the embryo/fetus, the amnion and the umbilical cord.

Week 2: after implantation

As the blastocyst lands on the spongy endometrium (wall of uterus) its placental cells are arranged as tiny projections called villi which burrow through the endometrium, connect with the mother's bloodstream and absorb oxygen, protein, sugars, minerals, vitamins and other essential nutrients. The chorion develops into an important fetal membrane in the placenta. The chorionic villi connect the blood vessels of the chorion to the placenta. The placenta anchors the developing fetus to the uterus and provides a bridge for the exchange of nutrients and waste products between mother and baby.

The blastocyst continues to develop, forming a structure with two cavities: the yolk sac and the amniotic cavity. The function of the yolk sac in humans is not a nutritive one, as in some animals, but includes the production of blood cells. The amniotic sac will protect the fetus. The allantois forms from a pocket of the hind gut embedded within the umbilical cord which is incorporated into the developing urinary

systems. The yolk sac develops on the ventral side of the embryonic disc and is important for the nutrition of the embyro while the uteroplacental circulation is forming. Its role in haematopoiesis (formation of blood cellular components) is taken over by the liver in the 6th week of development.

These changes are referred to as the *'rule of twos'* (Larsen 1993):

- Two germ layers have formed – the endoderm and ectoderm.
- Two trophoblastic layers have formed – the cytotrophoblast and the syncytiotrophoblast (these relate to placental development).
- Two waves of remodelling have occurred – the blastocyst into the primary and then the definitive yolk sac.
- Two novel cavities have formed – the amniotic cavity and the chorionic cavity.
- Two layers are formed from the extra-embryonic mesoderm.

The placenta

The placenta is essentially the fetus's support system and any problems with it may endanger the fetus's life and well-being. The placenta transfers nutrients and gases from the mother to the fetus and removes waste products from the fetus. Further, because by the end of pregnancy it is a well-vascularised organ, problems with the placenta can lead to haemorrhage, so may be life-threatening to the mother.

The placenta regulates hormones from early pregnancy. Placental cells produce hCG which signals the corpus luteum to continue producing progesterone and oestrogen to nourish the uterine lining. As the placenta grows, it gradually produces oestrogen and progesterone and the corpus luteum gradually shrinks until it is no longer needed.

It also has a protective function and acts as a barrier to the passage of most bacteria. However, most drugs and anaesthetic agents cross the placenta to the fetus and some have a teratogenic effect. It allows the transfer of the antibody IgG from the mother to the fetus in the later stages of gestation, giving the fetus a certain immunity to infection for the first few months of life.

The placenta acts as a 'radiator' with 85% of fetal heat production transmitted to the mother via the placenta (Fraser & Watson 1989, Lowe & Cunningham 1990, Schroder & Power 1997, Voigt et al 1990).

Placental development (Fig. 1.11)

The placenta develops in two main phases. During the first 12 weeks of pregnancy it is not immediately connected with the maternal circulation

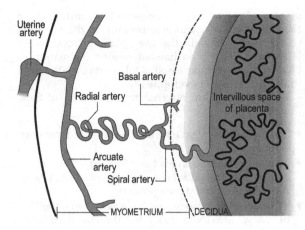

Fig. 1.11 The arterial supply to the placenta in normal pregnancy.

(Hustin & Schaaps 1987) but there is a second wave of development from 14 weeks onwards. It is during the second and third trimesters that the larger increases occur in uterine blood flow. In non-pregnant women uterine blood flow is approximately 40 ml/min which rises by around 10 ml/min in the first trimester. By the end of pregnancy uterine blood flow reaches over 800 ml/min (De Sweit 1991).

At term the placenta is about 18–20 cm across and 2–3 cm thick in the middle. On average it weighs about a sixth of the weight of the fetus (about 500 g). The umbilical cord is normally about 50–60 cm long as it gets progressively longer during pregnancy. If it is too short it can cause bleeding problems. If it is too long it may prolapse through the cervix or entangle with the fetus, possibly forming knots which could impede fetal circulation during delivery. Most umbilical cords are twisted but true knots appear in about 1% of all births (Moore & Persaud 1998). Two arteries carry blood from the fetus and one vein carries blood to the fetus.

Placental blood flow

It has been suggested that lack of fetal growth may be caused by 'placental insufficiency'. In fact the fetal placenta is rarely insufficient. Like all essential organs it has a considerable physiological reserve. It has been estimated that the placenta could lose 30–40% of its villi without affecting its function (Coad & Dunstall 2001: 169). Inadequate blood flow is probably due to incomplete conversion of the spiral arteries (the arteries which connect the maternal blood with the placenta) during the early stages of pregnancy.

Fetoplacental blood flow

As the source of oxygen for the fetus is blood from the placenta rather than the lungs, its blood largely tends to bypass the lungs. In order for this to happen, fetal circulation has some additional structures (the umbilical vein, Ductus venosus, the hypogastric arteries, Foramen Ovale, Ductus Arteriorus; Fig. 1.12).

Maternal uteroplacental blood flow

Maternal blood enters the intervillous space (where the placenta is attached to the uterus via the chorionic villi) via about 50–100 of the spiral arteries. An exchange of gases takes place but there is no direct exchange of blood between the mother and fetus.

One of the theories about pre-eclampsia is that it is due to partial failure of placentation resulting in an inadequate transformation of the early spiral arteries into uteroplacental vessels. Later in pregnancy, the spiral arteries fail to cope with the increased blood volume.

Uterine blood flow in pregnancy

The amniotic sac and amniotic fluid

The amniotic sac surrounds the fetus and is in contact with the chorion. The amniotic fluid surrounds the fetus protecting it by cushioning it from stresses. It allows for symmetrical fetal growth and movement and prevents parts of the fetus from adhering to each other or the amnion. It has bacteriostatic properties and maintains a constant temperature. Before 20 weeks when the fetal skin is keratinised, fluid and electrolytes can diffuse freely across the skin so the amniotic fluid is similar to fetal tissue fluid. Fetal urine and lung secretions form part of the fluid after this time. The fetus swallows as much as 20 ml of fluid per hour and the turnover is rapid. By term the amniotic fluid is between 500 and 1000 ml.

Development of the fetus (Fig. 1.13)

The first system to develop is the brain and nervous system, followed by the cardiovascular system. The last system to mature is the lungs.

First trimester (to week 12 for the mother, week 0 to week 10 for the fetus)

By the end of this trimester all the major structures of the baby have developed and the baby is over 5 cm long (crown–rump length).

Weeks 0–3: pre-embryonic period

This has already been described. After implantation, the pre-embryonic cells continue their rapid division.

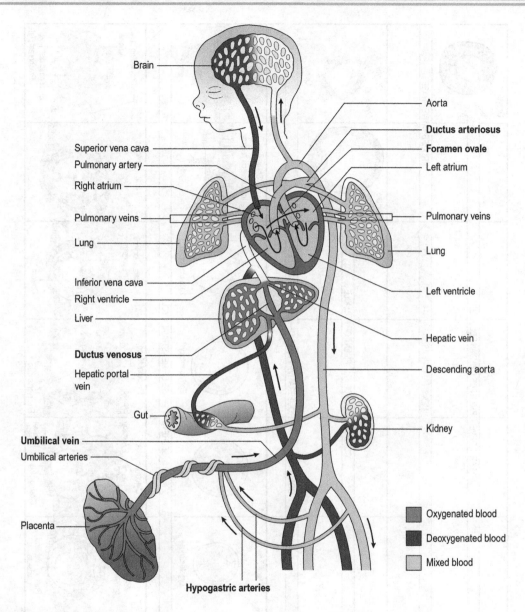

Fig. 1.12 Fetal circulation.

Week 3: gastrulation

By week 3 cells divide to form the primitive streak in the midline and then invaginate to spread between the epiblast and hypoblast layers. The bilaminar disc is then converted into a trilaminar disc consisting of the three germ layers – ectoderm, mesoderm and endoderm (Fig. 1.14).

The mesoderm is the middle layer of cells which will develop into connective tissue, smooth muscle, the cardiovascular system, blood, skeleton, reproductive and endocrine systems. The epiblast becomes the ectoderm which will develop into the epidermis, central and peripheral nervous systems and the retina. It is in contact with the amniotic cavity. The hypoblast becomes the endoderm from which epithelial linings and some glandular structures will form.

The endodermal prochordal plate is fused to the ectoderm forming the oropharyngeal membrane

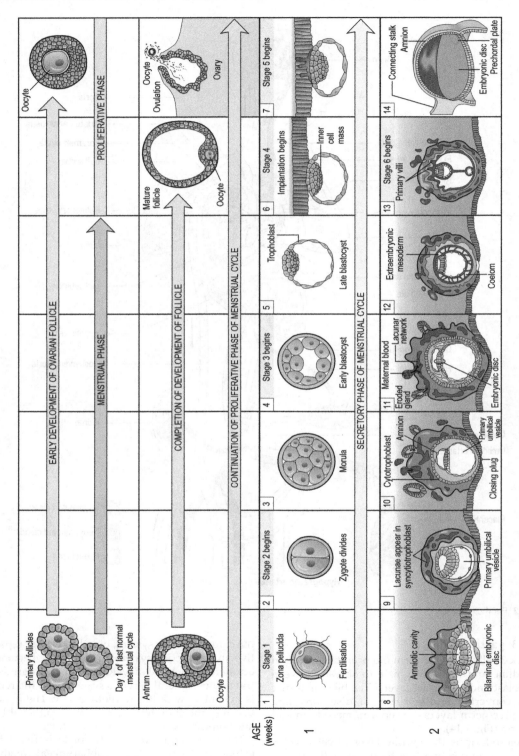

Fig. 1.13A and B Fetal development.

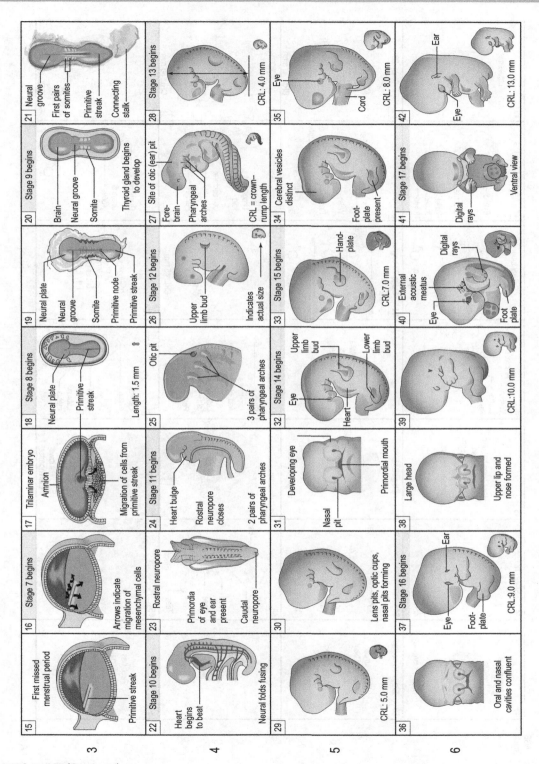

Fig. 1.13A and B (Continued)

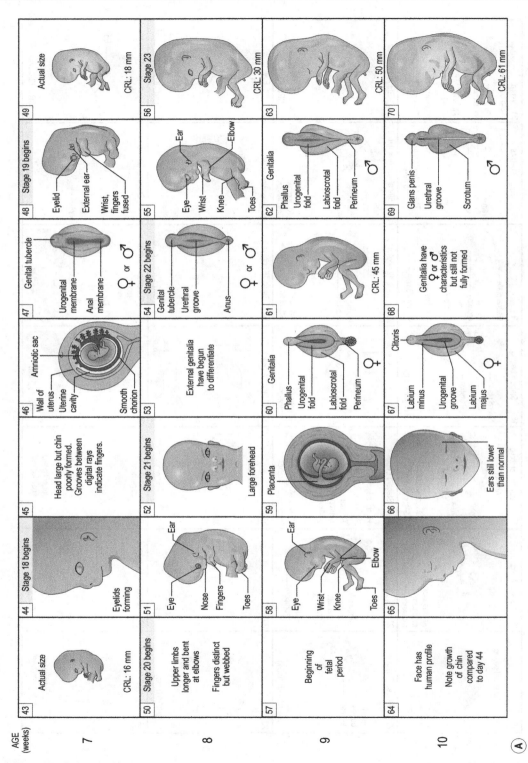

AGE (weeks)

7

8

9

10

(A)

Fig. 1.13A and B (Continued)

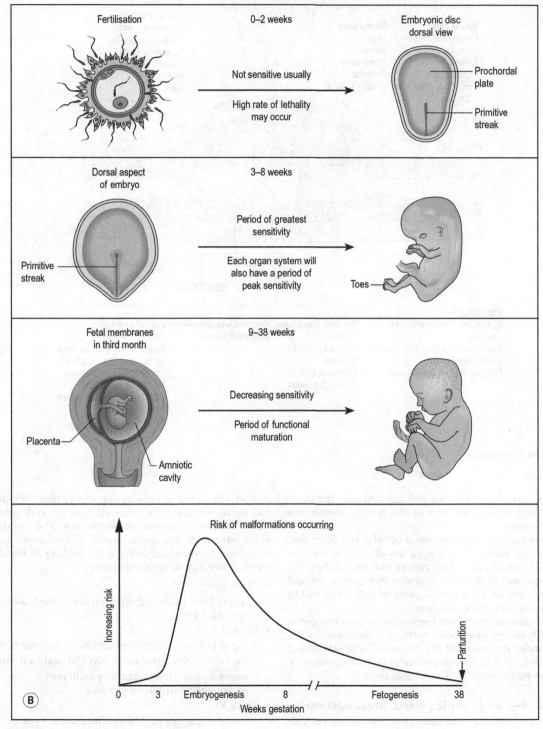

Periods of susceptibility to teratogenesis

Fertilisation — 0–2 weeks — Embryonic disc dorsal view

Not sensitive usually

High rate of lethality may occur

Prochordal plate

Primitive streak

Dorsal aspect of embryo — 3–8 weeks

Primitive streak

Period of greatest sensitivity

Each organ system will also have a period of peak sensitivity

Toes

Fetal membranes in third month — 9–38 weeks

Placenta

Amniotic cavity

Decreasing sensitivity

Period of functional maturation

Risk of malformations occurring

Increasing risk

Parturition

0   3   Embryogenesis   8   Fetogenesis   38

Weeks gestation

B

Fig. 1.13A and B (Continued)

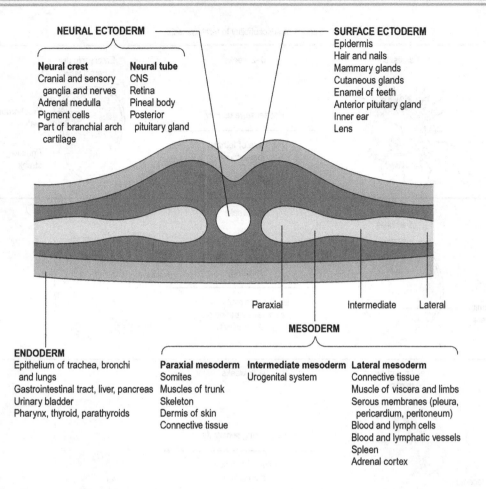

NEURAL ECTODERM

Neural crest
Cranial and sensory
 ganglia and nerves
Adrenal medulla
Pigment cells
Part of branchial arch
 cartilage

Neural tube
CNS
Retina
Pineal body
Posterior
 pituitary gland

SURFACE ECTODERM
Epidermis
Hair and nails
Mammary glands
Cutaneous glands
Enamel of teeth
Anterior pituitary gland
Inner ear
Lens

Paraxial   Intermediate   Lateral

MESODERM

ENDODERM
Epithelium of trachea, bronchi
 and lungs
Gastrointestinal tract, liver, pancreas
Urinary bladder
Pharynx, thyroid, parathyroids

Paraxial mesoderm
Somites
Muscles of trunk
Skeleton
Dermis of skin
Connective tissue

Intermediate mesoderm
Urogenital system

Lateral mesoderm
Connective tissue
Muscle of viscera and limbs
Serous membranes (pleura,
 pericardium, peritoneum)
Blood and lymph cells
Blood and lymphatic vessels
Spleen
Adrenal cortex

Fig. 1.14 Germ layers.

(future mouth). Below the primitive streak, the ectoderm and endoderm fuse at the cloacal membrane (future anus).

The notochord evolves into a cellular rod-like tube. If identical twins are going to develop there are two parallel notochords. The notochord establishes the development of the axial skeleton (bones of head and spinal cord) and the neural plate which gives rise to the primitive nervous system.

Gastrulation marks the beginning of the emergence and development of body form and structure. In the UK, under the terms of the Human Fertilisation and Embryology Act 1990 experimental manipulation of human embryos is legally obliged to stop.

Weeks 4–8: embryonic period, organogenesis

Organ systems are established and the embryo develops distinct human characteristics. This is a critical period where the processes are susceptible to external influence that can cause disruption and subsequent serious congenital abnormalities. The disc-like arrangement of the germ layers is converted in a recognisable vertebral embryo by folding in the 4th week. Some key developments are:

- Week 4
  - upper limb buds appear, then lower limb buds, and the heart.
- Week 5
  - rapid brain development and head enlargement
  - the heart beats from week 5 at 150 beats a minute
  - mesonephric ridges denote position of mesonephric (interim) kidneys.
- Week 6
  - joints of the upper limbs differentiate, eyes obvious, head large with neck

- bloodstream, digestive system; reflex responses to touch.
- Week 8
  - purposeful limb movements occur
  - ossification begins in lower limbs
  - head still disproportionately large (about half total embryo length)
  - embryo consists of 10 000 cells and resembles a human
  - startle reflex
  - external genitalia evident (but not distinct enough for sexual identification)
  - crown–rump length 27–31 mm.

Week 9 onwards: the fetal stage (weeks 11–26 second trimester for the mother)

The fetus grows rapidly and lays down fat.

Fetal weeks 9–12
- Growth in body length and limbs accelerates.
- Primary ossification centres develop in skeleton, notably skull and long bones.
- Intestines return to abdominal cavity and body wall fuses.
- Erythropoiesis (formation of red blood cells) decreases in the liver and begins in the spleen.
- Urine formation begins and there is fetal swallowing of amniotic fluid.

Weeks 13–16
- Rapid growth.
- Coordinated movements, not felt by mother.
- Active ossification of skeleton.
- Slow eye movements.
- Ovaries differentiated and contain primordial follicles.
- External genitalia recognisable.
- Eyes and ears closer to normal positions.

Weeks 17–20
- Growth slows down.
- Limbs reach mature proportions, the skin is covered with protective layer of vernix caseosa, held in position by lanugo (downy hair), brown fat is deposited.

Weeks 21–25
- Fetus gains weight, skin wrinkled, rapid eye movements begin, blink-startle responses to noise, surfactant secretion begins but respiratory system immature, fingernails are present, may be viable if born prematurely.

Week 26 onwards: third trimester

The fetus continues to grow and begins to settle into positions as it has less space. The position may be noted by primary caregiver.

Weeks 26–29
- Lungs are capable of breathing air, CNS can control breathing, eyes open, toenails visible, fat (3.5% bodyweight) deposited under skin so wrinkles smooth out, erythropoiesis moves from spleen to bone marrow.

Weeks 30–34
- Pupillary light reflex, skin pink and smooth, limbs chubby, white fat is 8% body weight, from 32 weeks survival is usual.

Weeks 35–38
- Firm grasp, orientates towards light.
- White fat is about 18% of body weight, 14 g fat gained per day.
- At term about 3400 g, crown–rump length is about 360 mm.

(After Coad & Dunstall 2001: 185–186.)

Summary of senses developed

Until relatively recently, the fetus was considered to be passive and not feel pain. In fact the senses develop progressively in utero and the importance of the prenatal environment on the future development of the child is now recognised. At birth it may help facilitate the transition of the newborn if there is an awareness of the newborn's responsiveness to the various senses and encouragement of continuity of activation through contact with the parents' touch, voice, smell and so on (with thanks to Pierre Deglon's notes from workshop, Switzerland, July 2007).

The development of the senses in all mammals is in the same order:

- Touch.
- Proprioception: perception of joint and body movement and the position of the body; tactile and vestibular receptors.
- Vestibular: balance and postural control.
- Chemoreception: smell and taste.
- Hearing.
- Vision/sight.

These senses were first shown by D. Hooker in work on terminated fetuses (Gorski et al 1987, Hooker 1952).

Touch

Touch entails contact with the amniotic fluid which is approximately body temperature and contact with body parts or the wall of the uterus. Skin receptors are developed around the mouth from 7 weeks, and from 11 weeks around the face, palm of hand and sole of foot (Vanhatalo & van Nieuwenhuizen 2000).

From 20 weeks they are developed in the whole of the body and muscles. For the rest of pregnancy they develop progressively. The baby develops senses by sucking their thumb, playing with the cord and with their feet.

Proprioception

This is interrelated with tactile and vestibular receptors.

Balance and postural control

This begins to develop from the eighth week and is regulated by the inner ear. It develops from both maternal and fetal movements. Maternal movement and buoyant amniotic fluid provide rich vestibular stimulation.

Chemoreception: smell and taste

Smell The nasal cells begin to differentiate at 4 weeks and from 8 weeks the structure resembles an adult. The nose is developed by smells which are passed from the mother's blood into the amniotic fluid. Responsiveness to odours is observed in pre-term infants from about 26 weeks. Newborns recognise smells they were used to in utero.
Taste Begins to develop from 13th week and reach adult numbers by term (Lecanuet & Schaal 1996).

Hearing

This is quite developed from 26 weeks (Peck 1994). The baby responds to music and to the mother's voice. These responses of recognition can be observed in the early postnatal period.

Sight

This is the last sense to develop. Although it gradually begins to develop from 30 weeks it is not until birth that the development of photoreceptors is completed.

Maternal and fetal tests

There are various tests which are done to check the development and well-being of both mother and baby (see for example MIDIRS information guides; http://www.midirs.org/).

1.11 Miscarriage

The medical term is 'spontaneous abortion' and it occurs before 24 weeks. After 24 weeks the delivery of a dead baby is called 'still birth'. There are some inconsistencies in the use of these terms and the term 'spontaneous abortion' can be quite upsetting for parents.

The miscarriage may be 'complete' – i.e. fetus, placenta and aminiotic sac are all evacuated. It may also be an 'incomplete miscarriage', so the woman may need surgical removal of the remaining contents as there is a possible risk of infection.

At least 15% of confirmed pregnancies end in 'spontaneous abortion' before 12 weeks. The true rate of pregnancy loss is likely to be much higher, as it often occurs earlier. It is more common in a first pregnancy (Lewis 2001).

Common causes

It is unlikely that a healthy fetus that is developing well will simply miscarry. Fetuses have been known to survive car accidents or attempts at home abortions, such as hot baths or throwing oneself downstairs. While some kinds of maternal illness at key critical times of development may cause a miscarriage, the majority of miscarriages are caused by genetic factors resulting in poor development of embryo or placenta. Often the pregnant woman wonders if there is something that she could have done to prevent miscarriage. The simple answer is: probably not.

The main causes of miscarriage include:

Maldevelopment of the conceptus

The fertilised egg not developing properly – defective conceptions.

Chromosomal abnormalities

Chromosomal abnormalities account for about 70% of defective conceptions (Lewis & Chamberlain 1990). These can cause problems with the developing embryo or with the development of the placenta. First trimester losses are often due to aneuploidy, a chromosomal abnormality. Genetic material from the sperm and egg do not fuse together appropriately or there are problems in cell division: the resulting embryonic cells do not develop properly. In other cases, a 'blighted ovum' occurs, where the placental cells develop but not the pre-embryonic cells.

In most cases chromosomal abnormalities are the result of a one-off genetic abnormality in the baby, which means that it is unlikely to occur in subsequent pregnancies – it is nature working according to the law of the survival of the fittest.

Less commonly there can be problematic genes in one or both of the partners; this can be tested for. Some abnormalities are so severe that there is no possibility of the fetus developing normally while others can cause conditions which a baby can survive, such as cystic fibrosis or Down's syndrome.

Rarely (about 3%), a chromosomal problem of one or both partners can lead to recurrent pregnancy loss although these clients can also deliver normal babies.

Defective implantation, *ectopic pregnancy* and *tubal pregnancy*, and *hydatiform mole* are all described in the high risk section (p. 367).

Medical disorders
These include diabetes, thyroid disease, renal disease and hypertensive disorders (Chamberlain 1995).

Maternal infection
This accounts for a small number of miscarriages. Any acute illness, particularly with a high temperature, may cause a miscarriage. This may be due to the general metabolic effect of a high fever or the result of transplacental passage of viruses. Influenza, rubella, appendicitis, pyelonephritis, pneumonia, toxoplasmosis, cytomegalovirus, syphilis and brucellosis are associated with increased pregnancy loss.
Genital tract infection Some unusual vaginal infections can cause recurrent miscarriages, although it appears that this is not common.

Endocrine abnormalities
Initially the corpus luteum produces progesterone necessary to maintain pregnancy. Towards the end of the first trimester the placenta plays a more significant role. Some doctors consider that this is a time of potential increased risk of pregnancy loss if the placental production of progesterone is suboptimal in amount or timing. Treatment is usually hormonal but is fraught with problems.

There can also be inadequate secretory endometrium and poor development of the corpus luteum.

Polycystic ovaries (PCOS) increase the risk of miscarriage.

Uterine abnormalities
A uterine malformation may cause about 15% of recurrent miscarriages as the fetus cannot grow appropriately. The diagnosis is made by X-ray or ultrasound of the uterus.

Fibroids
The presence of fibroids may increase the chances of abortion.

Retroversion of the uterus
This may not in itself cause an abortion but if it fails to rise into the abdomen then attempts to correct it may induce the abortion.

Cervical weakness

Autoimmune disorders and maternal immune response
Professor Hughes, head of the lupus arthritis research unit at St Thomas's hospital in London, has done research linking systemic lupus erythematosus (SLE) with high rates of miscarriage. His original investigations showed that many lupus sufferers also had a blood clotting syndrome which can be detected through the presence of antiphospholipid antibodies in the blood. Lupus sufferers get pregnant easily but have a high rate of miscarriage. This syndrome has now been called 'Hughes syndrome' or 'antiphospholipid syndrome' or 'sticky blood syndrome'. It is thought to trigger miscarriage either by causing blood clots to form in the placenta or because the antiphospholipid antibodies attack the cells of the placenta making implantation difficult. Hughes syndrome can sometimes be found in women who do not have SLE but have a history of recurrent miscarriage. It is also associated with pre-eclampsia, IUGR and placental abruption.

Professor Regan has pioneered work on antiphospholipid antibodies and miscarriages at the recurrent miscarriage clinic at St Mary's hospital in London. The treatment of choice for this condition is aspirin, which is surprising since previous studies have linked taking aspirin in pregnancy with children's heart diseases, brain malformation and cleft palates. The difference is that the dose is very low, only 75 mg daily, and is given prior to conception. Once the woman finds she is pregnant, she is given the anticoagulant drug heparin. Another possibility is to use vitamin E which can help thin the blood and prevent blood clots. A 1996 study in *The Lancet* showed that taking vitamin E reduced the risk of heart attack (Stephens et al 1996). Interestingly Hughes recommends taking long-chain essential fatty acids, such as found in oily fish, rather than vitamin E.

Environmental factors
Smoking
A number of studies have shown that cocaine and tobacco use are significant factors in spontaneous abortions among pregnant users, and that they contribute to a number of other threats to the health of the unborn.

Maternal age
Both women over 40 and teenagers are at higher risk.

Stress and anxiety, emotional factors
There is also evidence that there is an interplay between the emotions and the hormonal systems which regulate pregnancy and that stress can be a factor. Weil and Tupper (1960) write:

The pregnant woman functions as a communications system. The fetus is a source of continuous messages to which the mother responds with subtle psychobiological adjustments. Her personality, influenced by her ever-changing life situation, can either (1) act upon the fetus to maintain its constant growth and development or (2) create physiological changes that can result in abortion.

Paternal causes

Secondhand smoke appears to present an equal danger to the fetus, as one study noted that 'heavy *paternal* smoking increased the risk of early pregnancy loss'. One of the rotating warnings that cigarettes are required to display notes that smoking can lead to 'low fetal birth weight'.

Fertility drugs

Some of these can cause miscarriage.

Overweight or underweight

Can be a factor in miscarriage.

No cause

It is not considered unusual to experience one or two miscarriages and most doctors will only recommend an investigation after three or four losses.

Summary box of implications of miscarriage for bodyworkers

- Refer suspected cases of tubal pregnancy or hydatiform mole.
- Work with clients pre-conceptually where possible to support positive lifestyle.
- Be aware of issues which may increase the risk of miscarriage and support these women appropriately.
- Reassure women that regular moderate exercise and receiving bodywork do not increase the chances of miscarriage, as most causes are genetically based.
- The eastern view on miscarriage is that it is related primarily to the strength of the Jing and the energy of the Kidneys and the Extraordinary Vessels; this fits in with the genetic and endocrine basis for many miscarriages.

Reflective questions

- Why is it important to understand fetal development?
- What are the main causes of miscarriage?
- Consider how we might work with clients trying to conceive and with a history of miscarriage.
- Consider effects of changes in different systems on how we work with pregnant clients.

- Do you think pregnancy is a state of health or disease, and why?

References and further reading

Abel, E.L., 1983. Marijuana, Tobacco, Alcohol and Reproduction. CRC Press, Boca Raton, FL.

ACOG, 2006. Exercise during pregnancy and the postpartum period. ACOG Tech. Bull. 189 Feb 1994. International Journal of Gynecology and Obstetrics 1994; 45(1):65–76. Washington: ACOG, RCOG Statement No. 4 – January 2006.

Adams, D., Keegan, K.A., 1998. Physiological changes in normal pregnancy. In: Gleicher, N. (Ed.), Principles and Practice of Medical Therapy in Pregnancy, third ed. Appleton & Lange, Stamford, CT.

Albert, H.B., Godskesen, M., Westergaard, J.G., 2002. Incidence of four syndromes of pregnancy-related pelvic joint pain. Spine 27 (24), 2831–2834.

Aminoff, M.J., 1999. Neurologic disorders. In: Creasy, R.K., Resnick, R. (Eds.) Maternal Fetal Medicine, fourth ed. WB Saunders, Philadelphia.

Ances, I.G., Pomerantz, S.H., 1974. Serum concentrations of beta-melanocyte-stimulating hormone in human pregnancy. Am. J. Obstet. Gynecol. 119 (8), 1062–1068.

Andres, R.L., 1999. Social and illicit drug use in pregnancy. In: Creasy, R.K., Resnik, R. (Eds.) Maternal Fetal Medicine, fourth ed. WB Saunders, Philadelphia.

Andrews, C., 2008. Pelvic girdle pain in 3 pregnant women choosing chiropractic management: a pilot study. J. Assoc. Chart. Physiother. Women's Health 102, 12–24.

Arafeh, J.M., 1997. Disseminated intravascular coagulation in pregnancy: an update. J. Perinat. Neonatal Nurs. 11 (3), 30–45.

Baird, J.D., 1986. Some aspects of the metabolic and hormonal adaptation to pregnancy. Acta Endocrinol. (Suppl.) 277, 11–18.

Barker, D.J.P., 1998. Mothers, Babies and Health in Later Life, second ed. Churchill Livingstone, Edinburgh.

Bateson, P., Barker, D., Clutton-Brock, T., et al., 2004. Developmental plasticity and human health. Nature 430 (6998), 419–421.

Benedetti, J., 1990. Pregnancy induced hypertension. In: Elkayam, U., Gleicher, N. (Eds.) Cardiac Problems in Pregnancy: Diagnosis and Management of Maternal and Fetal Disease, third ed. Wiley-Liss, New York.

Blackburn, S.T., 2003. Maternal Fetal and Neonatal Physiology: A Clinical Perspective, second ed. Elsevier, St Louis, MO.

Blackburn, S.T., Loper, D.L., 1992. Maternal, Fetal and Neonatal Physiology: A Clinical Perspective. WB Saunders, Philadelphia, PA.

Bolt, R.J., van Weissenbruch, M.M., Lafeber, H.N., et al., 2001. Glucocorticoids and lung development in the fetus and preterm infant. Pediatr. Pulmonol. 32 (1), 76–91.

Bonapace Jr., E.S., Fisher, R.S., 1998. Constipation and diarrhea in pregnancy. Gastroenterol. Clin. North Am. 27 (1), 197–211.

Burke, M.E., 1993. Myasthenia gravis and pregnancy. J. Perinat. Neonatal Nurs. 7 (1), 11–21.

Burrows, T.D., King, A., Loke, Y.W., 1996. Trophoblast migration during human placental implantation. Hum. Reprod. Update 2 (4), 307–321.

Buster, J.E., Sauer, M.V., 1989. Endocrinology of conception. In: Brody, S.A., Ueland, K. (Eds.) Endocrine Disorders in Pregnancy. Appleton and Lange, Norwalk, CT.

Calais-Germain, B., 2000. Le périnée féminin et accouchement. Editions DésIris, Meolans-Revel, France.

Capeless, E.L., Clapp, J.F., 1989. Cardiovascular changes in early phase of pregnancy. Am. J. Obstet. Gynecol. 161 (6/1), 1449–1453.

Caulin-Glaser, T., Setaro, J.F., 1999. Pregnancy and cardiovascular disease. In: Burrow, G.N., Duffy, T.P. (Eds.) Medical Complications During Pregnancy, fifth ed. WB Saunders, Philadlphia.

Chamberlain, G., 1995. Obstetrics by Ten Teachers, sixteenth ed. Arnold, London.

Chesley, L.C., 1972, February 1. Plasma and red cell volumes during pregnancy. Am. J. Obstet. Gynecol. 112 (3), 440–450.

Christensen, D., 2000. Weight matters, even in the womb: status at birth can foreshadow illnesses decades later. Sci. News 158, 382–383.

Christensen, T., Klebe, J.G., Bertelsen, V., et al., 1989. Changes in renal volume during normal pregnancy. Acta Obstet. Gynecol. Scand. 68 (6), 541–543.

Clark, S.L., Cotton, D.B., Lee, W., et al., 1989. Central hemodynamic assessment of normal term pregnancy. Am. J. Obstet. Gynecol. 161 (6/1), 1439–1442.

Coad, J., Dunstall, M., 2001. Anatomy and Physiology for Midwives. Mosby, Edinburgh.

Coldron, Y., 2005. Margie Polden Memorial Lecture: 'Mind the gap!' Symphysis pubis dysfunction revisited. J. Assoc. Chart. Physiother. Women's Health 96, 3–15.

Comeglio, P., Fedi, S., Liotta, A.A., et al., 1996. Blood clotting activation during normal pregnancy. Thromb. Res. 84 (3), 199–202.

Culpepper, L., Jack, B., 1990. Prevention of urinary tract complications in pregnancy. In: Merkatz, I.R., Thompson, J.E. (Eds.) New Perspectives on Prenatal Care. Elsevier, New York.

Cunningham, F.G., Whitridge, W.J., 1997. Williams Obstetrics, twentieth ed. Appleton & Lange, Stamford, CT.

Davison, J.M., 1987. Kidney function in pregnant women. Am. J. Kidney Dis. 9 (4), 248–252.

Davison, J.M., 1997. Edema in pregnancy. Kidney Int. Suppl. (59), S90–S96.

Davison, J.M., Linheimer, M.D., 1999. Renal disorders. In: Creasy, R.K., Resnik, R. (Eds.) Maternal Fetal Medicine, fourth ed. WB Saunders, Philadelphia.

De Aloysio, D., Penacchioni, P., 1992. Morning sickness control in early pregnancy by Neiguan point acupressure. Obstet. Gynaecol. 80 (5), 852–854.

De Swiet, M., 1985. Thromboembolism. Clin. Haematol. 14 (3), 643–660.

De Swiet, M., 1991. The cardiovascular system. In: Hytten, F., Chamberlain, G. (Eds.) Clincial Physiology in Obstetrics. Blackwell, Oxford.

De Swiet, M., 1998. The cardiovascular system. In: Chamberlain, G., Broughton Pipkin, F. (Eds.) Clinical Physiology in Obstetrics, third ed. Blackwell, Oxford.

De Swiet, M., 1999. Pulmonary disorders. In: Creasy, R.K., Resnik, R. (Eds.) Maternal Fetal Medicine, fourth ed. WB Saunders, Philadelphia.

De Swiet, M., Fidler, J., 1981. Heart disease in pregnancy; some controversies. J. R. Coll. Physicians Lond. 15 (3), 183–186.

Donaldson, J.O., 1998. Neurologic complications. In: Burrow, G.N., Duffy, T.P. (Eds.) Medical Complications During Pregnancy, fifth ed. WB Saunders, Philadelphia.

Duvekot, J.J., Peters, L.L.H., 1998. Very early changes in cardiovascular physiology. In: Chamberlain, G., Broughton Pipkin, F. (Eds.) Clinical Physiology in Obstetrics, third ed. Blackwell, Oxford.

Duvekot, J.J., Cheriex, E.C., Pieters, F.A., et al., 1993. Early pregnancy changes in hemodynamics and volume homeostasis are consecutive adjustments trigged by a primary fall in systemic vascular tone. Am. J. Obstet. Gynecol. 169 (6), 1382–1392.

Elden, H., Ladfors, L., Olsen, M.F., et al., 2005. Effects of acupuncture and stabilising exercises as adjunct to standard treatment in pregnant women with pelvic girdle pain: randomised single blind controlled trial. Br. Med. J. 330 (7494), 761.

European COST Commission (ECC), 2004. Working group 4, pelvic girdle pain. <www.backpaineurope.org> (accessed 23 March 2009).

Fast, A., Weiss, L., Ducommun, E.J., et al., 1990. Low back pain in pregnancy: abdominal muscles, sit up performance, and back pain. Spine 15 (1), 28–30.

Faúndes, A., Brícola-Filho, M., Pinto e Silva, J.L., 1998. Dilatation of the urinary tract during pregnancy: proposal of a curve of maximal caliceal diameter by gestation age. Am. J. Obstet. Gynecol. 178 (5), 1082–1086.

Flaxman, S.M., Sherman, P.W., 2000. Morning sickness: a mechanism for protecting mother and embryo. Q. Rev. Biol. 75, 113–148.

Fraser, D.M., Cooper, M.A., 2003. Myles' Textbook for Midwives, fourteenth ed. Elsevier Churchill Livingstone, Edinburgh.

Fraser, R., Watson, R., 1989. Bleeding during the latter half of pregnancy. In: Chalmers, I. (Ed.), Effective Care in Pregnancy and Childbirth. Oxford University Press, Oxford.

Frienkel, N., Metzger, B.E., Nitzan, M., et al., 1972. Accelerated starvation and mechanisms for the conservation of maternal nitrogen during pregnancy. Israeli J. Med. Sci. 8, 426–439.

Gamble, J.G., Simmons, S.C., Freedman, M., 1986. The symphysis pubis: anatomic and pathologic considerations. Clin. Orthop. Relat. Res. 203, 261–272.

Garn, S.M., Ridella, S.A., Petzold, A.S., et al., 1981. Maternal hematologic levels and pregnancy outcomes. Semin. Perinatol. 5 (2), 155–162.

Garnica, A.D., Chan, W.Y., 1996. The role of the placenta in fetal nutrition and growth. J. Am. Coll. Nutr. 15 (3), 206–222.

Gates, S., 2000. Thromboembolic disease in pregnancy. Curr. Opin. Obstet. Gynecol. 12 (2), 117–122.

Gilleard, W.L., Brown, J.M., 1996. Structure and function of the abdominal muscles in primigravid subjects during pregnancy and the immediate postbirth period. Phys. Ther. 76 (7), 750–762.

Gitau, R., Cameron, A., Fisk, N.M., 1998. Fetal exposure to maternal cortisol. Lancet 352 (9129), 707–708.

Gitau, R., Adams, D., Fisk, N.M., et al., 2005. Fetal plasma testosterone correlates positively with cortisol. Arch. Dis. Child. Fetal Neonatal Ed. 90 (2), F166–F169.

Glinoer, D., Lemone, M., 1992. Goiter and pregnancy: a new insight into an old problem. Thyroid 2 (1), 65–70.

Gluckman, P.D., Hanson, M.A., 2004. Living with the past: evolution development and patterns of disease. Science 305 (5691), 1733–1736.

Goldenberg, R.L., Mercer, B.M., Miodovnik, M., et al., 1998. Plasma ferritin, premature rupture of membranes, and pregnancy outcome. Am. J. Obstet. Gynecol. 179 (6/1), 1599–1604.

Gorski, P.A., Lewkowicz, D.J., Huntington, L., 1987. Advances in neonatal and infant behavioural assessment: toward a comprehensive evaluation of early patterns of development. J. Dev. Behav. Pediatr. 8 (1), 39–50.

Graham Jr, J.N., Edwards, M.J., Edwards, M.J., 1998. Teratogen update: gestational effects of maternal hyperthermia due to febrile illness and result patterns of defects in humans. Teratology 58, 209–521.

Hathaway, W.E., Bonnar, J., 1987. Hemostatic Disorders of the Pregnant Woman and New Born Infant. Elsevier, New York.

Heckman, J.D., Sassard, R., 1994. Current concepts review: musculoskeletal considerations in pregnancy. J. Bone Joint Surg. 76, 1720–1730.

Heffner, L.J., Sherman, C.B., Speizer, F.E., et al., 1993. Clinical and environmental predictors of preterm labor. Obstet. Gynecol. 81 (5/1), 750–757.

Heinrichs, W.L., Gibbons, W.E., 1989. Endocrinology of pregnancy. In: Brody, S.A., Ueland, K. (Eds.) Endocrine Disorders in Pregnancy. Appleton and Lange, Norwalk.

Henderson, C., Macdonald, S., 2004. Mayes' Midwifery: A Textbook for Midwives, thirteenth ed. Baillère Tindall, Edinburgh.

Hertzberg, B.S., Carroll, B.A., Bowie, J.D., et al., 1993. Doppler US assessment of maternal kidneys: analysis of intranal resistivity indexes in normal pregnancy and physiologic pelvicaliectasis. Radiology 186, 689–692.

Hooker, D., 1952. The Prenatal Origin of Behaviour. University of Kansas Press, Lawrence, KS.

Hughes, R.V.G., 1998. Lupus Arthritis Research Unit, Rayne Institute, St Thomas's Hospital, London. Lupus UK News & Views, no. 55

Hustin, J., Schaaps, J.P., 1987. Echographic [corrected] and anatomic studies of the maternotrophoblastic border during the first trimester of pregnancy. Am. J. Obstet. Gynecol. 157 (1), 162–168.

Huxley, R.R., 2000. Nausea and vomiting in early pregnancy: its role in placental development. Obstet. Gynecol. 95 (5), 779–782.

Hytten, F.E., 1991. The alimentary system. In: Hytten, F., Chamberlain, G. (Eds.) Clinical Physiology in Obstetrics, second ed. Blackwell, Oxford, pp. 137–149.

Institute of Medicine, 1990. Nutrition During Pregnancy. Part I, Weight Gain; Part II, Nutrient Supplements. Committee on Nutritional Status During Pregnancy and Lactation, Food and Nutrition Board, National Academy Press, Washington, DC, 468 pp.

Ireland, M.L., Ott, S.M., 2000. The effects of pregnancy on the musculoskeletal system. Clin. Orthop. Relat. Res. 372, 169–179.

Jacobs, A., Miller, F., Worwood, M., et al., 1972. Ferritin in serum of normal subjects and patients with iron deficiency and iron overload. Br. Med. J. 4 (5834), 206–208.

Jewell, D., Young, G., 2000. Interventions for Nausea and Vomiting in Early Pregnancy. Cochrane Review. Cochrane Library Issue 2. Update Software, Oxford.

Kerr, M.G., 1965. The mechanical effects of the gravid uterus in later pregnancy. J. Obstet. Gynaecol. Br. Commonw. 72, 513–529.

King, J.C., 2000. Physiology of pregnancy and nutrient metabolisms. Am. J. Clin. Nutr. 71 (5 Suppl.), 1218S–1225S.

Klebanoff, M.A., Shiono, P.H., Selby, J.V., et al., 1991. Anemia and spontaneous preterm birth. Am. J. Obstet. Gynecol. 164 (1/1), 59–63.

Kristiansson, P., Svardsudd, K., Von Schoultz, B., 1996. Serum relaxin, symphyseal pain and back pain during pregnancy. Am. J. Obstet. Gynecol. 175 (5), 1342–1347.

Langman, J., Sadler, T.W., 2000. Langman's Medical Emybryology, eighth ed. Lippincott, Williams & Wilkins, Philadelphia.

Larsen, W.J., 1993. Human Embryology, second ed. Churchill Livingstone, New York.

Larsen, E.C., Wilken-Jensen, C., Hansen, A., et al., 1999. Symptom-giving pelvic girdle relaxation in pregnancy. I, Prevalence and risk factors. Acta Obstet. Gynecol. Scand. 78 (2), 105–110.

Lecanuet, J.P., Schaal, B., 1996. Fetal sensory competencies. Eur. J. Obstet. Gynecol. 68, 1.

Lee, R.V., McComb, L.E., Mezzadri, F.C., 1990. Pregnant patients, painful legs: the obstetrician's dilemma. Obstet. Gynecol. Surv. 45 (5), 290–298.

Lesage, J., Del-Favero, F., Leonhardt, M., et al., 2004. Prenatal stress induces intrauterine growth restriction and programmes glucose intolerance and feeding behaviour disturbances in the aged rat. J. Endocrinol. 181 (2), 291–296.

Leutwyler, K., 1998, January. Don't stress: it is now known to cause developmental problems, weight gain and neurodegeneration. Sci. Am., 28–30.

Lewis, G.T., 2001. Why mothers die, 1997–1999. In: Fifth Report of Confidential Enquiries into Maternal Deaths in the United Kingdom. CEMD with NICE and RCOG, London.

Lewis, T., Chamberlain, G., 1990. Obstetrics by Ten Teachers, fifteenth ed. Edward Arnold, London.

Lindsey, R.W., Leggon, R.E., Wright, D.G., et al., 1988. Separation of the symphysis pubis in association with childbearing. J. Bone Joint Surg. 70, 289–292.

Lockwood, C.J., 1999. Heritable coagulopathies in pregnancy. Obstet. Gynecol. Surv. 54 (12), 754–765.

Lockwood, C.J., Kuczynski, E., 1999. Markers of risk for preterm delivery. J. Perinat. Med. 27 (1), 5–20.

Lowe, T.W., Cunningham, F.G., 1990. Placental abruption. Clin. Obstet. Gynecol. 33 (3), 406–413.

Lu, Z.M., Goldenberg, R.L., Cliver, S.P., et al., 1991. The relationship between maternal hematocrit and pregnancy outcome. Obstet. Gynecol. 77 (2), 190–194.

Mabie, W.C., DiSessa, T.G., Crocker, L.G., et al., 1994. A longitudinal study of cardiac output in normal human pregnancy. Am. J. Obstet. Gynecol. 170 (3), 849–856.

McMurray, R.G., Katz, V.L., Meyer Goodwin, W.E., et al., 1993. Thermoregulation of pregnant women during aerobic exercise on land and in the water. Am. J. Perinatol. 10 (2), 178–182.

Malloy, M.H., Hoffman, H.J., Peterson, D.R., 1992. Sudden infant death syndrome and maternal smoking. Am. J. Public Health 82 (10), 1380–1382.

Manga, M., 1999. Maternal cardiovascular and renal adaptations to pregnancy. In: Creasy, R.K., Resnick, R. (Eds.) Maternal Fetal Medicine: Principles and Practice, fourth ed. WB Saunders, Philadelphia.

Maxwell, K.B., Niebyl, J.R., 1982. Treatment of nausea and vomiting of pregnancy. In: Niebyl, J.R. (Ed.), Drug Use in Pregnancy. Lea and Febiger, Philadelphia, pp. 11–19.

Meetze, W.H., Valentine, C., McGuigan, J.E., et al., 1992. Gastrointestinal priming prior to full enteral nutrition in very low birth weight infants. J. Pediatr. Gastroenterol. Nutr. 15 (2), 163–170.

Mikhail, M.S., Anyaegbunam, A., 1995. Lower urinary tract dysfunction in pregnancy: a review. Obstet. Gynecol. Surv. 50 (9), 675–683.

Miller, M.J., et al., 2002. Respiratory disorders in preterm and term infants. In: Fanroff, A.A., Martin, R.J. (Eds.) Neonatal and Perinatal Medicine: Diseases of the Fetus and Infant, seventh ed. Mosby, St Louis.

Milunsky, A., Ulcickas, M., Rothman, K.J., et al., 1992. Maternal heat exposure and neural tube defects. JAMA 268 (7), 882–885.

Moore, K.L., Persaud, T.V.N., 1998. Before We are Born: Essentials of Embryology and Birth Defects, fifth ed. WB Saunders, Philadelphia.

Mori, M., Amino, N., Tamaki, H., et al., 1988. Morning sickness and thyroid function in normal pregnancy. Obstet. Gynecol. 72 (3/1), 355–359.

Morton, M.J., 1991. Maternal hemodynamics in pregnancy. In: Mittelmark, R.A., Wiswell, R.A., Drinkwater, B.L. (Eds.) Exercise in Pregnancy, second ed. Williams & Wilkins, Baltimore, pp. 61–70.

Nathanielsz, P.W., 1999. Life in the Womb: The Origin of Health and Disease. Promethean Press, Ithaca, NY.

Nyman, M., Durling, U., Lundell, A., 1997. Chorea gravidarum. Acta Obstet. Gynecol. Scand. 76 (9), 885–886.

O'Connor, T.G., Heron, J., Golding, J., et al., 2002. Maternal antenatal anxiety and children's behavioural/emotional problems at 4 years. Report from the Avon Longitudinal Study of Parents and Children. Br. J. Psychiatry 180, 502–508.

O'Connor, T.G., Heron, J., Golding, J. et al., and the ALSPAC study team, 2003. Maternal antenatal anxiety and behavioural/emotional problems in children: a test of a programming hypothesis. J. Child Psychol. Psychiatry 44 (7), 1025–1036.

O'Connor, T.G., Ben-Shlomo, Y., Heron, J., et al., 2005. Prenatal anxiety predicts individual differences in cortisol in pre-adolescent children. Biol. Psychiatry 58 (3), 211–217.

Odent, M., 2002. Primal Health, second ed. Clairview Books, Forest Row, East Sussex.

Ostgaard, H.C., Anderson, G.B., 1991. Previous back pain and risk of developing back pain in a future pregnancy. Spine 16 (4), 432–436.

Ostgaard, H.C., Zetherstrom, G., Roos-Hansson, E., et al., 1994. Reduction of back and posterior pelvic pain in pregnancy. Spine 19 (8), 894–900.

Owens, K., Pearson, A., Mason, G., 2002. Symphysis pubis dysfunction – a cause of significant obstetric morbidity. Eur. J. Obstet. Gynecol. Reprod. Biol. 105 (2), 143–146.

Parry, E., Shields, R., Turnbull, A.C., 1970. The effect of pregnancy on the colonic absorption of sodium, potassium and water. J. Obstet. Gynaecol. Br. Commonw. 77, 616–619.

Peck, J.E., 1994. Development of hearing. Part II, Embryology. J. Am. Acad. Audiol. 5 (6), 359–365.

Pitkin, R.M., 1985. Calcium metabolism in pregnancy and the perinatal period: a review. Am. J. Obstet. Gynecol. 151 (1), 99–109.

Prentice, A., Goldberg, G., 1996. Maternal obesity increases congenital malformations. Nutr. Rev. 54 (5), 146–150.

Press Release 07, Pregnancy diet has life long effects for babies, PA37/06 March 07 2006.

Priddy, K.D., 1997. Immunologic adaptations during pregnancy. J. Obstet. Gynecol. Neonatal Nurs. 26 (4), 388–394.

Quilligan, E.J., Tyler, C., 1959. Postural effects on the cardiovascular status in pregnancy: a comparison of the lateral and supine postures. Am. J. Obstet. Gynecol. 78, 465–471.

Resnik, R., 1999. Anatomic alteration in the reproductive tract. In: Creasy, R.K., Resnick, R. (Eds.) Maternal Fetal Medicine, fourth ed. WB Saunders, Philadelphia.

Richardson, C.A., Jull, G.A., 1995. Muscle control – pain control. What exercises would you prescribe? Man. Ther. 1 (1), 2–10.

Rosa, F.W., Wilk, A.L., Kelsey, F.O., 1986. Teratogen update: vitamin A congeners. Teratology 33 (3), 355–364.

Rowe, J.W., Brown, R.S., Epstein, F.H., 1981. Physiology of the kidney in pregnancy. In: Freed, S.Z., Herzig, N. (Eds.) Urology and Pregnancy. Williams & Wilkins, Baltimore.

Royal College of Obstetricians and Gynaecologists (RCOG), 2006. Exercise in Pregnancy. RCOG statement no. 4, January 2006. RCOG, London.

Rubin, P.H., Janovitz, H.D., 1991. The digestive tract and pregnancy. In: Cherry, S.H., Merkatz, I.R. (Eds.) Complications of Pregnancy: Medical, Surgical, Gynecological, Psychosocial and Perinatal, fourth ed. Williams & Wilkins, Baltimore.

Sandman, C.A., Wadhwa, P.D., Dunkel-Schetter, C., et al., 1994. Psychobiological influences of stress and HPA regulation on the human fetus and infant birth outcomes. Ann. N. Y. Acad. Sci. 739, 198–210.

Sapolsky, R.M., 1997. The importance of a well-groomed child. Science 277, 1620–1621.

Scholl, T.O., Schroeder, C.M., 1999. High ferritin and very preterm delivery: influence of iron supplements during pregnancy. Ann. Behav. Med. 21, S087.

Schroder, H.J., Power, G.G., 1997. Engine and radiator: fetal and placental interactions for heat dissipation. Exp. Physiol. 82 (2), 403–414.

Shepherd, J., Fry, D., 1996. Symphysis pubis pain. Midwives 109 (1302), 199–201.

Sherwood, O.D., Downing, S.J., Guico-Lamm, M.L., et al., 1993. The physiological effects of relaxin during pregnancy: studies in rats and pigs. Oxf. Rev. Reprod. Biol. 15, 143–189.

Sichel, D., Driscoll, J.W., 1999. Women's Moods: What Every Woman Must Know about Hormones, the Brain and Emotional Health. Harper Collins, New York.

Skatrud, J.B., Dempsey, J.A., Kaiser, D.G., 1978. Ventilatory response to medroxyprogesterone acetate in normal subjects: time course and mechanism. J. Appl. Physiol. 44, 344–393.

Smithells, R.W., Sheppard, S., Schorah, C.J., et al., 1981. Apparent prevention of neural tube defects by periconceptional vitamin supplementation. Arch. Dis. Child. 56, 911–918.

Stein, Z., Susser, M., Saenger, G., et al., 1995. Famine and Human Development: The Dutch Hunger Winter of 1944/45. Oxford University Press, New York.

Steinlauf, A.F., Traube, M., 1999. Gastrointestinal complications. In: Burrow, G.N., Duffy, T.P. (Eds.) Medical Complications During Pregnancy, fifth ed. WB Saunders, Philadelphia.

Stephens, N.G., Parsons, A., Schofield, P.M., et al., 1996. Randomised controlled trial of vitamin E in patients with coronary disease: Cambridge Heart Antioxidant Study (CHAOS). Lancet 347, 781–786.

Stuge, B., Laerum, E., Kirkesola, G., et al., 2004. The efficacy of a treatment program focusing on specific stabilizing exercises for pelvic girdle pain after pregnancy: a randomised controlled trial. Spine 29 (4), 351–359.

Teixeira, J.M., Fisk, N.M., Glover, V., 1999. Association between maternal anxiety in pregnancy and increased uterine artery resistance index: cohort based study. BMJ 318 (7177), 153–157.

Theunissen, I.M., Parer, J.T., 1994. Fluid and electrolytes in pregnancy. Clin. Obstet. Gynecol. 37 (1), 3–15.

Thorp Jr., J.M., Norton, P.A., Wall, L.L., et al., 1999. Urinary incontinence in pregnancy and the puerperium: a prospective study. Am. J. Obstet. Gynecol. 181 (2), 266–273.

Thorpy, M., Ehrenberg, B.L., Hening, W.A. (National Heart, Lung, and Blood Institute Working Group on Restless Legs Syndrome, National Institutes of Health, Bethesda), et al., 2000. Restless legs syndrome; detection and management in primary care. Am. Fam. Physician 62, 108–114.

Tulchinsky, D., Hobel, C.J., 1973. Plasma human chorionic gonadotropin, estrone, estradiol, estriol, progesterone and 17 alpha-hydroxyprogesterone in human pregnancy. III, Early normal pregnancy. Am. J. Obstet. Gynecol. 117 (7), 884–893.

Uvnäs-Moberg, K., Francis, R., (trans.), 2003. The oxytocin factor. Da Capo Press, Cambridge, MA.

Van den Bergh, B.R., Mulder, E.J., Mennes, M., et al., 2005. Antenatal maternal anxiety and stress and the neurobehavioural development of the fetus and child: links and possible mechanisms. A review. Neurosci. Biobehav. Rev. 29 (2), 237–258.

Vander, A., Sherman, J., Lucian, D., 2000. Human Physiology: The Mechanisms of Body Function, eighth ed. McGraw-Hill, New York.

Vanhatalo, S., van Nieuwenhuizen, O., 2000. Fetal pain?. Brain Dev. 22 (3), 145–150.

Voigt, L.F., Hollenback, K.A., Krohn, M.A., et al., 1990. The relationship of abruptio placentae with maternal smoking and small for gestational age infants. Obstet. Gynecol. 75 (5), 771–774.

Weil, R.J., Tupper, C., 1960. Personality, life situation, and communication: a study of habitual abortion. Psychosom. Med. 22, 448–455.

Weinberger, S.E., Weiss, S.T., 1999. Pulmonary diseases. In: Burrow, G.N., Duffy, T.P. (Eds.) Medical Complications During Pregnancy, fifth ed. WB Saunders, Philadelphia, pp. 363–400.

Wilkening, R.B., Meschia, G., 1983. Fetal oxygen uptake, oxygenation and acid base balance as a function of uterine blood flow. Am. J. Physiol. 244 (6), H749–H755.

Wise, R.A., Polito, A.J., Krishnan, V., 2006. Respiratory physiologic changes in pregnancy. Immunol. Allergy Clin. North Am. 26 (1), 1–12.

Wolfe, L.A., Kemp, J.G., Heenan, A.P., et al., 1998. Acid–base regulation and control of ventilation in human pregnancy. Can. J. Physiol. Pharmacol. 76 (9), 815–827.

Young, G., Jewell, D., 2000. Interventions for preventing and treating backache in pregnancy. Cochrane Database Syst. Rev. 2000 (2) CD001139.

Chapter contents

Learning outcomes

- The physiological process of birth
- Optimal fetal and maternal positions to support labour
- The changes in maternal and fetal systems during labour
- The effects of place of birth on the process of labour

Introduction

'Labour' is the process by which the fetus is born. It is variable in its onset and duration for each woman. Term pregnancy is defined as 37–42 weeks. Dating by last monthly period (LMP) alone provides a reasonably accurate indicator of the length of gestation; however, an early ultrasound scan has been shown to provide a more accurate expected date of delivery (Crowley 2003).

There is an increased likelihood of neonatal complications if the fetus is born either earlier or later than this timeframe (RCOG 2001a). While most fetuses born after 42 weeks will be perfectly healthy, some may experience complications during the birthing process and primary care providers face complex situations in deciding whether to induce labour. Supporting 'nature' to take its course versus utilisation of medical intervention is also complex, and decisions occur in the context of many factors including the training and attitudes of the individual care provider and their team, the environment where the birth is taking place, and current obstetric policies and trends.

Due to increased technology, babies can now survive delivery at an earlier gestational age. Ethical issues arise in determining the appropriate antenatal and birthing care for a baby born in the range of 23–32 weeks, and decisions relating to the pregnancy and birth are made by parents in consultation with neonatal and perinatal specialists. Along with mortality concerns, there are short- and long-term consequences for an infant born in these earlier timeframes (McGrath et al 2000).

As well as considerable variation in the length of gestation, there are also variations in both the process and the length of labour. The duration of labour can vary from as little as 45 minutes or less to days.

Since the Second World War, there has been an increased medicalisation of the birthing process, and today most labours include various forms of medical care (Downe et al 2001, Department of Health 2005). Some of the interventions improve both maternal and fetal health and save lives and this is reflected in decreased maternal mortality rates in many countries. Medicine has helped women with pre-existing medical conditions in succeeding in bringing their pregnancy to term. However, this means that these women are more likely to need medical intervention. Increasing infertility, age and obesity rates also add medical complexity to pregnancies.

However, there is concern, even within the medical community, that medical care during pregnancy and birth has led to the utilisation of practices which may not improve maternal or fetal outcome. Sometimes, standards of care which may be relevant in a higher-risk pregnancy may be over-utilised in lower-risk situations. The current high mortality rate in some countries may be best addressed through appropriate support with issues such as nutrition and basic health care rather than increased use of technology (Wagner 1994).

Some practitioners have expressed concern that the process of birth, which for healthy women and babies should be essentially a 'natural' process, is being unnecessarily interfered with and that the natural variability of labour is becoming lost.

There is considerable need for ongoing research into the effects of specific practices such as the rise of caesareans, and commitment to such research presents challenges for everyone involved in the perinatal community. 'There is an urgent need for a systematic review of observational studies and a synthesis of qualitative data to better assess the short and long-term effects of caesarean section and vaginal birth' (Lavender et al 2006). Bodies of knowledge such as the Cochrane Database help to inform and challenge existing maternity care.

The importance of providing encouragement, and continuous emotional and physical support for women in labour has received worldwide recognition:

Given the clear benefits and no known risks associated with intrapartum support, every effort should be made to ensure all labouring women receive appropriate support, not only from those close to them but also from specially trained caregivers. This support should include continuous presence, the provision of hands-on comfort, and encouragement.

(Hodnett 1998)

This has led to an increased focus on the importance of midwifery care for lower-risk birthing women, and the existence of the growing field of labour support provision or doula care.

The ultimate responsibility for ensuring the woman and infant's health in labour lies in the hands of the maternity care provider, whether obstetrician, family physician or midwife. They make all medical decisions concerning their patient, while ideally providing them with information which underscores informed choice. Respect for this reality is crucial. It is also important that bodyworkers understand current medical practice and its effect on their pregnant and birthing clients and differing variations in different countries.

Even the generic term 'maternity care provider' has different connotations. For example, in countries such as the UK and Holland, midwives tend to be the primary maternity care providers for uncomplicated births, while in the USA and Canada, maternity care is most commonly provided by obstetricians regardless of the status of the woman's health history.

2.1 Physiological basis of labour

What starts labour?

There is no definitive answer to this question. What is known is that the onset of labour is a complex response triggered by hormones released by both the woman

and the fetus. For the fetus, these hormonal changes are related to the maturation of the fetal hypothalamic–pituitary–adrenal system. For the woman, levels of utero-tonic inhibitors decrease (the ratio of progesterone goes down while oestrogen, oxytocin and contraction association proteins (CAPs) increase). CAPs include gap junction proteins which allow the transfer of current carrying ions in labour. The position of the fetus also seems to be a factor in supporting the onset of labour and it is thought that a poorly positioned fetus may be a factor in contributing to delayed onset of labour.

Changes in the cervix

At the beginning of labour the cervix of a nulliparous women is usually a thick-walled canal of at least 2 cm in length. The cervix may, however, shorten and dilate before the onset of labour. This process is known as 'cervical ripening' and caregivers assess it using the *Bishop score* (1964) which rates:

- Cervical dilatation (from closed to 3+ cm).
- Cervical consistency (from firm to soft).
- Length of cervix (from 3 cm to 0 cm, as it shortens in labour).
- Position of cervix (from posterior to anterior).
- Station of the presenting part (usually the head of the fetus) (from −3 above ischial spines to 0).

There can be a 'bloody show'. This is when the mucous plug from the cervix is discharged. It is a mucousy, slightly bloody vaginal loss. This can happen a couple of days or weeks before labour begins, or during early labour itself.

The first contractions begin by stretching the lower segment of the uterus but the lower part of the cervical canal is initially unaltered. As labour progresses, the internal os is pulled open and the cervix dilates from the top downwards. It becomes shorter until no projection into the vagina is felt but only a more or less thick rim at the external os, the whole cervix being taken up and its cavity made one with that of the body of the uterus.

Prelabour

There are nearly always prelabour contractions which may or may not be perceptible to the woman. These prepare the woman and fetus for labour. They shape the cervix, help with the positioning of the fetus, may begin the process of effacement, and in multiparous women, sometimes the process of dilatation. Many nulliparae will feel prelabour contractions when the fetus engages. In multiparae it is not unusual for the fetus to engage at the onset of or during labour.

Rupture of the membranes

This may occur prior to labour or at any stage in labour, although it usually occurs towards the end of first stage. As the cervix starts to efface and the fetal head descends on to the cervix, the small bag of waters in front of the head (the forewaters) is separated from the remainder (the hindwaters). The forewaters help the early effacement of the cervix and dilatation of the os uteri. The hindwaters help to equalise the pressure in the uterus during uterine contractions and provide some protection to the fetus and placenta.

Changes in the uterus and the mechanism of contractions

All stages of labour are characterised by contractions of the uterus, which are slightly different for each stage of labour. A contraction is an experience which feels different for each woman. Some feel latent labour contractions intensely, others feel only slight discomfort. Some may not even be aware of contractions at all other than a hardening of the abdomen. Usually as labour progresses most women do feel their contractions and experience intense sensations, although a minority of women do not feel them much at all.

How contractions begin varies from woman to woman. Some women enter labour with strong contractions while other women have days of lighter contractions or perhaps several hours of strong contractions and then nothing for hours. It is not uncommon for multiparae to experience uterine contractions which are strong enough to be painful for some days or even weeks before real labour starts. These have been called 'false pains' but in fact they are part of the preparation for labour. Elizabeth Davis prefers to call them 'practice contractions' because otherwise women may feel that their body is deceiving them by being 'false'. These early contractions differ from labour 'pains' only in that they are less regular and less effective in dilating the cervix.

Myometrium contraction (Fig. 2.1)

The uterus is a smooth muscle and is mediated by the action of actin and myosin which is controlled by hormonal, biochemical, neurogenic and physical factors.

There is an intrinsic excitability of the uterine muscle which is dominated by hormonal influences during labour. This is due to the number and size of gap junctions. Gap junctions allow the transfer of current carrying ions and the exchange of second messengers between the cytoplasm of adjacent cells. Increased gap junction interaction will increase electrical impulses and therefore the contractility of the myometrium. Gap junctions are absent or infrequent in the non-pregnant myometrium and decline markedly within 24 hours of delivery.

The number and size of gap junctions increase to approximately 1000 per cell during labour (Benito-Leon & Aguilar-Galan 2001, Donaldson 1998, Garfield et al 1988). An increase in gap junctions has been reported in women with pre-term labour, and delay in formation is associated with prolonged pregnancy.

Neurological control of contractions is not critical due to this increase in gap junctions, which means that labour can occur in women with spinal injury. Contractions follow a cycle of activity of slow rhythmic fluctuation in the magnitude of electrical potential across the cell membrane.

What is physically happening is that the abdomen/ uterus is tightening. A normal uterine contraction spreads downward from the cornus (top of the uterus) within about 15 seconds. The contractile phase begins slightly later in the lower portion of the uterus but functional coordination is such that the contraction's peak is attained simultaneously in all portions during active labour. There is an increase in intrauterine pressure of approximately 10–12 mmHg which may increase to 30 mmHg with hypertonia (increased tightness of muscle tone). Contractions can be palpated abdominally with pressure greater than 10–20 mmHg and perceived by the woman at 15–20 mmHg.

A labouring woman generally perceives pain at pressure greater than 25 mmHg, although this varies. This means that the duration of a contraction assessed from palpation or a woman's perception will be shorter than the actual contraction, and the duration between contractions will seem longer.

The uterus is divided into segments. The upper part of the uterus, known as the upper uterine segment (UUS), contracts strongly, and with each contraction the smooth muscle fibres become shorter and thicker. These muscles not only contract but 'retract'. This means that when the active contraction passes the fibres re-lengthen, but not back to their former length. If they went back to their previous length, no progress would be made. Retraction means that some of the shortening of the muscle fibres is maintained and each successive contraction starts at the point where the previous one ended. With each contraction the uterine cavity becomes a little smaller. Retraction is a property of other muscles but is most marked in the uterus.

The powerful upper segment draws up the weaker, thinner and more passive lower segment and so the cervix dilates. During early pregnancy the lower segment is not clearly defined but by late pregnancy it is recognisable and corresponds with the lower limit of the firm peritoneal attachment to the uterus. Below this point the uterovesical peritoneum is loosely attached.

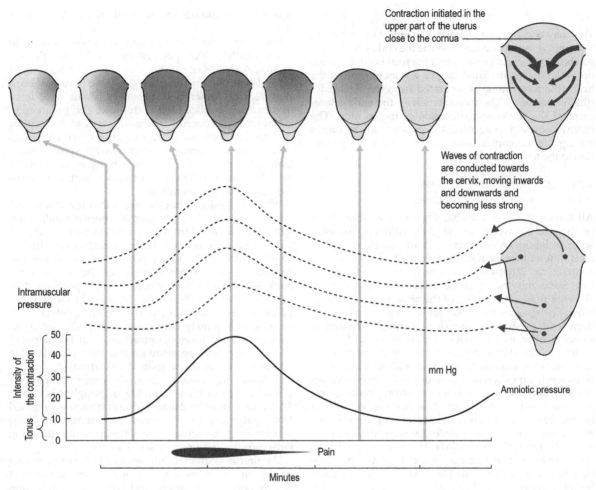

Contraction initiated in the upper part of the uterus close to the cornua

Waves of contraction are conducted towards the cervix, moving inwards and downwards and becoming less strong

Intramuscular pressure

Intensity of the contraction

Tonus

50
40
30
20
10
0

mm Hg

Amniotic pressure

Pain

Minutes

Fig. 2.1 Contraction and retraction of uterine muscle cells.

These two segments are not clearly formed until the end of the first stage of labour where they can be clearly seen. In labour, as the lower segment is drawn up, its shape changes from a hemisphere to a cylinder. If there is obstruction the restriction of the upper segment is even more pronounced.

In labour the lower uterine segment, cervix, vagina, pelvic floor and vulval outlet are dilated until there is one continuous birth canal. During the second stage the contractions of abdominal muscles and the diaphragm help the baby to be born.

Contractions are not continuous. This is extremely important for both the woman and the fetus. During a contraction blood circulation through the uterine wall is stopped: if the contraction were continuous the fetus would die of oxygen deprivation. The intervals between the contractions allow the placental circulation to be re-established. They also allow the woman time to recover both physically and emotionally from the contraction.

Ina May Gaskin describes the cervix as a sphincter along with the anus and vagina, and has theorised 'the law of the sphincters' (Gaskin 2003). She outlines the emotional factors which may contribute to the woman being able to relax and go with her contractions, rather than trying to resist, or block them out. If women are relaxed then dilatation happens. Gaskin also believes that women can go 'backwards' in dilatation if they are stressed and that dilation is not necessarily a forward linear process. Many doulas have noticed that if women visualise their cervix opening it can help it dilate. It must be recognised that there is no conscious control over the cervix, while there is over the anus and vagina. Physiologically, the vaginal 'sphincter' and anal sphincter are rich in muscle whereas the cervix hardly has any muscle and is mainly collagen. However, it may be that the emotions affect the cervix less directly through their effects on the neuroendocrine system.

Pain in labour

Even though labour is often experienced as painful and uncomfortable, there are some women who feel minimal discomfort, or who are able to use breathing, visualisations or other tools to positively perceive their contractions. Many birthing clients who have used bodywork to support them during labour report positive descriptions of contractions ranging from associating a positive experience of 'pain', to feelings of empowerment, or to finding labour an 'amazing' and even 'enjoyable' experience. There are recorded examples from women who have used hypnobirthing tools (Mongan method), or who refer to contractions as 'rushes' and even record feelings similar to orgasm (Gaskin 2002). More recently some women have referred to birth as 'ecstatic' (Buckley 2005) or 'beautiful' (Yates 2008). Grantly Dick-Reid (1984) was one of the first obstetricians to record his surprise at a woman in labour who did not feel pain but often the possibility of experiencing contractions in this constructive fashion may be met with scepticism by those who assume labour must be a painful experience.

The perception of pain is influenced by physiological, psychological and cultural factors. Anxiety will influence the course of labour, reducing pain toleration. Relaxation seems to play an important role in breaking this cycle (Jimenez 1983). Many writers attribute the naturally released hormones which are produced during labour as being to a large part responsible for experiencing birth in a positive way (Buckley 2005).

Discomfort or pain is experienced as either *visceral* (due to the contractions of the uterus and how this affects both the uterus and other organs and tissues of the body), or it can be *somatic* (due to the pressure of the fetus on the cervix and surrounding structures).

Visceral pain

Visceral pain is related to the contractions of the uterus and the dilatation of the cervix. Pain caused by the contraction of the uterus is transmitted by afferent fibres to the sympathetic chain of the posterior spinal cord at T10–T12 and L1. In early labour and during transition this is mostly between T10 and T11. Pain can be referred and may be experienced over the abdominal wall, between the umbilicus and symphysis pubis, around the iliac crest to the gluteal area, radiating down the thighs, and in the lumbar and sacral regions (Smith et al 2000; Fig. 2.2).

During second stage, pain is transmitted more through the posterior roots at S2, S3 and S4 and therefore may be experienced lower down, so is likely to be somatic pain.

Pain caused by the dilation of the cervix is usually stronger towards the end of first stage. Sensory impulses from the cervix probably enter the cord via the sacral roots. Pain at the end of the first stage is often referred to the sacral region.

Somatic pain

This is caused by pressure of the presenting part of the fetus on the cervix. It is more likely to be experienced during the second stage of labour.

Gate control theory

This theory postulates that the nervous stimuli can be inhibited at the level of the substantia gelatinosa and the dorsal horn of the spinal cord from reaching the thalamus and cerebral cortex (Melzack & Wall 1983).

The gate control theory is used as a basis for promoting the use of massage and strokes such as effleurage during labour. These modalities are considered to be a distraction from the pain messages that the brain is processing. The gate control theory has also been considered in the development of TENS machines for pain relief.

In simple terms there are thought to be 'gates' at the spinal cord. If these gates can be 'closed', then whatever pain stimulus arrives at the level of the spinal cord will not be allowed up the cord to the brain and therefore will not be experienced by the woman as pain.

(Dr J Barrett)

2.2 Stages of labour

Labour has traditionally been divided into three different stages, although the stages are not always clearly defined for the birthing woman. They may seem to flow into one another. Some writers have recently suggested that for this reason, it may be more useful to consider labour as a continuum from onset to completion, characterised by particular physiological and psychological behaviours at various points (Downe 2000).

This social model places an emphasis on the differences between individual women's experiences, and underscores the importance of trusting a woman's physiology to function optimally. This approach may have a positive impact on the woman's view of her labour, and tends away from imposing set time

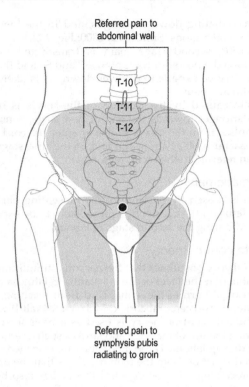

Referred pain to
abdominal wall

T-10
T-11
T-12

Referred pain to
symphysis pubis
radiating to groin

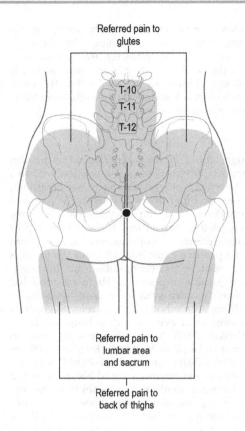

Referred pain to
glutes

T-10
T-11
T-12

Referred pain to
lumbar area
and sacrum

Referred pain to
back of thighs

Fig. 2.2 Pain sites in labour.

frames for different stages of labour (Gould 2000, Green et al 1998).

It is important to recognise that there can be differences between nulliparae and multiparae labours. There can also be differences in labours between women of different cultures and races. For example midwives have observed that, probably due to differences in the pelvis, with Afro-Caribbean women the fetus does not tend to engage before labour begins.

The following information relates to what happens in 'unmedicated' labours. In this section, as we consider what supports or impedes the process of labours, we are primarily considering treatment strategies which are within the bodyworker's scope of practice, including self-help activities for the client. It is important to differentiate this from the care given by the primary care provider. Their scope of practice may include similar tasks to bodyworkers such as providing supportive and encouraging words and behaviour towards their client, but also has the primary task of safe care of the woman and her baby. It therefore also includes medical interventions which are discussed under the medical approach to labour.

Latent and first stage labour

What is happening?

- Contractions serve to thin/efface the cervix from 0 to 100% and to dilate/open the cervix from 0 cm to 10 cm, which is considered full dilatation.
- Latent labour is the phase of labour which takes the longest amount of time and can vary most in its duration. For a nulliparae it may take several days but multiparae may skip the latent phase. Generally, this phase tends to be shorter for multiparae.
- Once the active phase begins then the cervix usually dilates at around 1 cm/h or more from 3 to 10 cm.
- Transition ends the first stage of labour with the cervix dilating from 7 (8) to 10 cm.

One of the most common questions for families to ask during the latter stages of their pregnancy is how to determine whether the woman is in labour or not. This may be challenging for a woman who has never experienced labour before.

Latent first stage labour

This is before labour is 'established'. It can last for days with irregular contractions, or may even pass unnoticed. It is sometimes known as the 'stop/start' phase of labour. The contractions do not get progressively stronger and closer together and can be sporadic in nature. There can be an hour or two of strong, close together contractions, which may even be quite painful, but then they stop. These contractions usually last about 30–40 seconds each, and vary from 3 to 20 minutes apart. What is happening is the uterus is contracting but the contractions are not co-ordinated. Some practitioners refer to them as 'warm up' contractions. Sometimes, if the fetus is not in the best position for birth, the contractions of the uterus help to better position the baby rather than dilating the cervix.

Active first stage labour

This is the 'established' phase and usually lasts around 10–12 hours in a nullipara, but can be as little as 1 hour or as much, or more, than 36 hours. The contractions get closer together and stronger and last longer than in the latent stage. Contractions can last for 40 seconds and are 3–4 minutes apart. They have a more regular pattern of interval and duration, and are progressively building in length and intensity. Eventually they can last for up to 1 minute or more and come every 1.5–3 minutes. After about 6cm they tend to get closer together and therefore seem more painful and longer as there is not as much time to rest in between. The woman will feel her abdomen hardening, as she may have in latent first stage; this is the uterus contracting. This will happen with more rhythm and strength as first stage progresses. As the baby's head is pushed deeper into the pelvis it flexes. The pressure of the head stimulates the cervix and perineum which in turn brings about stronger contractions. Although there is pressure from the presenting part there may not necessarily be much actual descent of the baby.

What can impede progress in the first stage of labour

The birthing environment, both 'within and without'

- Fear and anxiety.
- A location that is noisy, cold, overly bright, or busy.
- Mental activity, e.g. too much 'expectation'.
- Inertia – sometimes physical activity, such as a long walk, may help get labour established.

If these circumstances cause anxiety in the woman, there may be an increase in the release of adrenaline. This can inhibit the production of oxytocin and endorphins with a result that physiologically labour may become more painful. The release of adrenaline occurs as part of the 'fight or flight' mechanism. It has been observed that if an animal is under threat in labour, she may either give birth quickly (if she has progressed sufficiently along in her labour, i.e. late second stage) or the birthing process will actually cease until she finds a safe place.

The same is probably applicable to humans as stress and interruptions affect the birthing process. An example of this is shifting the location of labour from home to hospital. Regardless of whether women prefer to birth at home or in the hospital, ensuring the woman is in her preferred space in a timely and smooth fashion is important. A major concern related to choice of birthing location is safety, and this means different things to every woman and family. Some women prefer to be in a hospital setting, with medical staff and equipment close at hand. They, or their partners, would feel too anxious delivering within their home situation. However, many women look forward to a home birth because they find the hospital setting to be less familiar and even frightening. The comfort of being in their own home helps them cope better with labour.

Creating 'safe and comforting strategies' which help the woman attune to a more relaxed state is an important process in either environment.

Being stationary or immobilised

Ineffective positioning and immobility may make labour more prolonged and/or painful because there is less mobilisation of the pelvis and use of gravity which tend to encourage descent of the fetus. Lying down and static positioning are relatively new events in the birthing process, and may have an effect on the increased use of interventions to deliver babies. Prolonged or static positioning may also increase musculoskeletal discomforts such as low back pain.

Physical activities such as walking, swaying and remaining upright can literally help 'mobilise' the birthing process.

Exhaustion

Some women misinterpret the idea of 'active' birth to mean they have to be active and in motion from the moment they have their first contraction. If they have a long labour, this could result in exhaustion. It is important to rest and relax as much as possible, especially between contractions. Holding unnecessary physical tension may also tire the woman. Listening to one's body, staying calm and relaxed, being efficient in terms of energy output and type of physical activity, as well as staying as comfortable as possible is crucial. Exhaustion may slow labour down: as the woman gets tired, so may her uterus, and this can lead to a sense of discouragement and defeat.

Lack of nourishment

Labour can last many hours, and it is not appropriate to deprive a woman of nourishment. It is estimated that labour requires a similar caloric intake to someone engaged in strenuous sport. If there are no carbohydrates available for conversion to glycogen, body fat will be utilised and so the quantity of ketones in the tissue and blood may increase (Foulkes & Dumoulin 1983).

It is important for the woman to eat what she feels like eating, when she feels like it.

For a normal labour, and if the woman is able, it is recommended that she eat frequent, light meals which are low in fat and roughage and easy to digest. Fluids should also be taken to prevent dehydration (Ludka & Roberts 1993, Sharp 1997).

Instinctively, many women have no appetite for heavy meals that take energy and time to digest. Many care providers will leave food choices up to the woman. Some hospitals have policies restricting food intake in the event that the need arises for a general anaesthetic. However, fasting in labour does not ensure an empty stomach and anaesthetic techniques have improved so that aspiration of gastric contents is unlikely (Baker 1996, Johnson et al 1989, Tranmer et al 2005).

Self-doubt and/or giving up

Some women can be managing well in labour when a misplaced word or two from someone around them creates self-doubt about their progress. Everyone involved in the labour process, from care providers, to doula, to partner, needs to be aware of the words they use, their facial expressions, their body language and their attitudes. It is amazing how quickly women can shift from being positive, focused and coping well to feeling overwhelmed and ready to give up! This can occur with a vaginal examination when the woman finds out her cervix is not as dilated as she had hoped. Encouragement from the partner and care providers is vital in helping the labouring woman stay focused and well supported.

Full bladder

Along with feeling uncomfortable, 'bladder distension can result in uterine atony and affect its ability to contract' (Bobak & Jensen 1993: 507). The woman needs to empty her bladder at least every hour or two. This also helps to keep her mobilised. If the woman is unable to urinate, she may need to be catheterised.

What supports first stage labour

This is explored in practical labour (refer Ch. 10, section 10.4 p. 297).

Transition

What is happening?

This indicates the end of the first stage of labour with the body beginning to get ready for second stage. The cervix is completing its final stages of dilation (8–10 cm).

In this phase, contractions will be closer together, as frequent as every 2 minutes, and they will also be longer, lasting up to 60 seconds. Things are physically getting more intense. The woman may feel hot and cold, vomit or feel nauseous, have shaky legs, grunt, feel pressure in her anus or empty her bowels. Emotionally it can also be intense. The woman may feel angry, frustrated, or feel that she cannot go on. It is the point in labour when she may berate her partner, or ask for an epidural or caesarean, even though she may have been doing fine with no desire for interventions prior to this phase. She may feel very tired and need to rest. In fact, labour may appear to have stopped. Transition may be brief, a few minutes, or it may last up to an hour or more. The important thing for both woman and partner to remember is that all of this intensity is an indicator that her body is getting on with labour, the cervix is dilating, her body is preparing to give birth. It means things are moving along. If these can be seen as 'good' signs and accepted, it is easier to cope. 'Oh, this is that intense phase of labour!'

The woman may feel an urge to push because of the increased pressure of the baby's head low in the pelvis, but this can sometimes happen before the cervix is completely dilated. If so, it is usually best for the woman to try not to actively push, but to relax and breathe during the contractions to feel what her body is doing. Telling a woman not to push may be counterproductive because she may then feel confused about what her body wants her to do. Pant breathing, which is often advocated, may make the woman disconnect from her own breathing rhythm and may not be particularly effective in reducing the urge to bear down. It is often preferable to give the woman strategies such as encouraging her to shift into positions such as the knee to chest position, where her pelvis is higher than her head in order to reduce pressure on the cervix.

Sometimes when the cervix is fully dilated there can be a pause in the intensity of the labour. Some women may feel drowsy or like going to sleep, especially if it has been a long first stage. It is important to wait until the woman feels strong second stage contractions before bearing down because the baby may still need to adjust its position and bearing down may force it into the wrong position. Some midwives call it the 'rest and be thankful' stage. It makes sense for the body to have a little rest before going into the potentially more physically demanding second stage.

Some women become vigilant and awake (even chatty) which is a sign of an increase in catecholamines. Odent suggests a surge in catecholamines causes the 'fetal ejection reflex' (Odent 1992).

What can impede transition

- Exhaustion.
- Feeling unheard and/or unsupported.
- Being in an uncomfortable position.
- Lying supine.
- Feeling frightened.
- Feeling cold or overheated.
- Giving up.

What supports transition

See practical labour (refer Ch. 10, section 10.4 p. 297).

Second stage labour

What is happening?

The contractions are called expulsive contractions as they are now working to push the fetus down the birth canal and out into the world.

It is usually best for the woman to try to be patient and wait, and not to bear down actively until the desire to push is overwhelmingly strong. It is important to let the body take over and for the woman to be able to go naturally with what she feels. Some women do not need to bear down strongly and the baby comes out gently. Some women have strong physical contractions. Some babies are born within one or two contractions, others take their time. Like all phases of labour this can be very different for everyone. Pushing should not be about forcing the baby out, but letting the woman's body give birth. The woman may start to try to push because she thinks that is what should happen next rather than what her body is actually needing to do. It is important to encourage the woman to listen to the sensations of her body and work with what needs to happen. Studies have shown that women tend to do more effective bearing down when they are responding to their body rather than being told to push (Enkin et al 2000).

The ligaments provide stretch for the bones of the pelvis to move in order to allow this process to happen. This stretch helps give enough space for the delivery of the baby. The coccyx moves slightly out of the way. It is important to know that the bones of the spine and the pelvis move; they are not fixed. The more the woman can understand, envision, and allow this process of opening and stretching to happen, the easier the delivery can be.

With each contraction the presenting part of the baby is forced down on to the pelvic floor, facilitated by the action of the abdominal wall and the diaphragm. In between contractions, the pelvic floor can push the presenting part back up again. This is where uterine retraction is important, as progress is not completely lost. Eventually the presenting part is stationary at the end of the contraction. The baby's head gradually comes down. With a nullipara, the baby's head may become visible at the perineum before it exits.

When the widest diameter of the head appears this is what is known as 'crowning'. For a first time delivery this can be painful as the perineum stretches, and is sometimes described as a burning sensation. Perineal massage or hot compresses may support the process of stretching, while also providing some comfort.

In the second stage there is some moulding of the baby's head. The sutures of the baby's skull are not fused which allows movement of the bones to ensure the baby's head is sized in conjunction with the mother's pelvis.

There are four movements of the baby's head in this stage (Fig. 2.3): (i) internal rotation; (ii) extension; (iii) restitution; (iv) external rotation.

- *Internal rotation*: when the head meets the resistance of the pelvic floor the occiput rotates forward from the left occiput transverse (LOT) or left occiput anterior (LOA) position to lie under the subpubic arch.
- *Extension*: as the head advances it passes through the vulva by a process of extension. This causes the anterior part to stretch the perineum gradually until the moment of crowning when the greatest diameter slips through the vulva.
- *Restitution*: as the head descends the shoulders enter the pelvic brim. When the head has internally rotated it is twisted a little on the shoulder. Once it is born it resumes it natural position and this is called restitution.
- *External rotation*: as the shoulders descend one shoulder meets the resistance of the pelvic floor first and rotates to the front, and the head also rotates as the shoulders rotate.

Some maternity care providers help to control the exit of the baby's head as well as allowing for slow stretch of the perineum by providing direct hands-on contact with the perineum. This may include the application of pressure to the area, or perineal massage to help facilitate the stretch of the tissues and minimise tearing. Other maternity care providers rely on the efforts of the woman's pushing without any touch contact, allowing the head to be delivered and the perineum to stretch and adapt to the forces of the delivery.

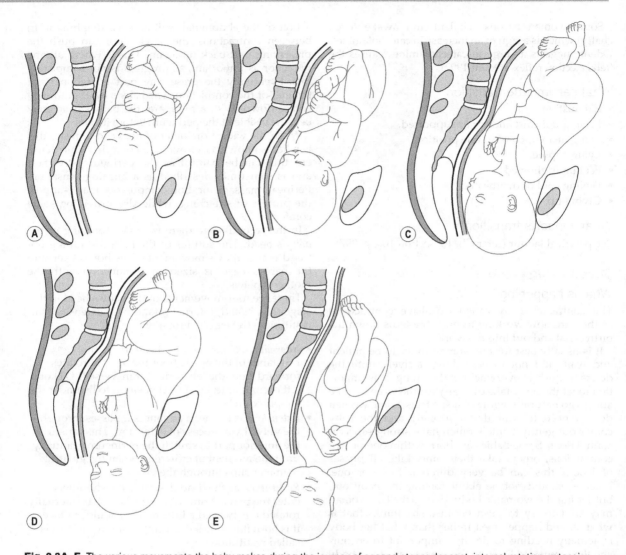

Fig. 2.3A–E The various movements the baby makes during the journey of second stage: descent, internal rotation, extension, restitution, external rotation.

It is helpful if the woman is in tune with bearing down and does not overpush at the moment of crowning because otherwise the perineum can tear and the baby may be born too rapidly.

When the head is born, the maternity care provider slips their fingers over the occiput to see if the cord is around the neck. If so, it must be freed, or a loop made large enough for the shoulders to pass through. The birth of the trunk should not be hurried and usually comes out with another contraction. Following restitution and external rotation of the head, the shoulders should be in the anteroposterior diameter of the pelvis. Then they can be delivered safely without the risk of perineal trauma.

This stage is shorter than first stage and actively bearing down would tend not to be more than 2 hours for a nulliparae, and for multiparae may be 15 minutes or less. The end of first stage does not, however, necessarily mean the beginning of second stage. It is important that second stage is measured from the actual start of it, i.e. when the woman experiences the urge to bear down, as otherwise unnecessary time limits may be imposed on the woman.

Sometimes women can be fully dilated but they do not have an urge to push and so there is a period of waiting between the phases.

What can impede the progress of second stage

If a woman does not feel a spontaneous urge to push, is unsure of 'how to push' or whether she is 'doing it correctly', feels rushed or forced to push, or has any fear related to the final exit of the baby from her perineal area, she may become anxious and tense, or panic. This can result in unproductive attempts to bear down. Further unproductive efforts may occur if there is tension in the upper body, particularly in the neck and shoulder regions, or if the woman is holding back from bearing down into her pelvis and perineum. Straining can be tiring and the woman may find that she runs out of energy.

Lying semi-supine may result in unproductive pushing and other positions such as upright forward leaning, standing or assisted semi-squatting can be encouraged. However, the most important factor is that the woman is as comfortable as possible.

A full bladder can also interfere with second stage by affecting the uterus and its contractility.

What supports second stage

See practical labour (refer Ch. 10, section 10.4 p. 297).

Third stage labour

What is happening? (Fig. 2.4)

This stage is the delivery of the placenta. If this stage proceeds without intervention (physiological third stage) then it takes about 15 minutes but may take up to 1 hour or longer (Prendiville & Elbourne 1988).

The third stage is similar to second stage, but usually not as intense. Uterine contractions continue so that the placenta is sheared off the wall of the uterus. The placenta is smaller than the baby with no bony structure so it is easier to deliver through the passage already created by the baby. The placenta may be delivered with one contraction. Separation of the placenta usually begins with the contraction which delivers the baby's trunk and is completed within the next two contractions. Most women feel a difference with these contractions. As there is no longer a head pushing

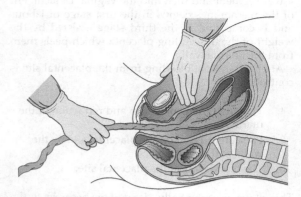

Fig. 2.4 Placental separation.

on the pelvic floor, they may feel the contractions as less urgent and intense. Some women, however, are surprised at the strength of contractions with this part of the delivery, particularly if they presumed they would not experience intense pain after the baby has been born.

As the baby is delivered there is a marked reduction in the size of the uterus due to the powerful contraction and retraction which takes place. The placental site reduces substantially in size. When the placental site is reduced by about one half, the placenta, being inelastic, becomes wrinkled and then is shorn off the uterine wall. It is tightly compressed by the contracted uterus. Some fetal blood is pumped back into the fetus's circulation and maternal blood in the intervillous spaces is forced back into the veins in the deep spongy layer of the decidua basalis. The blood in these veins cannot return to the maternal circulation because of the contracted and retracted state of the myometrium. The result is that the congested veins rupture and this small amount of extravasated blood is sheared off the villi from the spongy layer of the decidua basalis thereby separating the placenta from the uterine wall.

Bleeding is controlled by the action of the interlacing spiral fibres, named 'living ligatures', which contract around the torn maternal vessels to prevent further blood loss. This process happens rapidly. Brandt (1993) studied 30 women in third stage and found that in all cases the placenta had completely separated from the uterine wall within 3 minutes of delivery and was lying in the lower uterine segment.

When separation is complete the upper uterine segment contracts strongly forcing the placenta into the lower segment and then into the vagina. Detachment of the membranes begins in the first stage of labour and is completed in the third stage assisted by the weight of the descending placenta which peels them from the uterine wall.

After separation, bleeding from the placental site is controlled by:

1. The powerful contraction and retraction of the uterus.
2. Pressure exerted on the placental site by the walls of the uterus.
3. The blood clots at the placental site.

This stage is potentially dangerous because if the blood vessels which attached the placenta to the wall of the uterus do not close up, then there is a risk of haemorrhage. The woman's body is designed to deliver the placenta as well as the baby, and in a labour which has progressed without complication, and with a woman who has no history of haemorrhage in previous deliveries, there would be less likelihood of an indication for administration of drugs such as oxytocin.

In order to support a physiological third stage, the cord is not clamped immediately and is allowed to stop pulsating because the baby gets about 50 ml of blood from the placenta as the lungs expand with the first breath. It is best to keep the baby at the same level as the placenta or a little lower. If the baby is held high above the placenta (which may be inadvertently done in caesarean section) blood may run back into the placenta with the risk of hypovolaemia or subsequent anaemia in the fetus. It is also thought holding it lower may reduce the risk of haemorrhage for the mother (Yao & Lind 1969).

During the third stage of labour, supportive care is still essential. Creating an atmosphere of calmness and attention to the woman and her baby are essential. At this time, the high noradrenaline levels of the second stage, which may have kept woman and her baby wide-eyed and alert at first contact, will be decreasing. A warm and comforting atmosphere can counteract the cold, shivering feelings that a woman may have as her noradrenaline levels drop. If the environment is not well heated, and/or the woman is worried or distracted, continuing high levels of noradrenaline will counteract oxytocin's beneficial effects on her uterus. This, according to Michel Odent (1992), may increase the risk of haemorrhage.

Delivery of placenta with twins

Usually, even if there are two placentas they are both delivered after both twins have been born. If there is one placenta it is delivered after both babies have been born.

What can impede third stage

- Not promoting skin-to-skin contact whereby the baby can nuzzle at the mother's breast or latch when possible (thereby increasing the release of oxytocin hormones to help the uterus contract).
- Not emptying the bladder.
- Exhaustion.
- Giving up.
- Feeling cold.
- Worry – for example if the baby is taken away from the woman and she cannot see the baby or does not know what is happening.

What supports third stage

See practical labour (refer Ch. 10, section 10.4 p. 297).

Fourth stage
Immediately post birth

The fourth stage is essentially the rest of the woman's, the newborn's and the family's life. However, in the immediate period after birth it is important to give space for the initial bonding to happen between the woman and her baby, and for skin-to-skin contact and breastfeeding to begin.

The maternity care provider will check that the placenta is intact and therefore has completely separated, and that vaginal blood loss is within normal limits. If any of the placenta remains inside the uterus, it may cause excessive blood loss and/or infection. The perineum will be checked for tearing and suturing will be carried out if necessary.

What can impede the process of fourth stage

- If the woman has had drugs during the birthing process, particularly narcotics which may block the process (Bridges & Grimm 1982, Kinsley et al 1995, Stafisso-Sandoz et al 1998).
- Having the baby taken away unnecessarily.

This is the time for the support people to stand back and allow the woman and the baby's father/partner or other family members to be with their baby in a nurturing environment.

What supports fourth stage

Relaxation, reassurance, bonding time, providing a space to be together as a family (see postnatal practical, p. 313).

Summary of the implications of the stages of labour for bodyworkers

- Knowledge:
It is important to have a sound knowledge of what is happening physiologically as well as emotionally during the different stages of labour.
- Supportive comfort measures:
An understanding of what supports or may impede the progression of each stage in order to provide relevant and encouraging care for the woman and her family.
- The role of emotions and stress:
Understanding the role emotions play during all aspects of the birthing process, and the importance of reducing stress are fundamental elements of the bodyworker's supportive care.
Studies on doula care have indicated that comfort measures on a physical and emotional level can positively affect the outcome of labour. Stress has been shown to be a factor in women's perception of their ability to cope during labour and its relationship to birth outcome (Hodnett 2002).
- Environment:
The bodyworker needs to help create and maintain a calm space in the time before labour as well as during labour itself. Most women do need some form of emotional encouragement during labour.
- Pain relief in labour:
There is usually some degree of discomfort for the birthing woman. The following areas of the body are key areas to apply treatment modalities, whether massage, shiatsu, reflexology, etc.: T10–L1, the abdomen, especially between the umbilicus and pubic bone, the iliac crest to the gluteals and greater trochanter region, the lumbar and sacral areas, and the thighs.

2.3 Fetal position/presentation

This section examines the positions and growth of the fetus, fetal presentation, descent of the fetus and movement of the fetus during the birth process.

The 'position', 'presentation' and 'lie' of the fetus at the start of labour will influence the outcome of labour. The position of the fetus as well as the position of the birthing woman are key factors in the progression of labour.

Lie

The 'lie' means the relation which the long axis of the fetus bears to the uterus. It may be longitudinal, oblique or transverse.

Presentation

The 'presentation' refers to which part of the head or body is in or over the pelvic brim. When the head is first it is called 'cephalic' and if the head is flexed on the spine then the vertex presents. If the head is fully extended on the spine there is a face presentation, and if partly extended, a brow presentation. If the bottom presents first then it is called a 'breech' presentation.

If the fetus lies obliquely then the shoulder lies over the cervix and this is called a shoulder presentation. Any presentation other than vertex is referred to as a 'malpresentation'.

Position

The 'position' describes the relationship which a selected part of the fetus (the denominator) is in, in relation to the maternal pelvis. With a vertex presentation the denominator is the occiput. There are six presentations (Fig. 2.5):

- Left or right occiput anterior (LOA or ROA). Anterior means to the anterior of the woman's body, i.e. the back of the baby's head (occiput) and its spine are presenting at the front of the woman's body.
- LOP and ROP (left and right occiput posterior) are the opposite, i.e. the back of the baby's head (occiput) and spine are facing the direction of the woman's spine.
- LOT and ROT (left and right occiput transverse) mean the occiput lies in the transverse diameter of the pelvic brim.

The fetus makes various movements, twists and turns on its journey down the birth canal, and it is generally accepted (e.g. Henderson & Macdonald 2004, Lewis & Chamberlain 1990) that the position of the fetus which most supports this process is anterior cephalic.

The position of the first twin is an important consideration if a woman is having twins. The second twin is usually smaller and therefore it is easier to pass through the space already created by the first and larger fetus.

It is important to remember that as the fetus changes position during labour it may subtly move out of position, either due to the shape of the woman's pelvis or due to the position the woman is in. This can result in the use of interventions in the labour. Labour may slow down or be more painful for the woman if the fetus is stuck within the pelvis or not progressing down the birth canal.

Fetal position can be affected by other factors as well, such as: the shape of the woman's pelvis, the shape of the uterus, especially with uterine abnormalities, any blockages in the uterus such as fibroids

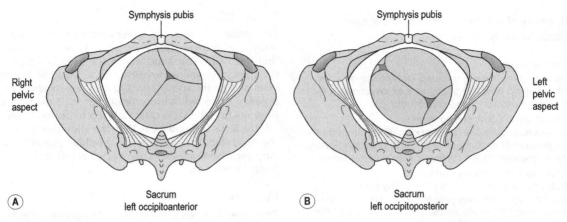

Fig. 2.5 A and B Different presentations; anterior and posterior.

or cysts, the tone of the abdomen, the size of the fetus, the position of the placenta, or issues related to the umbilical cord. Fetal position is also thought to be affected by the position of the woman both leading up to labour and during labour itself.

Traditionally the maternity care provider would assess fetal position from 28 weeks onwards. The UK NICE guidelines recommend assessment only after 36 weeks as prior to this the fetus can change position frequently. However, the fetus usually goes into spontaneous version between 30 and 34 weeks. While it is true that the fetus can change position right up to, and in, labour, and it is difficult to be sure of the position until 34–36 weeks, this aspect of antenatal care is often appreciated by the woman because it may help her to focus on her baby within. Many practitioners include assessing position as a way of supporting the woman's connection with her baby. It may also encourage the woman to be motivated in terms of practising forward leaning positions, which will not only help strengthen her body, but can also help prepare her for utilising upright birthing positions. From 34 to 36 weeks it is relatively easy to feel if a fetus is posterior or anterior, but harder to assess breech or cephalic. Even the maternity care provider may find it difficult to assess breech through palpation alone at this stage and if there is concern, ultrasound may be required to establish an accurate assessment.

Use of ultrasound for assessment of fetal position and fetal growth

In the third trimester ultrasound may be used for verifying fetal presentation if there is concern, for example in cases of suspected breech. It may also be used for rechecking the position of the placenta if it had been assessed as low lying during the second trimester scan, or if there is vaginal bleeding.

Engagement of presenting part

The other aspect assessed is fetal engagement. If the fetus is cephalic the assessment is how much the fetal head has engaged in the pelvic inlet (i.e. below the level of the pubic bone). This is measured in fifths, with a measurement of 4/5 meaning that 4/5 of the fetal head is palpable above the pubic bone and only 1/5 has engaged; 1/5 is therefore more engaged than 2/5 and 0/5 is fully engaged. In some countries engagement is assessed according to 'station' which is determined by vaginal examination (Fig. 2.6). This relates the head of the baby relative to the ischial spines of the woman's pelvis. This is assessed as −1, −2 and so on, i.e. how much the head is presenting below the level of the ischial spines. This is also used in labour itself to determine the further descent of the head which occurs during labour.

If the fetus is breech then the 'presenting part' is the buttocks, knees or feet.

The fetus tends to engage earlier in a primipara as opposed to multipara, probably due to the role of tighter abdominal muscles pushing the fetus down. It is also common for babies of Afro-Caribbean women to not engage before birth due to the differing shape of their pelvis (midwives' clinical observations and Homebirth.org). If the fetus is not engaged with a primapara in the weeks leading to term it may be possible that there is an issue such as cephalopelvic disproportion, low umbilical cord, low lying placenta, or poor fetal positioning such as posterior or transverse, although the last is rare.

During labour itself, the head descends further down into the pelvis and from the level of the ischial

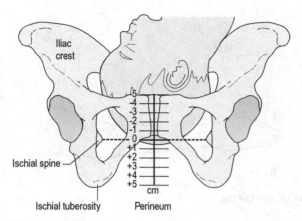

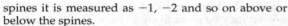

Fig. 2.6 Stations of the head.

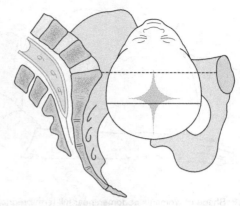

Fig. 2.7 Asynclitic head position.

spines it is measured as −1, −2 and so on above or below the spines.

At the onset of labour many fetal heads are asynclitic (Fig. 2.7). This means that the head is angled so that one parietal bone enters the pelvis first and the fetal biparietal diameter is not parallel to the plane of the inlet of the pelvis. As labour progresses and the head descends deeper into the pelvis it usually assumes the synclitic position.

If the baby's head remains asynclitic, progress of labour can be slowed. In some cases the head becomes arrested with its long axis in the transverse diameter of the pelvis, the degree of extension being such that neither the occiput nor the forehead is sufficiently advanced enough to influence rotation. This is called 'deep transverse arrest'.

Positions of the baby and how these affect labour

See Figure 2.8.

Anterior cephalic position

This is the 'ideal' position which most supports the normal process of labour. The head of the fetus is down, with its spine (and head) away from the woman's spine. The fetus is more often in the LOA position (left occiput anterior), probably due to anatomy (the woman's spleen and stomach are softer than her liver and gallbladder) and the shape of the pelvis. ROA (right occiput anterior) is less common (Henderson & Macdonald 2004).

An anterior position is not only more comfortable for the woman prenatally and in labour, as there is less pressure on her sacrum, but it also facilitates the descent of the head through the pelvis. The pelvic inlet is widest horizontally (side to side), the outlet widest

vertically (top to bottom). The baby's head in an anterior position tends to be more flexed and stimulates the cervix more. It will therefore pass more easily through the birth canal. The cardinal movements of fetal descent are described in the section on the second stage of labour (i.e. internal rotation, extension, restitution, external rotation) (Lewis & Chamberlain 1990).

Posterior presentation

The occiput posterior (OP) position is the opposite presentation to occiput anterior (OA). In this position, the back of the baby's head (occiput) and spine lie against the woman's spine and sacrum. Right occiput posterior (ROP) tends to be more common than left occiput posterior (LOP). It is the most common malposition of the fetus with a vertex presentation. It occurs in about 10–25% of pregnancies during the early stage of labour and in 10–15% during the active phase (Cunningham et al 1997).

Persistent fetal occiput posterior positioning at delivery has been reported in up to 6% of all deliveries (Gardberg & Tuppurainen 1998).

While most OP babies do turn in labour, the fact that they have to make an additional turn means that labour tends to be longer. In this case, the contractions are serving not only to dilate the cervix but also to position the fetus. One of the main issues is that the head tends to be deflexed which means it tends to be pushed downwards and forwards against the back of the symphysis pubis rather than directly downwards onto the cervix. Thus some of the effectiveness of the uterine contractions is lost. Cervical dilatation tends to be slow and labour is prolonged. The cervix may be compressed between the head and the pubis so that progressive oedema of the anterior lip of the cervix occurs, impeding dilatation.

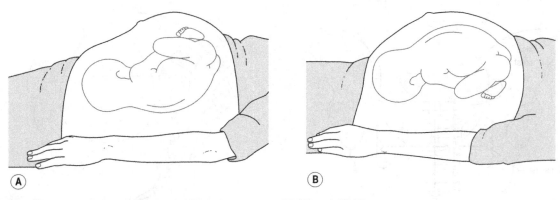

Fig. 2.8 Shape of woman's abdomen near full term pregnancy, OA (A) and OP (B).

A long first stage is likely to be followed by a long second stage because the woman is tired and the uterus may be less capable of continuing its strong contractions. However, if the baby rotates naturally during the course of labour, then second stage may be straightforward. This occurs in about 70% of cases (Clayton et al 1985: 183). In another 10% of cases the occiput undergoes short rotation so that delivery in the 'face to pubes' position can occur. In the remainder of cases assisted rotation will be required. This may be able to be performed manually but vacuum or forceps extraction may be used. If there is an 'arrest' of the labour or if the well-being of the fetus becomes compromised because of prolonged labour with excessive pressure on the head, a caesarean delivery may be carried out.

OP presentation is therefore associated with an increased incidence of prolonged painful labour, operative delivery, postpartum haemorrhage, vaginal trauma, maternal infection, and neonatal morbidity (Fitzpatrick et al 2001, Gardberg & Tuppuainen 1994, Pearl et al 1993, Ponkey et al 2003).

A recent study has also shown a significant association between occiput posterior position during labour and newborn encephalopathy (Badawi et al 1998).

Breech presentation

A baby is in a breech position when its head is superior to the lower half of its body, i.e. the buttocks or legs are down in the pelvis. The incidence of breech presentation at the time of delivery is 3–4% and spontaneous version occurred in 57% of pregnancies after 32 weeks and 25% after 36 weeks (Westgren et al 1985).

The cause of a persistent breech position may be due to uterine abnormalities (such as bicornuate uterus), oligohydramnios (low levels of amniotic fluid which may restrict the movement of the fetus), or polyhydramnios (Kean et al 1999). A bicornuate uterus or uterine septum may be associated with other issues such as low lying placenta, fibroids, contracted pelvis, fetal abnormalities or multiple pregnancy.

It has also been proposed that anxious and fearful women may be more likely to have a breech presentation (Founds 2007, Lowden 1998) and the principal author had found some evidence of this as a factor in her work. A study researching the impact of moxibustion for promoting cephalic version from breech positioning made reference to the emotional factors affecting women whose babies were in a breech position. The current pressure to have a caesarean section may cause increased anxiety and stress for the woman (Allen & Mitchell 2008).

There are different types of breech position (Fig. 2.9):

- *Complete breech*: buttocks and knees at cervix. This type is most common in multigravidae.
- *Frank or extended breech*: buttocks down at cervix but the legs are extended. This is the most common and frequent breech position in primigravidae. Their firmer uterine and abdominal muscles make it harder for the fetus to move.
- *Footling breech*: one or both feet are below the buttocks with hips and knees extended. This is quite rare.
- *Knee presentation*: one or both knees present below the buttocks with one or both hips extended and knees flexed. This is the least common breech position.

Risks of breech delivery There is an increased incidence at delivery of morbidity and mortality for both the mother and the baby when a breech presentation occurs (Cheng & Hannah 1993, Hofmeyr 1991). Some of this risk may be associated with the reasons associated with why the fetus is presenting in the breech position as listed previously, for example if a fetal abnormality exists. A frank breech with no other complications is the breech presentation which has the fewest issues for a potential vaginal delivery.

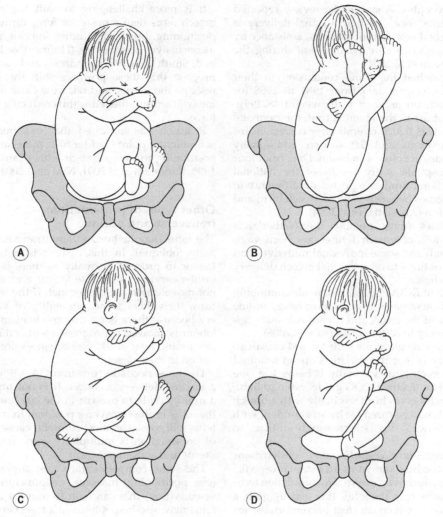

Fig. 2.9 Breech positions.

The main issue in breech deliveries is that as the larger head and shoulders are born after the buttocks, the head may get stuck in the pelvis. Other issues are that the fetus may inhale amniotic fluid as the sac may rupture with the delivery of the buttocks, or that the cord may be compressed, compromising oxygen to the fetus.

As well, especially with a complete or footling breech, there is a higher risk of cord prolapse. This is when the cord slips in between the fetus and the cervix if the amniotic sac breaks in a gush. This is a rare occurrence, but is a medical emergency. The woman would need to call an ambulance or go to the hospital immediately in a knee to chest position in order to minimise the risk of cord occlusion and hypoxia. The fetus would need to be delivered by caesarean section.

Until 2000, many caregivers attempted to deliver breech babies vaginally when possible. However the Term Breech Trial concluded that delivery by planned caesarean was safer for the fetus than planned vaginal delivery, and this resulted in a change in the recommended guidelines for breech deliveries (Hannah et al 2000).

Most countries now have a policy on elective caesarean section for breech. In the UK, 18% of all caesarean sections are carried out for breech (RCOG 2006). The effect of this policy change has been to markedly increase the caesarean section rate. This worldwide shift has not been without controversy, as some additional studies contradict the findings of the Hannah study (Hannah et al 2000). The issues involved in safe delivery are complex. A systematic review reported that most studies conclude that 'vaginal delivery is safe, given a good selection of patients, assistance by qualified staff, and careful management during the delivery' (Haheim et al 2004).

Reviewers reached the same conclusion in their analysis of Norwegian data from 1981 to 1998 for singleton breech births with birth weight >2499 g. In marked contrast to the Hannah trial, the perinatal mortality rate was 0.31% overall after correction for lethal malformations and 0.09% after additionally correcting for death before admission. Data from four Norwegian hospitals verify results of the national data analysis. Some studies reported no difference in perinatal outcomes between vaginal breech birth and caesarean section (Abasiattai et al 2004).

Some countries (most notably the Netherlands where about 40% of breech fetuses are born vaginally in hospital) and some individual midwives and obstetricians continue to offer vaginal breech delivery as a potential choice.

The most recent RCOG guidelines, while continuing to recommend caesarean section in most cases, outline the complexity of the issue, and do not rule out vaginal breech delivery in certain cases (RCOG 2006).

An unfortunate result of the shift toward caesarean section delivery is that the specific skill set required to deliver a breech fetus vaginally is being lost due to lack of practice. As the RCOG guidelines highlight, 'Any woman who gives birth vaginally with a breech presentation should be cared for by an attendant with suitable experience'. This is increasingly difficult to access.

Turning a breech into cephalic Some obstetricians carry out a procedure known as an external cephalic version (ECV), which is an external manipulation technique to manually turn the fetus. It is usually quite a physical technique which can feel uncomfortable for the woman and is carried out in conjunction with ultrasound to determine the location of the placenta. It is successful in 30–80% of cases. A systematic review of ECV suggests that ECV reduces the incidence of breech presentation at term by 60% (Hofmeyr & Kulier 2001a). Success rates range from 35% to 57% in primigravidas and 52% to 84% in multigravidas, although in 10–15% of cases the fetus returns to its former breech positioning (Lau et al 1997).

Research indicates that it is worth trying ECV and the RCOG guidelines (2006) recommend that all women with an uncomplicated breech pregnancy should be offered ECV at 36–37 weeks gestation to reduce their risk of caesarean section. There is an ongoing trial in Canada to determine when this is best performed (ECV2, results due 2009).

It is more challenging to shift the position of a breech fetus than a posterior fetus through maternal positioning, but some studies indicate promising, if inconclusive, possibilities (Hofmeyr & Kulier 2000a, b, d, Smith et al 1999). Andrews and Andrews (1983) propose that these postures shift the fetal weight, reshape the uterus, and relax the close fit of the uterine wall around the fetus, thus reducing the frictional force.

Research has indicated that moxibustion on the acupuncture point Bladder 67 is more successful than positioning to turn a breech fetus (Cardini & Weixin 1998, Kanakura et al 2001, Neri et al 2004).

Other types of presentation: transverse and oblique

The fetus may lie horizontally (transverse) or diagonally (oblique). In this case, it is not possible for labour to proceed normally as there is no pressure on the cervix to stimulate labour and the fetus cannot move down the birth canal. If the fetus does not turn, then there is no possibility of vaginal delivery because there is no true mechanism of labour. If labour is allowed to progress it will end in obstructed labour and fetal death. Caesarean section is the safest option in these cases.

The fetus needs to turn into OA, OP or breech for a vaginal delivery to occur. It is not uncommon for a multigravida to present in the last few weeks with the fetus in the transverse position. In most cases the fetus will turn. The most common cause for this type of presentation is multiparity associated with a lax uterus and abdominal wall.

The same complementary care support strategies (e.g. positioning, massage, acupuncture points and visualisation) that can help to move a breech or OP fetus may also help a fetus in a transverse or oblique position to turn.

A transverse or oblique lie may also be found with polyhydramnios or multiple pregnancy, or anything which interferes with the engagement of the fetal head such as a contracted pelvis, placenta praevia, a pelvic tumour or fibroids, or malformation of the uterus. In these cases it is not advisable to attempt to change fetal positioning.

Unstable lie Sometimes fetuses change their position frequently. This may be associated with polyhydramnios, placenta praevia, or a pelvic tumour, but is often due to lax abdominal muscles. Usually these fetuses will turn into a favourable position for birth.

Twins The position of the first twin is most important as this twin is usually bigger.

Implications of fetal position for bodyworkers

- If possible, the bodyworker should learn the fetal position, either from talking with their client or from the information provided to the pregnant woman from her primary caregiver.
- The therapist should learn strategies to support optimal fetal positioning.
- The bodyworker needs to understand the potential medical reasons why the fetus may not change position.
- The bodyworker needs to understand that one potential factor in fetal positioning is the effect of bone or soft tissue issues, such as tight ligaments or misalignment of the sacrum or pelvis. Relaxation of soft tissue hypertonicity and/or correct pelvic alignment may help in these situations.
- Given that a diagnosis of 'malpresentation' will impact on the woman's preparation for labour, the means of delivery used and her emotional state, the bodyworker can provide emotional support and techniques that helps her connect with her baby.

2.4 Maternal position

Optimal fetal positioning antenatally and the position of the woman in labour

The use of a stationary labour position in bed is said to have been initially introduced because King Louis XIV of France wanted to witness the birth of his son. While this may or may not be true, the aristocracy of France started to use the lying down position during birth, and it was considered 'undignified' and 'primitive' to use the commonly used birthing positions of squatting, standing or leaning forwards.

In birth, upright positioning allows more movement of the joints of the pelvis, giving more space for the fetus to move down the birth canal, and allows the effect of gravity to help facilitate fetal descent. Although the use of the supine or semi-reclining position tended to slow labour down, it became popular historically as barber/surgeons started taking over the role of delivery to the aristocracy. Supine positioning became an easier way to facilitate increasingly instrumental delivery.

A recent review by the Cochrane Database related to positioning during labour showed that the use of supine positioning during the first stage of labour compromised effective uterine activity, prolonged labour and increased the use of drugs to augment labour (Roberts 1989).

The dorsal and supine positions have been associated with adverse effects on maternal haemodynamics and fetal status including supine hypotensive syndrome. They also make it more difficult for the engagement and descent of the fetal head (Roberts 1980). The review showed that in the second stage of labour any upright or lateral position compared to supine or lithotomy (lying back with legs apart) positioning decreased the length of the second stage, reduced the need for forceps or episiotomy, and decreased severe pain and abnormal fetal heart rate. However, it also concluded that upright positions increased the risk of blood loss (especially with chairs and stools) and increased the risk of perineal tears (Crowley et al 1991, Gupta & Nikodem 2000). The authors have noted in their work that in order to reduce tears and blood loss, it is important that the woman is relaxed in the upright position and therefore is not straining into the perineum.

Upright positioning has been associated with a significantly increased number of spontaneous uterine contractions, as well as being associated with the release of the blocked venous return flow, and restoration of normal maternal haemodynamics (Schneider et al 1993).

Positioning which supports the 'physiological' process of labour

One of the main reasons given for the use of medical intervention is 'dystocia' or dysfunctional labour. The main causes are due to the size and shape of the uterus, and the size, position and presentation of the fetus.

Simkin and Ancheta (2000) outline strategies to reduce interventions which are primarily based on utilising maternal positioning and comfort measures. Positions which support the physiological process of labour utilise the following elements:

1. Optimal use of gravity.
2. Forward leaning postures.
3. Movement of the pelvis, especially of the sacrum and coccyx.

The main positions which support these aspects of effective labouring are:

- Standing: rocking, leaning against something.
- Squatting: full squat, supported squat or standing squat.
- Forward leaning – for example over a ball.
- Forward sitting.
- Lateral or side-lying positioning.

The goal of utilising these positions during labour is to encourage comfort and relaxation for the mother, to allow the fetus to have more space to move into the best position in the pelvis at different times in labour, and to allow labour to progress (Simkin & Ancheta 2000).

The lateral recumbent position is a good resting position as it reduces pressure on the maternal blood vessels and promotes venous return and cardiac output. It can be used with an OP fetus as an alternative position to all fours.

Squatting enhances engagement and descent of the fetal head and increases maternal pelvic diameters. The pelvic outlet increases by 28% with increased transverse (1 cm) and anteroposterior (0.5–2 cm) diameters.

Women who suffer from pelvic girdle dysfunction (PGD) with symphysis pubis diastasis (SPD) need to be careful regarding their choice of labouring position, so that they do not aggravate their instability. Since they need to minimise abduction and other leg movements, the all-fours birthing position may be best. Women with sacroiliac (SI) joint issues also need to avoid excessive strain and movement of the hips/pelvis. Choosing non-injuring positions may be challenging as it can be difficult to determine if discomfort is related to the position of the fetus, the birthing process or the patient's musculoskeletal condition.

Some midwives have identified another reason why supine and semi-recumbent positions are less effective labouring positions, especially during the second stage of labour. They suggest that a key role is played by the rhombus of Michaelis, an area in the lower back. This wedge-shaped area, which includes the lower three lumbar vertebrae, the sacrum and iliolumbar ligament, moves backwards during the second stage of labour. As it moves back it pushes the wings of the ilea out, increasing the diameter of the pelvis. The woman's response to this destabilisation of the pelvis is to arch her back and push her buttocks out, raise her arms up, reaching for something to hold on to, and extend her head backwards (Sutton & Scott 1996).

This phenomenon is what Sheila Kitzinger was describing when she recorded Jamaican midwives saying that the fetus will not be born 'till the woman opens her back' (Kitzinger 2000). Supine or semi-recumbent positions hinder this sacral movement because the maternal weight is resting on the sacrum (Burnett 1969, Sutton & Scott 1996).

The most important factor, however, is that the woman finds her own preferred positions. This tends to happen instinctively if the woman is in an environment which supports her own natural physical and emotional responses. It is helpful if the woman is able to practise a variety of positions in advance. Some women find they favour one position the most. Others find they need to change position more frequently. Changing position during labour tends to be effective because it encourages the fetus to move and so it is wise to encourage women to try a variety of positions.

Prenatal maternal positioning to support optimal fetal positioning

Puddicombe first introduced the maternal hands and knees exercise as a way of facilitating fetal rotation antenatally (Puddicombe 1955). Other authors have subsequently advocated its use both antenatally and in labour (Andrews 1981, Andrews & Andrews 1983, Biancuzzo 1991, Sutton & Scott 1996, Hofmeyr & Kulier 2000b).

Some of these authors suggest that there is a greater incidence of malpositioned fetuses due to increasingly sedentary lifestyles, although there is no statistical evidence to prove this. It is true that modern women are sitting at desks and driving cars, unlike their ancestors who would tend to be engaged in more physical activities. In sedentary positions, the bones of the pelvis are more compressed than when forward leaning or moving around, and the fetal spine is pushed against the sacrum. Further, with reclining positions the angle between the maternal spine and the pelvic brim is reduced, thus reducing space in the pelvis. Static reclining positions also tend to reduce maternal circulation and discourage fetal alteration of position. Long car journeys in particular seem to encourage the fetus to move into the OP position (Fig. 2.10A). Forward leaning and upright positions allow the bones of the pelvis to shift and move, take the weight of the fetus away from the sacrum, increase the angle between the pelvic brim and maternal spine, help utilise the supporting effects of gravity and increase space in the uterus (Fig. 2.10B). Due to these effects they tend to relieve sacral back ache and pelvic congestion. It is important to recognise that continued mobilisation and forward leaning positioning is needed during labour to keep this opening of the pelvis, not only for maternal comfort but to continue to encourage optimal fetal movement. Posteriorly positioned fetuses can turn right up to term, and even during labour itself.

A recent study was not able to prove that kneeling was an effective intervention for reducing the incidence of OP positioning in labour. However, clearly there are factors other than just maternal positioning involved in a fetus who is malpositioned and more studies are needed in this area (Kariminia et al 2004).

The fetus may present in the posterior position due to reasons such as the position of the placental site and pelvic shape, or existing fibroids. It is important to recognise that while maternal positioning can encourage good fetal positioning, it does not guarantee it.

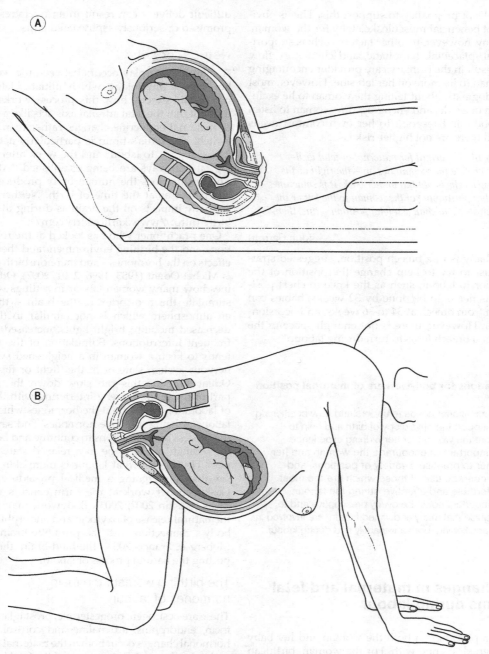

Fig. 2.10 (A) Fetus rotating to OP. (B) Fetus in OA. If the woman leans forward the fetus's back moves away from her back.

The course of labour should not be pre-judged, setting the woman up to 'fail' if the fetus is OP at the onset of labour. In many cases, vaginal delivery is still possible.

Some practitioners believe that lying more on the left side will tend to encourage LOA positioning. Some antenatal educators have argued that the woman should lie exclusively on her left side during the last few weeks of pregnancy to support this. This is obviously not beneficial musculoskeletally for the woman. There may, however, be other factors such as supporting renal, placental, lymphatic, and circulatory flow which result in the primary care provider encouraging the woman to lie more on her left side. However, most are not dogmatic about telling the woman to lie exclusively on one side, and encourage the woman to listen to her body and respond to her own comfort needs provided there are not higher-risk issues.

It is not really important for maternal or fetal well-being, which side the woman lies on – the right or the left, as long as she is not flat on her back. It is sometimes thought that positioning of the woman to the left or the right is advisable to change a fetal position – this, then, is acceptable.

(Jon Barrett)

If the baby is in a breech position, suggested strategies exist to try to help change the position of the baby prior to labour, such as the knee to chest position. This needs to be done by 32 weeks; babies can still turn from breech at 34 to 36 weeks, and occasionally later. However, there is not enough space in the pelvis for a breech fetus to turn during labour.

Implications for bodyworkers of maternal position

- The practitioner needs to understand how positioning can support the physiology of birth and help to prepare the woman for her birthing experience.
- It is important to encourage the woman and her partner to practise a variety of positions, and to encourage use of those which are the most comfortable and effective during the labour.
- It is important not to be overly prescriptive and to recognise that many and varied factors are involved in fetal positioning, both antenatally and during labour.

2.5 Changes in maternal and fetal systems during labour

Birth is a process that both the woman and her baby are designed to cope with. For the woman, birth can be both exhilarating and exhausting, and for the fetus, birth can be a stressful process. Both fetus and neonate can tolerate degrees of hypoxia (insufficient levels of O_2 in blood or tissue) and anoxia (reduced supply of O_2 in inspired gases, arterial blood or tissue) that would result in serious morbidity or mortality in an adult. However, it is a fine balance: prolonged or

difficult delivery can result in an overstressed, compromised or seriously asphyxiated fetus.

Neuroendocrine

A complex interplay occurs between the woman and her baby's physiology which initiates labour. It is not certain exactly how this process works, but it is thought that the fetal adrenal axis acts like a fine-tuner of maternal endocrine changes rather than an on–off switch. The fetus's brain is particularly active in the 2 weeks prior to labour and the week after as neurological pathways are being established. 'At no other time in life does the human body produce as much adrenaline as at the time of birth. Neither are there so many impacts on the brain as during the hours of birth' (http://www.karltonterry.com/).

One practitioner who has looked at the role of emotions and the birthing environment and their possible effects on the hormones – and therefore birth outcome – is Michel Odent (1983, 1996, 2001, 2007). Odent examines how many women labour in settings which may stimulate the neo-cortex of the brain – they are in an atmosphere which is not familiar to them, with decreased mobility, bright lights, increased noise and frequent interruptions. Stimulation of the neo-cortex tends to keep a woman in a heightened sympathetic nervous system state or in the 'fight or flight mode'. Odent suggests this can slow down the instinctive part of the brain, thereby interfering with the process of labour. He talks about the hormones which support labour as being 'the love hormones' and says that for the process of contractions to continue and be effective, the woman needs to be in a relaxed state of awareness. He suggests that labour is more akin to having sex than undergoing a medical procedure. Ina May Gaskin in her work at the Farm concurs with these ideas (Gaskin 2002, 2003). Bodywork may encourage the natural release of oxytocin and endorphins and the body's connection with the primitive brain (Unvnas-Moberg & Francis 2003), the hind-brain, thereby supporting the natural process of labour.

The birthing woman: the main hormones of labour

These are oestrogen, progesterone, prostaglandins, oxytocin, endorphins, adrenaline and cortisol. Complex hormonal changes occur both in the maternal neo-cortex and in local tissue. The pressure of the fetal head on the cervix releases prostaglandins and in turn stimulates the maternal neo-cortex.

Progesterone

Progesterone plays a major role in controlling the uterus and cervix and suppressing uterine contractions. There is not a significant fall in maternal serum progesterone but rather it is an increase in placental oestrogen which shifts the ratio so that in relation to oestrogen, there is proportionately less progesterone.

Oestrogen

Oestrogen levels start to rise from 34–35 weeks. This promotes the formation of gap junctions, increases oxytocin and oestrogen receptors in the myometrium, and stimulates prostaglandin production (by enhancing lipase activity and release of arachidonic acid). Together oestrogen and progesterone also activate opiate pain-killing pathways in the brain and spinal cord in preparation for labour (Russell et al 2001).

The two main types of hormones which stimulate the contractions of labour are oxytocin and prostaglandins.

Oxytocin

The role of oxytocin as a hormone has become understood relatively recently. It used to be thought of only in its role as the main hormone of childbirth and breastfeeding, but it is present at other times as well. It is considered to be a 'feel good' hormone – similar to endorphins. It is released through touch and other forms of nurturing contact and relaxation and not simply through breastfeeding. It has been called the hormone of love because of its connection with sexual activity and orgasm as well as with birth and breastfeeding. It is produced in social situations such as sharing a meal (Verbalis et al 1986).

Central stores of oxytocin are augmented in preparation for labour and breastfeeding. Oxytocin (OT) is produced by the posterior pituitary gland of both the woman and fetus as well as the myometrium, decidua, placenta and fetal membranes.

OT receptors in the uterus (myometrium) have increased by 300-fold at term (Zeeman et al 1997). OT stimulates the uterus to strengthen the strong, muscular labour contractions and is regulated by a positive feedback loop – once they have begun, uterine contractions push on receptors in the pelvis, which triggers the release of more OT, which pushes on the pelvic receptors, which stimulates more contractions, and so on. During the final uterine contractions there is a surge of oxytocin known as the Ferguson reflex (Dawood et al 1978).

After the birth of the baby, the contractions continue to some degree and help the uterus first to expel the placenta and then to return to its unstretched shape. High levels of oxytocin after birth, augmented by physical contact between mother and newborn, help to continue to contract the uterus and reduce the risk of haemorrhage. Oxytocin is likely to play a key role in supporting the bonding between mother and newborn.

The 'after birth' contractions (also known as 'after pains') are stimulated by breastfeeding as OT causes milk ejection from the breasts of lactating women. Milk cannot be removed by suckling until it has first been ejected into the ducts. Newborn suckling, mechanically and psychologically, increases OT levels which provides more milk. The action of the baby continuing to suckle further increases OT levels.

Some women in the first few days after delivery experience fairly strong after birth contractions (after pains), which are usually intensified with subsequent labours, and can increase if artificial hormones have been given to augment or induce labour.

If a woman is induced with an intravenous infusion it is artificial oxytocin which is used, Syntocinon (a synthetic oxytocin). These levels are much higher than those produced naturally by a woman in labour and are not received in the same pulsatile manner as naturally produced oxytocin. Similar synthetic preparations of oxytocin are given to augment labour if contractions slow down during labour. Failed induction and postdate pregnancies are associated with a decreased concentration of oxytocin receptors (Coad & Dunstall 2005: 291). Synthetic oxytocin does not work well as a labour stimulant before term, possibly due to the lack of adequate OT receptors.

The type of contraction initiated by the use of Syntocinon tends to differ from physiological contractions. Women may not experience a gradual build up of intensity, and they may experience discomfort as one long, continuous contraction with few breaks between them. This can make them harder to cope with. It is crucial that a minimal dose of oxytocin is given with a gradual increase in dosage in order to avoid the serious complication of excessive uterine contractions.

Prostaglandins

Prostaglandin F stimulates contractions. Prostaglandins are tissue hormones – they are produced in the tissue and diffuse only a short way to other cells in the same tissue. The first prostaglandin to be discovered was in semen, hence it gets its name from the prostate gland. It is in fact the seminal vesicles and not the prostate which secrete the prostaglandin. Prostaglandin in labour is produced by the pressure of the fetal head on the cervix which sends the message to the pituitary to release more OT. As the uterus contracts more, it releases more prostaglandins, which send the message to release more OT – another positive feedback mechanism.

Artificial prostaglandins are given in pessaries to stimulate contractions. These are prostaglandins E (PGE). The prostaglandins serve to soften and efface the cervix, which can be enough to trigger the onset of birth. If labour does not begin, then prostaglandin induction increases the chance of a successful induction of labour with oxytocin. It may be a less intense way of initiating labour than with an infusion of oxytocin, although some women do experience strong reactions and pain from PGEs. Women are sometimes advised to have sex as a way of introducing natural prostaglandins through semen, but the amount in semen is much less than is needed to stimulate labour. However, having an orgasm will produce oxytocin in women, and sometimes the combination of semen and an orgasm may help to trigger labour.

Endorphins and catecholamines (adrenaline and noradrenaline)

Endorphins are closely linked with the release of oxytocin. They are also 'feel good' hormones, released when we are feeling relaxed. They help women cope with pain in labour, acting as natural painkillers. Beta endorphin levels increase during labour allowing a labouring woman to transcend pain (Brinsmead et al 1985).

The hormones with the opposite effect are the catecholamines which include adrenaline, noradrenaline, cortisol and others. Adrenaline is released in stressful situations (the fight or flight hormones) and in Chinese medicine are linked with the Kidneys. Adrenaline levels are more responsive to psychological stresses such as pain and anxiety. High adrenaline in early labour can both slow down the process of labour and make it more painful as it works against the release of both endorphins and oxytocin. In most of the first stage of labour, high levels of circulating catecholamines cause maternal blood to be shunted away from the uterus and placenta which will slow uterine contractions (Lederman 1981b), and decrease the availability of blood to the fetus (Lederman 1981b). This explains the mechanism by which a woman in early labour, if feeling under threat, may stop labouring. However, catecholamine levels rise during a normal labour with noradrenaline increasing in response to the physiological work and during second stage there is a sudden increase in noradrenaline which activates the fetal ejection reflex. The woman experiences a surge of energy, is upright and alert, and strong contractions are initiated which will birth the baby quickly (Odent 1992).

The above helps explain why a woman's ability to cope with pain and her emotional state may affect the progress of her labour. Relaxation may therefore also affect labour by potentially reducing stress and physical tiredness, with an impact on hormonal activity. Further, if there is less stress and tension in the body, the woman will be more able to sustain supportive birthing positions.

Cortisol
This stimulates PG (prostaglandin) synthesis.

Hormonal changes in the fetus
The fetus responds to the stimuli of labour by showing a rise in catecholamine output from the adrenal medulla and from extramedullary cells – the adrenal hormones of dopamine, adrenaline and noradrenaline. Umbilical arterial concentrations are four times higher in vaginally delivered fetuses than those delivered by caesarean. These hormones stimulate the sympathetic nervous system and the subsequent mobilisation of glycogen and lipid stores helps to activate essential physiological mechanisms. They provide a variety of cardiorespiratory and metabolic adaptations during and after labour which result in an alert and active fetus at birth (Sweet 1997).

Corticotropin-releasing hormone (CRH), glucocorticoids (cortisol), and dehydroepiandrosterone (DHEAS)
Dehydroepiandrosterone (DHEAS) DHEAS is needed by the placenta to produce oestrogens, particularly estriol.
Cortisol Cortisol stimulates fetal lung maturation and placental CRH. This is in contrast to the effect of increased cortisol on the hypothalamus where it has an inhibitory effect. In the placenta, glucocorticoids stimulate CRH receptors and increase CRH production.
Corticotropin-releasing hormone (CRH) Placental levels increase by up to 50–100-fold in the last 6–8 weeks of gestation, paralleling the rise in fetal cortisol (Majzoub & Karalis 1999). CHR receptors are found on myometrium and it is thought that stimulation of these receptors may enhance myometrial contractility. CRH is thought to stimulate fetal ACTH which stimulates the fetal adrenal cortex to produce glucocorticosteroids such as cortisol and DHEAS.

Oxytocin
The fetus also releases large amounts of oxytocin from the pituitary during labour and there is some evidence that this may be transported back through the placenta into maternal circulation (Fuchs & Fuchs 1984), leading some researchers to hypothesise that fetal oxytocin may stimulate the uterus (Chard 1989).

Beta endorphins
The fetus secretes endorphins from the pituitary (Facchinetti et al 1989) and levels in the placenta at birth are higher than in maternal blood. This has led some researchers to speculate that early cord cutting may 'deprive mothers and infants of placental opioid molecules designed to induce interdependency of mothers and infants' (Kimball 1979).

Implications of hormonal changes in labour for bodyworkers

The therapist needs to be aware of the complex nature of hormonal changes for both the woman and the fetus, and note the potential importance of the fact that relaxation for the woman will not only probably help her during the birthing process but may also give support to the fetus. Stress and cerebral stimulation may interfere with this complex interplay.

Haematologic and haemostatic

Maternal changes

Circulatory changes prepare the woman to tolerate normal blood loss at delivery and prevent significant bleeding when the placenta separates. The amount of blood loss averages up to 500 ml for a vaginal delivery or 1000 ml with a caesarean section or with a vaginal twin delivery (Bassell & Marx 1981, Bonnar 2000). About half the RBC volume acquired in pregnancy is lost during delivery and in lochia over the first few postpartum days (Pritchard 1965). Haemoglobin levels tend to increase slightly during labour. The WBC count increases, which can complicate diagnosis of infection.

Haemostasis

Both the deciduas and the placenta are rich in thromboplastin and exposure or release of this during placental separation will activate coagulation.

Concentrations of clotting factors increase during labour. PT (prothrombin) shortens significantly, especially during the third stage with clotting at the placental site. Levels of fibrinogen and plasminogen may decrease as a result of increased utilisation after placental separation.

Fibrinolytic activity decreases during labour, enhancing the formation of clots at the placental site following separation. This promotes development of a haemostatic endometrial fibrin mesh over the wound. About 5–10% of total body fibrin is deposited at this site.

Levels of fibrin–fibrinogen degradation products (FDP) increase after delivery. This increases the risk of coagulation disorders in the immediate postpartum period by interfering with the formation of firm fibrin clots. The number of platelets falls about 20% with separation due to clotting at the placental site.

The hypercoagulable state of pregnancy is magnified during the intrapartum period. This protects the woman from haemorrhage and excessive blood loss at delivery by providing for rapid haemostasis following removal of the placenta. However, it also means that the risk of deep vein thrombosis (DVT) is at its highest during the immediate postnatal period. Postnatal DVT risk factors are: caesarean section, pre-eclampsia, assisted reproduction, abruptio placenta, and placenta praevia.

Cardiovascular

Cardiac output

There is a progressive rise in cardiac output in the first stage of labour. It rises even more in the second stage, and peaks following delivery (Manga 1999, Roberts 1989). This can be attributed to haemodynamic changes during a contraction but can also be attributed to a rise in stress. Supine positioning results in lower cardiac output, increased heart rate, and decreased stroke volume (Manga 1999, Roberts 1989, Ueland & Hanson 1969, Ueland & Metcalfe 1975).

Fetal changes

Fetal heart There is a slowing of the fetal heart rate during contractions, called deceleration, but this does not appear to affect umbilical circulation. The fetus can cope with dips in the heart rate and is quite resilient during uterine contractions. In some cases, however, it can go into 'compromise' (the term 'distress' tends to be less in use currently). This could occur in a prolonged labour, or if the cord is wrapped round its neck. There is more concern for the fetus if its heart rate does not react to contractions. A healthy sign during labour is a fluctuating fetal heart rate (FHR) that reacts to each contraction and returns to a normal rate between contractions. The deceleration has a uniform shape, with a slow onset that coincides with the start of the contraction and a slow return to the baseline that coincides with the end of the contraction. The normal FHR range is between 120 and 160 beats per minute (bpm). The woman should be moved into an upright position if the FHR is nonreactive to her contractions, as position changes can affect FHR reactivity. Medical interventions will be considered if the FHR becomes 'non-reassuring'.

Changes in cardiovascular system: implications for bodyworkers

- During labour, the main issue for the bodyworker is how maternal position affects cardiac output and this underscores the need to support the woman in upright positions.
- Therapists need to be aware of the increased risk of deep vein thrombosis (DVT) in the immediate postnatal period.

Musculoskeletal

Maternal

There are many changes in this system which has to allow the descent and delivery of the fetus. The uterus is a strong and powerful muscle. There are changes in the perineum and musculature of the pelvis, and the bones of the pelvis move during labour.

Importance of the pelvis in labour

Different types of pelvis The size of the pelvis is an important factor – if it is large enough then the fetus will pass through readily. The shape is more important if the pelvis is small in comparison to the fetal head. A diagnosis of cephalic pelvic disproportion (CPD) may be made, which means the pelvis is too small in relation to the head of the baby, but this is a subjective diagnosis which is commonly made for labours that do not fit the expectations of the care provider.

There are no agreed measurements, and it is generally concluded that even in situations of anticipated cephalopelvic disproportion (CPD) it is better to allow women to labour as in many cases normal delivery is possible (Ikhena et al 1999, Pattinson 2003, RCOG 2001b). The evaluation of the progress of labour is considered to be a more accurate indicator of cephalopelvic disproportion (Chhabra et al 2000).

In labour it is the 'true pelvis' (i.e. the lower part) which is the most important factor.

Landmarks of the pelvis (Fig. 2.11)

The brim or inlet The fetus has to descend here. It is almost round and its boundaries are:

- Promontory of the sacrum.
- Wings or alae of the sacrum.
- Right and left sacroiliac joints.
- Right and left iliopectineal lines.
- Right and left iliopectineal eminences.
- Upper inner borders of the superior pubic rami.
- Upper inner borders of the bodies of the pubes.
- Upper inner border of the symphysis pubis.

Pelvic cavity This extends from the brim to the outlet. It is shallow at the front and deeper at the back. It is circular and its anterior wall is 4.5 cm deep whereas the posterior wall is 12 cm. The fetus needs to move down through here in a curved path.

Its boundaries are:

- Hollow of the sacrum.
- Sacroiliac joints.
- Ischia and sacrospinous ligaments.
- Right and left upper and lower pubic rami.
- Bodies of the pubes and symphysis pubis.

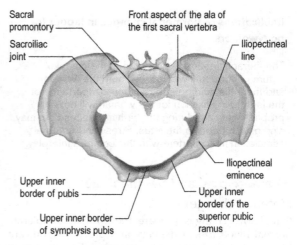

Fig. 2.11 Diagram of the pelvis.

Pelvic outlet This is ovoid or even diamond shaped and is partly bounded by the ligaments (sacrospinous and sacrotuberous). It is the lowest part of the pelvis and is divided into two levels: the upper and lower outlet. When it descends here, the fetus is constricted by bone on all sides. The coccyx extends lower than the lower outlet and has to move back during labour. The tuberosities are lower than the spines and slightly wider apart. Once the fetus has passed through the outlet it has no difficulty in emerging.

Borders of the outlet:

Upper outlet:

- Lower sacrum.
- Sacrospinous ligaments and ischial spines.
- Pubic arch.

Lower outlet:

- Tip of the coccyx.
- Sacrotuberous ligaments and ischial tuberosities.
- Pubic arch.

There are various diameters which can be measured.

Axis of the birth canal (Figs. 2.12, 2.13) The brim or inlet, the cavity and the outlet each slope at different axes. During labour, the fetus has to follow the axis of each plane. It descends in a straight line through the level of the pelvic brim and the plane of the cavity until it reaches the level of the ischial spines. At this point it is deflected by the pelvic floor and its pathway changes from downwards and backwards to downwards and forwards. The fetus essentially makes a curving movement through the pelvis.

Each of these three planes has different angles (see Fig. 2.13). When a woman stands, the pelvis slopes

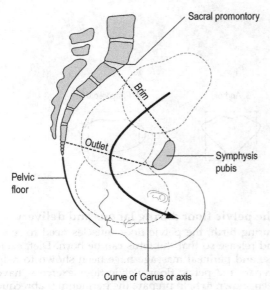

Fig. 2.12 Axis of the birth canal in the upright position.

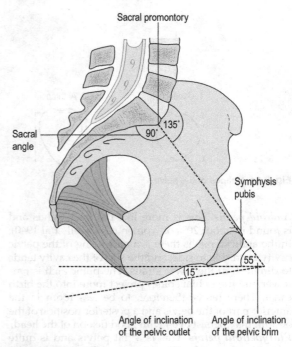

Fig. 2.13 Angles of the pelvis.

steeply. The anterior superior iliac spines are in the same plane as the symphysis pubis. The plane of the pelvic brim is 55° to horizontal. The plane of the cavity is the mid-point of the sacrum and pubis, and the plane of the outlet is at an angle of 15° and is almost horizontal.

The angle of the pelvis changes according to the position of the woman, and due to the more mobile joints and ligaments, the bones can move. Women can be encouraged to feel this. The supine position reduces the angle of the pelvic outlet as well as restricting the mobility of the bones. Squatting increases the angle of the pelvic outlet and along with small rhythmical movements commonly made by birthing women, helps increase the mobility of the pelvis (Woolley & Roberts 1996).

The shape of the pelvis (Fig. 2.14) Each woman's pelvis is slightly differently shaped and there are variations between different population groups. This can create variations in how women labour. However, more influential than genetic or hormonal factors in determining the shape of the pelvis is the role of long-term nutrition. This is not a significant factor in western culture but for therapists working in developing countries it may be. Women with a flatter pelvis (more challenging for childbearing) were of smaller stature and had a reduced intake of calcium, vitamin D, and protein during childhood. In the late 19th century and early 20th century the incidence of pelvic contraction, largely due to rickets and untreated infection in childhood and adolescence, was high. Sadly today this is still the case in many developing countries (Kwast 1992) and is one of the main reasons for difficulty during labour, contributing to the high rate of maternal and fetal mortality and morbidity in these countries.

The female pelvis is different from the male pelvis. The most common female pelvis (Caldwell et al 1940), found in over 50% of women, is known as the *gynaecoid pelvis*.

Gynaecoid pelvis The brim is round, the pelvis is shallow, the subpubic angle is wide (90° or more), the sacrosciatic notch is wide, and the transverse diameter of the outlet is 10 cm at least.

Anthropoid pelvis This shape is more like an ape's pelvis. It is found in about 25% of women (Caldwell et al 1940) and noted in unusually tall and well-built women. The brim is oval with an increase in the anteroposterior diameter and a decrease in the transverse diameter. The sacrum is long and narrow and may contain six vertebrae from the fusion of the fifth lumbar vertebra with the sacrum. This increases the inclination of the pelvic brim and is called high assimilation. It tends to hinder engagement of the fetal head.

During labour the head may engage in the anteroposterior diameter, sometimes with the occiput posterior. The head may descend through the pelvis in a persistently occiput posterior position and be born face to pubes. However, generally this pelvis is so large that labour tends to be straightforward.

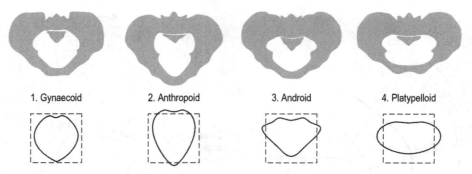

1. Gynaecoid   2. Anthropoid   3. Android   4. Platypelloid

Fig. 2.14 Shapes of the pelvis.

Android pelvis This is more like the male pelvis and is found in about 20% of women (Caldwell et al 1940). In the android pelvis there is a narrowing of the pelvic cavity from side to side, and the size of the cavity tends to diminish in the lower straits. The pubic arch is narrower and the ischial spines project more into the birth canal. There tends, therefore, to be less room in the anterior part of the pelvis and a posterior position of the occiput may persist even with good flexion of the head.

Platypelloid pelvis This is a flat pelvis and is quite rare, found in only 5% of women. The anteroposterior diameter is short, the sciatic notch is narrow, and the anterio-posterior narrowing of the pelvis continues in the cavity and outlet. During labour the head will engage in the transverse diameter of the brim, and rotation of the head may be restricted so that deep transverse arrest may occur.

Abnormalities of the pelvis These can occur due to:

1. Developmental abnormalities of the pelvic bones.
2. Disease or injury of the bones.
3. Abnormalities of the spine, hip joints or lower limbs.

This may cause what is known as a contracted pelvis, where one or more of the diameters is reduced and will interfere with labour.

- *Rachitic flat pelvis.* This is caused by rickets affecting a child in their second year. The softened bones are distorted as the child sits, and the promontory of the sacrum is forced forward to the symphysis pubis. It was once the most common form of pelvic deformity in developed countries but due to improved nutrition is rarely a factor. However, it is still an issue in many areas in developing countries.
- *Generally contracted pelvis.* Small in all diameters and found in women of small build.
- *Asymmetrically contracted pelvis.* This may occur after a disease such as polio or congenital dislocation of the hip following a car accident.

The pelvic floor during labour and delivery

During birth, the pelvic floor muscles need to relax and release so that the fetus can be born. Diet, exercise and perineal massage have been shown to help prepare the pelvic floor. Pelvic floor exercises have been shown to help prepare the perineum (Labrecque et al 2000, Mason et al 2001).

Over 85% of women who have a vaginal birth will sustain some form of perineal trauma and up to 69% of those will require stitches. These rates vary worldwide according to different obstetric and midwifery practices (McCandlish et al 1998). The rate of episiotomy ranges from 8% in the Netherlands, to 13% in the UK, to 43% in the USA, and 99% in Eastern European countries (Graham & Graham 1997, Graves 1995).

In the UK approximately 23–42% of women will have perineal pain and discomfort for up to 10–12 days following vaginal delivery and 7–10% of these women will have long-term pain up to 18 months postpartum (Glazener et al 1995, Gordon et al 1998, McCandlish et al 1998, Sleep et al 1984).

Many women suffer from stress incontinence in later life due to perineal trauma sustained through birth, although it is difficult to establish figures. Birth, with or without an episiotomy, is potentially traumatic for the pelvic floor.

Symphysis pubis diastasis (SPD)/pelvic girdle dysfunction (PGD) This does not necessarily present problems, more that the woman needs to be aware of the positions that she is labouring in so that she does not aggravate the instability of the pubic bone. Labouring for at least some of first stage in water may help to give support to the unstable pelvic girdle. Using an epidural for pain relief can present problems if the woman assumes positions which will aggravate the condition. Use of the lithotomy position and forceps or ventouse delivery should ideally be avoided as they will place more strain on the bones. If they become necessary then the lithotomy position should be closely monitored and the woman's legs abducted to the minimum and kept in this position for the minimum amount of time.

Fetus

The fetus responds to contractions in labour by adopting a more flexed position and moving lower down into the pelvis. As it meets the gutter-shaped angle of the pelvic floor muscles with each contraction, it is gradually nudged into a more anterior direction and when the vertex is presenting it becomes increasingly more flexed due to the downward pressure of contractions and the simultaneous upward pull of the dilating cervix. It is able to do this partly because the sutures of the skull are not yet fused and so the skull can move to a greater degree than in an adult. The initial position of the fetus at the start of labour will also influence its ability to navigate the various twists and turns of the pelvis. Its size will have some effect, but only if greater than 4500g (Jon Barrrett, contributor), and will be more of an issue with shoulder dystocia. Babies' heads mould, and so the head is usually born, but the shoulders may get stuck.

Implications of changes in the musculoskeletal system for bodyworkers

- If the therapist is working with disadvantaged groups or in developing countries where there are issues of malnourishment, then the size and shape of the pelvis may be a factor in obstructing labour.
- If the client and her partner are from different ethnic groups where the client is much smaller than the partner, delivery could also be a concern.
- For most women, the size and shape of the pelvis should be adequate to allow the fetus to be born.
- Position, relaxation and emotional support are important factors in helping labour to progress.
- Exercise and massage to encourage awareness of, and relaxation of, the pelvic floor is important.
- Awareness of position for women with pelvic girdle instability (PGI) is important.

Renal

The renin–angiotensin systems of the woman and fetus are altered during labour and delivery. At delivery maternal renin, plasma renin activity (PRA) and angiotensinogen as well as fetal renin and angiotensinogen levels are elevated (Lindheimer & Katz 1992, Lindheimer et al 1991).

Maternal

Prolonged straining in the second stage may lead to injury to the bladder. Changes in the renal system may affect handling and excretion of drugs so drug doses need to be carefully monitored.

Respiratory

Maternal

Breathing in labour is a crucial part of the process.

Fetal

During the last couple of days before labour begins the breathing activity of the fetus is reduced, and lung liquid is produced at a gradually decreasing rate. This is linked with the increase in catecholamines.

There is a difference in lung function between babies born vaginally and those born via caesarean (whether elective or emergency). If the woman has been in labour for some time before the caesarean section occurs, then the fetal lungs would have been stimulated to some degree. Higher levels of surfactant and more rapid elimination of lung liquid occurs in response to the stimulatory effects of vaginal labour (Strang 1991).

2.6 Place of birth: home, hospital or birth centre, waterbirth

Since the Second World War there has been a rapid shift worldwide from most births happening at home to majority of births happening in hospital, apart from some countries such as the Netherlands where the home birth rate remains high. This low rate can vary considerably from area to area within a country. The Albany Birth Group has raised the level of home deliveries in their area of London (Reid 2002). Sustained low levels are due to many factors including safety, availability of midwifery care, and distance from hospital maternity units. In 2002 the number of home deliveries in England and Wales was 2.9% (ONS 2004).

Although many professionals consider hospital birth to be safer (Peel Report 1970) there is increasing evidence that home deliveries or domino (spending most of labour at home) schemes for women with low-risk pregnancies are safe (Campbell et al 1994, Chamberlain et al 1997, Tew 1998). Many consider that for low-risk women in developed countries, living within a short distance from a hospital, there are likely to be fewer interventions at home. In 2006, Patricia Hewitt, UK Secretary of Health, suggested that healthy women with uncomplicated pregnancies should be encouraged to have their baby at home (UK Department of Health 2006).

It is important to distinguish between unplanned and planned home birth, and Chamberlain et al (1997) concluded that perinatal mortality for planned home births was low.

There are many reasons why women choose home birth:

- Family tradition.
- Personal control/privacy.
- Relaxed and familiar environment.
- Fear of hospital.
- Knowing the midwife.
- Intimacy with children and partners.
- Fewer limitations on who can be present.
- More freedom in choosing what and when to eat.
- Space for moving around freely.
- Emotional and physical spontaneity.

Women who give birth at home are less likely to require pharmacological analgesia when they labour and give birth in their own homes (Cronk & Flint 1989).

Some women feel more comfortable in hospital, knowing that the medical back up is there on hand if required. In some countries such as Britain and Australia, women can choose a half-way option of a birthing centre in order to have the best of both worlds. These can be midwifery led and based in the hospital or separate establishments. Only women considered 'low risk' would have that option.

For women in developing countries, or indeed women in a rural setting far from a hospital, the choices may be different. Often women make the trip to be nearer the hospital for the delivery. Antenatal care is the main factor here, being able to identify which women can safely give birth at home and who are likely to need the medical services provided in hospital.

Nancy Stewart of the Association for Improvement in Maternity Services (AIMS) sums it up nicely:

All of living involves some risk, and this applies to giving birth and being born, wherever the birth takes place. … It is important to go beyond the statistics to consider the real influences on safety for you and your fetus. Where to give birth is not a matter of physical safety versus feelings. They are inextricably wrapped up together and you can trust the wisdom of your feelings in choosing where your fetus is to be born.

(Thomas 1998)

The use of water during birth

The use of water during labour, such as having a bath or shower, has always been a popular choice among women for pain relief. However, since the late 1980s some people have pioneered its use for the actual delivery of the baby. This is controversial and more popular in some countries than others. In some countries, such as the UK, birthing pools are widely available both in hospitals and for home births. However, in other countries, for example in Canada and the USA, this option is not widely available. Even where pools are available many women do not choose to give birth in the pool but rather use the water for pain relief during labour.

The movement began in Russia in the 1960s, where Igor Tjarkovsky did some initial work with animals (Lines 1992). He installed a glass tank in his home in Moscow and many women gave birth in it. From the 1970s onwards women began to use pools and even, during the hot summer month of August, to go to the Baltic Sea to give birth (Tonetti 2007). In France, Michel Odent installed a water pool in the maternity unit in Pithviers in 1977. Also in France, Fredrick Leboyer encouraged the use of a bath for the new-born immediately after the birth.

Protocols vary. Some hospitals only support the use of water for first stage, primarily for pain relief. Some hospitals are happy for it to be used during second stage. Others find that if the woman is in the pool it is difficult for the care giver to observe the perineum and control the delivery – which may then result in significant tearing for the woman. Additionally it may be difficult to see the fetus. It is recommended that the third stage is conducted out of the water because of the theoretical risk of water embolism (Odent 1983).

In the UK, the Royal College of Midwives' paper (UKCC 1996) recommends that the pool should only be used from 37 weeks, in cases where there is no sedation, for singleton birth, and if the membranes have not been ruptured for more than 24 hours before labour begins.

Women are not usually allowed in the pool if:

- The fetus is not cephalic.
- Labour is not well established (often this is defined as from 4–5 cm).
- The fetus is considered at risk, or if narcotics have been administered in the previous 4 hours, or if the fetus is in distress.
- The woman has a raised temperature, if there is bleeding, if the woman has HIV or hepatitis. In some situations women having a vaginal birth after caesarean (VBAC) are allowed in water, but usually not.

There are varying guidelines on the temperature of the water, but the consensus amongst experienced waterbirth practitioners is not to be too rigid and to be guided by the woman's comfort levels (Anderson 2004).

Essentially the same maternal positions which support labour tend to be comfortable in water, although the effects of gravity on the opening of the pelvis are different. The woman can lie back and float as the pelvis will not be compressed. Most women tend to use forward leaning or squatting positions. Squatting is much easier in the water as the body is supported and does not have the forces of gravity acting on it in the same way as on land. Water can provide excellent support to women who have joint problems, especially PGD issues, although obviously care needs to be taken in supporting the woman to get in and out of the pool so that she minimises abduction of her legs. It can be helpful to have some inflatable plastic pillows and rubber rings on hand for aiding comfort. Plastic cushions can be placed over the rim of the pool to make it more comfortable to lean on or they can be taken inside the pool.

Some practitioners consider that it is important not to get into the pool too early (before 'established' labour, 3 cm) as it can slow labour down, but others say wait until 5 cm. There is no clear evidence for this. Others say that if labour stops then the woman was not ready to go into labour. Some women like to save the water for when they really need it, others like to get in earlier and come in and out. It is important to support women in whatever feels right for them. However, sometimes if labour is not progressing getting out of the water and the change of position combined with the different effects of gravity help move things on.

Some partners like to get into the water with the woman, others not. The hospital advise the partner to wear swimming trunks. For other labour support people, due to health and safety considerations, it is inappropriate to get in the pool: this means that any bodywork needs to be done more on the neck and upper body while the woman is in the pool.

Elementally water can be a beneficial medium for some women. Some people believe its popularity is due to being able to create a more restful space in a medical setting. However, it does not suit everyone and some birthing facilities do not have the facilities or the rules for its usage.

Possible benefits

There is no hard research, but advocates of this method suggest that it enhances relaxation which may therefore lead to relief of pain and potentially enhanced cervical dilatation. Some argue that due to the support of water there is less chance of perineal tearing, while others disagree as the woman may suddenly bear down.

Possible disadvantages

- Infection of woman or fetus.
- Rupture of membranes if there is meconium in the fluid.
- Water embolism.
- Difficulties for care provider in supporting second stage.
- Possible dehydration because of warmth and lack of drinking.

Implications for bodyworkers on labour/birth in water and place of birth

- It is important to support clients to access the wisdom of their feelings and to support them in the decisions that they make rather than try to influence their choices based on the therapist's own biases.
- Encourage the woman to be flexible in her desire to labour or give birth in water as it may not be appropriate in all cases and in all settings.
- Be aware of the factors which may limit the woman being in the pool.
- Support the woman in the different positions.
- Do not get into the pool (infection risk), adapt techniques.

References

Abasiattai, A.M., Etuk, S.J., Asuquo, E.E.J., et al., 2004. Perinatal outcome following singleton vaginal breech delivery in the University of Calabar Teaching Hospital, Calabar: a 10-year review. Mary Slessor J. Med. 4, 81–85.

Allen, K., Mitchell, M., 2008. An exploratory study of women's experiences and key stakeholders views of moxibustion for cephalic version in breech presentation. Complement. Ther. Clin. Pract. 14 (4), 264–272.

Anderson, T., 2004. Time to throw the waterbirth thermometers away. MIDIRS 14 (3), 370–374.

Andrews, C.M., 1981. Nursing intervention to change a malpositioned fetus. Adv. Nurs. Sci. 3 (2), 53–66.

Andrews, C.M., Andrews, E.C., 1983. Nursing, maternal postures, and fetal position. Nurs. Res. 32 (6), 336–341.

Andrews, C.M., Andrews, E.C., 2004. Physical theory as a basis for successful rotation of fetal malpositions and conversion of fetal malpresentations. Biol. Res. Nurs. 6 (2), 126–140.

Badawi, N., Kurinczuk, J.J., Keogh, J.M., et al., 1998. Intrapartum risk factors for newborn encephalopathy: the Western Australian case-control study. BMJ 317, 1554–1558.

Baker, C., 1996. Nutrition and hydration in labour. Br. J. Midwifery 4 (11), 568–572.

Bassell, G.M., Marx, G.F., 1981. Physiological changes of normal pregnancy and parturition. In: Cosmi, E.V. (Ed.), Obstetric Anesthesia and Perinatalology. Appleton Century Crofts, New York.

Benito-Leon, J., Aguilar-Galan, E.V., 2001. Recurrent myotonic crisis in a pregnant woman with myotonic dystrophy. Eur. J. Obstet. Gynecol. Reprod. Biol. 95, 181.

Biancuzzo, M., 1991. The patient observer: does the hands-and-knees posture during labour help to rotate the occiput posterior fetus? Birth 18 (1), 40–47.

Bobak, I., Jensen, M., 1993. Maternity and Gynecologic Care: The Nurse and the Family, fifth ed. Mosby, St Louis, p. 507.

Bonnar, J., 2000. Massive obstetric haemorrhage. Baillières Best Pract. Res. Clin. Obstet. Gynecol. 14, 1–18.

Brandt, M.L., 1993. The mechanism and management of the third stage of labour. Am. J. Obstet. Gynecol. 25, 662–667.

Bridges, R.S., Grimm, C.T., 1982. Reversal of morphine disruption of maternal behaviour by concurrent treatment with the opiate antagonist naloxone. Science 218 (4568), 166–168.

Brinsmead, M., Smith, R., Singh, B., et al., 1985. Peripartum concentrations of beta endorphin and cortisol and maternal mood states. Aust. N. Z. J. Obstet. Gynaecol. 25 (3), 194–197.

Buckley, S.J., 2005. Gentle Birth, Gentle Mothering. One Moon Press, Brisbane.

Burnett, C.W.F., 1969. The Anatomy and Physiology of Obstetrics: A Short Textbook for Students and Midwives, fifth ed. Faber and Faber, London.

Caldwell, W.E., Moloy, H.C., D'Esopo, D.A., 1940. The more recent conceptions of the pelvic architecture. Am. J. Obstet. Gynecol. 40 (4), 558–565.

Campbell, R., McFarlane, A., 1994. Where to be Born? The Debate and the Evidence, second ed. Oxford National Perinatal Epidemiology Unit, Oxford.

Campbell, R., Davies, I.M., Macfarlane, A., et al., 1984. Home births in England and Wales, 1979: perinatal mortality according to intended place of delivery. Br. Med. J. (Clin. Res. Ed.) 289 (6447), 721–724.

Cardini, F., Weixin, H., 1998. Moxibustion for correction of breech presentation. JAMA 280 (18), 1580–1584.

Chamberlain, G., Wraight, A., Crowley, P., 1997. Home births. Report of the 1994 confidential enquiry by the National Birthday Trust Fund. Parthenon, Carnforth pp. 107–113.

Chard, T., 1989. Fetal and maternal oxytocin in human parturition. Am. J. Perinatol. 6 (2), 145–152.

Cheng, M., Hannah, M., 1993. Breech delivery at term; a critical review of the literature. Obstet. Gynecol. 82 (4 pt 1), 605–618.

Chhabra, S., Gandhi, D., Jaiswal, M., 2000. Obstructed labour – a preventable entity. J. Obstet. Gynecol. 20 (2), 151–153.

Clayton, S.G., Lewis, T.L.T., Pinker, G., 1985. Obstetrics by Ten Teachers, 14th ed. Edward Arnold, London.

Coad, J., Dunstall, M., 2005. Anatomy and Physiology for Midwives, second ed. Churchill Livingstone, Edinburgh.

Cronk, M., Flint, C., 1989. Community Midwifery: A Practical Guide. Heineman Medical Books, London.

Croughhan-Minhane, M.S., Pititi, D.B., Gordis, L., et al., 1990. Morbidity among breech infants according to method of delivery. Obstet. Gynaecol. 75, 821.

Crowley, P., 2003. Interventions for Preventing or Improving the Outcome of Delivery at or Beyond Term. Cochrane Review, Cochrane Library Issue 3, Update software, Oxford.

Crowley, P., Elbourne, D., Ashurst, H., et al., 1991. Delivery in an obstetric birth chair: a randomized controlled trial. Br. J. Obstet. Gynaecol. 98 (7), 667–674.

Cunningham, F.G., MacDonald, P.C., Gant, N.F., et al., 1997. Williams Obstetrics, 20th ed. Appleton and Lange, Stamford, CT.

Davies, E., 2004. Heart and Hands: A Midwife's Guide to Pregnancy and Birth, 4th ed. Celestial Arts, Berkeley.

Dawood, M.Y., Raghavan, K.S., Pociask, C., et al., 1978. Oxytocin in human pregnancy and parturition. Obstet. Gynecol. 51 (2), 138–143.

Department of Health, 2005. NHS Maternity Statistics England 2003–4. DoH, London.

Dick-Read, G., 1984. Childbirth Without Fear: The Original Approach to Natural Childbirth, fifth ed. Harper & Row, New York.

Donaldson, J.O., 1998. Neurology of Pregnancy, second ed. WB Saunders, Philadelphia.

Downe, S., 2000. A proposal for a new research and practice agenda for birth. MIDIRS Midwifery Dig. 10 (3), 337–341.

Downe, S., McCormick, C., Beech, B.L., 2001. Labour interventions associated with normal birth. Br. J. Midwifery 9 (10), 602–606.

Duff, T.P., 1999. Hematological aspects of pregnancy. In: Burrows, G.N., Duffy, T.P. (Eds.), Medical Complications During Pregnancy, fifth ed. WB Saunders, Philadelphia.

Enkin, M., Keirse, M.J.C., Neilson, J., et al., 2000. A Guide to Effective Care in Pregnancy and Childbirth, third ed. Oxford University Press, Oxford.

Facchinetti, F., Lanzani, A., Genazzani, A.R., 1989. Fetal intermediate lobe is stimulated by parturition. Am. J. Obstet. Gynecol. 161 (5), 1267–1270.

Fitzpatrick, M., McQuillan, K., O'Herlihy, C., 2001. Influence of persistent occiput posterior position on delivery outcome. Obstet. Gynecol. 98 (6), 1027–1031.

Foulkes, J., Dumoulin, J.G., 1983. Ketosis in labour. Br. J. Hosp. Med. 29 (6), 562–564.

Founds, S.A., 2007. Women's and providers' experiences of breech presentation in Jamaica: a qualitative study. Int. J. Nurs. Stud. 44 (8), 1391–1399.

Fuchs, A.R., Fuchs, F., 1984. Endocrinology of human parturition: a review. Br. J. Obstet. Gynaecol. 91 (10), 948–967.

Gardberg, M., Tuppurainen, M., 1994. Persistent occiput posterior presentation – a clinical problem. Acta Obstet. Gynecol. Scand. 73, 45–47.

Gardberg, M., Tuppurainen, M., 1998. Intrapartum sonography and persistent occiput posterior position: a study of 408 deliveries. Obstet. Gynecol. 91, 746–749.

Garfield, R.E., Blennerhassett, M.G., Miller, S.M., 1988. Control of myometrial contractility: role and regulation of gap junctions. Oxf. Rev. Reprod. Biol. 10, 436–490.

Gaskin, I.M., 2002. Spiritual Midwifery, fourth ed. Book Publishing Company, Summertown, TN.

Gaskin, I.M., 2003. Ina May's Guide to Childbirth. Bantam, London.

Glazener, C.M., Abdalla, M., Stroud, P., et al., 1995. Postnatal maternal morbidity: extent, causes, prevention and treatment. Br. J. Obstet. Gynaecol. 102 (4), 282–287.

Gordon, B., Mackrodt, C., Fern, E., et al., 1998. The Ipswich childbirth study. 1, a randomised evaluation of two stage postpartum perineal repair leaving the skin unsutured. Br. J. Obstet. Gynaecol. 105 (4), 435–440.

Gould, D., 2000. Normal labour: a concept analysis. J. Adv. Nurs. 31 (2), 418–427.

Graham, I.D., Graham, D.F., 1997. Episiotomy counts: trends and prevalence in Canada 1981/2 to 1993/4. Birth 24 (3), 141–147.

Grant, A., Gordon, B., Mackrodt, C., et al., 2001. The Ipswich childbirth study: one year follow up of alternative methods used in perineal repair. Br. J. Obstet. Gynaecol. 108, 34–40.

Graves, E.J., 1995. The 1993 Summary National Hospital Discharge Survey. Adv. Data 24 (264), 1–11. Centers for Disease Control and Prevention. National Center for Health Statistics.

Green, J., Coupland, V., Kitzinger, J., et al., 1998. Great Expectations: a Prospective Study of Women's Expectations and Experiences of Childbirth. Cambridge Child Care and Development Group. Cambridge University, Cambridge.

Gupta, J.K., Nikodem, V.C. 2000 Women's Positions During Second Stage of Labour. Cochrane Review, Cochrane Library Issue 4, Update software, Oxford.

Haheim, L.L., Albrechtsen, S., Berge, L.N., et al., 2004. Breech birth at term: vaginal delivery or elective cesarean section? A systematic review of the literature by a Norwegian review team. Acta Obstet. Gynecol. Scand. 83 (2), 126–130.

Hannah, M.E., Hannah, W.J., Hewson, S.A., et al., for the Term Breech Trial Collaborative Group 2000 Planned caesarean section versus planned vaginal birth for breech presentation at term: a randomised multicentre trial. Lancet 356(9239):1375–1383.

Henderson, C., Macdonald, S., 2004. Mayes' Midwifery: A Textbook for Midwives, 13th ed. Baillère Tindall, Edinburgh.

Hodnett, E.D., 1998. Support from Caregivers During Childbirth. Cochrane Review, Cochrane Library Issue 2, Updated software, Oxford.

Hodnett, E.D. 2002. Caregiver Support for Women During Childbirth. Cochrane Reviews, Cochrane Library Issue 4. Update software, Oxford.

Hofmeyr, G.J., 1991. External Cephalic version at term: how high are the stakes? Br. J. Obstet. Gynaecol. 91, 1–3.

Hofmeyer, G.J., Kulier, R. 2000a. External Cephalic Version for Breech Presentation at Term. Cochrane Library Issue 2, Update software, Oxford.

Hofmeyr, G.J., Kulier, R., 2000b. Hands and knees posture in late pregnancy or labour for fetal malposition (lateral or posterior). Cochrane Database Syst. Rev. (2), CD001063.

Hofmeyr, G.J., Kulier, R., 2000c. Cephalic version by postural management for breech presentation. Cochrane Database Syst. Rev. (2), CD000051.

Hofmeyr, G.J., Kulier, R., 2000d. Cephalic version by postural management for breech presentation [update]. Cochrane Database Syst. Rev. (3), CD000051.

Ikhena, S.E., Halligan, A.W.F., Naftalin, N.J., 1999. Has pelvimetry a role in current obstetric practice? J. Obstet. Gynaecol. 19 (5), 463–465.

Impey, L., O'Herlihy, C., 1998. First delivery after caesarean delivery for strictly defined cephalopelvic disproportion. Obstet. Gynecol. 92 (5), 799–803.

Irion, O., Hirsbrunner Almagbaly, P., Morabia, A., 1998. Planned vaginal delivery versus elective caesarean section: a study of 705 singleton term breech presentations. Br. J. Obstet. Gynaecol. 105, 710–717.

Jimenez, S.L.M., 1983. Application of the body's natural pain relief, mechanisms to increase comfort in labour and delivery. NAACOG Update Series 1 (1), 1.

Johnson, C., Keirse, M.J.N.C., Enkin, M., et al., 1989. Nutrition and hydration in labour. In: Chalmers, L., Enkin, M., Kierse, M.J.N.C. (Eds.), Effective Care in Pregnancy and Childbirth, vol. 2. Oxford University Press, Oxford.

Kanakura, Y., Kometani, K., Nagata, T., et al., 2001. Moxibustion treatment of breech presentation. Am. J. Chin. Med. 29 (1), 37–45.

Kariminia, A., Chamberlain, M., Keogh, J., et al., 2004. Randomised controlled trial of effect of hands and knees posturing on incidence of occiput posterior position at birth. Br. Med. J. 328 (7438), 490.

Kean, L.H., Suwanrath, C., Gargari, S.S., et al., 1999. A comparison of fetal behaviour in breech and cephalic presentations at term. Br. J. Obstet. Gynaecol. 106 (11), 1209–1213.

Kimball, C.D., 1979. Do endorphin residues of beta lipotropin in hormone reinforce reproductive function? Am. J. Obstet. Gynecol. 134 (2), 127–132.

Kinsley, C.H., Morse, A.C., Zoumas, C., et al., 1995. Intracerebroventricular infusions of morphine, and blockade with naloxone, modify the olfactory preferences for pup odors in lactating rats. Brain Res. Bull. 37 (1), 103–107.

Kitzinger, S., 2000. Rediscovering Birth. Little Brown, London.

Kwast, B.E., 1992. Obstructed labour: its contribution to maternal mortality. Midwifery 8 (1), 3–7.

Labrecque, M., Eason, E., Marcoux, S., 2000. Randomized trial of perineal massage during pregnancy: perineal symptoms 3 months after delivery. Am. J. Obstet. Gynecol. 182, 76–80.

Labrecque, M., Eason, E., Marcoux, S., 2001. Women's views on the practice of perineal massage. Br. J. Obstet. Gynecol. 108, 499–504.

Lau, T.K., Lo, K.W.K., Wan, D., et al., 1997. Predictors of successful external cephalic version at term: a prospective study. Br. J. Obstet. Gynaecol. 104 (7), 798–802.

Lavender, T., Hofmeyr, G.J., Neilson, J.P., et al., 2006. Caesarean section for non-medical reasons at term. Cochrane Database Syst. Rev. (3), CD004660.

Lederman, E., Lederman, R.P., Work Jr, B.A., et al., 1981a. Maternal psychological and physiologic correlates of fetal newborn health status. Am. J. Obstet. Gynecol. 139, 956–958.

Lederman, E., Lederman, R.P., Work, B.A., et al., 1981b. Relationship of psychological factors in pregnancy to progress in labour. Nurs. Res. 25, 94–98.

Lewis, T., Chamberlain, G., 1990. Obstetrics by Ten Teachers, fifteenth ed. Edward Arnold, London.

Lindheimer, M.D., Katz, A.I., 1992. Renal physiology and disease in pregnancy. In: Seldin, D.W., Giebisch, G. (Eds.), The Kidney: Physiology and Pathophysiology, second ed. Raven Press, New York, pp. 3371–3431.

Lindheimer, M.D., Barron, W.M., Davison, J.M., 1991. Osmotic and volume control of vasopressin release in pregnancy. Am. J. Kidney Dis. 17 (2), 105–111.

Lines, M., 1992. Waterbirth, What I Need to Know. Self-published.

Lowden, G., 1998. Breech presentation: Caesarean operation versus normal birth. Aims J. 10 (3), 5. (http://www.aims.org.uk/Journal/Vol10No3/breechCSvsNormal.htm).

Lowe, S.W., House, W., Garrett, T., 1987. A comparison of outcome of low risk labour in an isolated general practitioner maternity unit and a specialist maternity hospital. J. R. Coll. Gen. Pract. 37 (304), 484–487.

Ludka, L.M., Roberts, C.C., 1993. Eating and drinking in labour: a literature review. J. Nurs. Midwifery 38 (4), 199–207.

McCandlish, R., Bowler, U., van Asten, H., et al., 1998. A randomised controlled trial of care of the perineum during second stage of normal labour. Br. J. Obstet. Gynaecol. 105 (12), 1262–1272.

McGrath, M.M., Sullivan, M.C., Lester, B.M., et al., 2000. Longitudinal neurological follow up in neonatal intensive care unit survivors with various neonatal morbidities. Pediatrics 106 (6), 1397–1405.

Majzoub, J.A., Karalis, K.P., 1999. Placental corticotrophin-releasing hormone: function and regulation. Am. J. Obstet. Gynecol. 180, S242–S246.

Manga, M., 1999. Maternal cardiovascular and renal adaptations to pregnancy. In: Creasy, R.K., Resnik, R. (Eds.), Maternal Fetal Medicine: Principles and Practice, fourth ed. WB Saunders, Philadelphia.

Mason, L., Glenn, S., Walton, I., et al., 2001. The instruction in pelvic floor exercises provided to women during pregnancy or following delivery. Midwifery 17, 55–64.

Melzack, R., Wall, P.D., 1983. The Challenge of Pain. Basic Books, New York.

National Institute for Health and Clinical Excellence (NICE), 2007. Intrapartum care: management and delivery of care to women in labour. Online. <www.rcog.org.uk/> (accessed 15.12.07).

Neri, I., Airola, G., Contu, G., et al., 2004. Acupuncture plus moxibustion to resolve breech presentation: a randomized controlled study. Journal of Maternal-Fetal and Neonatal Medicine 15 (4), 247–252.

Newton, N., 1987. The fetus ejection reflex revisited. Birth 14 (2), 106–108.

Odent, M., 1983. Birth under water. Lancet 2 (8365–8366), 1476–1477.

Odent, M., 1992. The fetus ejection reflex. In: The Nature of Birth and Breastfeeding. Bergin & Garvey, London, Chapter 5.

Odent, M., 1996. Why birthing women don't need support. Mothering 80, 46–51.

Odent, M., 2001. The Scientification of Love, revised ed. Free Association Books, London.

Odent, M., 2007. Birth and Breastfeeding. Clairview Books, Forest Row, East Sussex.

ONS, 2004. Birth Statistics, Maternities: Age of Mother, Occurrence within/outside Marriage Number of Previous Live Born Children and Place of Confinement. 2003 series. FM1 no. 30, Table 8.1, p. 38. HMSO, London.

Pattinson, R.C., 2003. Pelvimetry for Fetal Cephalic Presentation at Term. Cochrane Review, Cochrane Library Issue 1, Update software, Oxford.

Pearl, M.L., Roberts, J.M., Laros, R.K., et al., 1993. Vaginal delivery from the persistent occiput posterior position: influence on maternal and neonatal morbidity. J. Reprod. Med. 38, 955–961.

Peel Report, 1970. Standing Maternity and Midwifery Advisory Committee. Domiciliary midwifery and maternity bed needs: report of a sub-committee. HMSO, London.

Ponkey, S.E., Cohen, A.P., Heffner, L.J., et al., 2003. Persistent fetal occiput posterior position: obstetric outcomes. Obstet. Gynecol. 101 (5/1), 915–920.

Prendiville, W.J., Elbourne, D., 1989. Care during the third stage of labour. In: Chalmer, L., Enkin, M., Kierse, M.J.N.C. (Eds.), Effective Care in Pregnancy and Childbirth, vol. 2. Oxford University Press, Oxford.

Pritchard, J.A., 1965. Changes in the blood volume during pregnancy and delivery. Anesthesiology 26, 393–399.

Puddicombe, J.F., 1955. Maternal posture for correction of posterior fetal position. Int. Coll. Surg. 23 (1/1), 73–77.

RCOG, 2001a. Induction of Labour. Evidence Based Clinical Guideline no. 9. RCOG Press, London.

RCOG, 2001b. Pelvimetry – Clinical Indications. Green top Guidelines no. 14. RCOG Press, London.

RCOG, 2006. The management of breech presentation. RCOG guidelines no. 20b, December 2006.

Reid, B., 2002. The Albany midwifery practice. MIDIRS Midwifery Dig. 14 (1), 118–121.

Roberts, J., 1980. Alternative positions for childbirth. Part 2, Second stage of labour. J. Nurs. Midwifery 25 (5), 13–19.

Roberts, J.E., 1989. Maternal positioning during the first stage of labour. In: Chalmers, I., Enkin, M., Keirse, M.J.N.C. (Eds.), Effective Care in Pregnancy and Childbirth. Oxford University Press, Oxford.

Robson, S.C., Hunter, S., Moore, M., et al., 1987. Haemodynamic changes during the puerperium: a Doppler and M mode echocardiographic study. Br. J. Obstet. Gynaecol. 94, 1028–1039.

Romond, J.L., Baker, I.T., 1985. Squatting in childbirth: a new look at an old tradition. J. Obstet. Gynecol. Neonatal Nurs. 14 (5), 406–411.

Rovinsky, J.J., Miller, J.A., Kaplan, S., 1973. Management of breech presentation at term. Am. J. Obstet. Gynecol. 115 (4), 497–513.

Royal North Shore Hospital, 1996. Labour Ward Statistics, Ninth Annual Report. Royal North Shore Hospital, Sydney.

Russell, J.G., 1969. Moulding of the pelvic outlet. J. Obstet. Gynaecol. Br. Commonw. 76, 817–820.

Russell, J.A., Douglas, A.J., Ingram, C.D., 2001. Brain preparations for maternity – adaptive changes in behavioural and neuroendocrine systems during pregnancy and lactation: an overview. Prog. Brain Res. 133, 1–38.

Schneider, K.T.M., Bung, P., Weber, S., et al., 1993. An orthostatic uterovascular syndrome – a prospective, longitudinal study. Am. J. Obstet. Gynecol. 169 (1), 183–188.

Sharp, D.A., 1997. Restriction of oral intake for women in labour. Br. J. Midwifery 5 (7), 408–412.

Simkin, P., Ancheta, A., 2000. Labour Progress Handbook. Blackwell Science, Oxford.

Sleep, J., Grant, A., Garcia, J., et al., 1984. West Berkshire Perineal Management Trial. Br. Med. J. (Clin. Res. Ed.) 289 (6445), 587–690.

Smith, C., Crowther, C., Wilkinson, C., et al., 1999. Knee–chest postural management for breech at term: a randomised controlled trial. Birth 26 (2), 71–75.

Smith, R.P., Gitau, R., Glover, V., et al., 2000. Pain and stress in the human fetus. Eur. J. Obstet. Gynecol. Reprod. Biol. 92, 161–165.

Stafisso-Sandoz, G., Polley, D., Holt, E., et al., 1998. Opiate disruption of maternal behavior: morphine reduces and naloxone restores c-fos activity in the medial preoptic area of lactating rats. Brain Res. Bull. 45 (3), 307–313.

Strang, L.B., 1991. Fetal lung liquid: secretion and reabsorption. Physiol. Rev. 71 (4), 991–1016.

Sutton, J., Scott, P., 1996. Understanding and Teaching Optimal Foetal Positioning. Birth Concepts, Taraunga, New Zealand.

Sweet, B., 1997. Mayes Midwifery, nineth ed. Ballière Tindall, London.

Tew, M., 1998. Safer Childbirth: A Critical History of Maternity Care, third ed. Free Association Books, London.

Thomas, P., 1998. Choosing a Home Birth. AIMS Information Booklet. Association for Improvements in the Maternity Services, UK.

Thurmann, I.M., (trans.) Hetherington. P. 2005. Healing from the very beginning: Karlton Terry's therapeutic work with birth trauma. Healing Waters, Glastonbury. Online. <http://healing-waters.co.uk/resources/tips/1/art/19/> (accessed 25.03.09).

Tonetti, E., 2007. Birth as we know it. DVD, <www.Birthintobeing.com/>.

Tranmer, J.E., Hodnett, E.D., Hannah, M.E., et al., 2005. The effect of unrestricted oral carbohydrate intake on labour progress. J. Obstet. Gynecol. Neonatal Nurs. 34 (3), 319–328.

Ueland, K., Hanson, J.M., 1969. Maternal cardiovascular dynamics. II, Posture and uterine contractions. Am. J. Obstet. Gynecol. 103, 1–7.

Ueland, K., Metcalfe, J., 1975. Circulatory changes in pregnancy. Clin. Obstet. Gynecol. 18 (3), 41–50.

UKCC, 1996. Water Births: The Current Position. UKCC, London.

Uvnas-Moberg, K., (trans.) Francis, R., 2003. The Oxytocin Factor. Da Capo Press, Cambridge MA.

Verbalis, J.G., McCann, M.J., McHale, C.M., et al., 1986. Oxytocin secretion in response to cholecystokinin and food; differentiation of nausea from satiety. Science 232 (4756), 1417–1419.

Wagner, M., 1994. Pursuing the Birth Machine: The Search for Appropriate Birth Technology. Ace Graphics, Camperdown, Australia.

Waldenstrom, U., Gottvall, K., 1991. A randomised trial of birthing stool or conventional semirecumbent position for second stage labor. Birth 18 (1), 5–10.

Westgren, M., Edvall, H., Nordstrom, E., et al., 1985. Spontaneous cephalic version of breech presentation in the last trimester. Br. J. Obstet. Gynaecol. 92 (1), 19–22.

Woolley, D., Roberts, J., 1996. A second look at the second stage of labor. J. Obstet. Gynecol. Neonatal Nurs. 25 (5), 415–423.

Yao, A.C., Lind, A.J., 1969. Effect of gravity on placental transfusion. Lancet 2 (7619), 505–508.

Yates, S., 2008. Beautiful Birth: Practical Techniques to Help You Achieve a Happier and More Natural Labour and Delivery. Carroll and Brown, London.

Zeeman, G.G., Khan-Dawood, F.S., Dawood, M.Y., 1997. Oxytocin and its receptor in pregnancy and parturition: current concepts and clinical applications. Obstet. Gyncecol. 89, 873–883.

Websites

http://www.albanymidwives.org.uk/ReportsAndArticles/albanyMP1.pdf

http://www.rcog.org.uk/resources/Public/pdf/green_top20b_breech.pdf

http://www.statistics.gov.uk/downloads/theme_population/FM1_32/FM1no32.pdf

CHAPTER **3**

Western approach to the postpartum

See book on baby massage (e.g. Schneider 2000, Walker 2000)

For more information on:

Work with newborns and paediatrics

See labour Chapters 2, 6 and 13 and practical section Chapter 10

For more information on:

Effects of birth

Learning outcomes

- Define the postpartum period for the mother
- Describe the main changes in the different maternal physiological systems
- Discuss the main issues relating to breastfeeding
- Define the different emotional states and be able to identify signs of depression and puerperal psychosis
- Describe the implications for bodywork of these changes

3.1 Definition of postpartum period and overview of changes

It is a matter of debate how long the postnatal period actually is. Traditionally the 'puerperium' means the period belonging to the child, and medically it is defined as the 6 weeks following the delivery of the placenta. This is the time during which the pelvic organs return to their normal condition and most of the anatomical and physiological changes of pregnancy and birth are reversed. Many of the changes occur within 10–14 days after delivery. These first few weeks are potentially dangerous. There is the risk of infection due to the open placental site and blood loss. Fever, and in rare cases death, can ensue. There is also a risk of thrombosis developing. (See CEMACH 2006 for UK figures.)

The rate of these changes varies considerably from woman to woman. Recovery depends on the fitness of the mother, her general medical condition pre-, during and post-pregnancy and the kind of birth she has experienced. Recovery from instrumental or surgical delivery is longer as the mother has to recover from the surgery as well as the physiological processes. Some women may experience *involution* of the uterus within 4 weeks and for some of the systems in the body it can take 10–12 weeks or longer for structures to heal. The changes in the musculoskeletal system are slowest to recover and, if she does not care adequately for herself, the mother may experience long-term patterns of weakness in the areas of the body which had to make the most changes in pregnancy and labour, notably the abdomen, lower back and pelvic floor.

Both immediate and longer-term recovery is dependent on what the mother does, how she looks after herself, the balance she achieves between work and rest. These days, with the increasing demand for mothers to return early to work outside the home, women often have little time to rest and look after themselves and we have yet to see the effects on the long-term health of women of these recent changes in working and childrearing practices.

Midwives' care (in the UK) for the postpartum period is defined as 'a period of not less than ten and not more than 28 days after the end of labour, during which time the continued attendance of a midwife on the mother and baby is requisite' (UKCC 1998). Most northern and western European countries have home-based postpartum visits for up to the first 6 weeks (Kamerman & Kahn 1993). In the Netherlands women receive daily visits from a specially trained helper called the *Kraamverzorgester* (De Vries et al 2001) and many Chinese mothers have home-based support for the first month (Lee et al 2004). In the USA and Canada postpartum care is less extensive (Cheng et al 2006). A major component of current postnatal care consists of vaginal examination and contraceptive education. One third of women interviewed in a study felt that this was not sufficient and wanted more physical and emotional support and for a longer period (Declercq et al 2002). Postnatal care is being reviewed in many countries and there are recommendations by some that postpartum care could be extended to 1 year (Walker & Wilging 2000).

Many people have argued that the postpartum period should be considered as longer than it has been and include the first year. After 1 year more than 50% of women said they still suffered from fatigue (Saurel-Cubizolles et al 2000).

In many traditional cultures the period of full recovery was considered to be much longer and in ancient Japan and China women were sometimes advised to wait 5–7 years to have another child. Recent research suggests that it is better for women to wait for at least 2 years. Naturally for each mother the recovery will be different, depending on age, number of pregnancies, level of support on so on. It also depends on how long the mother is going to breastfeed. In modern cultures the tendency is more towards 3–6 months, whereas in traditional cultures it was 2–3 years. With the age of childbearing increasing, delaying future pregnancies may not be a viable option but pregnancies close together, especially when older, do tend to place more demands on the mother.

Not only is the body recovering from pregnancy but there are also the changes of labour and initiating lactation, if the mother is breastfeeding. The woman is processing major physical changes, including major hormonal changes which may affect her moods. Emotionally there are also major psychological and social changes to accommodate as she begins to assume care of her new child and integrate him or her into the family system as well as, increasingly these days, to balance work outside the home with family responsibilities. She may also be processing feelings resulting from her labour. The rate of depression at this time is relatively high.

For these reasons, we have chosen here to consider the whole of the first year as the postnatal period. By the end of the first year, the mother is more emotionally stable and longer-term patterns of good or poor health are beginning to be laid down. The completion of the first year often marks the infant's first steps and the beginning of a new phase of independence for the child. During this year, however, some women will conceive and so then they will be dealing with postnatal and pregnancy changes simultaneously.

For many women, long-term health patterns are poor (MacArthur et al 1991a, b). This could be due to changes in the pregnancy or birth, or to the physical, emotional and lifestyle changes consequent on accommodating a new baby in one's life. The McArthur et al study, conducted in Birmingham, UK (MacArthur et al 1991a, b) obtained information on the health problems of 11 701 women between 1 and 9 years after child birth. One of the main aims of the study was to investigate childbirth-related health problems and so the analysis was restricted to symptoms not previously experienced before the birth and starting within 3 months of it. Almost half the women (47%) reported one symptom which lasted for longer than 6 weeks. There have been other studies (Brown & Lumley 2000, Glazener et al 1995, Kahn et al 2002, Saurel-Cubizolles et al 2000) which have also examined health after birth. The types of symptoms identified are rarely life threatening but can have an effect on the quality of life.

Poor health issues in the postpartum

Urinary stress incontinence, haemorrhoids, faecal incontinence and other bowel problems, perineal pain and dyspareunia (i.e. pain during intercourse), backaches, headaches, depression and fatigue.

They are also concerning because poor maternal health has been related to poor children's health (Kahn et al 2002).

Often these changes are not reported to the medical carers. This can be an area where the bodyworker can play a huge role and offer immense support. Postnatal health lays the foundations for a woman's health for the rest of her life (WHO 1998).

3.2 The female reproductive system

The major hormonal changes of the early postnatal period support rapid changes in the reproductive system. The uterus returns to its pre-pregnant size as early as 4 weeks after a vaginal birth. After a caesarean birth recovery is longer and scar pain may still be felt years later. The pelvic floor recovers within a couple of weeks after a natural birth and up to 4–6 months after an episiotomy. Pregnancy may have a beneficial effect on conditions such as menstrual pain and endometriosis. However, long-term weakness often remains, with stress incontinence and haemorrhoids being common. If the woman is not breastfeeding her breasts return to their normal size and the menstrual cycle will resume within 15 weeks. If the woman is breastfeeding, the breasts will remain altered and fertility will resume usually within 9 months unless nutrition is poor and the mother is feeding frequently. Contraception is an issue as there can be a return to fertility before the first period.

Involution of uterus

Involution means the return of the uterus to normal size, tone and position. During this process the lining of the uterus (decidua) is cast off in the lochia and later replaced by new endometrium. After the birth of the baby and the expulsion of the placenta the muscles of the uterus constrict the blood vessels to reduce the blood circulating in the uterus: vasoconstriction. Oxytocin released from the posterior pituitary induces the strong myometrial contractions. During the first 12–24 hours these contractions ('after-pains') are relatively strong, gradually diminishing in intensity and frequency over the next 4–7 days. They tend to be stronger in multiparous women. They can also be stimulated by oxytocin released during breastfeeding.

About an hour after delivery the myometrium relaxes slightly but further active bleeding is prevented by the activation of blood clotting mechanisms which are altered greatly in pregnancy to facilitate a swift clotting response. This is why there is an increase in DVT in the early postpartum period. The primary caregiver will check that there are no 'retained products' such as pieces of the placenta, because these may impede the contraction of the uterus and cause abnormal bleeding. They can also cause secondary postpartum haemorrhage as they become the focus of infection.

Redundant muscles, fibrous and elastic tissue have to be broken down. The phagocytes deal with fibrous and elastic tissue but the process of phagocytosis is usually incomplete and some elastic tissue remains so that a once pregnant uterus never totally returns to its nulliparous state. Muscle fibres are digested by proteolytic enzymes in a process known as *autolysis*. The lysosomes of the cells are responsible for this process. The waste products then pass into the bloodstream to be eliminated by the kidneys.

The decidual lining of the uterus is shed in the lochia. The new endometrium grows from the basal layer, beginning to be formed from around the 10th postnatal day, and is completed in about 6 weeks.

The process of involution takes at least 6 weeks to complete (Fig. 3.1). Immediately after delivery the uterus weighs about 900–1000 g. By 24 hours postpartum the size is similar to its size at 20 weeks (Monheit et al 1980, Resnik 1999). The rate of involution can be assessed by the rate of descent of the uterine fundus. On the first day the height of the fundus above the symphysis pubis is just over 12 cm (Howie 1995). The height of the fundus usually decreases by about 1 cm per day so that by 3 days the fundus lies 2–3 fingers' widths below the umbilicus, or slightly higher in multigravidas. Primary caregivers feel the uterus each day to note the decrease in size, although the practice of recording and charting the fundal height is decreasing.

At about 5–6 days the uterus weighs about 500 g and the cervix is reforming and closing and will admit one finger. Usually by about 10 days the uterus has descended into the true pelvis.

The rate of involution varies from mother to mother and is usually slower in the following cases:

- Multiparous women.
- Multiple gestation.
- Infections.
- Delivery of a large infant.

Involution may be slower if there is retention of placental tissue or blood clot, particularly when this has caused an infection.

It is important if the bodyworker has any concerns to refer for medical help, especially if there is an increase in bleeding or pain or tenderness over the uterus.

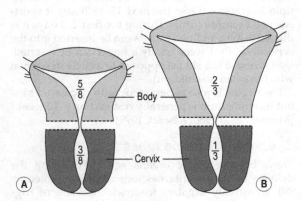

Fig. 3.1A and B Return of uterus to size. **A** is nalliparous; **B** is parous.

Discharge of lochia

Lochia is the name given to the discharge coming from the placental site. The normal pattern is for red discharge in the first 3 or 4 days: lochia rubra or red lochia. It consists mainly of blood mixed with shreds of decidua. This becomes lighter (more brownish) and eventually serous after about 5 or 6 days: lochia serosa or serous lochia. This is altered blood and serum and contains leucocytes and organisms. The final discharge is known as lochia alba, yellowish-white lochia, in which there is little blood. It is mostly white blood cells, cervical mucous and organisms. Discharge decreases in amount as the site heals. The average time for lochia to become colourless is about 3–4 weeks.

Lochia that remain red and abundant for longer than usual may indicate delayed involution of the uterus, which may be due to retention of a piece of placenta within the uterus and/or to infection. If placental tissue is retained the uterus remains enlarged and this may show on an ultrasound scan. Lochia with offensive odour may indicate infection. It is possible for red lochial discharge to still be present at 6–8 weeks. It is more common also after instrumental delivery. Seek medical help if concerned.

Cervix, vagina, ligaments and pelvic floor

The vagina, the ligaments of the uterus and the muscles of the pelvic floor also return to their pre-pregnant state. If the ligaments and pelvic floor do not return and are permanently weakened, a prolapse may occur later. Pre-pregnancy fitness is a factor in supporting the strength, as is fitness during pregnancy and postnatal exercises as well as avoiding constipation and coughing.

Cervix and vagina

After a vaginal delivery the cervix hangs into the vagina and is thin, bruised and oedematous with multiple lacerations. Over the next 12–18 hours it shortens and becomes firmer. During the first 2–3 days it is dilated 2–4 cm and two fingers can be inserted into the cervical os. By 1 week barely a finger can be inserted. By 4 weeks it is a slit (as opposed to a circle in women who have had no children).

The vagina is also oedematous with decreased tone but its epithelium is generally restored by 6–10 weeks (Monheit et al 1980, Resnick 1999).

Ovaries and uterine tubes

These become pelvic organs again. Following the delivery of the placenta, oestrogens and progesterone fall. Eventually negative feedback mechanisms trigger off the ovarian menstrual cycle.

The perineum

The perineum has to recover from stretching during birth and can be damaged during delivery as well as the stretching and additional work of pregnancy. Even after a caesarean, recovery and rehabilitation is necessary.

It is common to feel some soreness in the first few days but some women experience more intense pain. This can be relieved by the use of icepacks. However, especially after deeper tearing and stitches, more pain relief may be needed and women may need to be referred back to their primary caregiver to be prescribed oral analgesics such as paracetamol.

It is important for the mother to exercise the muscles, even if only very gently, within 24 hours of delivery, to promote blood circulation and strengthen the tissue. Pelvic floor exercises need to be gradually increased as the muscles heal, and carried on for the rest of the mother's life. If there is extensive damage she may need to see a physiotherapist and use ultrasound therapies to rehabilitate the muscles (Glazener et al 1995).

Episiotomies were once thought to limit perineal pain by limiting tearing. However, the most recent studies (Carroli & Belizan 2001) showed that there is little evidence to justify this.

Perineal damage

Types of perineal tear   These are classified according to the severity:

- *Superficial* – grazes, no treatment, a bit sore.
- *First degree* – tear in skin, often will heal on its own.
- *Second degree* – skin tears involve perineal muscle damage; usually these wounds are sutured.
- *Episiotomy* – a surgical incision falling into same category as second degree tear.
- *Third degree* – here the muscle of the anal sphincter is involved. Obstetric repair is essential so that the sphincter activity of the muscle is restored, thus avoiding problems of faecal incontinence at a later time.
- *Fourth degree* – when the tear is extensive and the anal sphincter may become completely divided and the tear continues through the rectal mucosa. Specialist surgical repair is required to ensure the resumption of normal anal function.

Damage to the perineum is associated with problems such as pain, infection, alterations in urination, faecal problems including incontinence, third degree laceration and dyspareunia (painful intercourse) (Brown & Lumley 2000, Glazener et al 1995). Initial healing takes about 2–3 weeks but the site may take 4–6 months to heal completely.

Mammary changes

In women who do not breastfeed, breast involution occurs. With no stimulation by suckling, prolactin levels decrease, milk production ceases and glandular tissue returns to a resting state over the next few weeks. Cold flannels can be used on the breast of non-lactating women to reduce the flow of colostrum. For women who breastfeed many changes occur in the breasts in the early postnatal period.

Physiology of lactation

Breastfeeding and fertility

Breastfeeding delays the recovery of the ovarian–pituitary axis. In non-breastfeeding women body temperature measurements and the first menstrual bleeding suggest that the earliest ovulation may occur at 4 weeks after delivery but is usually delayed to 8–10 weeks (Gray et al 1987). Most non-breastfeeding women have resumed normal menstrual patterns by 15 weeks. The first menstrual cycle is often anovulatory or associated with an inadequate luteal phase, but most cycles are ovulatory by the third cycle. About 50% of non-lactating women who do not use contraception conceive within 6–7 months so contraception needs to be discussed (Coad & Dunstall 2001: 357).

In lactating women menstruation and ovulation return more slowly. Lactational amenorrhoea may last from 2 months to 4 years and its variability seems related to a number of factors, of which the most important is frequency of feeding. In developing countries breastfeeding prevents more pregnancies than all other methods combined. Night-time feeds seem important in suppressing fertility (Howie & McNeilly 1982). Poor nutrition also suppresses fertility when combined with longer breastfeeding patterns (Rogers 1997). Women who have less optimal nutrition can breastfeed their babies but they secrete milk more slowly so infants feed more often and for longer, raising circulating prolactin levels.

Ovarian activity usually resumes before the end of lactational amenorrhoea and so conception can occur before the resumption of menstruation. Between 30% and 70% of first cycles are ovulatory. Neither ovulation nor menstruation usually occur within 6 weeks but about half of all non-contraceptive-protected breastfeeding mothers conceive within 9 months, 1–10% during lactational amenorrhoea.

The precise mechanisms involved in lactational amenorrhoea are not clear but it is due to high prolactin levels blocking the effects of luteinising hormone (LH) and follicle stimulating hormone (FSH) and it may possibly affect libido.

Sexual function

Resumption of sex can be uncomfortable for women, especially after an instrumental delivery, such as episiotomy or caesarean section, as there can be pain in the scars. Both emotionally, as well as physically, it may take several months for the mother to feel comfortable having sex again. In some cultures and religions there are taboos on having sex for the first few months.

Some mothers may not feel comfortable with sex for longer after a birth, even a year later, and this may create tension in their relationships.

Lack of oestrogen can aggravate the pain and the use of topical oestrogens may be advised.

Implications for bodyworkers of changes in the reproductive system

- Lochial discharge: be aware during the first 4–6 weeks to ask if there is still lochial discharge.
- While there is lochial discharge, work on the abdomen should be more gentle and care needs to be taken with exercises to not place too much pressure on the abdomen and there is an increased risk of infection.
- Refer if there is any concern re abdominal or pelvic floor pain or bleeding (lochial discharge or discharge from incisions).
- Note that after-pains may be experienced in the first few days, which may cause discomfort for the mother. Abdominal work will need to be adjusted accordingly.
- Sexuality: women may want to talk about their feelings about sex, which is often an issue: e.g. when to have sex, feelings about not wanting sex, the changes in the relationship with partner. While not being sexual counsellors, it may be helpful for bodyworkers to allow the woman space to express her feelings.
- Note that menstruation is not an indicator of fertility and the mother needs to be aware of contraceptive issues and be referred for appropriate follow-up.

Referral issues

- Refer if there is any concern over bleeding or pain, tenderness over the uterus.
- Be alert to any signs of possible infection in the first few weeks and refer to the primary caregiver.

3.3 Neuroendocrine system

Major and rapid changes happen in the hormone levels and many postulate that depression can be in part

Table 3.1 A comparison of prolactin and oxytocin (after Coad & Dunstall 2001)

	Prolactin	**Oxytocin**
Source	Anterior pituitary gland	Posterior pituitary (synthesised in hypothalamus)
Primary control	Lifting of dopamine inhibition	Neural pathway
Modulating factors	Positively stimulated by oestrogen, TSH, VIP	Neurotransmitters
Peak response	30 min	30 s
Stimulus	Suckling	Suckling, sound, sight and thought of baby
Target cell	Alveolar cell	Myoepithelial cell
Effect	Milk synthesis	Milk ejection

TSH = thyroid stimulating hormone; VIP = vasoactive intestinal polypeptide.

explained by this. As hormones have both blood and neural pathways they will impact on the mother's physical and emotional state of being.

Changes occur mostly after birth with the delivery of the placenta and due to changes in prolactin secretion. In general most peptide hormones, enzymes and other circulating proteins reach non-pregnant levels by 6 weeks postpartum.

If the mother is breastfeeding then the two most important hormones are prolactin and oxytocin and her hormone levels remain different from the non-lactating and pre-pregnant woman. These hormones aid with bonding and relaxation and support the process of breastfeeding.

Oestrogens and progesterone

As the placenta is the main source of oestrogens and progesterone, they tend to disappear rapidly following delivery. Plasma oestradiol (an oestrogen) reaches levels that are less than 2% of pregnancy values by 24 hours.

By 1–3 days oestradiol levels are similar to those found during the follicular phase of the menstrual cycle and oestrogen levels continue to fall until day 7, when they gradually increase to follicular phase levels over the next few weeks.

Progesterone levels fall rapidly at delivery (Dooley 1984). Generally progesterone levels similar to those found in the luteal phase of the menstrual cycle are reached by 24–48 hours and follicular phase levels by 3–7 days. Ovarian production of oestrogen and progesterone is low during the first 2 weeks. The levels gradually increase with the resumption of gonadotropin secretion by the pituitary and ovary (Liu & Yen 1989, Tulchinsky 1994).

These rapid changes are likely to affect mood swings.

Pituitary gonadotropin

This is suppressed during pregnancy. FSH and LH remain low during the first 2 weeks postpartum in

both lactating and non-lactating women then gradually increase over the next few weeks, more quickly in non-lactating women.

Prolactin and oxytocin

These are the two main hormones which regulate breastfeeding (Table 3.1).

Prolactin

Its levels are increased during pregnancy, although its effects are suppressed by oestrogen. During pregnancy it promotes the development of the mammary alveoli and duct system in preparation for breastfeeding. Its levels vary diurnally and increase during sleep. It increases with stress, anaesthesia, surgery, exercise, nipple stimulation and sexual intercourse (Lawrence & Lawrence 1999).

As labour begins prolactin levels fall, increasing immediately after delivery and peaking about 3 hours postpartum. Postnatally its secretion is triggered by the newborn suckling. In non-lactating women levels fall by 7–14 days to the high end of the non-pregnant range.

If the newborn suckles then levels of prolactin begin to rise within 10 minutes. They result in a complex neuroendocrine response. Levels peak about 30 minutes after initial stimulation and fall back to basal levels within a further 3 hours. Areolar stimulation is necessary for prolactin release.

Levels of prolactin are much diminished after 6 weeks at a rate dependent on suckling frequency and duration (Johnston & Amico 1986). There are higher circulating levels during sleep.

Oxytocin

Oxytocin is probably the main hormone which promotes 'mothering' feelings and emotions as well as supporting breastfeeding. Odent refers to it as 'the Love hormone' (Odent 2001, Pederson et al 1992). Uvnäs-Moberg (2003) refers to it as 'the hormone of calm, love and healing', the mirror hormone of adrenaline, the 'calm and connection system'. It is linked with intimacy and communication, bonding.

Oxytocin increases during labour. It plays a critical role in the ejection of milk. Putting the infant to breast immediately after delivery many enhance uterine involution (Neville & Neifert 1983). These 'after-pains' are experienced as a cramping pain in the abdomen. They usually only last for a few days and seem to be worse if the mother has received syntometrine and with each subsequent pregnancy.

After a caesarean there are less oxytocin impulses. It is not known if this is due to the mode of birth, the effects of delayed skin-to-skin contact, the pain and stress caused by surgery, or the effects of anaesthesia and analgesics (Nissen et al 1996).

Oxytocin helps the body store nutrients and promotes the differentiation and effectiveness of the body's storage systems. There has to be a balance in the body between nursing and the conservation of energy for the mother. This explains why some nursing mothers lose weight and others gain.

The milk ejection reflex is responsible for transfer of milk from the breast to the baby. It is independent from prolactin. It is released in short-lived bursts of less than a minute immediately in response to stimulus. The largest response is to the baby crying before feeding so maximum release is likely before suckling is started. Covering breasts and use of warm flannels can help with the release of oxytocin.

Unlike prolactin it can be conditioned. It is produced by continuous physical contact with the child and sensitive to inhibition by physical or psychological stresses such as emotional tiredness, embarrassment and worry. The limbic system which coordinates the body's response to emotions is involved in oxytocic release.

Implications for bodyworkers of changes in the neuroendocrine system

- It is common for the mother to feel emotional in the first week or two due to the huge changes in oestrogens and progesterones in addition to the life changes she is undergoing.
- Be aware of how breastfeeding mothers release high levels of oxytocin – the love hormone. This may help explain why breastfeeding mothers can find the adaptation to the postnatal period easier.
- The tissue remains soft in the early postnatal time as relaxin levels are still quite high.

It helps maintain a state of calmness and relaxation. Blood pressure can drop and cortisol levels drop. More seems to be released during sleep.

Relaxin

Levels fall rapidly after delivery but significant amounts remain for the first 6–8 weeks postnatally. It is still important to be aware of laxity in the pelvic girdle postnatally.

Thyroid

The enlarged thyroid gland regresses to its former size and the basal metabolic rate returns to normal.

3.4 Haematological, haemostatic and cardiovascular systems

The major changes in these systems happen in the first few weeks. The hypercoagulable state of pregnancy is increased in the early postnatal period and during the first 6 weeks the risk of thromboembolic disorders is high. Changes in these systems can lead to an increased risk of infection due to the placental wound site and the lochia, which provides ideal culture conditions for micro-organisms. There is additional risk with instrumental deliveries and the extra incision. Anaemia can also be a cause of infection. Further, the mother can be prone to anaemic conditions if she does not eat adequately, especially if she is breastfeeding.

Haemostasis

There are some changes in the haemostatic system during labour itself, in order to prepare the woman to tolerate the normal blood loss at delivery and prevent significant bleeding with the separation of the placenta. Haemoglobin levels increase slightly during labour and concentrations of clotting factors also increase. This means that the hypercoagulable state of pregnancy is increased in the early postnatal period, in order to protect the mother from haemorrhage and excessive blood loss.

Blood loss

Blood loss at delivery averages around 500 ml with vaginal delivery and 1000 ml with caesarean section or twins. It is more than compensated for by the increase in blood volume in pregnancy. This loss, along with the lochial discharge of the early weeks, accounts for about half of the increased RBC volume acquired during pregnancy (Chesley 1972).

Plasma volume decreases, reaching non-pregnant levels by 6–8 weeks or earlier (Chesley 1972). Increased RBC production ceases early postpartum and means haemoglobin levels decrease slightly in the first 24 hours after delivery and then rise to day 14. Haematocrit values follow a similar pattern and return to non-pregnant levels by 4–6 weeks. However, haemoglobin levels tend to be low postnatally even though they are not routinely tested. As many as 7% of women with no previous low HB have anaemia between 2 and 18 months after birth (Glazener et al 1993). This will contribute to the feelings of tiredness commonly experienced by women.

WBC increases in labour and the immediate postpartum then falls and returns to normal value by 6 days and can complicate diagnosis of infection (Kilpatrick & Laros 1999).

Fibrinolytic activity is maximal for the first 3 hours after delivery although it may return to normal ranges as early as 1 hour and reflects the removal of the fibrinolytic inhibitors produced by the placenta. Clotting factors slowly decrease reaching their lowest levels by 7–10 days. The haematological system returns to its non-pregnancy state 3–4 weeks postpartum. Changes in flow velocity and diameter of the deep veins may take up to 6 weeks to return to pre-pregnant levels. This means that during the first 6 weeks the risk of thromboembolic disorders is high (Hathway & Bonnar 1987).

Thromboembolic disorders

These represent some of the major causes of maternal death.

DVT: risk of thrombosis

Mobilisation after birth is essential to optimise venous return in order to avoid stasis within the vascular bed and reduce the risk of deep vein thrombosis (DVT) formation. Women who are unable to mobilise or at increased risk, owing to obstetric complications such as a lower segment caesarean section (LSCS), are given prophylactic anticoagulant treatment. Women are encouraged to report any discomfort or swelling of the lower legs as this may indicate DVT formation. It has been observed clinically that there is an increased risk of DVT in the left leg especially after caesarean section because blood flow velocity is reduced to a greater extent. Intimal vessel injury (damage to the inner lining of the vein injury) may occur during caesarean section delivery which could conceivably trigger a pelvic vein thrombosis.

Risk factors

Risk factors include: increased maternal age, parity, dehydration following delivery and delivery by caesarean section, previous history of thromboembolic problems, pregnancy-induced hypertension, artificial heart valve, operative delivery (Weiner 1985).

Pulmonary embolism

Pulmonary embolism (PE) is an obstetric emergency that may arise in the postnatal period as well as pregnancy and though rare, it is one of the main causes of maternal death.

Cardiovascular system

Despite the amount of blood loss, cardiac output is significantly elevated above pre-labour levels for up to 1–2 hours postpartum (Pritchard et al 1962). There are minimal changes in blood pressure and pulse. Stroke volume and cardiac output remain elevated for at least 48 hours after delivery, probably due to increased venous return with loss of uterine blood flow. Cardiac output decreases by 30% by 2 weeks postpartum and gradually decreases to non-pregnant values by 6–12 weeks in most women. Most of the other changes in the cardiovascular system resolve by 6–8 weeks postpartum. Left atrial size and heart rate reach pre-pregnancy values by 10 days postpartum. For 20% of women there is a systolic murmur which persists beyond 4 weeks postpartum.

Blood loss, and the mechanisms which compensate for it, render the cardiovascular system transiently unstable after delivery. During the first week after delivery, many women experience headaches due to this unstable fluid balance. Vascular remodelling persists for at least a year after birth and is enhanced by second and subsequent pregnancies (Clapp & Capeless 1997). This means stroke volume remains relatively high, causing reduced heart rate. It is normal for puerperal women to exhibit a reduced pulse rate. A raised pulse may indicate severe anaemia, venous thrombosis or infection.

During the first week after delivery there is an increase in diuresis which needs to happen in order to dissipate the increased extracellular fluid. Sometimes with women in pre-eclampsia or heart disease there may be no diuresis and so pulmonary oedema can result.

Blood volume returns to its pre-gravid levels and blood regains its former viscosity. Smooth muscle tone in the vessel walls improves and cardiac output returns to normal and the blood pressure to its usual level.

Varicose veins

These often regress after pregnancy, but usually become worse with each successive pregnancy and can become permanent.

Summary of implications for bodyworkers of changes in the cardiovascular system

- Most of the blood changes are in the early period (6–8 weeks).
- There is a possibility of infection in the early weeks while wound healing occurs, e.g. bleeding from vagina, from caesarean section scar.
- There is an increased risk of thrombosis in the first 6 weeks, especially the first week or so. Encourage mobilisation.
- Tiredness can be due to anaemia rather than simply sleep deprivation and stress.
- There is an increased incidence of varicose veins in women who have had children.
- Raised pulse may indicate severe anaemia, thrombosis or infection.

Referral

- Infection.
- Raised pulse.
- Oedema.
- Fever.

3.5 Musculoskeletal system

These systems take longest to recover and without appropriate exercises and self-care, some weakness may remain long term. While some women regain their fitness and health levels quickly, especially after one pregnancy, for others pregnancy can signal the beginning of patterns of weakness. If the weakened abdominal wall and pelvic floor are not exercised, then this may cause weakness in the pelvic area, leading to lack of support for the internal organs as well as problems with the lower back. Issues with pelvic girdle weakness overlaid on a body which is feeding and lifting young children often cause imbalance in the hip and the shoulders. The softness of the tissue can remain for a few months postnatally, especially if the mother is still breastfeeding as prolactin levels couple with relaxin and maintain the softened tone.

The multiparous breastfeeding mother may have ongoing pubic symphysis instability, anterior uterine strain as ligaments are engorged, coupled with increased lumbar lordosis for several months. There may also be adhesions within the abdominal and pelvic cavities due to the fascial stretching during pregnancy, and so postpartum resolution may take the first 12 months to clear if breast feeding.
(A. Morgan, personal communication, 2008)

Sometimes this muscular weakness, especially in the pelvis, can be triggered during the menstrual cycle.

Pelvic floor

Due to stretching during birth, these may be bruised or swollen and tender to pressure both externally (thighs, buttocks) or internally (coughing, laughing or sneezing). If there has been instrumental delivery, then there will be a need to recover from stitches. Previously it was thought that episiotomy was 'better' than a tear but now it is understood that torn tissue heals better, as it can knit together better. Most women suffer from some degree of tearing of the perineum.

After caesarean births women can have pelvic floor dysfunction as much as women who have experienced vaginal births because a lot of the additional strain on the pelvic floor is sustained during pregnancy.

Pelvic floor exercises help to pump blood back to the area and aid healing. Exercise can gradually become more intense. Long-term strength and support will help prevent issues such as stress incontinence and haemorrhoids. Bladder control can be improved (Cardozo & Cuter 1997) and the uterus supported, reducing the incidence of prolapse. Other benefits of strengthening pelvic floor muscles may be to help the mother feel more at ease with that area of her body and help in resuming sex. Sex in turn is good for the pelvic floor.

Abdominal muscles

The recti muscles usually close within a couple of weeks with primaparous women, provided that the separation was less than two fingers. If the mother was pregnant with twins, had a large baby or put on a lot of weight and they separated more, they take longer to close.

It is hard to give a time scale of how quickly this happens. 'Closing' is defined as less than two finger widths separation. For some women the muscles knit back, for others a gap of one finger may remain so that the connective tissue can be felt.

With each subsequent child the muscles separate a little more, take a little longer to 'close' and do not knit back together so much. If the muscles are separated more than four fingers, then extreme care needs to be taken with the exercises and physiotherapist referral may be needed. Initial treatment is usually with ultrasound. If this fails, then surgery may be required with an internal mesh inserted to knit the muscles back.

Remember that the recti muscles are simply the outer layer of the abdominal wall and their closure is only the first stage of healing. The transverse and oblique also need to be strengthened. This may take some time and there is a need for the rest of the mother's life for her to continue to exercise her abdominal muscles, especially if she had a caesarean.

Back problems

One study showed that 14% of women, who had not previously had backache, complained of backache post delivery which lasted more than 6 weeks. This rises to 23% when women who had backache previously were included (Grove 1973).

Two-thirds of these women still had backache 1–9 years later. Reasons are varied but are largely due to postural stresses due to lifting and carrying the baby and household tasks, combined with weak abdominal muscles and pelvic floor. In modern cultures women tend to lift and engage in physical activity too early after delivery.

Epidural anaesthesia during labour has been found to be closely associated with long-term backache (MacArthur et al 1990, Russell et al 1993) except where the epidural was given for elective section.

Arm problems

Often women report feelings of pain and weakness in the arms. Some of this can be due to strains experienced during pregnancy and delivery (MacArthur et al 1993). However, there is an increased incidence of carpal tunnel due to tension caused by carrying and lifting and feeding the baby.

The incidence of pain in the arms has been reported four times as often among the Asian community compared with Caucasian women (MacArthur et al 1993). This could be due to vitamin D deficiency, commonly found among the Asian community in the UK (Brooke et al 1980).

Joints and ligaments

The softened joints and ligaments gradually return to normal, in most cases, over a period of about 3 months, but this is dependent on whether the woman is breastfeeding or not. The skeletal system of parturient women is vulnerable to long-term injury because of the laxity of ligaments resulting from effects of relaxin.

SPD/pelvic girdle instability

This may be caused by labour, especially an instrumental delivery which has used the lithotomy position. Symphysis pubis diastasis (SPD) caused by the pregnancy may persist into the postnatal period.

Headaches

These are experienced fairly frequently. They can be posturally caused, especially holding the baby awkwardly for long periods or feeding and lying awkwardly during the night. They can also be due to stress or the side-effects of epidural anaesthesia.

Implications for bodyworkers on changes in the musculoskeletal system

- These are longer-term changes; key system for support with body work.
- Weakness may become more apparent as the baby gets heavier.
- Postural considerations must involve the baby and awareness of lifting, carrying and feeding and other children especially toddlers.
- Lifestyle issues: due to lack of support in carrying out tasks and emotional support.
- Backache may be due to epidural anaesthesia: care when working where needle was inserted.
- Awareness of caesarean section scar when working the abdomen, weakness or numbness here.
- Awareness of effects of caesarean section on rest of body muscles, e.g. hip pain, leg pain, weak lower back.
- SPD may be caused by birth or by pregnancy.
- Note continued laxity of joints and tissue in breastfeeding women.

3.6 Respiratory system

This returns rapidly to its pre-pregnant state. Full ventilation of the basal lobes of the lungs is possible again since they are no longer compressed by the enlarged uterus. Changes in rib cage elasticity may remain for months after delivery. However, most anatomical changes and ventilation return to normal 1–3 weeks postnatally. The reduction in progesterone restores pre-pregnant sensitivity to carbon dioxide so partial pressures return to pre-pregnancy levels.

Implications for bodyworkers on changes in the respiratory system

Changes are fairly minimal here. Good to encourage continued deep breathing patterns which have hopefully been adopted during pregnancy.

3.7 Renal system, urinary tract, bladder

The kidneys, as key organs for maintaining fluid and electrolyte balance in pregnancy, have to make

major readjustments. Post-delivery there is a redis-
tribution of body fluid and reduction of blood volume and they no longer regulate fetal waste. These
adjustments take place mostly during the first
couple of months and are usually easily accommodated. However, for women with pre-existing kidney
issues, or who developed eclampsia or hypertensive disorders during pregnancy, long-term damage may have been caused to the kidneys. Changes
in the bladder also occur in the postpartum. It may
have been injured during labour and a weakened
pelvic floor may lead to long-term patterns of stress
incontinence.

Urinary tract

There are changes in the hormone levels such as
plasma renin and angiotensin, reversing the sodium
and water retention of pregnancy. There is a rapid
and sustained *natriuresis* (excretion of sodium) and
diuresis (increased urination) after delivery which
lasts about 2–3 days (Davison 1985). Fluid and electrolyte balance is generally returned by 21 days postpartum and often earlier (Hill 1990). The decrease in
oxytocin contributes to diuresis. A normal voiding for
the postpartum woman may be 500–1000 ml, which
is several times greater than normal (Dahlenburg
et al 1980, Malinowski 1978, Paller 1999). Water
may also be lost through night sweats (Blackburn &
Loper 1992).

Renal plasma flow, GFR, plasma creatinine and
BUN (blood urea nitrogen) return to non-pregnant
levels by 2–3 months postpartum (Andriole &
Patterson 1991, Krutzén et al 1992, Lafayette et al
1999, Lindheimer & Katz 1992). Urinary excretion of
calcium phosphate, vitamins and other solutes generally returns to normal by the end of the first week
but hyperfiltration may be maintained for up to
4 weeks due to decreased glomerular oncotic pressure (Christensen et al 1989, Kwee et al 2000). Urinary
glucose excretion returns to non-pregnant patterns
by 1 week and pregnancy-associated proteinuria is
resolved by 6 weeks (Beydoun 1985, Davison 1987,
Rowe et al 1981).

Women with pre-eclampsia may become hyper-
volemic as water accumulated in the interstitial space
returns to the vascular compartment. If the renal
function remains impaired, diuresis may be delayed
and the woman may develop congestive heart failure
or pulmonary oedema. This means that oedema postpartum needs to continue to be monitored seriously.

The dilatation of the urinary tract of pregnancy
resolves and the renal organs gradually return to
their pre-gravid state. For most women they return to
their non-pregnant state by 6 weeks though in some

women they may persist for 12–16 weeks or longer.
The kidneys themselves return to the pre-pregnant
size by 6 months.

Bladder

The decreased tone, oedema and mucosal hyperaemia (blood flow) of the bladder can be aggravated
by prolonged labour, forceps delivery, analgesia or
anaesthesia (Beydoun 1985). Pressure of the fetal
head on the bladder in labour can result in trauma
and transient loss of bladder sensation in the first
few days or weeks postpartum. This can lead to over-
distension of the bladder with incomplete emptying
and an inability to void. Stress incontinence may be
experienced, although it is usually a continuation
of pregnancy issues. After a vaginal delivery there
is decreased urine flow and 1.7–17.9% of women
report urinary retention. It is more common after a
first vaginal delivery, epidural anaesthesia, caesarean section, instrumental delivery, prolonged delivery and catheterisation prior to delivery (Saultz
et al 1991). Retention is also due to the continuing
bladder hypotonia (low muscle tone) after delivery
without the weight of the pregnant uterus to limit its
capacity.

Urinary stress incontinence

It is difficult to determine the exact incidence of this
problem but the Wilson et al (1996) study found that
24% of 1505 women in New Zealand reported stress
incontinence. MacArthur and colleagues (1991a, b)
reported 15% of women had stress incontinence for
the first time after giving birth, persisting for more
than 6 weeks. Over a third of these still had stress
incontinence symptoms a year later but only 10% had
consulted a doctor about this.

Causes

It is probably largely due to pelvic floor innervation
damage sustained at labour and more common after
a longer second stage and delivery of a bigger baby.
It is less common after caesarean but this only applies
for up to two caesareans (MacArthur et al 1991a). It is
likely that pelvic floor exercises, if done properly, will
help (Mørkved & Bø 1996).

Urinary tract infections (UTIs)

These are more common postpartum due to pregnancy-
induced changes in the bladder that may have been
aggravated by delivery. Incomplete voiding will contribute. They are more common after a caesarean and
catheterisation.

Implications for bodyworkers in renal system

- Reassure women of the normality of early changes: increased natriuresis and diuresis, night-time sweats.
- Encourage proper voiding of the bladder.
- Encourage the mother to start or continue pelvic floor exercises on a daily basis to avoid long-term stress incontinence problems.
- Encourage women to drink sufficient liquid, to be aware of the importance of perineal hygiene to reduce UTIs.

Referral issues

- If there is continuing oedema refer to primary care provider, especially women who suffered from pre-eclampsia or hypertension in pregnancy, as it may indicate that there is an on-going problem with the renal system.
- Suspect UTI, refer to primary care provider.

3.8 Other systems: gastrointestinal and hepatic, nervous, immune, sensory, integumentary

Gastrointestinal and hepatic

After birth, with the decline of progesterone, smooth muscle tone gradually improves through the body and the organs can reposition themselves. Constipation may continue to be troublesome for the first few days. This can be due to inactivity and reflex inhibition of defecation by a painful perineum along with some decrease in gastrointestinal (GI) muscle tone and motility. Combined with the relaxation of the abdominal musculature this may result in some gaseous distension 2–3 days postpartum. Bowel movements usually resume 2–3 days after birth with resumption of normal bowel patterns by 8–14 days.

Haemorrhoids are common and some women experience faecal incontinence. Constipation is experienced in 15–20% of cases and is more common after instrumental delivery than vaginal or caesarean (Glazener et al 1995).

Heartburn usually improves quickly and gingivitis often disappears. Gallbladder volume returns to normal by 2 weeks postpartum and its contractility is enhanced. This means that it will expel microgallstones which may have developed during pregnancy (Van Thiel & Schade 1986). Liver enzymes return to non-pregnant levels within 3 weeks (Resnik 1999). The appendix returns to its usual position by 10 days (Steinlauf & Traube 1999).

Women experience varying degrees of weight loss. On average women lose 4.5–5.8 kg (10–13 lb) after birth. Most women steadily lose weight over the next 3–6 months with most weight loss in the first 3 months. Usually lactating women lose more weight. Most women do not lose all of their pregnancy weight gain, with an average retention of 1 kg per pregnancy. Women who are overweight or normal weight are more likely to retain weight (Crowell 1995).

Nutrition

Good nutrition is important to support the body's recovery. It is particularly important if the mother is breastfeeding.

Nervous system

Paraesthesias in the legs, buttocks and lower back have been reported as side-effects of epidural anaesthesia (Kitzinger 1987).

Immune system response

Risk of infection

Women are at increased risk of infection, particularly associated with the genital tract, urinary system, breast and any site of thrombophlebitis. The lochia provides ideal culture conditions for micro-organisms.

Sensory systems

Changes to the eyes resolve. Sensitivity of the cornea returns to normal within 6–8 weeks (Mogil & Friedman 2000, Weinreb et al 1987). Ptosis and subconjunctival haemorrhages disappear spontaneously. Nasal congestion, ear stuffiness and laryngeal changes usually disappear within a few days (Ellegard & Karlsson 1999, Schatz 1998).

Integumentary system

Some of the changes of skin pigmentation and melasma fade but some remain, especially in women with darker skin and hair. After birth, stria gravidarum and spider nevi fade and capillary haemangiomas, varicosities and skin tags regress but may not completely disappear (Chanco Turner 1999, Rapini 1999).

There may be hair loss due to the influence of oestrogen on slowing the rate of hair growth. Most women experience hair loss beginning 4–20 weeks after delivery. Usually complete regrowth occurs by 6–15 months although hair may be less abundant (Schiff & Kern 1963).

Implications for bodyworkers of changes in the gastrointenstinal, hepatic, immune and sensory systems

- Nutrition is of fundamental importance in supporting the postnatal changes.
- Constipation: good diet, abdominal massage.
- Hair loss is common.
- Haemorrhoids: importance of pelvic floor.
- Stretch marks may not disappear.

3.9 Infant feeding

Breastfeeding

Lactogenesis: initiation of lactation

The initiation of lactation involves a complex neuroendocrinal process with the interaction of several hormones. The initial stage begins mid-pregnancy as the mammary glands begin to secrete milk. Only small amounts are secreted due to the inhibition of the placental hormones. The second stage begins at birth and takes about 4 days to complete. After birth, milk protein and lactose synthesis and secretion increase rapidly. The major increase in milk volume is not until 2–3 days postpartum.

The predominant hormone which stimulates milk production is prolactin and this is secreted by the anterior pituitary gland. Levels of prolactin increase during pregnancy. After birth progesterone and oestrogen levels fall abruptly but prolactin levels continue to increase, stimulating milk secretion from the glandular epithelial cells within the breast. Once lactation has begun, it is maintained by the baby suckling.

Oxytocin stimulates the ejection of milk. An increase in the concentration of oxytocin contracts the cells around the alveoli and milk ducts, raising the intra-alveolar pressure that propels milk along the ducts. Its release may be experienced as a tingling sensation in the breast. It also stimulates contraction of the uterus and, during the first few days, after-pains can be worse when breastfeeding. The mother may experience breast engorgement in the first few days, as milk supply is controlled by supply and demand and often there is over-production until the baby regulates their particular milk supply.

Decreased frequency of feeding will decrease milk production. The regulation of the volume is thought to be controlled by milk protein feedback inhibitor (feedback inhibitor of lactation, FIL) which will accumulate if the milk is not completely removed from the breast (Wilde et al 1995). For mothers with pre-term babies, increasing the frequency of breast pumping will help establish the supply.

Galactopoiesis: maintenance of lactation

This is the maintenance of established milk secretion. It is dependent on periodic suckling and removal of milk and on an intact hypothalamic–pituitary axis regulating prolactin and oxytocin levels.

Involution

After ceasing lactation, involution takes about 3 months. Milk secretion is suppressed by the mechanical action of milk accumulating in the alveoli and ducts which causes distension and atropy of the epithelial cells. Gradually the alveolar lumens decrease in size and may disappear and the alveolar lining changes. If breastfeeding is stopped suddenly the process is more intense and painful. Breasts remain larger after lactation as deposits of fat and connective tissue are increased. These changes are different from the breast changes which occur after menopause due to the changes in oestrogen (Coad & Dunstall 2001: 355).

Energy requirements for milk production

It has been estimated that mothers who are lactating need a minimum of an additional 750 kcal a day to support lactation (Lawrence & Lawrence 1999, Worthington Roberts et al 1985). Approximately 900 kcal of energy are required to produce a litre of milk (Dewey 1997). Some of these additional calories come from maternal fat stores. During the first 3 months women use 2–4 kg of body fat stored during pregnancy to provide about 200–300 kcal/day. The rest of the calories need to be made up through their diet (approximately 500 kcal per day).

Human milk

Composition of human milk

Colostrum is the initial substance produced by the alveolar secretory cells. It appears in early second trimester and is produced in the first few days after delivery. It is transparent and derives its yellow colour from its high carotene content. It is higher in protein than mature milk and lower in carbohydrate, fat and calories. A *transitional* form of milk gradually replaces colostrum and this contains large quantities of fat, lactose and calories. Mature *milk* is produced over the first 1–2 weeks and as lactation progresses volume, potassium, lactose and fat content increase whereas protein, secretory IgA, lactoferrin, sodium, carotenoids and chloride content decrease (Kunz et al 1999, Rodriguez Palermo et al 1999).

Human milk optimally fulfils the nutritional requirements of the human neonate. It has a unique composition that is particularly suitable for the rapid growth and development of the infant born with immature digestive, renal and hepatic systems. Unique features of human milk are able to compensate for the under-developed neonatal capability. Human milk contains not only the macronutrients, vitamins and minerals but also non-nutrient growth factors, hormones and protective factors.

Immunological properties of human milk

Human milk has many important immunological properties including leukocytes, immunoglobulins and other proteins (Blackburn 2003: 478). Colostrum is especially rich in these properties.

Human milk may provide protection against infection and the development of allergies in the pre-term infant.

Benefits of breastfeeding

The World Health Organisation recommends 'exclusive breastfeeding for six months with the introduction of complementary food and continued breastfeeding thereafter ' (WHO 2002) due to its wide range of benefits for the baby. There are also many reported benefits for the mother.

Typically as countries have become industrialised breastfeeding rates have declined. For example in Japan the rate of women breast feeding during the first 1–2 months declined from 70.5% in 1960 to 44.8% in 2000 (Maternal and Child Health Statistics of Japan 2001). The length of time that women breastfeed has also declined. In the UK in 2007 the breastfeeding rates were shown to have increased for the first time since the 1970s, rising from 69% in 2000 in women initiating breastfeeding to 76% in 2005 (Department of Health National Infant Feeding Survey). The rate of women initiating breastfeeding had remained fairly static from 65% in 1980 to 68% in 1995 (Foster 1997). This was probably due to a greater awareness of the importance of breastfeeding and more cultural acceptance. In the first 2 weeks 20% of women discontinue breastfeeding, citing several reasons: the baby's failure to suck or rejection of the breast (31%), insufficient milk (29%), and painful breasts (27%). All these difficulties could potentially be overcome with appropriate support. It is often lack of support and other pressures, causing the women to feel tired and wanting a break from the intensity of feeding.

Breastfeeding support groups

The La Leche League is a peer support group which was first introduced in the UK from the USA in the early 1990s. It has given a lot of support to women.

Sure Start has also set up paid peer support groups in the UK (RCM et al 2000). Bodyworkers, even if not specially trained, may be able to offer some degree of support to women, giving them a space to relax, de-stress and talk about their feelings, as well as giving them appropriate relaxation and basic body awareness tools which may support the breastfeeding process. Of course, if these types of interventions prove ineffective, then the bodywork can refer to trained breastfeeding counsellors.

Artificial feeding

Many women choose to artificially feed, perceiving it as more convenient. Breastfeeding demands a commitment to spend significant time with the baby to keep up the supply and demand, especially at certain growth spurt times. The mother needs both emotional and physical support in order to be able to continue to breastfeed.

There are some women who may not be able to breastfeed. Women who are HIV positive in the UK are advised against breastfeeding because there is an increased risk of vertical transmission (Baby Milk Action 2001, RCM & Department of Health 2000). Certain drugs may pass through the breast milk and the mother may be advised not to breastfeed while she is taking those (e.g. antipsychotics, anticarcinogenics or iodides). Smoking reduces the volume of breast milk.

The mother may want to breastfeed but be unable to. For these women the first few weeks of trying and then failing to breastfeed can be difficult emotionally and physically and they may feel guilty about having 'failed'. This can be dependent on many factors. The mother may develop mastitis or simply not feel comfortable or relaxed. She may have lack of support, she may be tired, develop infections, be suffering from depression, or there may be issues with the baby. Each time they feed their newborn they can feel discomfort and so it may start to affect the bonding process.

Important factors in supporting breastfeeding

Early initiation and skin-to-skin contact

UNICEF advises early initial skin-to-skin contact to support early bonding and breastfeeding (UNICEF UK Baby Friendly Initiative 1998a, b). Interestingly a recent Cochrane review of early initiation of breastfeeding showed there is no statistical evidence to suggest the duration of breastfeeding will be shortened if a mother does not feed her baby immediately after the birth (Renfrew et al 1999) but that the mother–infant interaction is beneficial. This can be especially important after a caesarean section and many hospitals do encourage this early infant–mother contact in contrast to the older practice of separating mothers and babies at birth and placing the newborn in a nursery.

Positioning of baby: correct attachment

If the baby is not attached properly this may contribute to difficulties with breastfeeding such as: ineffective milk removal, sore and cracked nipples, obstruction of milk flow, mastitis and infrequent feeding. These are some of the most common causes for women giving up lactating as many of them cause discomfort and even infection as well as a dissatisfied infant.

Elements of good positioning

- Bring the nose to nipple to ensure the rooting reflect is triggered, causing the mouth to gape (RCM 2002).
- Bring the baby to the breast quickly rather than bringing the breast to the baby.
- If the baby is attached correctly there should be no friction of the tongue or gum on the nipple and no movement of the breast tissue.

Problems with feeding

Obstruction of milk flow

This may be caused by a combination of any of the following:

- Blocked duct.
- Compression from tight clothes.
- Holding the breast too tightly while feeding.
- Poor position of baby.
- Restrictive feeding.

Sore/cracked nipples

- The most common cause of sore nipples is incorrect attachment. This is usually because the neonate does not take in enough of the nipple and compresses the end of the nipple against the hard palate. It can cause extreme discomfort for the mother.
- *Candida* infection can also be a cause of sore nipples – this is usually treated by antifungal creams (Amir et al 2002).
- The use of moisture to aid the healing of the nipple in the form of hydrogel, lanolin, paraffin or gauze dressing (Cable et al 1997) is now the treatment of choice. Exposing the breasts to the air and using breast milk may also help.
- A break in the nipple skin increases the risk of mastitis as bacteria enter the breast through the break.

Engorgement

- This is defined as when oedema causes poor milk flow by constricting the milk ducts. It is caused by infrequent, ineffective milk removal and is preventable by good positioning and attachment.
- It is likely to peak around 3–6 days postnatally and may last for 48 hours. The woman is at risk from developing mastitis and subsequent breast abscesses (Aureback 1990).
- Warm flannels or a hot shower or bath help to improve milk flow by increasing blood supply around the alveola. Hand or pump expression will release milk and increase its flow.
- The Cochrane review noted that cabbage leaves or cabbage leaf extract, oxytocin and cold packs had no demonstrable effect (Snowden et al 2002).
- If problems continue then advise medical carer.

Mastitis/abscess

If there is obstruction with milk flow or sore nipples then the mother could develop mastitis or an abscess. This is inflammation of the breast ranging from a localised area to the whole breast. It can include pyrexia, rigors and flu-like symptoms.

There are two types:

1. *Infective*: caused by bacterial invasion usually via a cracked nipple. Staphylococci or streptococci are the most common. These act on the milk forced outside the alveoli into the surrounding cells. There are flu-like signs and symptoms and pyrexia. A reddened area appears around the infected breast or segment and if untreated may give rise to an abscess. Treatment is usually with antibiotics.

2. *Non-infective*: usually caused by milk stasis increasing pressure in the alveoli due to non-removal of milk. When pressure builds up milk is forced out into the surrounding tissues. It is associated with increased levels of stress and blocked ducts in women with other children, restriction from tight clothing and nipple pain (Fetherstone 1998).

Other causes of poor lactation

- Certain *drugs* reduce lactation, including oral contraceptives, as do smoking and alcohol (Horta et al 1997, Mennella 1997).
- *Anaemia*.
- *Breast surgery* where the ducts have been severed, as in breast reduction (Neifert et al 1990), but breast enhancement involving silicone implants does not normally cause nerve and duct damage.
- *Medical disorders* such as hyper- or hypothyroidism.
- *Insufficient milk*. Most of the time it is the woman's perception that she is not producing enough milk, rather than the reality. Woolridge has suggested

that true milk insufficiency occurs in as few as 2% of women (common myths; Woolridge 1995).

- *Drugs and viruses.* These can enter the breast milk although it is not clear how much they affect the infant.
- *Inverted nipples.* Antenatal preparation for inverted nipples is now known to have little bearing on the success of breastfeeding (McCandlish et al 1992) and this has led to a discontinuation of antenatal breast examination. This is a shame since it offered an opportunity for showing the woman how to

examine her breasts and become more comfortable with her anatomy.

3.10 Psychological state and postnatal depression

When we consider the major hormonal changes involved, the effects of birth, adjusting to being a mother with all that entails (sleep deprivation, emotional adjustment, feeding) and recovering from the physical demands of pregnancy, it is not surprising that women tend to experience major emotional changes in the early postnatal period. In many traditional cultures women would be supported and not be expected to engage in normal life as it is recognised that they need time to recover both emotionally and physically. Often what might be described as 'depression' may in fact simply be tiredness. These days, with the emphasis on 'getting back to normal' even within a few days, it is no wonder that many women experience pressure and feel that these emotional changes are in some way abnormal.

For some women the patterns can be more extreme and they may experience longer-term feelings of 'depression'. This could be at a low level or develop into more extreme psychosis. If women develop mental health issues in the postnatal period they are more likely to suffer in later life.

It is now also being recognised that maternal depression has implications for the child. Depressed mothers have less interaction with their babies (Righetti-Veltema 2003). This has been shown to have a longer-lasting impact on the mother/child relationship (Cogill et al 1986).

It is not clear why some women develop depression and others do not but it is likely to be related to many factors such as poor nutrition, housing, lack of sleep, financial, marital or other family pressures, low social support and socioeconomic deprivation (O'Hara & Swain 1996).

It is a matter of some controversy as to which of the hormones is likely to most contribute to depression. Some authors argue it is progesterone (Dalton 1980), others oestrogen (Brace & McCauley 1997) while others that it is cortisol and endorphins (Harris et al 1996). The reality is that it is likely to be the complex interplay between them all. Some authors suggest that breastfeeding isolates the mother and affects cortisol levels, but oxytocin seems more likely to promote well-being. It is our culture which tends to isolate breastfeeding mothers and not give them enough support. Exercise has been found to decrease depression (Koltyn & Schultes 1997).

Implications for bodyworkers for supporting women in their feeding choices

Supporting breastfeeding

- Correct position: baby is brought to the breast and there is no movement of breast tissue while feeding.

Be aware of the basic factors which may inhibit breastfeeding:

- Obstruction of milk flow and infrequent feeding.
- Compression from clothes, tight feeding.

Encouraging relaxation while feeding may be helpful. Offer safe space to explore physical relaxation with baby and to express feelings, but be aware of limitations.

Breastfeeding support

- Advise comfort and massage measures re engorgement.
- Be aware of the importance of nutrition for breastfeeding mothers.
- Think of the many issues involved in supporting women to breastfeed and be able to support appropriately, especially with regard to posture and relaxation.

Supporting women who have to stop breastfeeding

- Allow woman space to explore her feelings.
- Explore other ways of bonding with her child.
- Be aware of guilt issues.
- Be sensitive to different cultural realities of each mother and do not impose view.

Referral issues

- If basic support re positioning and relaxation does not help refer to breastfeeding advisor.
- If there is infection, refer to primary caregiver.

Patterns of emotional adjustment in the postnatal period

1. 'Baby blues' – 'normal'; affects most women in some way, even if just being more emotionally sensitive.
2. Depression – longer-term effects with more cause for concern; affects around 10–15% of women.
3. Puerperal psychosis – serious psychosis; affects a small number of women (2–3 per 1000 births).

Normal patterns of emotional adjustment postnatally

0–3 days The woman is often in a state of euphoria, restlessness, excitement due to the rise of adrenal hormones and oxytocin. She may not take enough rest in the day or sleep well enough at night, especially as her newborn is likely to be in unsettled sleeping patterns. As she feels so well, she may minimise the effects of birth and do too much, e.g. pop out to do some shopping, collect other children from school.

The bodyworker can advise the mother to rest and not to take over domestic tasks too soon. For the first week at least the mother should try to get some help for family tasks so that she can just focus on being with the baby and recovering. In the Netherlands home help is provided for the first 10 days (De Vries et al 2001).

3–10 days 'Blues' may occur anytime between day 3 and day 10. Although sometimes called the 'third day blues' they most likely happen on day 5. It is a normal reaction to birth and affects 70–80% of all mothers. It is the 'low' after the 'high' of birth and reflects the changes in hormones but it also coincides with the milk coming in for breastfeeding mothers, breast engorgement, perineal pain and wound discomfort. The mother is likely to feel tearful and sensitive and the blues are described as a transient, self-limiting condition with no known serious after-effect (Kumar 1985). Although most women recover from the blues in a day or two it is thought that a serious episode may be an important predictor of postnatal depression (Cox 1986, Cox et al 1982). Postnatal depression is a serious condition that may last for months or even years.

Post 10 days For much of the first year the woman may feel quite emotional due to the new demands of caring for a baby, feeding, altered and often insufficient sleep, fatigue. She may also be juggling work with caring for her baby.

The bodyworker can reassure the mother that this emotionally sensitive time is part of a 'normal' adjustment. However, if the mother feels emotional for longer it is important to ensure that she has the appropriate support.

Depression

As many as 16% of women suffer from some form of postnatal mental illness (O'Hara & Swain 1996, Romito 1990).

Signs of severe postnatal depression

- Depressed mood.
- Sleep disturbance not related to discomfort and infant wakening.
- Unable to cope – feelings of guilt or failure.
- Thoughts of harming self or baby, including suicide.
- Rejection of baby.
- Altered libido.
- Anxiety.
- Loss of energy and enjoyment.
- Lack of interest.
- Impaired concentration.

Puerperal psychosis

A small number of women (2–3 per 1000 births) develop a more serious mental illness which is known as puerperal psychosis. This term covers a group of illnesses which are characterised by delusions, hallucinations and an impaired perception of reality. Conventional treatment is to give sedatives, phenothiazines or butyrophenones for a few days and then to continue with either electroconvulsive therapy (ECT) or antidepressants.

The causes of this extreme depression are numerous but one factor may be the major changes in the levels of steroid hormones, especially the drop in oestrogen. It is thought that high-risk women develop a hypersensitivity of the central D2 receptors and this may be related to the effect of the drop in the oestrogen levels

---

Summary of implications of emotional changes for body workers

- Be aware that many women will experience emotional mood swings in the first few weeks postnatally.
- Reassure that these changes are 'normal' but be alert to signs of this developing into more extreme psychosis and refer accordingly.
- Learn the signs of severe postnatal depression listed as above.

Referral issues

- Refer if concerned that mother is showing signs of more extreme depression.

on the dopamine system. Another theory is that it is related to the drop in progesterone which occurs after delivery. Nearly one third of women who develop puerperal psychosis will develop another manic depressive illness at some later stage in their life.

These women are at risk of harming both themselves and their baby. This is an extreme condition and appropriate medical support must be sought.

3.11 Summary and implications

Infection

The risk of infection is high in the early postnatal period. The bodyworker needs to be alert to this possibility and refer. Conventional medical treatment is antibiotics but these can be transferred to the infant. Prevention is better, and good health care, cleanliness and good nutrition are of fundamental importance in the early postnatal period.

Causes of infection include changes in many systems:

- Genital tract.
- Urinary system.
- Breast.
- Site of thrombosis.
- Placental wound site.
- Lacerations and incisions of the perineum.
- Lochia provide ideal culture conditions for micro-organisms.

Other preconditions include:

- Anaemia.
- Fatigue.
- Malnutrition.
- Traumatic delivery.
- Presence of retained tissue in the uterus.

Tiredness

This can be due to: lack of sleep, anaemia, inadequate nutrition, stress.

Effects of birth

The type of birth a woman has, especially if it is not the one she wanted, will have an effect on her recovery.

Long-term patterns of good or poor health established

This is a vital period for establishing long-term health patterns for both mother and infant. Breastfeeding is an ideal way of supporting this, but respect needs to be shown for a mother who chooses otherwise. Bodywork can play a crucial role in this early period.

Reflective questions

Q. What changes are the most important in the early postnatal period and how can we support them?

Q. What affects the emotional well-being of the mother in the postnatal period?

Q. How can we best support the postnatal mother in establishing long-term patterns of good health?

References and further reading

Amir, R., Liu, C.N., Kocsis, J.D., et al., 2002. Oscillatory mechanism in primary sensory neurones. Brain 125 (2), 421–435.

Andriole, V.T., Patterson, T.F., 1991. Epidemiology, natural history and management of urinary tract infections in pregnancy. Med. Clin. North Am. 75 (2), 359–373.

Aureback, K.G., 1990. Breastfeeding fallacies: their relationship to understanding lactation. Birth 17 (1), 44–49.

Baby Milk Action., 2001. HIV and Infant Feeding – Issue Paper. Baby Milk Action, Cambridge.

Beydoun, S.N., 1985. Morphologic changes in renal tract in pregnancy. Clin. Obstet. Gynecol. 28 (2), 249–256.

Blackburn, S.T., 2003. Maternal, Fetal and Neonatal Physiology: A Clinical Perspective. WB Saunders, St Louis, MO.

Blackburn, S.T., Loper, D.L., 1992. Maternal, Fetal and Neonatal Physiology: A Clinical Perspective. WB Saunders, Philadelphia.

Brace, M., McCauley, E., 1997. Oestrogens and psychological well being. Annals of Medicine 29 (4), 283–290.

Brooke, O.G., Brown, I.R., Bond, C.D., et al., 1980. Vitamin D supplements in pregnant Asian women: effects on calcium status and fetal growth. Br. Med. J. 280 (6216), 751–754.

Brown, S., Lumley, J., 1998. Maternal health after childbirth: results of an Australian population based survey. Br. J. Obstet. Gynaecol. 105, 156–161.

Brown, S., Lumley, J., 2000. Physical health problems after childbirth and maternal depression at six to seven months postpartum. Br. J. Obstet. Gynaecol. 107, 1194–1201.

Cable, B., Steward, M., Davis, J., 1997. Nipple wound care: a new approach to an old problem. J. Hum. Lact. 13 (4), 313–318.

Cardozo, L., Cuter, A., 1997. Lower urinary tract symptoms in pregnancy. Br. J. Urol. 80, 14.

Carroli, G., Belizan, J., 2001. Episiotomy for Vaginal Birth. Cochrane Review, Cochrane Library Issue 4. Update software, Oxford.

CEMACH, 2006. [Perinatal mortality reports. Confidential enquiries into maternal deaths in the UK; most up-to-date figures for maternal and fetal deaths.] www.dh.gov.uk

Chanco Turner, M.L., 1999. The skin in pregnancy. In: Burrow, G.N., Duffy, T.P. (Eds.) Medical complications in pregnancy, fifth ed. WB Saunders, Philadelphia.

Cheng, C.Y., Fowles, E.R., Walker, L.O., 2006. Continuing education module: postpartum maternal health care in the United States: a critical review. J. Perinat. Educ. 15 (3), 34–42.

Chesley, L.C., 1972. Plasma and red blood cell volumes during pregnancy. Am. J. Obstet. Gynecol. 112 (3), 440–450.

Christensen, T., Klebe, J.G., Bertelsen, V., et al., 1989. Changes in renal volume during normal pregnancy. Acta Obstet. Gynecol. Scand. 68 (6), 541–543.

Clapp, J.F., Capeless, E., 1997. Cardiovascular function before, during and after the first and subsequent pregnancies. Am. J. Cardiol. 80 (11), 1469–1473.

Coad, J., Dunstall, M., 2001. Anatomy and Physiology for Midwives. Mosby, Edinburgh.

Cogill, S., Caplan, H.L., Alexandra, H., et al., 1986. Impact of maternal postnatal depression on cognitive development of young children. Br. Med. J. 292, 1165–1167.

Cox, J.L., 1986. Postnatal Depression: A Guide for Health Professionals. Churchill Livingstone, Edinburgh.

Cox, R.A., Arnold, D.R., Cook, D., et al., 1982. HLA phenotypes in Mexican Americans with tuberculosis. Am. Rev. Respir. Dis. 126 (4), 653–655.

Crowell, D.T., 1995. Weight change in the postpartum period: a review of the literature. J. Nurse–Midwifery 40 (5), 418–423.

Dahlenburg, G.W., Burnell, R.H., Braybrook, R., 1980. The relation between cord serum sodium levels in newborn infant and maternal intravenous therapy during labour. Br. J. Obstet. Gynaecol. 87 (6), 519–522.

Dalton, K., 1980. Depression after Childbirth. Oxford University Press, Oxford.

Davison, J.M., 1985. The physiology of the renal tract in pregnancy. Clin. Obstet. Gynecol. 28 (2), 257–265.

Davison, J.M., 1987. Kidney function in pregnant women. Am. J. Kidney Dis. 9 (4), 248–252.

De Vries, R., Benoit, C., van Teijlingen, E. (Eds.), et al., 2001. Birth by Design: Pregnancy, Maternity Care, and Midwifery in North America and Europe. Routledge, New York.

Declercq, E.R., Sakala, C., Corry, M.P., et al., 2002. Listening to Mothers: Report of the First National U.S. Survey of Women's Childbearing Experiences. Maternity Center Association, New York.

Dewey, K.G., 1997. Energy and protein requirements during lactation. Annu. Rev. Nutr. 17, 19–36.

Dooley, M., 1984. MMS Thesis NUI thesis. A study incorporating salivary progesterone measurement in monitoring the treatment of premenstrual syndrome with oral micronized progesterone.

Ellegard, E., Karlsson, G., 1999. Nasal congestion during pregnancy. Clin. Otolaryngol. 24, 307.

Fetherstone, C., 1998. Risk factors for lactation mastitis. J. Hum. Lact. 14 (2), 101–109.

Foster, K., 1997. Infant Feeding 1995: A Survey of Infant Feeding Practices in the United Kingdom. Stationery Office, London.

Glazener, C., Abdalla, M., Rusell, I., et al., 1993. Postnatal care: a survey of patients' experiences. Br. J. Midwifery 1, 67–74.

Glazener, C.M., Abdalla, M., Stroud, P., et al., 1995. Postnatal maternal morbidity: extent, causes, prevention and treatment. Br. J. Obstet. Gynaecol. 102 (4), 282–287.

Gray, R.H., Campbell, O.M., Zacur, H.A., et al., 1987. Postpartum return of ovarian activity in non-breastfeeding women monitored by urinary assays. J. Clin. Endocrinol. Metab. 64 (4), 645–650.

Grove, L.H., 1973. Backache, headache and bladder dysfunction after delivery. Br. J. Anaesth. 45 (11), 1147–1149.

Harris, B., Lovett, L., Smith, J., et al., 1996. Cardiff puerperal mood and hormone study III: postnatal depression at 5 to 6 weeks postpartum, and its hormonal correlates across the peripartum period. Br. J. Psychol. 168 (6), 739–744.

Hathway, W.E., Bonnar, J., 1987. Hemostatic Disorders of the Pregnant Woman and Newborn Infant. Elsevier, New York, chapter 1.

Hill, L.L., 1990. Body composition, normal electrolyte concentrations and the maintenance of normal volume, tonicity, and acid-base metabolism. Pediatr. Clin. North. Am. 37 (2), 241–256.

Horta, B.L., Victora, C.S., Menezes, A.M., et al., 1997. Environmental tobacco smoke and the breastfeeding duration. Am. J. Epidemiol. 146, 128–133.

Howie, P.W., 1995. The physiology of the puerperium and lactation. In: Chamberlain, G. (Ed.), Turnbull's Obstetrics, second ed. Churchill Livingstone, Edinburgh, p. 749.

Howie, P.W., McNeilly, A.S., 1982. Effect of breastfeeding patterns on human birth intervals. J. Reprod. Fertil. 65 (2), 545–557.

Johnston, J.M., Amico, J.A., 1986. A prospective longitudinal study of the release of oxytocin and prolactin in response to infant sucking in long term lactation. J. Clin. Endocrinol. Metab. 62, 653–657.

Kahn, R.S., Zuckerman, B., Bauchner, H., et al., 2002. Women's health after pregnancy and child outcomes at age 3 years: a prospective cohort study. Am. J. Public Health 92 (8), 1312–1318.

Kamerman, S.B., Kahn, A.J., 1993. Home health visiting in Europe. Future Child 3, 39–52.

Kilpatrick, S.J., Laros, R.K., 1999. Maternal hematologic disorders. In: Creasy, R.W., Resnik, R. (Eds.), Maternal Fetal Medicine, fourth ed. WB Saunders, Philadelphia.

Kitzinger, S., 1987. Some Women's Experiences of Epidurals: A Descriptive Study. National Childbirth Trust, London.

Koltyn, K.F., Schultes, S.S., 1997. Psychological effects of an aerobic exercise session and a rest session following pregnancy. J. Sports Med. Phys. Fit. 37 (4), 287–291.

Krutzén, E., Olofsson, P., Bäck, S.E., et al., 1992. Glomerular filtration rate in pregnancy: a study in normal subjects and in patients with hypertension, pre-eclampsia and diabetes. Scand. J. Clin. Lab. Invest. 52, 387–392.

Kumar, R., 1985. Pregnancy, childbirth and mental illness. Prog. Obstet. Gynaecol. 5, 146–159.

Kunz, C., Rodriguez-Palmero, M., Koletzko, B., et al., 1999. Nutritional and biochemical properties of human milk, part 1; general aspects, proteins and carbohydrate. Clin. Perinatol. 26, 307.

Kwee, A., Graziosi, G.C., Schagen van Leeuwen, J.H., et al., 2000. The effect of immersion on haemodynamic and fetal measures in uncomplicated pregnancies of nulliparous women. Br. J. Obstet. Gynaecol. 107, 663–668.

Lafayette, R.A., Malik, T., Druzin, M., et al., 1999. The dynamics of glomerular filtration after Caesarean section. J. Am. Soc. Nephrol. 10 (7), 156–1565.

Lawrence, R.A., Lawrence, R.M., 1999. Breastfeeding: A Guide for the Medical Profession, fifth ed. Mosby, St Louis.

Lee, D.T., Yip, A.S., Leung, T.Y., et al., 2004. Ethnoepidemiology of postnatal depression: prospective multivariate study of sociocultural risk factors in a Chinese population in Hong Kong. Br. J. Psychiatry 184, 34–40.

Lindheimer, M.D., Katz, A.I., 1992. Renal physiology and disease in pregnancy. In: Seldin, D.W., Geibisch, G. (Eds.), The Kidney: Physiology and Pathophysiology, second ed. Raven, New York.

Liu, J.H., Yen, S.S.C., 1989. Endocrinology of the postpartum state. In: Brody, S.A., Ueland, K. (Eds.), Endocrine Disorders in Pregnancy. Appleton and Lange, Norwalk, CT, p. 161.

MacArthur, C., Lewis, M., Knox, E.G., et al., 1990. Epidural anaesthesia and long term backache following childbirth. Br. Med. J. 301, 9–12.

MacArthur, C., Lewis, M., Knox, E.G., 1991a. Health After Childbirth. HMSO, London.

MacArthur, C., Lewis, M., Knox, E.G., 1991b. Health after childbirth. Br. J. Obstet. Gynaecol. 98 (12), 1193–1195.

MacArthur, C., Lewis, M., Knox, E.G., 1993. Comparison of long term health problems following childbirth in Asian and Caucasian women. Br. J. Gen. Pract. 43, 519–522.

McCandlish, I.A., Cornwell, H.J., Thompson, H., et al., 1992. Distemper encephalitis in pups after vaccination of the dam. Vet. Rec. 130, 27–30.

Malinowski, J., 1978. Bladder assessment in the postpartum patient. JOGN Nurs. 7 (4), 14–16.

Maternal and Child Health Statistics of Japan, 2001. Decline of Breastfeeding in Japan. Maternal and Child Health Statistics of Japan, Tokyo.

Mennella, J.A., 1997. Infants' suckling responses to the flavor of alcohol in mother's milk. Alcholism. Clin. Exp. Res. 21, 581–585.

Mogil, L.G., Friedman, A.H., 2000. Ocular complications of pregnancy. In: Cohen, W.R., Cherry, S.H., Merkatz, I.R. (Eds.), Cherry and Merkatz Complications of Pregnancy, fifth ed. Lippincott Williams & Wilkins, Philadelphia.

Monheit, A.G., Cousins, L., Resnick, R., 1980. The puerperium: anatomic and physiologic readjustments. Clin. Obstet. Gynecol. 23 (4), 973–984.

Mørkved, S., Bø, K., 1996. The effect of post-natal exercises to strengthen the pelvic floor muscles. Acta Obstet. Gynecol. Scand. 75, 382–385.

Neifert, M., DeMarzo, S., Seacat, J., et al., 1990. The influence of breast surgery, breast appearance, and pregnancy-induced breast changes on lactation sufficiency as measured by infant weight gain. Birth 17, 31–38.

Neville, M.C., Neifert, M.R., 1983. Lactation; Physiology Nutrition and Breastfeeding. Plenum Press, New York.

Nissen, E., Uvnäs-Moberg, K., Svensson, K., et al., 1996. Different patterns of oxytocin, prolactin but not cortisol release during breastfeeding in women delivered by caesarean section or by the vaginal route. Early Hum. Dev. 45 (1–2), 103–118.

Odent, M., 2001. The Scientification of Love, revised ed. Free Association Books, London.

O'Hara, M.H., Swain, A.M., 1996. Rates and risk of postpartum depression – a meta analysis. Int. Rev. Psychol. 8, 37–54.

Paller, M.S., 1999. Renal diseases. In: Burrow, G.N., Duffy, T.B. (Eds.), Medical Complications During Pregnancy, fifth ed. WB Saunders, Philadelphia.

Pederson, C.A., Caldwell, J.D., Jirikowski, G.F. (Eds.), et al., 1992. Oxytocin in Maternal, Sexual, and Social Behaviors, vol. 652. New York Academy of Sciences, New York, pp. 70–82.

Pritchard, J.A., Baldwin, R.M., Dickey, J.C., et al., 1962. Blood volume changes in pregnancy and the puerperium. II: Red blood cell loss and changes in apparent blood volume during and following vaginal delivery, caesarean section and cesarean section plus total hysterectomy. Am. J. Obstet. Gynecol. 84 (10), 1271–1282.

Rapini, R.P., 1999. The skin and pregnancy. In: Creasy, R.K., Resnick, R. (Eds.), Maternal Fetal Medicine, fourth ed. WB Saunders, Philadelphia.

Renfrew, M.J., Lang, S., Martin, L., et al., 1999. Interventions for influencing sleep patterns in exclusively breast fed infants. Cochrane Review, Cochrane Library (2), CD000113.

Resnik, R., 1999. The puerperium. In: Creasy, R.K., Resnik, R. (Eds.), Maternal Fetal Medicine, fourth ed. WB Saunders, Philadelphia.

Righetti-Veltema, M., Bousquet, A., Manzano, J., 2003. Impact of postpartum depressive symptoms on mother and her 18-month-old infant. Eur. Child. Adolesc. Psychiatry. 12 (2), 75–83.

Rodriguez-Palmero, M., Koletzko, B., Kunz, C., et al., 1999. Nutritional and biochemical properties of human milk. II: Lipids micronutrients, and bioactive factors. Clin. Perinatol. 26, 335–359.

Rogers, I.S., 1997. Lactation and fertility. Early Hum. Dev. 49 (Suppl), S185–S190.

Romito, P., 1990. Postpartum depression and the experience of motherhood. Acta Obstet. Gynecol. Scand. 69 (154), 7–19.

Rowe, J.W., Brown, R.S., Epstein, F.H., 1981. Physiology of the kidney in pregnancy. In: Freed, S.Z., Hersig, N. (Eds.) Urology in Pregnancy. Williams & Wilkins, Baltimore.

Royal College of Midwives (RCM), Position paper 25: home birth 2002. RCM Midwives J. 5 (1), 26–29.

Royal College of Midwives, Department of Health, 2000 HIV and infant feeding. Report of a seminar, 30 June 2000. RCM, London.

Royal College of Midwives (RCM), National Childbirth Trust, Royal College of Nursing, 2000 Barriers to breastfeeding. Conference report. Department of Health, London.

Russell, R., Groves, P., Taub, N., et al., 1993. Assessing long term back ache after childbirth. Br. Med. J. 306, 1299–1303.

Saultz, J.W., Toffler, W.L., Shackles, J.Y., 1991. Postpartum urinary retention. J. Am. Board Fam. Pract. 4 (5), 341–344.

Saurel-Cubizolles, M.J., Romito, P., Lelong, N., et al., 2000. Women's health after childbirth: a longitudinal study in France and Italy. Br. J. Obstet. Gynecol. 107 (10), 1202–1209.

Saving Mothers 2003–5 Online. Available at: <http://www.cemach.org.uk/Publications.aspx (accessed 29.03.09)

Schatz, M., 1998. Special considerations for the pregnant woman and senior citizen with airway disease. J. Allergy Clin. Immunol. 101 (2/2), 5373.

Schiff, B.L., Kern, A.B., 1963. Study of postpartum alopecia. Arch. Dermatol. 87, 609–611.

Schneider, V., 2000. Infant Massage: A Handbook for Loving Parents. Bantam, New York.

Snowden, H.M., Renfrew, M.J., Woolridge, M.W., 2002. Treatments for Breast Engorgement During Lactation. Cochrane Library, Issue 1. Update software, Oxford.

Steinlauf, A.F., Traube, M., 1999. Gastrointestinal complications. In: Burrow, G.N., Duffy, T.P. (Eds.), Medical Complications During Pregnancy, fifth ed. WB Saunders, Philadelphia.

Tulchinsky, D., 1994. Postpartum lactation and resumption of reproductive function. In: Tulchinsky, D., Little, B. (Eds.), Maternal Fetal Endocrinology. WB Saunders, Philadelphia, PA, pp. 172–191.

UNICEF UK Baby Friendly Initiative, 1998a. Implementing the 10 Steps to Successful Breastfeeding: A Guide for UK Maternity Services Providers Working Towards Baby Friendly Accreditation. UNICEF UK BFI, London.

UNICEF UK Baby Friendly Initiative, 1998b. Breastfeeding your Baby. UNICEF UK BFI, London.

United Kingdom Central Council for Nursing, Midwifery and Health Visiting (UKCC), 1998. Midwives Rules and Code of Practice. UKCC, London.

Uvnäs-Moberg, K., 2003. The Oxytocin Factor. Da Capo Press, Cambridge, MA.

Van Thiel, D.H., Schade, R.R., 1986. Pregnancy: its physiologic course, nutrient cost and effects on gastrointestinal function. In: Rustgi, V.K., Cooper, J.N. (Eds.), Gastrointestinal and Heptatic Complications in Pregnancy. John Wiley, New York.

Walker, P., 2000. Baby Massage for Beginners. Carroll and Brown, London.

Walker, L.O., Wilging, S., 2000. Rediscovering the 'M' in 'MCH': maternal health promotion after childbirth. J Obstet. Gynecol. Neonatal Nurs. 29 (3), 229–236.

Weiner, C.P., 1985. Diagnosis and management of thromboembolic disease during pregnancy. Clin. Obstet. Gynaecol. 28, 107–117.

Weinreb, R.M., Lu, A., Key, T., 1987. Maternal ocular adaptations during pregnancy. Obstet. Gynecol. Surv. 42, 471.

Wilde, C.J., Addey, C.V., Boddy, L.M., et al., 1995. Autocrine regulation of milk secretion by a protein in milk. Biochem. J. 305 (1), 51–58.

Wilson, P.D., Herbison, R.M., Herbison, G.P., 1996. Obstetric practice and the prevalence of urinary incontinence three months after delivery. Br. J. Obstet. Gynaecol. 103 (2), 154–161.

Woolridge, M.W., 1995. Breastfeeding: physiology into practice. In: Davies, D.P. (Ed.), Nutrition in the Normal Infant: Nutrition in Child Health. Royal College of Physicians, London, ch 2, pp. 13–30.

World Health Organisation (WHO), 1998. Report from WHO Consultation on the Needs of Women and their new born During Postpartum Period. WHO, Geneva.

World Health Organisation (WHO), 2002. Infant and Young Child Nutrition: Global Strategy on Infant and Young Child Feeding. Fifty-fifth World Assembly A55/15 16th April, Geneva.

Worthington-Roberts, B.S., Vermeersch, J., Williams, S.R., 1985. Nutrition During Pregnancy and Lactation. Mosby, St Louis.

CHAPTER 4

Introduction to the eastern approach

Chapter contents

Introduction

The body is a dynamic energy field – it is constantly changing, not static.

Eastern terms

- Blood – nutritive energy; blood flows in blood vessels but also in meridians and vessels.
- Extraordinary Vessels – core meridians which regulate Jing and Qi.
- Jing/Essence – fluid-like substance which is the source of life. The most dense material manifestation of Qi.
- Meridians – energy pathways in the body which circulate Qi and organ energy.
- Qi – invisible energy in the body, creative principle, life's animating force.
- Shen – the spirit of a person.
- Tao – the whole.
- Tsubos – points along the meridians.
- Yin and Yang – the two main forces in the universe:
  - Yin – earth, night, more inward moving, resting/ forming, contraction
  - Yang – heaven, day, more outward moving, active/transforming, expansion.

Refer to the many texts on Chinese medicine, including Suzanne Yates's *Shiatsu for Midwives* (2003), for more detail on key concepts. As many texts, especially bodywork ones, do not consider the Extraordinary Vessels in detail and as they are so fundamental to the maternity period, we are going to describe them here.

4.1 Key theoretical concepts in eastern bodywork, including the importance of the Extraordinary Vessels in maternity care

Qi

There are different forms of Qi.

1. Original Qi: this is the ancestral Qi, transmitted by the parents at the time of conception. This fits in with knowledge of how the health of the parents has long-term effects on the health of the child.

2. Yuan Qi: endowment of primordial Yin and Yang and comes from Jing. It is the representation of heaven and earth imprinted on to Jing at the time of conception. Yuan Yang is similar to Shen and Yuan Yin is similar to Jing.

3. Air Qi: this comes from the breath. Exercise, massage and shiatsu all promote the development of good breathing, which is important for relaxation and good health of both mother and child.

4. Food Qi: this comes from food and drink. Diet has long been recognised as important and recent research has shown that poor diet in pregnancy does not just affect a baby at birth, but affects organs and body systems for the rest of the baby's life. We are now finally trying to understand why some bodies are built like Rolls Royces and others like cheap cars.

Essence: Jing

This is the substance that underlies all organic life and is the source of organic change. It is thought of as fluid-like; it is supportive and nutritive, and is the basis for growth and development including sexual maturation, conception and pregnancy. It is on the edge between energy and matter. It is stored in the

Kidneys and is circulated through the body in the Extraordinary Vessels. It is important throughout the maternity period.

It does not change quickly as it flows in long cycles – 8 years for men and 7 years for women. It comes from two sources: the 'Pre-Heaven Essence' and the 'Post-Heaven Essence'. The blending of the sexual energies of the man and the woman at the time of conception form the 'Pre-Heaven Essence' of the baby. This Essence then nourishes the baby through the pregnancy. It is dependent on nourishment derived from the mother's Kidneys. It determines each person's basic constitutional energy. It is 'fixed' in quantity and its quality can only be affected within certain limits, but good exercise and bodywork, a good balanced lifestyle without excessive work, and breathing will all have a positive effect on it.

The 'Post-Heaven Essence' comes from food. Since Essence flows in such long cycles, changing diet just before conception will not have much of an effect on the Essence, although it will affect the Qi. It is longer-term health patterns which effect the Essence. Since the Essence is drawn upon in pregnancy, some schools of eastern thought say that the mother should wait 5–7 years between children, to allow the Essence to renew.

Qi and Essence are mutually dependent: Qi emerges out of Essence since prenatal Essence is the source of life. Qi helps transform food into postnatal Essence, maintaining and expanding that life. The better Qi a person has, the less they need to draw upon their Essence. Qi is more Yang and Essence is more Yin.

The meridian pathways

Both Qi and Essence flow through the body along meridian pathways which contain important points known as 'tsubos'. The 12 main meridians in the body are divided into Yin/Yang pairs and they circulate Qi on a day-to-day basis. The eight Extraordinary Vessels, most of which share points of other meridians, formed first and are overall regulators of energy, including Jing. Four of these Extraordinary Vessels are of particular importance in the maternity period. These are the Conception Vessel (Ren Mai), the Governing Vessel (Du Mai) the Penetrating Vessel (Chong Mai) and the Girdle Vessel (Dai Mai). The other four – Yin and Yang Ankle (Yin and Yang Qiao) and Yin and Yang Linking (Yin and Yang Wei) – also have some relevance.

The Extraordinary Vessels in maternity care

These circulate the Essence, and are linked with Kidney energy. They represent a level of treatment at the constitutional energy, tapping into both the Jing (Essence) and Yuan Qi (Original Qi). They are about sexual energy, how we maintain and contain our lineage, how we adapt to our environment and the unfolding of cycles of life. They are the link between the Pre-Heaven and the Post-Heaven Qi. In writing about them I have drawn upon my own experience and the writings of Maciocia (2006), Low (1983) and Yuen (2005).

They relate to:

- The brain and spinal cord and hormonal control.
- The skeletal system.
- The genitalia.
- The circulatory system and formation of blood cells.
- The hepatic and circulatory system (Low 1983: 145).

Reservoirs

They act as a reservoir for the other 12 meridians in the body which are considered to be like the streams flowing from the main reservoir. In times of shock, or major change, they can either send out more energy to the meridian network or absorb energy from it. This is a particularly relevant aspect in the maternity period. They link the 12 primary channels.

- Governing Vessel (GV) (Du Mai) links all the Yang channels at GV 14.
- Conception Vessel (CV) (Ren Mai) links all the Yin channels.
- Penetrating Vessel (Chong Mai) links Stomach and Kidney and strengthens the link between CV and GV.
- Girdle Vessel (GDV) (Dai Mai) binds the 12 primary channels PV and CV and especially LV, KD and SP.
- Yin Heel (Yin Qiao) connects Kidney and Bladder and promotes quietness.
- Yang Heel (Yang Qiao) connects Bladder, Gall Bladder, Small Intestine, Large Intestine and Stomach channels and promotes activity.
- Yin Linking (Yin Wei) connects Spleen, Kidney and Liver and Conception Vessel and dominates the interior of the body.
- Yang Linking (Yang Wei) connects Bladder, Gall Bladder, Three Burners, Small Intestine, Stomach and GV and dominates the exterior of the body.

Protecting the body

Conception, Penetrating and Governing Vessels circulate defensive Qi over the chest, abdomen and back. They help protect the body from exterior pathogenic factors.

Link with curious organs

They have a link with the extraordinary organs; of particular relevance in maternity work is the link between the Brain and the Uterus. The Gall Bladder provides a link with the 12 organs.

Hormonal and nervous system control

This is postulated by Low (1983), and I tend to agree that they have a profound effect on these systems. He suggests:

- Hormonal: Yang and Yin Ankle and Girdle and Penetrating Vessel.
- Nervous: Du, Ren, Yang and Yin Linking.

There are eight Extraordinary Vessels. Different authors postulate different theories about their order. Everyone agrees that Chong, Ren and Du are the fundamental circuit. Many say Du and Ren are the first to form with Chong third. Jeffrey Yuen talks about them flowing in a sequence beginning with the Chong, the Ren and then the Du, flowing into the Yin Wei and Yang Wei and then the Yin Qiao and Yang Qiao and finally into the Dai Mai (Yuen 2005).

Energetic dynamics of the Extraordinary Vessels (Fig. 4.1)

- Governing, Conception (Directing) and Penetrating Vessels; three branches with the same origin from the space between the Kidneys.

- Penetrating Vessel; centre of vortex.
- Governing and Conception Vessels define back and front.
- Yin and Yang Ankle Vessels; define Left and Right (of Yin and Yang).
- Yin and Yang Linking Vessels; define interior and exterior.
- Girdle Vessel: defines above and below.

Basic fundamental circuit: first ancestry (Yuen 2005)

The Conception Vessel, the Governing Vessel and Penetrating Vessel

These meridians are the reservoirs of energy for the other 12 meridians. They form the basic cellular energy of the body and are the first meridians to develop in the fetus. Essentially they form one circuit, connect the Uterus with the Kidneys, Heart and Brain, and from a western perspective represent the hypothalamus–pituitary–ovarian axis which is responsible for ovulation. Both meet on head at GV 20 –100 points of meeting.

They originate from deep within the body and pass through the kidneys and then the uterus in women. They all emerge on the perineum, at CV1. The Governing Vessel runs up the centre of the spine, up the neck, over the top of the head and down towards the mouth, where it then goes inside the body, back to

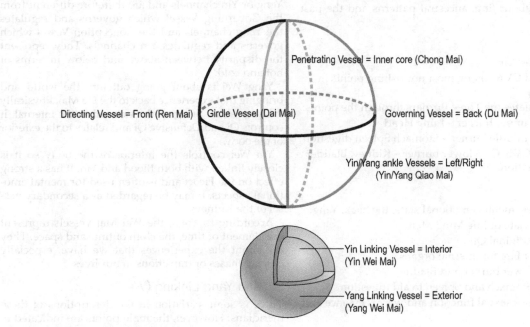

Fig. 4.1 Vortex of Extraordinary Vessels.

the kidneys. The Conception Vessel runs up the centre of the front of the body, to the mouth, where it then goes down inside back to the kidneys. The Penetrating Vessel runs up the front of the body half a thumb-width lateral to the Conception Vessel, on the abdomen and two thumb-widths lateral on the chest, up to the collar bone. It then goes up through the throat into the mouth and inside the body. It also has a pathway which goes from CV 1 up the centre of the spine, flowing along with the Governing Vessel and another pathway which flows down the legs. All three meridians connect the Uterus with the Kidneys, Heart and Brain.

- The CV – the sea of Yin Channels.
- The GV – the sea of Yang Channels.
- The PV – the sea of Blood.

Yuen (2005) argues that the Chong is first because it brings about form. It is the 'ancestral blue print' providing a connection between the pre- and postnatal energies. It links the Shen of the Heart, our individual destiny, with the Zhi, Will, our ancestral energy, of the Kidneys. Low also says 'somehow, deep inside, I feel Chong Mai is possibly the most important vessel in the body' (Low 1983: 154). I tend to concur. It gives birth to the Yin 'Vessel of bonding', the Ren, before flowing into the Yang Du. Du Mai is about 'separation from the maternal matrix': individuality. Yang provides the structure which puts everything together and enables us to go out into the world.

These first three vessels begin in the abdomen and are more about Jing, ancestral patterns and the past (Fig. 4.2).

CV

- Regulates: Yin.
- CV 4 and CV 6 among most nourishing points in the body.
- CV regulates the Three Burners through the points:
  - CV 17 upper burner – Lung Heart
  - CV 12 middle burner – Stomach Spleen digestion
  - CV 6, CV 5, CV 3 lower burner – Kidney, Bladder elimination.

GV

- Regulates: mental emotional state, the back, Yang.
- GV and Gate of Life Ming Men.
- Root or original Qi.
- Source of Fire for internal organs.
- Warms lower burner and Bladder.
- Warms Stomach and Spleen to aid digestion.
- Harmonies sexual function and warms essence and uterus.
- Assists Heart in housing the mind.

PV

- It is known as the 'Sea of Blood' because of its links with Blood and Menstruation. It is also known as the 'Sea of the Twelve Meridians' because of its many connections with the tendino-muscular meridians , particularly in the chest and the abdomen.
- The Pre-Heaven Chong is essentially one meridian which runs through the centre of the body. The one we work with is the Post-Heaven PV pathway, the Kidney meridian in the torso and the leg branches and into the neck.
- Points: CV 1, ST 30, KI 11–27, CV 23, GV 4 in leg, LV 3, SP 4, KI 1.

Second ancestry (Yuen 2005): Linking (Wei) and the Ankle (Qiao) Channels

Most sources concur that this core energy is then moved to the rest of the body, flowing into the Linking (Wei) and the Ankle (Qiao) Channels. Yuen says that these vessels are about how the archetypal Kidney Qi is expressed through the individual. He refers to these as the 'second ancestry' vessels, representing the individual choices we make in our lives.

Yin and Yang Wei Mai Linking

They usually relate to patterns of deficiency and so in the maternity period tend to be used more postnatally. They facilitate the movement of Qi between the Yang or Yin channels and are therefore different from the Governing Vessel which governs and regulates the Yang channels and the Conception Vessel which governs and regulates Yin channels. They represent the disparity between above and below in terms of hot and cold.

Yang Wei is about going out into the world and bringing that experience back to the Du Mai. Physically it is also about bringing the external to the internal. It controls Qi and Defensive Qi and relates to the exterior of the body.

Yin Wei controls the interior of the body so it is closely linked with both Blood and Yin. It has a strong effect on the Heart and is often used for mental emotional aspects. It may be regarded as a secondary vessel of the Kidneys.

According to Yuen, the Wei Mai vessels represent the element of time, the cloth of time and space. They are about the experiences that we have, especially crucial phases or transitions in our lives.

Yin and Yang Linking (Wei)

There is some variation in the descriptions of these meridians. However, the main points are indicated in Figs 4.3 and 4.4.

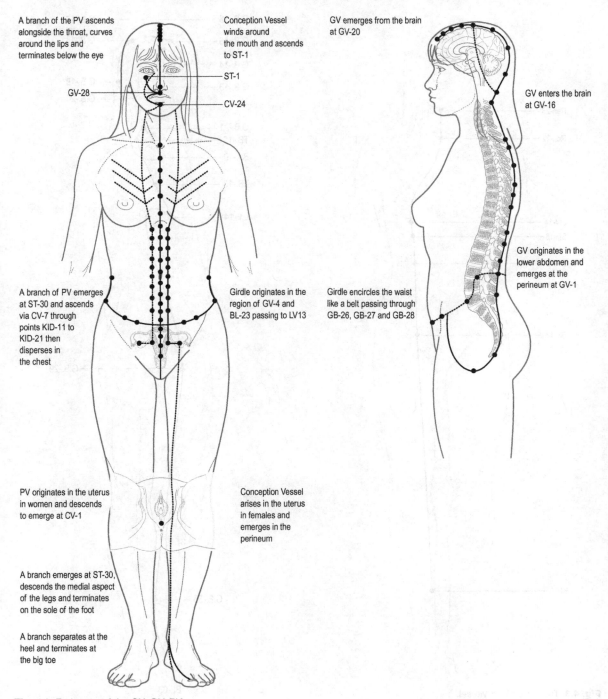

A branch of the PV ascends alongside the throat, curves around the lips and terminates below the eye

Conception Vessel winds around the mouth and ascends to ST-1

GV emerges from the brain at GV-20

ST-1

GV-28

CV-24

GV enters the brain at GV-16

GV originates in the lower abdomen and emerges at the perineum at GV-1

A branch of PV emerges at ST-30 and ascends via CV-7 through points KID-11 to KID-21 then disperses in the chest

Girdle originates in the region of GV-4 and BL-23 passing to LV13

Girdle encircles the waist like a belt passing through GB-26, GB-27 and GB-28

PV originates in the uterus in women and descends to emerge at CV-1

Conception Vessel arises in the uterus in females and emerges in the perineum

A branch emerges at ST-30, descends the medial aspect of the legs and terminates on the sole of the foot

A branch separates at the heel and terminates at the big toe

Fig. 4.2 Pathways of the CV, GV, PV.

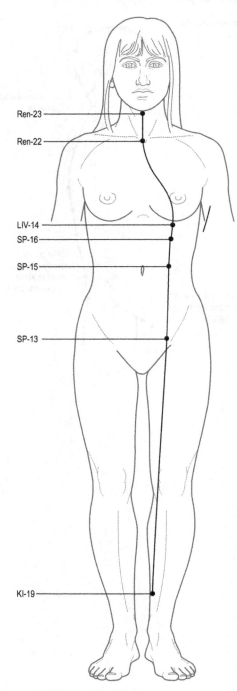

Ren-23
Ren-22

LIV-14
SP-16

SP-15

SP-13

KI-19

Fig. 4.3 The Yin Linking Vessel.

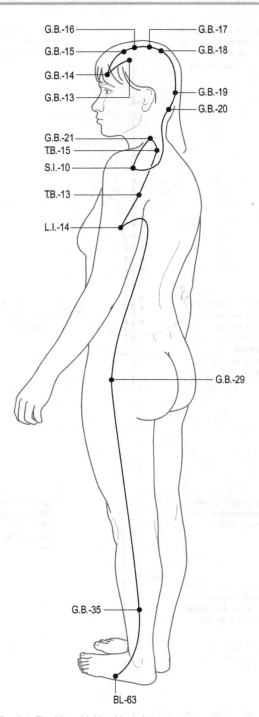

G.B.-16
G.B.-15
G.B.-14
G.B.-13

G.B.-17
G.B.-18

G.B.-19
G.B.-20

G.B.-21
TB.-15
S.I.-10

TB.-13

L.I.-14

G.B.-29

G.B.-35

BL-63

Fig. 4.4 The Yang Linking Vessel.

Yin/Yang Qiao Ankle

These two vessels form a balanced couple. They tend to relate more to excess energy and reflect moment to moment adjustments that are being made in the body. Often there is left and right Yin tightness along the medial aspect of body and Yang tightness along lateral aspect. There is a similarity and complementarity to these vessels. Although they are separate pathways they come together in neck and head.

They absorb excesses of Yin and Yang and tend to be used more in the antenatal period than the Linking, for clearing blockages and excess energy. Royston Low (1983) argues there is a relationship between BL1 and hormonal control through the pituitary gland and that they represent metabolism as expressed through the Stomach/Small Intestine. They are also said to harmonise Yin and Yang, respecting the cyclical nature of the seasons. They often relate to addictive patterns of behaviour.

- Yang Qiao – vessel of reactivity, stance in the world, structure.
- Yin Qiao – self-reflection, meditation. Excessive Yin (Yuen).

According to Yuen, the Qiao vessels are also about time but more about the current moment, the ability to be fully present in each moment. The quality of their energy in an individual represents how much that person has been living in the present as opposed to living in the past or projecting into the future.

See Figs 4.5 and 4.6.

Girdle Vessel – organ of the pelvis

The eighth vessel is the Dai Mai or the Girdle – 'the vessel of latency'. Yuen refers to Dai as the closet where things go that are no longer wanted or that we are unable to process. It is essentially about stagnation, the absorption of excess from the postnatal environment, and where deeply held sentiments and violations may be stored. It also acts as a link between the lower and upper body.

As with all the Extraordinary Vessels, there are some variations in points included. GB26, GB27 and GB28 are included in all descriptions. Many sources include GV4, BL23, and Yuen also includes CV8, KI16, ST25 and BL52. I link it very much to coming round to CV2 at the front and with the CV between the ribs and the navel with CV8 being an important point. These points represent the mid-line of the belt, the binding together of the energies.

This is the only horizontal meridian in the body and binds the vertical paths of all twelve meridians as well as the Penetrating Vessel and Conception

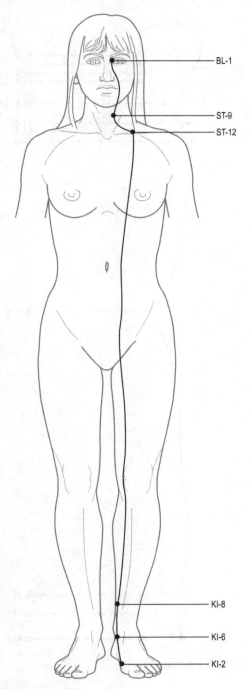

Fig. 4.5 Yin Ankle Qiao.

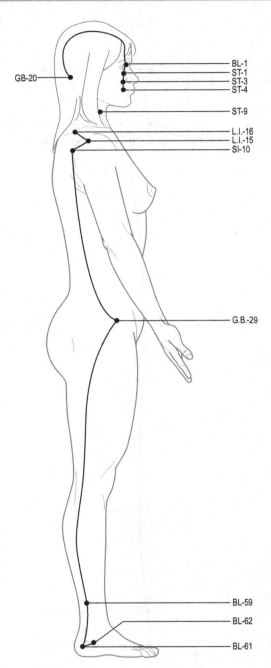

GB-20

BL-1
ST-1
ST-3
ST-4

ST-9

L.I.-16
L.I.-15
SI-10

G.B.-29

BL-59

BL-62

BL-61

Fig. 4.6 Yang Ankle Qiao.

Vessel. It particularly connects the Spleen (muscles), Liver (blood and sinews) and Kidney (bones) meridians and passes through points associated with them. It has a strong structural support element to it.

Its pathway is like a belt, rather than a thin line connecting these points. Indeed, I consider it to be like a pantie-girdle, linking into the pelvic floor. It originates from the space between the kidneys (GV 4) and passes under the rib cage, down the side of the body, over the anterior iliac spines to gather round the front of the body above the pubic bone. It affects both the bones and muscles of the pelvis, including the sacroiliac joint, the symphysis pubis, internal and external obliques, transverse abdominal muscles, deep and superficial muscles of the pelvic floor, muscles of the lower back, erectae spinae and quadratus lumborum, and gluteus and piriformis.

Clinical applications

- It guides and supports the Qi of the Uterus and the Essence. Ideally it should be relaxed yet supportive.
- It is about central physical support and how one is emotionally anchored in the world.
- It harmonises connections between the upper and lower body. If it is too tight then energy cannot pass between them. If it is too slack then energy fails to circulate properly.
- It harmonises Liver and Gall Bladder, especially LV, and is often associated with patterns of Liver Qi stagnation, including headaches.
- It is used for pelvic structural issues, as well as stagnation, including dampness in lower burner and emotional holding patterns in the abdomen.

Uterus and the Kidney–Uterus and Heart–Uterus meridians

The Uterus includes the uterus itself as well as the fallopian tubes and the ovaries. There are two special meridians which connect the Uterus with the Kidneys and the Heart. The Kidney–Uterus meridian nourishes the Uterus with Jing. The Heart–Uterus meridian nourishes the Uterus with Blood.

Some people argue that they are branches of the CV GV PV circuit.

Heart–Uterus meridian – Bao Mai

There is a direct connection between the Heart and the Uterus via this meridian. It nourishes the Uterus with Blood energy sent down from the Heart. It provides a link between Fire and Earth elements. There can be disturbance in this meridian if there is stress on the mother's Heart (for example through mental agitation or emotional frustration) which will affect the baby in the womb emotionally.

The Kidney–Uterus channel – Bao Luo

There is a channel which connects the Kidneys with the Uterus. This nourishes the Uterus with Essence. It provides a link between the Water and Earth elements. Overwork and exhaustion, as well as fertility treatment which over-stimulates the Essence, all deplete its energy.

References

Low, R., 1983. The Secondary Vessels of Acupuncture. Thorsons, Northamptonshire.

Maciocia, G., 2006. The Channels of Acupuncture. Churchill Livingstone, Edinburgh.

Yates, S., 2003. Shiatsu for Midwives. Books for Midwives, Oxford.

Yuen, J.C., 2005. The Eight Extraordinary Vessels. New England School of Acupuncture, Boston, MA.

Eastern approach to pregnancy

Chapter contents

Learning outcomes

- Have an overview of the main changes in energy for both the woman and fetus during pregnancy
- Have a specific understanding of the changes in the Extraordinary Vessels and the 12 meridians for woman and fetus
- Describe the main treatment principles for working

Introduction

Historically, the Chinese considered pregnancy to be an important time in any woman's life. Because of alterations in Jing, Blood and Qi, they felt that it offered the possibility of positive change. At this time a woman's health can be either strengthened or weakened.

Pre-conceptual health was considered to be fundamental. The quality of energy of both the mother and fetus is dependent on how the mother has looked after herself before the pregnancy, as well as the type of energy that she has inherited from her mother and father.

They also considered pregnancy to be an important time for the fetus and had a concept of 'fetal' education (*Tai Kyo*). The mother needs to eat good foods and have a balanced emotional and physical lifestyle to support the fetus's physical and emotional development. A calm atmosphere was generally emphasised, although if a woman wanted a boy she was advised to attend archery contests during certain months.

With much of Chinese medical theory, different and sometimes contradictory ideas are presented in different texts.

Some of the earliest texts (Huainanzi, 3rd century BC, translation by Major 1993) were written before the systematisation of the five elements, and therefore different resonances and correspondences are made between the elements and the organs. Some later texts, such as the Qipolun (11th century), emphasise the more esoteric aspects of pregnancy. Despite these differences the basic aspects of foetal development are quite consistent.

(Sandra Hill)

I have drawn upon various sources and linked this with my own knowledge. I have primarily included information which supports a relatively consistent model for the practitioner and so not all descriptions are included. I would suggest that the reader interested in a more detailed analysis of the classical texts look at the work of Elisabeth Rochat de la Vallée or Jean-Marc Eyssalet who both refer to the traditional texts. Many of these texts are only in Chinese or Japanese, but I have included the English references given by Rochat de la Vallée at the end of her text. I have also included some ideas from Jeffrey Yuen's work which sometimes give a slightly different perspective.

Pregnancy was defined as 10 lunar months. Ten is a number which expresses the perfection of human nature and a unity for the Chinese (Suwen *c.* 100 BC). The natural duration for life is given as 100 years (10 × 10). Pregnancy is seen as being predominantly a time of Yin energy. In traditional Japan and China, indeed in many pre-industrial societies, pregnancy was a time when women were encouraged to take more care of themselves and would follow special diets and lifestyle changes.

5.1 General energy patterns for the mother

Pre-conception and fertility

The most important energy for supporting both fertility and pregnancy is Jing. Having a weak Jing would be considered to be one of the primary causes of infertility and miscarriage (Fu Qing Zhu and Tang Zong Hai). It is generally considered that the optimum time for conception is before 35 years of age. This represents five cycles of 7 years. Some writers think 21–29 years is the optimum time and others (Kawada 2006) consider 29–35 to be better because the mother is more emotionally mature. After 35 years the quality and amount of the mother's Jing is declining. This affects both her ability to build the child and the child's coding for its own growth. It does not mean all women over 35 have poor pregnancies and weak children but good pregnancy outcomes are dependent on a strong inherited Jing and healthy lifestyle.

GV, PV and CV are the basis for follicle maturation, ovulation and corpus luteum development and are always involved with fertility. Anything, physical or emotional, which weakens the Uterus or the GV, PV and CV and Blood will reduce fertility, especially exposure to Cold. Excessive consumption of greasy foods and dairy products may lead to dampness in the lower burner which may prevent fertilisation. Liver Qi stagnation affects the CV and PV; this may correspond in western terms to tubal obstruction.

Miscarriage

The main cause of early miscarriage is also likely to be considered due to weakness of Kidney Jing which cannot support the growth and development of the fetus. This is linked with the quality of the DNA from a western viewpoint and corresponds to genetic factors being main causes of miscarriage. From a Chinese point of view the 'DNA' is not just about physical patterns passed through the generations but also about mental and emotional aspects.

Miscarriage can also be due to weakness in any of the energies which are needed to nourish the fetus. It may be due to weakness of Spleen or Girdle Vessel failing to hold the energy of the fertilised egg in the uterus. It can be linked in with dampness in the lower burner.

The energetics of conception

The eastern view of conception includes a philosophy on the purpose of manifesting as an individual and the destiny of that individual. Much of this aspect of Chinese medicine was either recorded in the oral traditions or

lost during the Maoist Cultural Revolution but there are some references to it in the Neijing, Ling Shu and Dang Zhunyi, and Lonny Jarrett writes about it in *Nourishing Destiny* (Jarrett 1998).

Conception is the moment of destiny; the initial movement from the Tao, the one, undifferentiated, formless energy, to move into differentiation and form making the first step on the journey of forming an individual energy. The Jing of the two parents and the Blood of the mother unite and determine the energetic quality of the rest of the pregnancy (Ling Shu, *c.* 100 BC, Ch. 30).

Jeffrey Yuen (2005: 17) and others talk about the five elements flowing in reverse prenatally, reflecting the fact that prenatal life is like a mirror of our soul, showing where we come from. This movement therefore begins with Water and ends with Wood. As Water moves into form it passes through Metal. Most authors agree that the Soul is captured by the Po of the mother, which is stored in the Lungs. Po is the Corporeal Soul, that aspect of the soul which is expressed through the body. The quality of the mother's Lungs in drawing energy into the body mirrors the importance of the health of the mother's basic Qi, drawn into her body through the breath and expressed in her physical form.

Other energies present are the Yuan Qi. This is the representation of Heaven and Earth imprinted onto Jing at the time of conception, the Qi of the Universe, primordial Yin and Yang. Yin and Yang Qi energies are also present, the cultural and historical period, season, time of day in which a fetus is conceived. This is the basis of Chinese Nine Star Qi theory and astrology, and indeed of western astrology.

At the moment of conception the Jing (Earth) and the Shen (Heaven) mingle at the point of Ming Men 'gate of destiny'. (GV 4)

Mingmen contains and focuses the infusion of our inheritance of primordial Yin and Yang (the Yuan Qi) which at our core joins each of us to the primordial Dao.

(Larre et al 1986)

The interaction of this authentic water and fire conforms to the deep inner nature of each individual. The authentic self

(Larre & Rochat de la Vallée 1985)

The inherited constitution intermingles with the acquired constitution and the Shen is interacting with the Jing. During pregnancy the Yuan Qi guides the differentiation of the embryo and fetus. During life it is the inner fire which fuels developmental processes such as making blood, the growth of bones, emotional and psychic development and the ascent of spirit.

Shen is our purpose in life that provides us with the capacity to return to original nature by focusing our intention inwardly toward the Jing. The heavenly aspect of inborn nature is Shen, the earthly aspect is Jing. Humans must establish their Zhi (human will) as a conduit for Shen (heaven) to interact with Jing (earth).

(Jarrett 1998: 59)

5.2 Main energy changes and patterns during pregnancy for the mother

To support the growth of the fetus, there is a change in the flow of energies in the mother's body. The mother needs to have enough Jing, Qi and Blood to nourish the fetus and they need to be able to flow freely to the Uterus.

Although the fetus is drawing on the mother's energies, pregnancy need not necessarily weaken a woman. The mother's body is designed to be able to pass Jing on to her fetus, to be able to reproduce. Indeed for some women, the activation of these functions can strengthen and stimulate her body; for some women pregnancy is one of the healthiest, happiest times of her life. However, if any of the energies are insufficient, problems may arise with the growth and development of the fetus and the successful completion of gestation. The mother may also become weakened through the pregnancy.

The main focus of work is to maintain the best, most balanced production and flow of Qi, Blood and Essence.

Yin and Yang aspects of pregnancy

Pregnancy as a state of Yin/Water

At conception, Yang is the sperm which provides the spark of energy to begin the process of transforming the Yin egg into the embryo. The development of the being takes place in the watery environment of the womb–Yin energy in relation to conception and birth. The cessation of menstruation means that more Blood energy is available, mirroring what we know physiologically about the maternal increase in blood volume. Blood energy and body fluids are part of Yin fluids. The fetus is nourished, especially in the first trimester, by the mother's Jing, which is stored in her Kidneys.

Yang aspects of pregnancy

Yin cannot exist without Yang. The absence of periods leads to an accumulation of Fire heat in the body and heat needs to be supplied to the fetus. This is how the Chinese viewed the rise in core body temperature in pregnancy.

During pregnancy there are more of all energies, Yang included.

If there is insufficient Yin, then there can be too much Yang. Excess Yang energy tends to rise. This can be the energetics behind migraine and even pre-eclampsia.

Changes in Qi, Blood and Jing

Jing

On one level Jing represents the huge hormonal changes the mother undergoes. These changes are most marked in the first trimester both energetically and physically. On another level it is about how the early stages of growth and development unfold for the fetus. It is of particular importance in the first trimester as the organ systems are being formed.

It relates mostly to the energy of the Kidneys, which store the Essence, and the Extraordinary Vessels of Governing Vessel, Conception Vessel, Penetrating Vessel, Girdle Vessel, Yin and Yang Heel and Linking, which circulate the Essence. It also relates to the Kidney–Uterus meridian which is responsible for the flow of Essence to the Uterus.

It is not possible to increase the amount of Essence which someone has, but it is possible to balance how it is moved around the body through working these meridians, especially in making sure that it gets to the fetus as well as the mother. The quality of Essence is affected by its interaction with the energy of food, processed mainly by Stomach and Spleen. Work with these meridians will be important, as will attention to proper diet and physical nourishment.

Stress and overwork particularly affect the Essence.

Flow and production of Qi: CV, GV and the 12 meridians

In the first trimester there are subtle changes in Qi flow in the body as Qi needs to be directed to the Uterus to nourish the placenta and the fetus but the fetus is still physically minute.

As the pregnancy progresses the fetus essentially blocks the flow of Qi in the mother's abdomen, which affects Qi flow through the rest of the body. Furthermore the fetus is increasingly drawing upon the mother's Qi to support its own growth and development.

The Conception Vessel and Governing Vessel are the regulators of Yin and Yang Qi in the body, especially in times of change, but ultimately all the 12 meridians are affected in different ways as they circulate different types of Qi, all of which are important for the fetus.

As the fetus grows, the abdomen distends and pressure is put on the abdominal organs and meridians, especially Heart–Uterus, Penetrating Vessel and Conception Vessel. The development of the linea nigra indicates some women's response to the changes in the Conception Vessel. Both Qi and Body fluids find it more difficult to flow up and down the body. Energy is blocked in the Three Burners as the fetus prevents energy from moving between them. Blocked energy in the middle burner affects digestion. Energy flow into the upper burner also becomes blocked, affecting the flow into the arms and chest, influencing energy flow to the Heart and Lung. Blocked energy in the lower burner affects Bladder and Kidney and the flow of energy down to the mother's legs, blocking especially the Yin meridians of Spleen, Liver and Kidney.

The increasing weight of the fetus tends to place strain on the back creating lordosis and affecting the flow of the Governing Vessel.

Flow and production of Blood

The extra Blood in the body tends not to be held in the uterus in the first trimester as the tiny embryo does not need it and so it may rise up the mother's torso causing feelings of heat and Fire. This may cause morning sickness, breast fullness and emotional unsettledness. From the second trimester the fetus needs more blood and the placenta regulates hormones and blood flow to the fetus and feelings of heat settle at that time; the Penetrating Vessel energy becomes more settled.

After conception, Blood is gradually being transformed to Milk, in preparation for breastfeeding, and some of this Blood transfers its location from the lower to the upper burner. This will also contribute to morning sickness and the general feeling of heat above and distension of the breasts.

By the third trimester, the fetus needs a lot of Blood to support the rapid weight gain and laying down of fat. The mother may tend to be anaemic. The mother is not really suffering from typical Blood deficiency as overall there is still more Blood in the system. However, the composition of Blood has changed due to the 'addition' of Jing through menstrual Blood and the transformation into Milk.

The Penetrating Vessel is the Sea of Blood. Other important meridians are the Spleen which produces the Blood energy, the Liver which stores the Blood energy, and the Heart which rules the Blood energy. Heart–Uterus sends Blood energy and emotional energy to the Uterus.

Maternal changes in the different trimesters – five elements, 10 lunar months and dominant meridians

Over the centuries theories have developed referring to patterns of a dominant organ/meridian energy in the mother which nourishes the fetus during the different months (Ling Shu quoted in Eyssalet 1990; Zhubing Yuanhou Lun quoted in Rochat de la Vallée 2007). Some schools say that the dominant meridian for the mother in the month should not be worked (Eyssalet 1990, Maciocia 1998: 28). However, most therapists today would not avoid using the meridians. Indeed by understanding which meridian is nourishing the fetus during any month, it may be helpful to work that meridian in the mother with the focus on supporting the energy flow to the fetus. Zhubing describes points on the meridians to work.

In over 20 years of working with pregnant women, I have not specifically avoided working any of the meridians. Indeed I have often worked meridians which correspond to the month, to no ill effect. The schema can, however, provide a useful way of understanding which energies in the mother may tend to go out of balance at particular stages of pregnancy and indeed sometimes it is useful to work with the energies of the dominant meridian in order to support the mother (Suzanne Yates).

The Huainanzi text became the basis of many later descriptions, one of the most well known being the Zhubing Yuanhou Lun (6th century CE). This text gives a detailed account of the changes within both the mother and foetus during the 10 months of pregnancy, presenting the dominant meridian in the mother, the kind of food she should eat, the behaviour she should adopt. Within the mother the meridians are given in order as: liver, gall bladder, pericardium, triple heater, spleen, stomach, lungs, large intestine and kidney; the functions of these meridians as governing the development of blood, essences, vital spirits, the six fu, the four limbs, the mouth and eyes, skin and body hair, the nine orifices and the vital circulation within the foetus.

(Sandra Hill)

Dominant meridians for each month of the 10 lunar months of pregnancy are:

1. Liver (LV).
2. Gall Bladder (GV).
3. Pericardium (HC/HP).
4. Triple Heater (TH).
5. Spleen (SP).
6. Stomach (ST).
7. Lungs (LU).
8. Large Intestine (LI).
9. Kidney (KD).
10. Bladder (BL).

(Rochat de la Vallée 2007).

Energies of the different trimesters

Conception: Water > Metal
First trimester: Earth – months 1–3

The fertilised egg embeds in the wall of the uterus (Earth), putting down roots and beginning to grow and develop.

Common symptoms for the mother in the first trimester are of Spleen and Stomach not being harmonised (e.g. bloating, nausea, sickness, emotional ungrounding).

Changes in Blood predominate here and this aspect represents close links with the Earth and the energy of nourishment. Blood is no longer lost each month. A woman needs to keep a good balance of energy between her Qi and Blood and it is important that she has good-quality food to nourish her. There is a need to increase stores of Blood, and this is done through the Liver.

Dominant meridians

- **First month** – Liver. This represents the beginnings of creation. Blood gathers in the Uterus. Sun Si Miao (Rochat de la Vallée 2007) says that in the first month the mother should not move too much as Blood will go to the muscles rather than be gathered in the Uterus. He suggests that it is better to be quiet and rest.
- **Second month** – Gall Bladder. This represents the movement of Blood as it gathers more strongly in the Uterus.
- **Third month** – Heart Protector. This completes the action of enriching the Blood with the Spirit. It is at this point the fetus is considered to exist.

Second trimester: Fire – months 4–6

The mother begins to develop more of an emotional connection with the fetus as she feels movements. Fetal education begins. During the fifth month the fetus receives the Essences of Fire. Physically the changes in the Blood will support the continued growth of the fetus.

Often the mother feels more at ease and settled both physically and emotionally. The texts now recommend that she moves and spends time outside.

Dominant meridians

The dominant organs here are those connected with the continued growth and development of the fetus.

- **Fourth month** – Triple Heater. This continues the process of Blood moving through the body and the blood and blood vessels. It is also about the movement of water, fluids and Qi through the body.
- **Fifth month** – Spleen. The mother's Blood nourishes the growing fetus as it lays down more fat.
- **Sixth month** – Stomach. Continues the giving of nourishment to fetus as well as defensive Qi. However, it was considered important in this month that the mother should not eat too much food. This is often the month that the mother may begin to experience heartburn and needs to start to eat smaller amounts of food, maybe at more frequent intervals through the day.

Third trimester: Wood – months 7–10

If the mother continues to exercise and move physically, then the free flow of Wood energy prepares her for the physicality of birth and caring for a new baby. If she rests too much, then frustration, worry and feelings of control may build up and she may find birth difficult, both physically and emotionally.

In old Chinese traditions, during the last 3 months of pregnancy (Eyssalet 1990, quoting Lin Shu J in ch. 10, article 2) the mother would be in a separate room so that she did not have contact with the father. This was to bring about a more feminine contact and bond between mother and fetus and in preparation for birth and for breastfeeding. The husband would be purifying himself through abstinence in preparation for meeting his child.

- **Seventh month** – Lungs (Metal). Nourish the Wood of the fetus. Lungs affect the exteriorisation of the energy.
- **Eight month** – Large Intestine. The Yang of Metal is fixing limits. Breathing of the mother is considered especially important during these last months. Her skin is lustrous.
- **Ninth month** – Kidney energy supports the fetus for the completion of the ancestral plan.
- **Tenth month** – Bladder. The Yang aspect of Water, preparing for birth moving into the Yang energy of Wood for birth.

5.3 Energy patterns for the fetus

For the Chinese, at birth we are already 1 year old. This may even represent the idea that the spirit of the fetus is present in the few months before conception.

There are theories about the development of the meridians in the fetus and what is happening at each month (Matsumoto & Birch 1988: 153–156). The most important energy shift is along the midline of the body – the development of the Extraordinary Vessels, which is discussed on p. 123.

In eastern philosophy, by contrast with western where it is now known that the fetus is mostly developed in the first few months, the fetus develops more gradually as the pregnancy progresses and different aspects of the soul come into the body.

Mother and child interactions: fetal education

Fetal education (*Tai Kyo*) begins from the third month when the fetus is formed: 'The beginning of the person is the beginning of the heart/mind and the ability to receive influences at the mental level. So what the mother thinks and sees can influence the formation of the child's mind' (Rochat de la Vallée 2007: 48). One writer, Chao Shi Lin, (quoted in Essaylet) provides a prescription of each month such as:

if you want a boy take a bow and arrows
if you want a girl wear round Jade
if you want a beautiful infant wear white jade
and admire peacocks (paon)

Other writers and other descriptions are elaborated in the texts.

Music was considered especially important for developing the heart and Shen of the fetus. Good-quality food was considered important for strengthening the Jing of the fetus and in the Zhubing Yuanhou Lun (quoted in Essaylet) specific foods are suggested for each month of pregnancy.

There was, however, also the idea that the child is able to separate from the mother and have his/her own individual characteristics. Eyssalet links this with the idea of the earthly spirits, the Gui as opposed to the heavenly spirits of the Shen (Eyssalet 1990: 214). The Gui are points linked more with the separation of a separate and distinct energy of the fetus. Points linked with the Gui are: LI 1, LI 10, LI 11, Lung 5, Lung 9, Lung 10, ST 36, ST 6, SP 1, HC 5, HC 7, GV 22, GV 23, GV 26, GV 16, BL 62, CV 24. We could consider using these points with a focus on connecting with the individual nature of the fetus.

Yin and Yang in the developing fetus

There can be imbalances of Yin or Yang in the developing fetus. Congenital defects can be seen as too much consolidation of Yin without the ability to disseminate Yang. CV is in state of excess and GV is in state of deficiency. This can be seen in cases of dwarfism, Down's syndrome, mental retardation, or where the body is truncated with the head close to the shoulders and lots of padding around the neck. The legs and hands are sometimes clubbed. All this represents excessive Yin.

Too much Yang would be infantile seizures and convulsions, or heat presiding over damp.

Changes in Qi, Blood and Jing

Jing

This is the essential building block which forms the fetus, as the Jing of the mother and father unite. It is the DNA, the ancestral blueprint. The mother's Jing continues to nourish the fetus during gestation.

Qi

The Qi in the fetus is not said to flow independently as the source for the Qi (Air and Food) comes via the mother. Once the egg is fertilised Qi starts to flow. As the egg develops so too does Qi. There are references to Qi flowing through the meridians, which are developing during each lunar month of gestation. Qi can be said to flow with Blood – Qi is mediated by Blood as it comes to the fetus via the placenta.

The source of Qi is considered to be the Ming Men and Qi first flows along the axis of the CV and GV, which regulate Yin and Yang Qi and PV which regulates Blood. As the limbs develop and the meridians therefore form, then Qi starts to flow out from this mid-line. This fits in with the idea of the Extraordinary Vessels being older energies and the 12 meridians being more recent.

There is also the idea of Yuan Qi guiding the differentiation of the embryo and fetus fuelling developmental processes such as making blood, the growth of bones, emotional and psychic development.

Blood

The nourishing quality of Blood is important for the fetus. The fetus receives nourishment directly through the Blood which is flowing into it via the placenta and thus the PV of the mother is important. As the fetus grows and lays down fat it starts to need more Blood, so that by the end of the pregnancy this is one of the main energies which is nourishing it.

Embryological development

One interesting view of fetal development put forward by Michio Kushi (1979) is viewing fetal development as mirroring the whole period of human evolution (the human being as the microcosm of the universe, which is the macrocosm) from our time in water to the time of volcanic shifts and eruptions, through to the evolution of reptilian and mammalian life on earth. The total period of 280 days of pregnancy represents a repetition of the evolutional process of biological life in the ocean of the earth until the time of the rise of land upon the surface of the water. It repeats at least 2.8 billion or nearly 3 billion biological years. The ancients therefore considered that the average speed of growth is 10 million biological years per 24 hours.

This means each day of life in utero represents a considerable amount of human evolution and this was why the Chinese felt that the influences upon the fetus in the womb in pregnancy had such a profound effect.

The Chinese texts detail many aspects of fetal development. Rochat de la Vallée says that the

building starts with the most internal composition, the water, the ability to take a form, the five zang and the five constituent parts of the body and then moves from the depths outwards to the surface and the nine orifices (Guanzi Ch 39 and Lingshu Ch 10) . . . The sense organs . . . are able to perceive not only big and obvious things but also that which is not seen or heard directly. The production of a human being implies a destiny not just to comprehend the obvious, but to use the fullness of blood and qi and spirits and all the sensory faculties to go further than what is easily perceptible. The heart or mind can be used to think about what is really important in life and what is the subtle mystery of life.

(Rochat de la Vallée 2007: 14, 15)

And Sandra Hill says:

The earliest text on the development of the foetus is found in Chapter 7 of the Huainanzi, a compilation of Daoist philosophical writings from the 3rd century BCE. Chapter 7 is called Jing Shen, vital spirit, or essence spirit; the development of the foetus follows directly after a well known quotation from the Dao De Jing – the dao gives rise to the one, the one gives rise to the two, the two give rise to the ten thousand beings . . .

At 1 month it is a bulge; at 2 months it is a paste; at 3 months it is foetus; at 4 months it has flesh; at 5 months it has sinews; at 6 months it has bones; at 7 months it is complete; at 8 months it moves; at 9 months it quickens; at 10 months it is born.

In other texts, the development of the foetus is expressed as in the first month, the beginning of form; the second, the beginning of the rich paste; the third, the beginning of the foetus; and at the fourth month there is a change from the Huainanzi text to present a rotation of the elements through water, fire, metal, wood and earth, and ending in the tenth month with stone.

(Sandra Hill)

Summary of changes (Eyssalet 1990)

Jean-Marc Eyssalet summarises the changes for the fetus presented in eight traditional texts (Hua Tai Jing Zhong Ji Jing (A); Chao Shi (B); Wu Zang Lun (C); Lu Xin Jing (D); Qian Jin Lin (E); Yi Jing Mi Lu de Hua Tuo (F); Huai Nan Zi (G); Rgyud Bzi du Thibet (H)).

I have selected some of the most important to give an idea. (For the full table see Eyssalet 1990: 169–173.)

Month 1 – takes the breath (A), blood and sperm fix (D).

Month 2 – seizes the Ling (A).

Month 3 – contains changes (A) (D) Yang spirit gives the three Hun.

Month 4 – fixes the vital principle: Jing (A), takes on corporeal form (C), takes on the Yin and the seven Po (D).

Month 5 – takes on the substance of the head (A), tendons and bones formed (C), five movements of the subtle organs (D).

Month 6 – hair and skin formed (C), six rules (Lu) fix and bones and tendons (E) (G).

Month 7 – Shen covers everything (A), the Hun start beating (C), the vital principle opens the main orifices and communicates with a clear light (D), the being is formed (G).

Month 8 – takes possession of individual spirit.

Month 9 – takes the voice (A), turns the body three times (C).

Month 10 – takes order of the destiny and is born (A), five organs and spirits are equipped (B), takes on sufficient breath of sufficiency (C).

Fetal changes during the trimesters with the energies from Water–Wood

Conception: Water > Metal

For the fetus this is the moment of destiny. There is the Cosmic Qi, the Yuan Qi, the vibration of the universe, which is the energy field from which the fetus differentiates itself. At this moment the Corporeal soul, Po, comes into the body, the Po through the Lungs. This is the aspect of our spirit which is contained within the physical body. At death it is said to descend through the anus to the earth and, as it were, fertilise the soil. The first breath is the way the fetus enters into the earthly world from the mother's womb. The breath is the last energy to leave the body at death, as we let go of our hold on life. This also represents the mouth/nose–anus connection – the basic tube of taking in and letting go which is the energy of metal. Birth and death are interconnected.

There is an interesting connection here with the ghosts of the earth. When someone dies a violent death or does not want to leave their physical body they hold on to the Po and do not let it go. They therefore remain trapped on the earth in a more ephemeral way, as a ghost.

First trimester: Earth

This is about the embodiment of the corporeal soul. Rochat de la Vallée (2007: 101) emphasises the first 3 months as being about 'the creation of a form, or the rich paste of the embryo'. A healthy nourishing environment needs to be provided for the fertilised egg to implant in the soil of the uterus.

- **First month:**

In the first month the conceived being is called 'embryo' (some ancient doctors called it 'dew'); in the second month fat ('gao') in the third month 'fetus' (bao). In the third month there is the presence of blood and vessels.

(Sun Si Miao 652)

- **Second month:** the essences of the child are formed and become its own.
- **Third month:** there is the presence of the fetus which is male or female and the education begins.

Second trimester: Fire

This is about the fetus connecting with the sovereign purpose of its existence and becoming the individual and connecting with the individual destiny through the Shen.

- The fetus receives Blood and Qi in the fourth and fifth months. In the fifth month Fire is said to predominate. In the sixth month muscular forces and bones develop (Rochat de la Vallée 2007: 101). Sun Si Miao:

- In the fourth month it acquires a body shape; in the fifth month it can move; in the sixth the sinews and bones are formed.
- In the sixth month the fetus receives the essences of Metal.

Third trimester: Wood

This is about the organisation of events and the time for experience.

The Hun (spirit of Wood) starts to beat. The Hun is the

evolutionary spirit that is raised in virtue as we strive toward manifesting the highest which heaven has placed within. Upon death the Hun exits through the extremity of the liver meridian at GV 20 ... (where) it reports to the spirits that preside over destiny on the degree to which each of us has cultivated virtue during our lifetime.

(Jarrett 1998: 236)

In a sense, experiences in life have been programmed and are needed so that one can transcend ... that is the idea of Harmonisation. The idea is that, if I can't get over it in this lifetime, well I'm going to have to go through the same thing all over again. ... try to transcend it right now, in this life, rather than wait for another life ... so that we can willfully die, with no regrets left!

(Yuen 2005)

Sun Si Miao:

- In the seventh month the skin and hair are formed.
- In the eighth month the organs are fully formed and the fetus receives the essences of earth.
- In the ninth month the food Qi enters the stomach.
- In the 10th month the Shen is fully established and childbirth occurs.

5.4 Changes in the Extraordinary Vessels

Mother

These vessels provide the link between the changes in flow and production of Essence and Qi which they all regulate and Blood which the Penetrating Vessel regulates.

They are about how ancestral patterns are transmitted. Often the mother herself becomes more aware of her own connections with her family. Women who have not had a good relationship, or had a distant relationship with their parents, may seek the opportunity of pregnancy to reconnect or heal old patterns. Shifts often happen within the family. It is not uncommon for close family members to become ill or even die during the time of the pregnancy or fairly soon afterwards. Sisters or other relatives may be pregnant at the same time. From a Chinese view the whole energy field of the family is affected by the new life within. Even western psychotherapy now recognises these effects and supports families to look at the impact of changes on the whole network of family relationships (Pierre Deglon workshop, Beau Site, Switzerland, summer 2007).

Physically these vessels reflect the changes in the core of the body – mid-line energies in the back and front and especially the abdomen. As these vessels are so affected by the physical changes, they naturally change energetically. If they are weak then the mother is more likely to experience issues with weakness in the lower back or abdomen, which could be connected with feelings of lack of support, especially from the family. If they are strong, the mother can move with confidence, both physically and emotionally, through the changes she is experiencing.

As overall regulators of change they support the 12 organs and meridians to make the many and varied adaptations they need to make. Again if they are strong, the mother will find that she is able to adapt well during the pregnancy. If they are weak then they may fail to support all or some of the organs and the mother may experience pregnancy as a more difficult time in her life.

As reservoirs of Qi and Blood they support the specific changes in these energies. Again, they are designed to support the process of pregnancy and if they are strong the mother will feel well and enjoy her pregnancy. If they are weak then she may well feel tired and drained by the experience.

Penetrating Vessel

Chong is considered the 'architect of creation' (Yuen 2005). It is the link between the Pre-Heaven and the Post-Heaven energy. It can be thought of as the ancestral blueprint: Spirit conveyed through Blood.

In the first trimester it sends some of the increased Blood in the system downwards to the Uterus to nourish the development of the blastocyte, into embryo and fetus and to establish the placenta and amniotic sac. Until the placenta is established it is more difficult for this energy to be physically held and it tends to rise up the chest, creating feelings of suffocation and heat in the upper body, sometimes causing feelings of anxiety. Changes in the breasts are often the first sign of changes the mother notices in her body during pregnancy: PV is the main meridian regulating the breasts.

As Kidney and Penetrating Vessel are closely linked, this rising Penetrating Vessel energy, 'Running Piglet Qi', may drain Kidney energy and lead to it becoming depleted in the lower burner area of the lower abdomen and back. This may lead to feelings of tiredness, weakness and even pain in these areas. Other symptoms include abdominal distension and cold feet.

Stomach energy works with Penetrating Vessel. It needs to flow down to keep Penetrating Vessel anchored in the lower abdomen. If Stomach is weak and fails to do this during the first trimester, the upward movement of the Penetrating Vessel will be aggravated, creating feelings of nausea and sickness. If the Liver meridian also flows upwards, due to weak Stomach failing to control it, there will be patterns of more extreme vomiting and sickness which may even develop into hyperemesis.

Emotionally during the first trimester, as the PV is unsettled so too tend to be the emotions of the mother. She may be immediately 'bonded' with her fetus or it might take some time for feelings of connection to be established. She may feel very unsettled and emotionally 'all over the place'.

Once the placenta is established by the end of the first trimester, essentially anchoring the Penetrating Vessel, PV energy tends to settle down again. Emotionally the mother begins to feel more settled and morning sickness tends to decline. Usually during the second trimester the mother will have a 'blooming' complexion, feel her Blood energy is flowing well and be more contented and settled. However, if the patterns of weak Stomach and upward flowing Liver are extreme, the result may be that nausea or even hyperemesis continues, sometimes throughout pregnancy.

By the end of the third trimester, the fetus is drawing more again on the Penetrating Vessel energy to support its rapid weight gain. This is why the mother can begin to feel more tired and tend towards anaemia. She may also feel anxious, especially about the impending birth, and feel weakness in the lower back and dragging down feelings along the PV pathway.

The PV anatomically flows through the rectus abdominis muscle which is known as the ancestral muscle. As pregnancy progresses the recti tend to separate. Minor separation is a normal part of the changes in the body enabling it to accommodate the expansion of the uterus. Excessive separation (more than two fingers) may lead to less support for the mid-line energies.

The leg branch of the vessel has an important role in regulating the energy of the legs. The points KD 11, ST 30, ST 37 and SP 6 are useful for working with restless leg syndrome and also for supporting the flow of Blood in the legs.

Heart–Uterus

This is closely linked with the energy of the Penetrating Vessel. Some sources even say that it is a branch of the PV. It is about Blood and emotional energy being settled or unsettled in the body. In the first trimester, the fetus may not make full use of Blood sent to it and this can be a cause of nausea and anxiety in the mother. As the fetus begins to grow more, it makes use of the Blood energy and the mother becomes less anxious and more emotionally connected with her fetus. Heart–Uterus is about the combination of Fire and Fire energy: the Uterus being the soil for the seed and the Heart being the Shen/Blood connection to the Uterus.

Conception Vessel

This represents the Yin aspect of the Kidneys and provides Yin energy to the Uterus, fetus and placenta. A lot of the mother's creative energy is focused on creating new life and she finds her focus of creativity may switch to activities concerning her new fetus such as nest-building. With so much Yin energy focused on the fetus, the mother may find she lacks enough for herself. CV contains the two seas of Qi (CV 6 and CV 17) which provide the basis for Yang. The balance between Yin and Yang is important: if too many demands are placed on the mother to focus her energies outside this may lead to relative depletion of both CV and Kidney Yin. Liver Yang or Liver wind may then start to rise. This is the pattern with aggravation of migraine in some women or even pre-eclampsia/eclampsia.

The mother may feel tired, exhausted and have problems with breathing and digestion. This links closely in to the pattern described with energy not moving in the chest and the three burners. CV regulates, along with GV, the energy of the three burners.

The lower burner

This regulates urination and has a link with hormonal energy and so CV is a useful meridian to work with in cases of excessive urination, frequent urination and generally regulating changes in urination.

As CV flows through perineum and governs the genital and urinary orifices, it can be used in cases where there is pain in the perineum which may or may not be due to a specific cause. The beauty of shiatsu is that work can be done to support the perineum, without working directly on it. Points above and below can be utilised to support the flow of energy. This may help the mother connect with her perineum and aid with pelvic floor exercises.

Since CV is linked with regulating issues of the abdomen and uterus, it can be used where the following are present: haemorrhoids, vulva or vaginal pain or varicosities, diarrhoea with cold pain, abdominal pain, difficult urination, weak rectus muscles, digestive issues and food stasis. Since weakness in the front of the body can also lead to weakness in the back it can be a useful meridian to work with cases of lower backache.

The middle burner

This is about issues to do with digestion, such as heartburn and the movement of food.

The upper burner

CV regulates the Lungs and breathing. Often mothers find it hard to breathe fully and there can be issues with breathlessness. Work with the CV and its opening point of L7 support this. Breathing and the CV can also be used to support prenatal bonding.

Along with Stomach and PV, it governs the rectus (ancestral) muscles of the abdomen and needs to be strong to minimise their natural softening and to support the abdomen.

Governing Vessel

The Yang aspect of Kidney energy is important as a source of support for the mother and also to provide Yang energy to the fetus, often in the form of heat and warmth.

It is related closely to the spine through which it flows and so is responsible for the basic structural support of the body. Many women suffer from backaches and lack of Yang energy in pregnancy. It is especially linked with chronic lower back pain due

to Kidney deficiency, especially when pain is experienced along to the mid-line.

Forgetfulness and a lack of focus, especially related to responding to the external stimuli, are a sign of weakened energy. The mother may find it hard to keep up with demands unrelated to her focus on the fetus. Excessive focus on the Yang can lead to depletion of the Yin leading to depletion of the Conception Vessel and Kidney Yin.

Internally it flows through the Heart and influences the Brain so is often used for depression and anxiety. GV 11 can be used to support the Heart in mental emotional issues. It helps to strengthen the Mind and the Shen as well as the Zhi of the Kidneys and willpower. This is useful to support women during the emotional changes of pregnancy. Some women may experience feelings of depression in pregnancy and GV can be used in these cases.

Girdle Vessel – vessel of the Pelvis

It links Spleen, Liver and Kidney energies. It offers strong structural support through the links with the bones of the pelvis (Kidney), with the muscles (Spleen) and blood flow (Liver). It is also important in supporting the Yang energy of the pelvis through its links with the Gall Bladder meridian. All these energies need to support the fetus in the Uterus and the Uterus in the abdomen and the pelvis with Essence and Qi.

If it is not strong it may fail to give adequate support. This can be a cause of miscarriage. This is related to its role in regulating Blood and Jing flow to the pelvis which are essential.

Later on, Qi flow can be blocked in the uterus/pelvis for the mother and there can be an inadequate flow of energies to the fetus. This can be caused by it either being too slack or too tight. Imbalances in the GDV will affect the flow of energies between the mother's upper and lower body. This pattern can be linked with the Chong Mai as Blood may not reach the fetus. This may express itself as the mother not connecting emotionally with her baby or the fetus being insufficiently nourished by the Blood. This will then affect the fetus's emotional and physical growth and development.

For the mother, if Qi and Blood are not flowing in the pelvis there can be patterns of dampness or holding on. Dampness, especially in the lower burner, can lead to difficulty in urination or issues such as fibroids increasing in size during pregnancy. Stagnation of Liver Qi in the Girdle Vessel can lead to headaches.

Structurally it offers an important source of support during pregnancy. Along with the Conception Vessel it supports the abdominal muscles, especially the transverse and internal and external obliques and the pelvic floor. It is closely linked with the ancestral muscle, binding the CV and PV points together at the front. CV8 is an important point. As the fetus increases in size, slack or weak energy can lead to problems with these supporting muscles, as well as the ligaments and joints of the pelvis such as the sacroiliac and the symphysis pubis. Lower back or hip ache, pelvic girdle instability, including patterns of symphysis pubis instability (SPI) are often linked with weak GDV.

If the Girdle Vessel energy is weak it may not hold the fetus in a good position, so letting the fetus 'fall out' into the transverse or oblique position. On the other hand the energy may be excessive so that the girdle feels too tight, and the fetus may be held in an unfavourable position such as breech, or the mother may find it difficult to give birth and let the fetus be born.

It also harmonises structural balance between the upper and lower body. If it is too tight then energy may not flow between the two and the mother may experience extreme patterns of imbalance such as weakness in the upper body and tightness in the legs. Or she may experience a disconnection with the pregnancy or an inability to connect with the fetus.

Kidney–Uterus

The fetus draws on the Essence supplied to it via this meridian. This means that the mother may feel coldness in the Kidneys, suffer from lower backache and feel tired. It is closely linked with effects on Kidney energy and with all the Extraordinary Vessels as they share this internal pathway.

Kidney–Uterus is about the combination of Earth and Water energy.

Yin and Yang Linking/Wei Mai

These are mostly used in deficiency conditions which are less common in pregnancy as overall there is more Yin, Yang and Blood. However, they can be used to support cases where there is deficient Yin or Yang. They also support the defensive Qi and can be used to support changes in the immune system.

Yin Wei

This links into the Heart, Blood and Yin and the interior of the body. It can be used to support the changes in the mental emotional aspect. It can also be used where the Blood is not strong such as in cases of anaemia or Blood not flowing to the fetus.

Yang Wei

This is often used to support structural and exterior issues. It is also used in cases of backache, especially when it involves more than one Yang channel, particularly Gall Bladder and Bladder. This is a fairly common scenario in pregnancy.

Yin and Yang Ankle Qiao

These are mostly used in excess conditions. There is a similarity and complementarity to these two vessels. They are often used for structural issues. They can be used for tightness in the legs and are useful to use with restless legs syndrome.

Yin Ankle

This can be used in cases of too much Yin, which is often the scenario in pregnancy. They are helpful with oedema and excessive dampness, especially in the legs. Emotionally they can be linked with the emotional pattern of being too sunk into one's self, so that there is a sense of lethargy.

It can be linked with diabetes which is relatively common in pregnancy. There is a connection with the eyes and so they can be used with sleep disturbances, especially when there is an excess energy such as with insomnia. They are also used for excess patterns of lower burner and tightness in abdomen. Women often experience this in pregnancy due to the fetus in the abdomen. They are also used for Full Blood conditions – again this is common in pregnancy.

Yang Ankle

These are used for hip and back pain, especially sciatica and when there is excess Yang. They can be used with restless leg syndrome. They can be used for urinary problems. They control tightness in the legs. They are also used for breast abscesses, so can be useful if there is fullness of the breasts antenatally.

Fetus

Extraordinary Vessels

These are said to be the first vessels which develop in the fetus, from the moment that the egg is fertilised. This is why they are considered to be such fundamental vessels. Ancient Chinese doctors would not have understood fetal development in the way that we do, but the functions they ascribe to the vessels do mirror how they develop.

The moment that the sperm enters the ovum it determines a ventral and dorsal surfaces which are the Governing and Conception Vessels. Their energy emanates from the space between the Kidneys (GV4 – Ming Men). The PV is at the centre of this vortex and distributes its Qi and Blood over the body.

The egg begins to develop into the ectodermal and endodermal layers. The middle layer forms along a ridge which is the centre line or polar axis at the tail or caudal end of the embryo; the primitive streak. A rapid proliferation of cells pour in from the ectodermal layer and pass in all directions between the ectodermal and endodermal layers to form the intraembryonic mesoderm. At the cranial end of the streak a small node called the primitive node later becomes the neurenteric canal. It is the point from which the mesodermal tissues proliferate to become the notocord which later helps make up the vertebral column. Ming Men may be related to this node. These three primitive germ layers can be related to the GV, PV and CV.

- *Ectoderm* – gives rise to the nervous system (brain, spinal cord), parts of eyes, epithelium of nose, mouth and anus, surface of body. This relates to Yang areas and GV.
- *Endoderm* – gives rise to epithelial lining of most of the alimentary canal, larynx, trachea, bronchi and parts of the epithelium of bladder (interior portions of body) – Yin and CV.
- *Mesoderm* – gives rise to connective tissues, virtually all muscles of the body, the blood and lymph vessels, the heart, the cartilage and skeletal systems, most of the urogenital system including the kidneys, the mesothelial linings of the pericardial, pleural and peritoneal cavities, almost all of the mesenchyme, all connective tissues and fasciae of the body.

Virtually the whole of the system that becomes the medium for the meridian systems is derived from the intraembryonic mesoderm. This relates to the PV, the three burners and the immunological role of Triple Heater (TH).

As the cell continues dividing and the fetus develops, the other five Extraordinary Vessels develop. These are related more to the limbs of the body which develop after the central core: spine and digestive system. The left and right side are the Yin and Yang Ankle vessels. The exterior of the body is determined by the Yang Linking Vessel and its interior by the Yin Linking Vessels. The last vessel to develop is the Girdle Vessel which binds all the vessels together horizontally.

The eight Extraordinary Vessels are the primary energetic forces along which the body and all other channels are formed. They relate to the hormonal and neurological systems:

- GV – medulla and cerebrum.
- Heel vessels – motor nerves.
- PV – adrenals and their cortex.
- CV – ovaries.

Kidney Uterus (Bao Luo) and Heart Uterus (Bao Mai)

These vessels can be considered as branches of the Extraordinary Vessels and are about the connection of the Jing flow to the fetus and the Blood flow to the genital area. For boy babies, rather than the Uterus it is the Gong.

5.5 Changes in the twelve organs and meridians

Mother

Kidneys and Bladder – Water

Water is the main energy of pregnancy, relating to Yin, Jing and Body fluids. Emotionally water energy is linked to the mother's ancestral or family energy. In cultures which do not have this sense of family connection the mother may feel isolated and is more prone to stress, and may even experience feelings of rejection towards her fetus, or that it is a burden too great to bear on her own.

If the mother can tune into the watery state of pregnancy and 'go with the flow', resting as she needs to and not pushing herself too hard, she can feel quite well. It is the tension set up by always being on the go, and especially being in stressful situations which draw upon adrenal energy, which will cause tension in the Kidney and Bladder meridians.

Kidney

These are in a sense the most important of the organs/meridians as they are linked with Yin, Essence and Body Fluids.

Excessive physical work and overwork may weaken Kidney Yang energy which will fail to transform and excrete fluids, so that they accumulate under the skin causing oedema. Weak Kidney Yang may also lead to stress and other conditions to do with the flow of fluids such as urine, urinary tract infections, cystitis, blood flow.

Weak Kidneys can affect the Lungs as the Kidneys help bring down the energy of the Lungs, so in Chinese medicine there is a close relationship between the two. BL13 is the back transporting point of Lungs and restores descent of LU Qi. Moderate physical work is considered to be beneficial and would probably minimise oedema by helping Kidney and Lung energy to flow. Hypotension and hypertension can both be linked with Kidney.

Bladder

The Bladder energy relates to the normal functioning of the Uterus and autonomic nervous system as well as supporting the spine through the erector spinae muscles. Weakness and backaches are often linked with low Bladder or Kidney energy. BL23 is a powerful tonic for the Kidneys and is frequently used to strengthen the lower back. Work with Bladder can help address all aspects of the back from neck tension/weakness to mid-back as well as the lower back.

There are more fluids in the body in pregnancy and the body has to work hard to process them all. Bladder affects the urinary system and can be used to support the changes here. The points in the face are beneficial for clearing nasal congestion which pregnant women often suffer from. It can be a useful energy to work along with Kidney in cases of oedema. It is also helpful for tightness in the calves and cramps in the leg along its pathway.

Emotionally, as it is in the back, it can be thought of as providing basic back-up and 'support'. Lack of support and back-up may well affect Bladder energy, and lead to it not being able to support the mother's energies physically.

Spleen/Stomach – Earth

Earth is the energy of first trimester: the seed (fertilised egg) putting down its roots (establishing the placenta) in the soil (wall of the uterus). Earth energy is important throughout pregnancy; providing physical and emotional nourishment for the fetus and grounding energy for the mother.

In traditional societies, the mother would draw support from her family. It would often be her mother or grandmother who would act as the midwife. The importance of this type of family support cannot be overestimated and is an expression of Earth energy. The mother needs to be nourished emotionally, 'mothered', surrounding herself with people who will take care of her needs in practical ways, especially cooking her food.

She needs to have good physical nourishment, so she can enjoy the roundness and fullness of pregnancy – Earth energies. It is interesting that in many traditional cultures, where women lived in connection with the land and had a good diet, there was no mention of nausea or sickness. In modern culture many women are disconnected from the land and may not be eating healthy foods, so it makes sense that so many women suffer from nausea. Additionally there is pressure for a woman to appear not to be pregnant but to remain slim and slender rather than round and curvy. While it is important not to put on too much additional weight, many mothers worry about any additional weight. This creates tension and may cause the mother to feel disconnected from her real needs and frustrated with the pregnancy. If she does put on too much weight, especially by eating too much sugar or drinking iced beverages, both of which affect the Spleen, she may feel stuck and burdened down emotionally as well as physically.

Spleen

Extra demands are placed on the Spleen due to the Yin state of pregnancy. There are more fluids, including Blood. Since Spleen generates and transforms the Blood, the increased demand for Blood after conception to nourish the fetus may result in the Spleen's function of promoting transportation and transformation declining. This can lead to problems of puffiness and oedema, especially in the legs, as well as digestive problems. Poorly functioning Spleen may be a cause of gestational diabetes or blood sugar problems. Faulty diet, especially eating greasy or dairy foods, worry, excessive thinking and fatigue all weaken the Spleen and aggravate these conditions.

As the fetus grows, it tends to block the mother's energy in her groin, which prevents the Spleen meridian flowing in the legs, placing further demands on it. Conditions such as varicose veins in the legs, or vulval varicosities or haemorrhoids are related to Spleen failing to be able to hold the blood in the blood vessels.

The changes in the size of the mother and the stretching of the flesh, especially along the midline of the body, mean that Spleen has to work hard at its function of keeping organs in place. If it fails then there may be prolapse of any abdominal organ. Heavy, dragging down feelings in any muscle, but especially in the abdomen, often relate to Spleen.

As the blood volume increases through the pregnancy, the Spleen has increased demands placed on it. The mother may become anaemic. In pregnancy, this cannot be said to be caused by a deficiency of Blood – there is more blood as menses has ceased. This links with the western viewpoint of haemodilution. Anaemia is often resolved by improving the diet – that is to say nourishing Stomach and Spleen so they can make Blood.

Excessive consumption of dairy and greasy foods injures Spleen and leads to formation of Phlegm – this may settle in Lungs and prevent proper descent of Lung Qi. This can be a pattern all the way through pregnancy, depending on the quality of the mother's Spleen energy.

Stomach

Stomach is about taking food into the body and the first stage of digestion. Due to the hormonal/Jing changes in the first trimester which affect the Penetrating Vessel, Stomach has to work harder. Spleen weakness can mean that the energy of the Stomach which needs to go down to help digestion and grounding, rises up. This aggravates the rising of the Penetrating Vessel energy in the first trimester and is an underlying cause of nausea.

Later in pregnancy, if Stomach Qi fails to descend, stagnant food may accumulate in the stomach. It may lead to problems with digestion such as heartburn.

Changes in the breasts in pregnancy will also affect the Stomach which flows directly through the midline of the breasts and helps to support the Penetrating Vessel.

The three main organs involved with the counter-flow of Stomach are Spleen, Liver and Kidneys. If any of these are out of balance then they will affect the Stomach.

Stomach helps ground the mother's energy and support her in the changing body shape and needs. If the energy is balanced she can adapt to the changes in the food she needs to eat and her relationship to her body.

Heart and Small Intestine – Fire

This is the energy of the second trimester when the mother begins to bond more with her baby. Fire is the ruler of all emotions and linked with the Shen (Spirit). It is the Yang energy of pregnancy. If the mother feels happy with her pregnancy, she can focus on her positive bond and developing relationship with her fetus, as well as her changing relationship with her partner. She needs to be able to express her feelings about what is going on, her joys and sadnesses, to feel emotionally supported so Fire energy can flow.

Heart

Ideally the mother should feel safe from anxiety in pregnancy. Unfortunately in modern culture, the incidence of violence against women increases in pregnancy, partly because the partner's Heart energy is also likely to be affected by the changing relationship (Andrews & Brown 1988, Bohn 1990, Sweet 1997: 351). This will then affect the mother's Heart energy and can lead to depression, either antenatally or post-natally. Severe shock can also weaken the constitution of the fetus, as well as creating an emotional and physical predisposition to anxiety.

Physically the Heart has to work harder in pregnancy because of the increased blood volume and so it may be less stable emotionally. This is why the Chinese and Japanese would advise that the mother would stay in peaceful situations and not be emotionally disturbed. Now even from a western point of view, the emotional state of the mother is considered to be one of greatest causes of emotional and physical damage in the womb. The mother's emotional response affects neurohormones which affect the fetus (cross to placenta), creating emotional and physical predisposition to anxiety.

Of course it is not always possible to be completely stress-free and this desire may even create more stress in women. Some amount of emotional disturbance in pregnancy is natural. It is long-term, continuous stress which is the most damaging. The most important thing is, regardless of the stress, to encourage the mother to communicate her feelings with her baby. Babies can cope with a certain amount of stress, as long as the mother is able to send love and have times of being calm and happy.

Stagnation of Qi often turns into Fire which affects the Heart, Fire harasses downwards and disturbs the PV and CV. Sadness and overwork also weaken Heart energy. If Heart Qi rebels upwards then it impairs the descending of Lung Qi. Worry agitates the Heart and Emperor Fire fails to move and communicate with the Kidneys.

The mother may feel overly hot or ungrounded and unstable. Excessive consumption of hot, spicy foods can turn into Fire and disturb the Mind (Shen). Sadness and overwork weaken Heart energy, as does not sleeping well. The main Fire meridians are in the arms and are regulated by the upper burner.

Small Intestine

This is an important organ for assimilating nourishment and has to work hard due to the changes in the digestive system. As it has a close link with the Blood and can move Blood in the pelvis, it can be used to support Spleen in cases where there are issues with the Blood. It has close links with the Heart and the Bladder and can affect urination and fluid balance in the body.

Mentally it is about sorting the pure from the impure, so it is about the capacity for making decisions and clarity of mind.

SI points in the shoulder can relieve much of the shoulder tension the mother may suffer from during pregnancy due to changes in the breasts. It has close direct links with the breasts and SI points are often used to control disorders of the breasts.

It also has a link with the hormonal/Jing changes in the body and the flow of Yang energy as SI3 is the opening point of the GV.

Triple Heater and Heart Protector – supplemental Fire

Emotionally these are about how the mother integrates the changes of the pregnancy, especially Heart Protector. They are related to the overall flow of energy through their connections with the fascial system, particularly the immune and lymphatic systems and the regulation of body temperature. Flowing in the arms, they are often involved with carpal tunnel syndrome or oedema, along with the Lung. They also affect the mother's sensitivity to her environment, which is going to be changing at the end of pregnancy.

Triple Heater

As the pregnancy progresses the three burners' energy tends to get blocked by the growing fetus in the womb (lower burner area). This affects elimination functions and movement of energy in the lower abdomen as well as affecting digestion (middle burner) and respiration (upper burner).

In pregnancy, it plays an important role because:

1. It is closely linked with Kidney energy. Its source is seen as the moving Qi between the Kidneys and messenger of the source Qi. Therefore TH Yu (BL 22) point is just above KI Yu (BL 23) and 3 *cun* lateral is Huang Men (BL 51) – space between organs, bones and flesh, through which the Yang Qi streams. It sends energy to the source points on meridians. It moves Jing from the Kidneys to the upper *dantian* (situated between eyebrows) and Shen from the heart to the lower *dantian* (between CV 6 and CV 4). Middle *dantian* is related to the heart and on chest near heart. Therefore it is linked with the PV, the Heart, the Uterus and the Kidneys.

2. It has a strong relationship to CV/GV/PV as all arise in the same place, and shares a connection with the Uterus. Important points for regulating the Three Burners lie along the CV – CV 3/4 for regulating the lower burner, CV 12 the middle burner and CV 17 the upper burner.

3. Of the energy shift from lower to upper burner which happens in pregnancy. The Triple Heater controls normal mucus secretion in the Uterus and dampness in the lower burner can be a cause of infertility. Excessive dampness in the lower burner can lead to issues with excessive amniotic fluid, growth of fibroids and so on.

4. Its role in regulation of fluids, lymph (relationship here also with PV as ST 30 close to lymph nodes). Fluid levels increase in pregnancy and so it has to work harder. It is useful for regulating odema.

5. Of its relationship to fascia – many sources say that TH rules the fascia. During pregnancy there are many changes in the fascia: changes in position of abdominal organs, movement of fascia and so on.

6. It has important immune functions:
   - the upper warmer relates to thymus gland
   - the middle to pancreas and spleen
   - the lower relates to lacteal ducts, especially cistern chyli, lies level with Lumbar 1 and Lumbar 2 collecting sac of lacteal ducts.

In pregnancy there are changes in the maternal immune system response and a healthy TH energy will not only support the mother but also aid the development of the fetus's immune system.

Heart Protector

The Heart Protector supports the changes in the Heart and helps the mother adapt to her new relationships with other people and with her baby. Additionally the mother is in effect acting as the Heart Protector for the fetus who does not regulate their own heating system and does not have direct contact with the outside world.

Liver and Gall Bladder – Wood

Wood energy is about growth and new life and needs physical activity to keep it flowing. In modern culture, many women are not engaged in physical activity and this tends to block Wood energy which gathers in the neck, jaw, head and shoulders causing emotional and physical tension. This is aggravated by sitting at a desk where the shoulders are often held stiffly. Rising Wood energy creates heat and headaches. Blocked Wood energy causes feelings of frustration – unexpressed emotion. This links in with the patterns of Fire energy rising and may create explosive emotional outbursts of frustration.

Wood energy likes to be in control and have an overview of the situation. The mother wants to know all the time what is happening with the fetus and may feel that she is being taken over by someone else.

Liver

Liver stores the Blood and has a close relationship with the Penetrating Vessel – the Sea of Blood. In early pregnancy, when menstruation ceases, Blood energy and Qi tend to gather in the Liver and then its excess energy flows up the body. This aggravates the upward flow of the Penetrating Vessel, making the patterns of nausea more extreme, sometimes resulting in vomiting and hyperemesis.

Progesterone and relaxin affect the ligaments/tendons which are ruled by the Liver, and the instability of many of the major joints in the body can be said to be linked to Liver not supporting them. In the case of symphysis pubis diastasis, this may be linked to Liver's relationship to the Girdle Vessel and excessive physical activity in the past which has caused the ligaments and tendons to become overstretched.

Because of the relationship of the Liver and Stomach described by the five phase theory, if Liver Qi counterflows, it vents itself horizontally on the Stomach causing it to counterflow upwards as well. Women with a tendency to Liver Qi stagnation are prone to this scenario. It may also arise as a result of emotional stress in the first trimester. This will mean that the mother is likely to suffer from sickness which may last through much of the pregnancy. This pattern can also lead to migraines, headaches and even pre-eclampsia in the second and third trimesters.

Liver is responsible for the storage and distribution of Blood and Qi. Liver Yang provides heating to the fetus. If Liver Qi accumulates and becomes depressed this depression may transform into Fire and excess Heat.

Blood and Yin deficiency can often lead to Liver rising.

Gall Bladder

Gall Bladder has a close link with the Extraordinary Vessels. As the 'lieutenant' it has to work hard to make moment-to-moment decisions which are many in pregnancy due to the changes that are happening. This links with its relationship with the bile which is a pure fluid and therefore said to help support clarity in mental thinking. Often mothers find it harder to be clear, especially around things which are less immediately to do with the pregnancy.

Disharmony in the Gall Bladder often expresses itself in neck and shoulder tightness along the sternocleidomastoid (SCM) and trapezius muscles. It is about supporting physical action and activity. Many women these days are engaged in sedentary deskbound jobs where a lot of neck and shoulder tension can build up. Some women believe that in pregnancy they should not do much exercise. In fact achieving the right amount of exercise is important to allow the Gall Bladder energy to flow.

It also affects the eyes and often in pregnancy women experience changes in the eyes and their vision. Emotionally that sense of vision and seeing beyond the present and coming to terms with a phase of new growth is going to be altered because of the new sense of direction and purpose that a new baby is going to bring into the mother's life.

Lung and Large Intestine – Metal

Emotionally Metal relates a lot to sense of self and to how we perceive ourselves in the world. Basic identity is often challenged in pregnancy and work with these meridians can help the mother to process these changes. The Metal type can be emotionally detached – quite incisive and clear but often cold. It is the movement towards Yin energy. Women with imbalanced Metal may find it hard to form close, emotional friendships so they may lack support or be unable or unwilling to express their emotions. As becoming a mother brings up new emotions, they may find this time of life difficult to relate to – especially as it often brings with it a certain amount of letting go and lack of order, both of which the

Metal type finds hard to cope with. They may find it hard to connect emotionally with their baby and may even feel that their space is being invaded by the fetus. At the end of pregnancy they may find it hard to open up for birth.

Physically Metal types are often quite angular type people and may find the roundness of pregnancy uncomfortable – they may be the kind of people who do not appear to be pregnant until quite late on.

Lung

The Lung has to work harder as respiration needs to expand in order to increase oxygenation, elimination and take in more Qi. Furthermore the upper burner may become blocked by the blockage of energy in the lower burner and the increased size of the breasts blocking energy flow in the upper burner. Lung energy may become blocked, affecting the arms, sometimes creating carpal tunnel syndrome or oedema. Deep breathing and shiatsu and exercise to open the chest will help Lung energy to flow better.

Large Intestine

The Large Intestine performs its role less effectively because of the compression from the growing fetus and the effects of relaxin. The traditional Large Intestine meridian has no points on it which directly affect the Large Intestine but the Masunaga Zen Shiatsu extended branch is an excellent meridian for supporting issues to do with constipation or diarrhoea in pregnancy, especially since LI 4 can not be used before 37 weeks.

The classical Large Intestine can be used for releasing tension in the neck and shoulder which can build up with the upper burner being more blocked.

Emotionally Large Intestine is about letting go and accepting change. If its flow is blocked then women find the huge emotional changes brought on by pregnancy harder to process.

Fetus

Eastern theory has not developed such detailed or consistent theories for the development of the meridians in the fetus. Indeed in the Ling Shu there is an implication that the Qi and Blood and thus the meridians do not start circulating until after birth (Matsumoto & Birch 1988: 154). However, other writers believe that the meridians do start circulating in the fetus in the womb, albeit in rudimentary form. This mirrors what we know from western embryology that the organs form and mature at different rates in utero.

I have extrapolated from what we know about fetal development from a western viewpoint, how the meridians might develop in utero.

Lung/Large Intestine – Metal

The Chinese idea is that, even from conception, the fetus does have a sense of self/identity as separate from the mother: the corporeal soul. However, the fetus does not exist as a completely separate individual and the first breath at birth establishes a different level of separateness of identity which is less closely linked with that of the mother.

Lung

This is the last organ to mature, as the fetus does not need its own air supply. This shows the close link of the fetus's Lungs with the mother's and their interdependence. The fetus does not have direct contact with the Air Qi; it bypasses the Lungs and is brought directly into the fetus's body through the Blood via the placenta. This underlies the importance of good-quality Blood in pregnancy and the mother taking in and circulating good Air Qi. Energetically this is about the emotional interdependence and sensitivity of the fetus to the mother's emotional well-being. From a Chinese point of view smoking, with all its effects on Lung, would certainly be discouraged.

Large Intestine

The fetus is digesting blood and so the Large Intestine is functioning in some way, although not through excreting waste through the bowels. This maturation of its function only begins at the end of pregnancy. The first bowel movement is usually soon after birth, the meconium. If the fetus opens its bowels before birth, this is considered in western terms to be a sign of distress. Energetically this could be seen as the fetus opening up too soon or becoming anxious about the impending separation from the mother.

Stomach and Spleen

The first trimester in Chinese medicine is about taking on physical form embedding in the wall of the uterus: Earth. Physically the fetus is putting on more weight during the second and third trimesters and needs more physical nourishment. Stomach and Spleen will be active through these trimesters. In the sixth month Metal Jing is accepted and the Stomach meridian nourishes the development of the leg muscles. The Earth Jing is accepted during the eighth month and skin is composed (Chao Yuan Fang, quoted in Matsumoto & Birch 1988: 154).

Spleen

This is more active during pregnancy once the placenta is more established (from about week 9 of fetal growth) and the fetus's Spleen needs to start processing the Blood.

Stomach

This functions differently in utero as no food comes through the mouth directly to the Stomach. In a way we could say that the Stomach is bypassed as food comes directly through the Blood in the fetus. However, the fetus is growing and developing and laying down muscles so it is active in the womb.

The fetus sucks its thumb and activates the Stomach meridian in the womb.

Heart and Small Intestine – Fire

Heart and Small Intestine are one of the first systems which develop. The fetal heart beats from the fifth week and a rudimentary circulation is established. During the fifth month the fetus is influenced by Fire and in the second trimester connects with the sovereign purpose of existence as well as developing more of an emotional connection with the mother.

Heart

This is developed in the fetus and regulates Blood flow and supports the emotional connection with the mother. There is a direct link with the Blood through hormones and the mother's feelings can be felt on a physical level in the Blood through these chemical changes. There is the influence of the Shen and Heaven.

Small Intestine

This separates the pure from the impure and is working to support the Heart.

Triple Heater and Heart Protector

The TH and HC energy of the mother provides these functions when the fetus is in the womb. The fetus is not relating directly to others, the heating system is immature, the immune system is not having to process defensive Qi, as there is no direct contact between the fetus and the outside world. TH and HC only really start functioning at birth.

Triple Heater

The mother regulates the temperature of the fetus so it is kept constant. She also provides immune protection and protection from the external environment.

Heart Protector

The fetus does not relate directly to people other than through the mother, although it begins to respond to voices and touch of other people.

Bladder and Kidney – Water

Both these energies are functioning from the beginning of the pregnancy. Jing is especially important in early embryological development. The mid-line energy is the first to develop and the early structures of the spine are among the first to form. From the second trimester the fetus is in the amniotic sac and is in a Water environment.

Kidney

Weeks 9–12 – urine formation begins and it is excreted into the amniotic fluid, which the fetus swallows and then may hiccup.

Bladder

The spine is one of the first structures to develop in the fetus in rudimentary form from week 3. Development issues with the spine will affect the whole of fetal development. There are links with the nervous system. This is one meridian which can be worked directly on the fetus in the womb, once the spine can be felt, through GV, Yu and Bladder points. This can support fetal development and work with supporting the fetus with genetic issues.

Liver/Gall Bladder

Wood is the first meridian in the mother which nourishes the fetus and Blood flow to the fetus in the first trimester is important. Purposeful movements in the limbs occur as early as 8 weeks. Wood energy is the energy of the third trimester and is stimulated during birth and the movement out of the womb.

Liver

Week 7 – Liver prominent and Liver functions in utero. It governs movement.

Gall Bladder

Relates to eyes which start to be sensitive to light from third trimester and physical movement.

5.6 Summary of main treatment principles

Ultimately the mother and fetus are one energetic system and it is not possible to work the energies of either one separately. Most of the work will be focusing on the mother which will indirectly support the fetus. If the fetus has specific issues (such as congenital problems) then work can be done with the relevant meridian for the fetus by working that meridian in the mother. It is obviously difficult to be specific with working points on the fetus. However, in the last trimester it may be possible to distinguish particular parts of the fetus's body, especially the spine.

Work to support the Jing

This is the underlying energy which supports all other energies. The main way of working this is through the eight Extraordinary Vessels and the Kidneys.

Work to support the balance of Yin and Yang

Although pregnancy is predominantly Yin it is important to have a balance between Yin and Yang. There can be too much or too little Yin or too much or too little Yang. Too little Yin can lead to too much Yang.

Work can be done with Conception and Governing Vessels and the Yin and Yang Heel and Linking vessels to regulate this balance as well as the meridians which are most out of balance.

Stagnation of Qi

Many of the issues of later pregnancy are to do with the 'Obstruction' caused by the fetus preventing proper ascending and descending of Qi in the middle burner.

Work is done to support the movement of Qi and eliminate stagnation.

Phlegm – weakness of Spleen

This is particularly important to support.

Work with the Girdle Vessel

This is the vessel of the pelvis and as there are so many changes here on both a structural and energetic point of view this is relevant through the whole of the pregnancy.

Supporting the connection with the fetus and working with the fetus directly

Work can be done to support this connection. This is work with the:

- Heart–Uterus.
- Heart and the Shen.
- Heart Protector.

There can be a focus on abdominal work. During the first trimester this is on more of an energy and Jing focus and through the mother. In the second and third trimesters there can be more of a physical focus and work can be done more directly with the baby.

Focus of work by trimester

Trimester one

Support Blood, Qi and Jing to the uterus to promote good development of the embryo, amniotic sac and placenta. Ground and settle the mother's Earth energy so that the seed embeds.

This would include work with:

- Girdle Vessel: to hold energy in.
- Spleen: to support the holding up energies and the Blood. Work would tend to be along the direction of the traditional pathway (i.e. up the legs avoiding deep work over SP 6).

- CV and PV: to support the change of energy to the more Yin state of pregnancy. Include opening and associated points.
- PV: to support changes in Blood.
- Heart–Uterus: to support emotional changes.
- Liver, Heart, Spleen: to support Blood.
- Work to support changes in the flow of Jing: Kidney–Uterus, Kidney, Extraordinary Vessels.
- KD9 and KD3: to support fetal development.
- Lung: to support Metal.
- The mother's connection with the fetus.

Trimester two

Support the transition of energies from first trimester to the third. Support the more settled energies.
   This would include:

- Continue work to allow Qi, Blood and Jing to flow.
- First trimester and third trimester approaches as appropriate.

Trimester three

Allow a good flow of Qi, support bonding with the fetus and working with postural issues for the mother.
   This would include work to:

- Ensure a good flow of Qi between the three burners.
- Support the flow of Qi into the limbs, addressing specific meridian blockages.
- Support the flow of Qi, Jing and Blood to the Uterus.
- Work to support the abdominal muscles – CV, ST, Girdle Vessel, PV.
- Work to support the lower back – BL/SI, GV, Yang Stepping.
- Extraordinary Vessels for hormone support and balancing – especially CV and PV.
- Work to ensure good flow of energy in the pelvis and abdomen. This would especially include work with the Girdle Vessel and Spleen, Liver and Kidney.
- Support energy flow in the sacrum. The sacral points become more relevant to work as the fetus puts more pressure on this area, blocking the flow of energy here.
- Work with encouraging mother's emotional connection with the fetus, especially through meridians such as the Heart–Uterus and the Chong Mai.
- Work directly with an awareness of the fetus – work with the fetal spine, the mother's Bladder, the physical connection of therapist with fetus, positioning work.

Birth preparation work and late third trimester work

Towards the end of this trimester, from week 37, work can begin to focus on preparing the mother and fetus for the upcoming birth. This involves work with the Extraordinary Vessels, especially CV, GV and GDV and regulating hormonal flow.

- Supporting the movement of energy of Yin pregnancy to Yang labour.
- Work with 'labour focus' points as indicated.
- Sacral release work and work to support good energy flow in the pelvis: this would be especially work with the Girdle Vessel.
- Working directly with the energy of the fetus especially through meridians such as Bladder.

Avoidance of points

In Japan SP6 is often used throughout the third trimester as a good uterine tonic point. It may be that it is indicated for some mothers, but it would be unwise to use it routinely as a kind of shiatsu 'raspberry leaf tea tonic'.
   It is wise to avoid deep stimulation of the 'labour focus' points until the fetus is mature. It is most important to avoid work on them in the first trimester while the pregnancy is still unstable. However, from 37 weeks the body is preparing for birth and these points can then be worked quite safely without any fear of inducing premature labour.

Reflective questions

Q. What is the most important energy to consider in pregnancy work for mother and fetus and why?
Q. How does our work change from trimester to trimester?

References

Andrews, B., Brown, G.W., 1988. Marital violence in the community: a biographical approach. Br. J. Psychiat. 153, 305–312.

Bohn, D.K., 1990. Domestic violence and pregnancy: implications for practice. J. Nurse Midwifery 35 (2), 86–98.

Chao Shi Lin quoted in Rochat de la Valtee 2007.

Chou, C., 1968. The Complete Works of Chuang Tzu. Translations from the Asian Classics (B. Watson, Trans.). Columbia University Press, New York.

Eyssalet, J-M., 1990. Le secret de la maison des ancêtres. Editions Trédaniel, Paris.

Fu, Q.Z., 1973. [Fu Qing Zhu (1607–1684); first published 1827] Fu Qing Zhu's Gynecology ('Fu Qing Shu Nu Ke'). Shanghai People's Publishing House, Shanghai, p. 27.

Fu, Q.Z., 1995. Fu Qing-zhu's Gynecology (S.-Z. Yang, D.W. Liu, Trans.), second ed. Blue Poppy Press, Boulder, CO.

Guanzi: Allyn Rickett, W., 1998. In Political, Economic and Philosophical Essays from Early China. (Guanzi, Trans.). Princeton Library of Asian Translations. Princeton University Press, Princeton, NJ.

Harper, D., 1998. Early Chinese Medical Literature: The Mawangdui Medical Manuscripts. Kegan Paul, London.

Huainanzi, Chapter 3 ('Tianwen'), in Major 1993, p. 123.

Jarrett, L.S., 1998. Nourishing Destiny: The Inner Tradition of Chinese Medicine. Spirit Path Press, Stockbridge, MA p. 59.

Kawada, 2006. Workshop in Vienna attended by Suzanne Yates.

Kushi, M., 1979. The Book of Dō-In: Exercise for Physical and Spiritual Development. Japan Publications Trading Co., Tokyo.

Larre, C., Rochat de la Vallée, E., 1985. The Secret Treatise of the Spiritual Orchid. J. Chin. Med., 46. Monkey Press, Cambridge.

Larre, C., Schatz, J., Rochat de la Vallée, E., 1986. Survey of Traditional Chinese Medicine. Traditional Acupuncture Institute, Columbia, MD.

Ling Shu. The Heavenly Ordance In Pre Ch'in In China, 1 Dao De Jing, ch 30. Cited in Rochat de la Vallée 2007.

Ling Shu quoted in Essaylet 1990.

Ling Shu Jin, 1981. Spiritual axis. People's Health Publishing House, Beijing [first published c.100 BC].

Maciocia, G., 1998. Obstetrics and Gynecology in Chinese Medicine. Churchill Livingstone, Edinburgh.

Maciocia, G., 2006. The Channels of Acupuncture: Clinical Use of the Secondary Channels and Eight Extraordinary Vessels. Elsevier, Churchill Livingstone, Edinburgh.

Major, J.S., 1993. Heaven and Earth in Early Han thought: Chapters Three, Four and Five of the Huainanzi. SUNY Series in Chinese Philosophy and Culture. State University of New York Press, New York.

Matsumoto, K., Birch, S., 1988. Hara Diagnosis: Reflections on the Sea. Paradigm Publications, Brookline, MA.

Quipolon 11th century AD.

Rochat de la Vallée, E., 2007. Pregnancy and Gestation in Chinese Classical Texts. Monkey Press, Cambridge.

Sun Si Miao AD 652 Thousand Golden Ducat Prescriptions of the Tang Dynasty, cited in Luo Yuan Kai, 1979. Gynecology in Chinese medicine. Nanjing College of Traditional Medicine, Nanjing. Quoted in Maciocia G 1998.

Su, Wen., 1979. The Huang Di Nei Jing Su Wen – Yellow Emperors Classic of Internal Medicine: Simple Questions. People's Health Publishing House, Beijing [first published c.100 BC].

Yuen, J.C., 2005. The Eight Extraordinary Vessels. New England School of Acupuncture, Boston, MA.

Zhubing Yuanhou Lun.

Further reading

Legge, F.M.M.J., 1899. The Sacred Books of China. Oxford University Press, Oxford.

Look at the Chinese texts quoted and discussed in works by Jean-Marc Eyssalet and Elisabeth Rochat de la Vallée.

Neijing, Ling Shu, Dang Zhunyi (T'ang Chu-cited in, Japanese Philosophy and Culture 1962 East and West, 12;29–49).

CHAPTER 6

Eastern approach to labour

Our birth is but a sleep and a forgetting: The Soul that rises with us, our life's Star, Hath elsewhere its setting, And cometh from afar: Not in entire forgetfulness, and not in utter nakedness, But trailing clouds of glory do we come

(William Wordsworth, *Ode, Intimations of Immortality from Recollections of Early Childhood*, 1807)

You are assisting at someone else's birth. Do well without show or fuss. Facilitate what is happening rather than what you think ought to be happening. When the baby is born, the mother will rightly say: we did it by ourselves

(Lao Tzu, The Tao of Leadership, 5th century BC)

Chapter contents

Learning outcomes

- Have an overview of the main changes in energy for both mother and baby during the birth process
- Have a specific understanding of the changes in the Extraordinary Vessels and the 12 meridians for mother and baby
- Describe the main treatment principles for working during the different stages of labour

Introduction

There is not so much written about supporting a mother during birth in Chinese medicine. More attention was paid to the moment of the baby's arrival and to ensuring a calm atmosphere. This extends to the support people as well as the mother herself and the environment. Maybe this is because birth was in the female domain and most of the ancient writers were men. The type of conditions which were addressed were more to do with ensuring the safe delivery of the baby than with providing pain relief or supporting the process for the mother. Shiatsu and acupuncture have only been written about in terms of pain relief since the 1970s, although traditional midwives in China and Japan probably have always supported women with touch.

Difficult or delayed labour was a major concern as this was the main cause of maternal or fetal death. There was minimal surgical intervention during birth, so it is a realm which has changed considerably. Working alongside a western medical approach to birth has become a necessity for anyone in the field and it is important to understand the energetics not only of physiological birth but also of the effects of interventions on the process for both mother and baby.

Much of the theory in this section has come from my own experience of working in the field since 1990. Lea Papworth and Jacky Bloemraad-de Boer have also kindly contributed comments.

Traditionally during the time leading up to birth, a woman was apart from her husband so that the feminine connection could be built up. Old advice to the mother approaching labour includes:

- Sleeping in a separate room from her husband.
- Washing hair regularly in the last month to avoid breech births – an interesting link to the Water energy.
- Avoiding the presence of people in mourning or those who are emotionally disturbed in any way.

False labour was considered the baby playing and so was not necessarily seen as of concern. 'This is probably referring to the increased intensity of Braxton Hicks contractions occurring towards term, or niggling pre-labour, rather than true premature labour' (Lea Papworth).

Although the birth process was considered to be a journey for the mother, the Chinese particularly emphasised those aspects of the journey for the baby: 'Waking up from a dream, the child is capable of rotating their body, opening up the envelope and finding their path. They follow the amniotic fluid and descend' (Xu Chun Fu, from Ming period, quoted in Eyssalet 1990).

If the baby is not breathing well at birth, then it was considered that they had not woken up from their dream. The first cry and the first gestures of the baby were taken seriously. The music master who had accompanied the mother in the last few months would determine the note of the cry. The cook would work out which of the five tastes would correspond to the baby. The time of the moment of birth and the placement of the stars would help identify the Nature of the child (Xing) and their line of destiny (Ming). Modern distortions of this include women planning their caesareans to coincide with what they consider to be an auspicious time.

The main pattern of energy in labour is the movement from Yin to Yang; the movement from Water to Wood. This is the five element movement and is followed by Fire, the energy of bonding.

It is important to have an understanding of the energy of the different phases of labour, so that any work can be geared individually to the mother and her response to these patterns. Work can be done on the meridians and approaches which are most relevant to her. It is important not to have preconceived ideas. Sometimes the changes in energy can be surprising. For example a very Yin woman may move without difficulty into Yang energy. Furthermore the process of labour is different for different women. A 'quick' 10-hour labour for one woman may seem a slow labour for a woman who labours in 2 hours. For another woman a 2 hour labour can feel quite shocking.

6.1 Main energy changes during birth: mother

Yin and Yang: the fundamental shift

Birth is a movement of energy from Yin, the state of pregnancy with the fetus on the inside in water, to Yang, bringing the baby out into the world. The most Yin energy is Water and the most Yang is Fire. To move

from Yin to Yang, following the five phase movement of elements, means to move into the season of spring, to the Wood energy of growth and transformation. Wood is the movement of energy in the second stage of labour.

With the beginning of labour, there is a Yang, active impetus, caused by changes in the Governing Vessel. From a western perspective this represents the hormonal shifts. The Yin to Yang shift continues to build. The first stage of labour is more Yin in relation to second stage. The more Yin type person will tend to find the first stage of labour easier as Yin energy still predominates. As labour progresses to second stage she may find this shift more difficult to assimilate. It is the opposite for the Yang type person, who tends to find first stage of labour more difficult than second stage.

This correlates to the Western approach: a woman who is more able to shift into connecting with the primitive brain, the hind-brain, is generally a Yin type of person and tends to ease into labour whereas someone who stays in the neo-cortex mode is more Yang and will struggle to move into the first phase of labour.

(Jacky Bloemraad-de Boer)

Once the baby is born, they begin to form relationships with people other than the mother and this is more to do with Fire, the most Yang energy. The mother also has to draw on her Fire to relate to the baby in a different way and on her Metal to let go of the identity she had formed of her baby and relate to it as a separate person.

Yang wood energy – the spiritual aspect of the Hun

This movement to Yang is linked with a movement of Wood energy. Wood is about birth, new life and the baby coming into the world and beginning its journey. Hun resides in the Liver. It is to do with the word, imagination, Yang energy and the spirit, and to some extent the breath.

Changes in flow of Qi, Blood and Jing

All of these energies change dramatically over a short period of time. As well as CV and GV being important, PV and the other five Extraordinary Vessels play a role. Any blockage during labour for mother or baby can ultimately be caused by any of the energies in the body being out of balance.

Qi

There is a big movement of Qi with the baby moving from being inside the mother to outside. The biggest movement is at the moment of birth when there is a large surge of the mother's Qi.

This is seen when an exhausted mother makes the final push that delivers the baby, and she takes her child in her arms.

At this point, her Shen reignites. Considering the digestive functions slow to minimal activity in labour, a women relies on her reserve (Pre-Heaven) Qi as well as her Jing.

(Lea Papworth)

Blood

This is important throughout the labour as the baby needs to keep receiving nourishment, especially during the contractions when Blood flow is restricted. If the labour is long, maternal position will be important to ensure good Blood flow. For a woman lying on her back, even in the semi-recumbent position which is often favoured now, the free flow of breath, Qi and Blood tends to be blocked. At the moment of birth there are huge changes in Blood as the placenta stops providing the Blood to the baby and the baby has to start producing its own Blood. For the mother also there are big changes in the flow of Blood as the placenta detaches and the blood vessels start healing over.

Jing

This supports the whole process with changes in hormonal energy initiating labour for both mother and baby and the changes in the early postnatal period. As the flow of Qi slows then Jing and Yuan Qi are drawn upon to provide the energy to support the birth process.

Stages of labour: the movement of the five elements

All elements are present, supporting each other, but the overall movement is from Water to Wood.

First stage: water Yin to Yang, opening up and letting go

This is the first stage of the movement from Yin to Yang. It involves a shift from the Yin to the Yang aspect of Water, from Kidney Yin to Kidney Yang and then to Bladder. As the first stage progresses women often connect with images and visualisations of water, and may even want to get into water. The image of the wave gets stronger as the contractions become more intense. As the first stage culminates with transition many women exhibit fear or anger. This indicates the emotions connected with the shift from Water (fear) to Wood (anger) which the mother is passing through.

I often ask a mother who is struggling during the latent phase if there is any 'stuck' anger in her. This very strange question almost always results in a resounding YES and a dam of anger bursting. Once this has happened the mother usually moves right along into good latent and then active labour! I have to mention though that I usually have a close relationship to these clients and choose the moment very carefully.

(Jacky Bloemraad-de Boer)

The latent phase is Kidney Yin and during the active phase there is a shift to Kidney Yang and Bladder.

Opening up Metal and CV/GV

This is expressive of LI/LU energy: the movement of the out-breath and letting go both emotionally and physically. There is an interesting connection between the jaw being open and the cervix being open. The mouth to anus connection represents the beginning and end of Metal energy as well as the basic GV/CV circuit. Often women experience sickness or diarrhoea before or during labour and LI4 is a point which can reduce these symptoms and enable this energy to support the opening up process.

When supporting a woman in labour take note of her lips. A woman pursing her lips is tensing with her contractions, particularly tensing her abdominal muscles, often pulling up her shoulders as well. Encouraging her to let go assists her to relax and seems to increase the effectiveness of natural painkillers – endorphins.

(Lea Papworth)

Going with the flow – Water

With the onset of labour there is a Yang impetus as energy shifts from Kidney to Bladder. Often BL and KD points are used to support first stage, for example BL67 and BL60, KI1, sacral BL points and KD6 and BL62. It is well accepted that fear increases pain. KD1 helps calm fear.

Muscular contractions – Earth

The uterine muscles contract but they also need to relax. The process of retraction means that the upper uterine muscle contracts and then partially relaxes resulting in their bulking and shortening. The lower uterine muscles and cervix relax and lengthen. Spleen/Earth (SP6, ST36) supports this process. If the mother uses too much muscular contraction in other parts of her body and does not nourish herself adequately she can get tired and this can lead to tiredness in the uterus and ineffective contractions, thus tending to prolonged labour.

Relaxation of the sinew and tendons – Wood

The cervix relaxing is related to the Wood energy of the sinews. GB34 is often used to relax a tight or scarred cervix and points such as GB30, LV3, GB21 help the Wood to flow.

Shoulders being pulled up is a sign of Liver Qi stagnation (Gall Bladder 21) and so in relation to that shift from Water to Wood it is important to ensure a woman relaxes her shoulders during and between contractions.

(Jacky Bloemraad-de Boer).

Transition – the movement from Yang Water to Wood

The mother may get stuck here. How she gets stuck reflects the balance of the elements within her. It could express itself as either a physical or emotional block.

It could be Earth not moving, a phase of withdrawal expressing through tiredness and lack of energy, feelings of being stuck, or feelings of lack of nourishment, either physical or emotional.

It could be Wood not flowing, in which case there is often a lot of anger and physical holding on, especially in the jaw and shoulders.

It could be Water not flowing. Water could be Bladder or Kidney energy but it could also be Extraordinary Vessel energy. The mother may go to sleep, switch off, or simply pause at the pivotal moment of the shift between the Water and Wood. There could be trembling, tiredness and exhaustion. The mother could feel very fearful.

If Metal is not flowing there can be feelings of sickness or holding on emotionally or expressed physically through being constipated.

If Fire is not flowing there can be panic or emotional disconnection. The mother could feel very cold.

Second stage – Water to Wood and the moment of birth

The predominant energy here is of Yang energy rising. This is Wood. It is a much shorter phase relative to first stage involving a more dynamic physical shift of Qi.

The contractions change in their energy flow from dilating to expulsion so there is a strong downward movement of energy as the baby moves down the birth canal. Governing Vessel as overall regulator of Yang predominates at this phase. The Chinese advised against pushing too strongly. The most important thing was to allow Wood to flow like a general marshalling his troops. It is difficult to assess what 'too strongly' is as it is different for different women and is probably related to cultural traditions. Mediterranean women are known for vocalising in their labours and asking them to breathe out quietly and bear down gently can inhibit and annoy them or make them feel ashamed of their need to express. Amish women in North America, by contrast, often make no sound at all. The main principle is to assess that Wood energy is flowing and that the bearing down is not full of tension. If the mother is tense, she may think she is bearing down but the energy is often stuck in the upper body and her mouth and jaw are likely to be tight. GB21 is a powerful point to release this energy and allow it to flow to the cervix to facilitate productive bearing down. At the moment of the actual delivery the mother may feel that she is breathing the baby out. At this stage women sometimes open their eyes to bring more of an outward energetic focus to the process.

Blocks to the flow of Wood

Blocks in the flow of Qi in any element or meridian will block the flow of Wood.

It can be hard for the Wood to flow if the Water is exhausted because Water is the mother energy of Wood. If first stage has gone well then there is more likely to be a natural flow into Wood. Stuck Water could be indicated by a full bladder which can block the process of the second stage. It is interesting that often physiologically the amniotic sac (waters) break at the beginning of the second stage of labour, facilitating the movement into Wood. If Water is not flowing the mother may be afraid of the pressure on the perineum and hold back through fear.

Metal can block the movement of Wood by not allowing it to flow. If the mother is unable to open her jaw, relax, soften her shoulders, open the cervix and let go both physically and emotionally, then Wood can become blocked. She may be slightly constipated. Again it is interesting that often at this stage women feel the urge to defecate and indeed sometimes small amounts of faeces are released. If Metal is over-controlling Wood it is usually expressed as tension in the neck and shoulders and unproductive pushing utilising the upper body rather than allowing the energy to flow down. The mother may feel quite angry. GB21 and release work to the shoulders can often unblock this pattern but LI4 can also be useful.

If the Earth energy is exhausted then the mother may not have the energy for second stage, or it may be that the baby is exhausted.

Lack of Fire could lead to emotional exhaustion.

Third to fourth stage – Wood to Fire and bonding

Fire is the predominant energy here as the mother begins to bond with her baby outside the womb and the baby begins to make new relationships.

The third stage has very similar energy to the second stage but is less intense. It is still about the downward movement of Wood to deliver the placenta. If this does not happen, then the placenta may be retained. However, there is already a shift of movement from Wood to Fire which happened with the birth of the baby, and the mother's and baby's energy is more expansive. This is the energy of the fourth stage – the beginning of the bonding process between the mother and her baby.

It also correlates to keeping a woman warm (Fire) after the second stage so that high amounts of adrenaline (needed for the "fetal ejection reflex") can drop. Otherwise the production of oxytocin needed to release the placenta is blocked'.

(Jacky Bloemraad-de Boer).

Fourth stage – Fire and bonding

This is postnatal energy and is about the relationship between Fire and Metal as the bonding is closely linked with the process of separation of mother and infant. There is the continuation of the hormonal changes and changes in the flow of Blood and Qi which need to happen for both mother and baby.

6.2 Main energy changes during birth: baby

Yin and Yang: moving from Water to Wood and Earth

The process of the birth for the baby is about moving from the Yin Water environment of the womb to the Earth outside and from being dependent on the mother's Qi, Blood and Essence for nourishment to making the transition to producing its own energies. The circuit of the Extraordinary Vessels is important in regulating this process of change. In the fetal position, the Governing Vessel surrounds the Conception and Penetrating Vessels. During labour, they are stimulated through compression and then undergoes changes at birth as the baby's spine is extended and the head and shoulders rotate. At birth there is a gradual opening and unfolding which continues in the early days and weeks as the baby opens up its body and the Yin channels come into more direct contact with the outside and become the front as opposed to the inside of the body.

The baby is considered to be vulnerable in the early days. The Shen is open. To protect the Shen, the baby is in immediate and direct contact with the mother's abdomen. To protect the Jing of the baby, birth would be in a darkened room and strong voices and shocks and contact with metal would be avoided where possible.

In old China, and indeed in many traditional cultures, there were some traditions where the baby would pass the first 3 days of life on the ground on their abdomen without food so that they can connect with the Earth. There would be rites of purification before the infant would have first milk. This is an example of a traditional practice which is not helpful and underlies the importance of not slavishly following ancient writings. It can be understood energetically but skin-to-skin contact and breastfeeding are better ways of supporting

the Earth. The pre-milk, colostrum, contains important minerals and immunological properties so it is important for the baby to feed from the breast as soon as it can. Feeding also encourages involution of the uterus. Energetically the mother has been the infant's Earth for 9 months and continues to provide that continuity of support. In some cultures the mother would hold the baby for most of the first 6 months.

Another eastern view (Kushi 1979; see Ch. 5) sees birth as representing the occurrences on earth about 400 million years ago. As land masses formed and creatures moved from the sea to the land there were repeated catastrophes in land formation and large scale flooding. This is like the baby moving from water to earth. In order to adapt to the new expanded atmospheric environment the baby must first experience contraction by being compressed through the birth canal and breathing out excessive substances through the contraction of the lungs. Babies who are born by caesarean miss out on this process of contraction and may need additional support to make the transition.

Changes in flow of Qi and Blood and Jing

As with the mother there are big changes in all these energies.

Qi

There is a big shift in Qi as the baby makes the journey down the birth canal through the process of movement involving various twists and turns. The Qi and limbs are compressed. The moment of birth represents the movement when the baby starts making its own Qi, separate from the mother's. The first breath opens the lungs and Air Qi comes directly into the baby's body. Shortly afterwards the baby will suckle, taking in Food Qi. In this way the organs each become activated as they start to assume their functioning outside the womb.

Blood

There is a need for an adequate supply of Blood, particularly during the contractions themselves as Blood flow is restricted. At birth it is important that the flow of Blood continues. It was considered important not to cut the cord and thus allow Blood to continue to flow while the baby makes the transition to form its own Blood. If there is not a good flow of Blood then the baby can become emotionally distressed and disturbed.

Jing

The mother's Jing continues to support the baby during labour and there are hormonal shifts for the baby. The baby is connecting with the will of the earth and coming into the realisation of his/her destiny. After birth the Jing is vulnerable and it is important to continue to support the baby's Jing through the breast milk and colostrum. This is one of the reasons why the baby and mother would remain in a quiet, stress-free environment for some time after birth.

Stages of labour: the movement of the five elements

First stage – Yang Water

The baby is moving from Water propelled by the Yang energy of the mother. Sometimes the waters break before labour begins, sometimes during labour and sometimes not at all. These differences show how different babies relate differently to Water. The change of energies is less dramatic when the waters break later in labour or the baby is born into water. Water is also about the hormonal changes which the baby is going through. The hormonal changes for the baby are more on the adrenal level, which is related to the Yang aspect of the Kidneys. However, there is a fine line between Yang stimulation and stress and fear. Sometimes the baby can go into an unbalanced as opposed to a supporting stress response and this is when it can become 'compromised'.

Earth

The baby feels the energy of contractions around its body. These muscular forces represent the strong containment of Earth. However, they are gradually moving the baby away from the womb home towards a new experience of Earth. The mother's Earth which contained them is now the very force which is propelling them out from their home. The baby may resist this emotionally or even on a physical level if they have poor muscle tone. They may want to stay in the womb home and not move on. This can slow down or block the process of labour.

Transition

The energies of first stage become stronger and more intense as there is more physical compression. The baby may resist by becoming stuck and not wanting to make that big shift before the final stage of the journey.

Second stage – downward movement of Yang

This is the time when the baby experiences the more Yang energy of Wood. It is a physical phase of movement and change. The baby needs Blood to support the movement. There needs to be a free flow of Liver energy. The baby will begin to be pushed down and will undergo various movements due to the force of the contractions, the shape of the perineum and pelvis. The baby's position at the start of labour, as well as the shape of the mother's pelvis, will influence whether or not this is an easy process or whether the baby gets stuck. The Yang energy of the mother is the driving force behind moving the baby out of the womb. The baby is probably involved in some way in this process although the exact mechanism is not clear.

It is interesting to consider water birth from the baby's point of view. There is a less dramatic shift from the womb to the earth and less intense Wood energy.

Third stage

The baby feels direct contact with the Earth for the first time. As it moves out it also starts to take in Food Qi fairly soon after birth. It will make skin-to-skin contact with the mother and especially her breasts and therefore connect with the Earth.

There can also be big shifts in the Fire Heart and the Shen which begin to happen as the baby starts to make its own Blood and to separate from the mother.

The Chinese considered that it was not so good to cut the cord with metal. This was considered to be too brutal a separation. They preferred cutting it with teeth (Sun Si Miao, Traité valant mille pièces d'Or, in Eyssalet 1990). There is already a big separation which happens naturally and the Chinese felt it should be as gentle as possible.

Fourth stage

The Fire energy becomes more active as the baby continues the bonding process with the mother and Blood is being made within the baby's own body as opposed to coming via the placenta. Within this closeness of Fire there is also the separation of Metal. This can be made more extreme by separating the mother from the baby and placing the baby elsewhere, for example in a nursery or on the ground.

6.3 Changes in the Extraordinary Vessels: mother and baby

Mother

As birth is a time of great change which involves strong movements of the mother's Qi and Jing, the overall process is said to be regulated by the Governing and Conception Vessels. They regulate the hormonal changes, send energy to the relevant meridians and support the shift from Yin to Yang energy. Girdle Vessel regulates changes in the pelvis and Penetrating Vessel in the Blood.

Governing Vessel

As Governing Vessel is related to the neocortex and labour is initiated by the release of oxytocin produced by the posterior pituitary gland which relates to Governing Vessel, GV represents the energy of birth. As the mother progresses to the more Yang second stage she may well begin to assume upright positions and engage the Yang energy of the Governing Vessel. This is the surge of catecholamines which happens in late first stage to cause the 'fetal ejection reflex' (Odent 1992).

If the woman is lying on her back during birth, then this tends to physically block the flow of energy in the GV, especially in the lower back and the coccyx area. This can interfere with the strong mind focus required especially in the second stage.

Energy needs to move down to the perineum for the second stage and this is connected with the lower pathways of the Governing Vessel and Conception Vessel. Governing Vessel energy needs to flow freely to allow the coccyx to move and for the Yang impetus for birth.

Conception Vessel

Yin energy needs to support the Yang. Especially in a long labour, the mother may need to be encouraged to have time to connect with the more Yin aspects – to rest and to pause allowing the Yin energies to build up so that they can support the Yang. Often, with the focus on the 'progress of labour', this aspect can be neglected in the more medical environment.

Conception Vessel relates to Yin energy and the old, instinctive aspects of the brain. If women are allowed to take instinctive positions in early labour, they find the most comfortable positions. They are often leaning over forward on all fours with the Conception Vessel more protected by the Governing Vessel on the outside. If the mother is protected then she may feel more able to be in her own space and to breathe more easily.

In a more medicalised birth the Yin vessels can be more exposed and less protected, for example the mother is often lying on her back with the CV exposed. This may make her feel more passive and less connected, more vulnerable emotionally and physically. Many of the drugs administered in labour have a sedating effect which can build up too much Yin. The CV needs to be supported in these situations.

CV can be used to support the connection with the perineum and help if there is pain or discomfort here. It can also be used if there is urinary retention which may block the progress of labour.

At delivery, placing the baby on the mother's chest stimulates and reinforces the connection with the CV and with the Yin energy from where the baby has come and helps to support the transition.

Heart-Uterus and Kidney-Uterus

Heart-Uterus needs to send Blood and Kidney-Uterus needs to send Jing to the Uterus. Heart-Uterus has a strong link with PV. A tired or ineffectively contracting Uterus can be supported with these energies, as well as enabling the baby to have these energies for its journey. They both help to settle the mother's and baby's emotions to help them process the huge changes which are happening for them and to help the mother stay connected with her baby. This focus is often particularly useful in the current climate of birth where so much emphasis is placed on coping with the pain of labour rather than supporting the baby in labour. Women often find this shift of focus helpful and they may even enjoy giving birth.

The Girdle Vessel

It is probably the first vessel that needs to open up for labour as it is the last one in the sequence (Yuen 2005) and the one where experience is stored. In order to move on, the past needs to be released. Girdle Vessel supported the baby in the womb and needs to make a shift and open up in order for the baby to be birthed. Many women find this transition difficult. They may not necessarily be afraid of labour, but have become so used to holding on to and nurturing their baby within their body, that it is hard for them to make the emotional and structural shift in order to let go and give birth.

It is a key vessel for promoting the initiation of labour or prolonged labour. It helps with the movement and position of the baby, especially in promoting descending.

As it affects changes in the pelvis, if it is too loose then the contractions may be ineffective and fail to dilate the cervix. If it is too tight then the baby may get stuck. There can be a big difference in its energy between front and back. Sometimes, with ineffective contractions, there can be too much energy in the lower back and not enough flowing round to the Uterus. This may cause or be caused by the fetus being in a less favourable position or in deep transverse arrest. Sometimes the pattern can be the reverse and then the mother would feel excessive pain in her abdomen/uterus.

Through its links with the ancestral muscle and pelvic floor it can help direct the energy of the abdomen, particularly the deep abdominal muscles, to assist with bearing down in the second stage. Again at the moment of delivery the energy needs to shift to allow the perineum to open up and the baby to be born.

A flexible yet strong GDV will support and facilitate the birth process. A GDV which is too tight or too loose may slow it down. As it continues to support the mother postnatally, especially if she has had a caesarean section, then thought needs to be given to how it is affected in different positions. Any instrumental delivery with the mother in the lithotomy position will tend to result in either excessive pressure on the symphysis pubis (and may be a cause of pelvic girdle dysfunction (PGD) issues postnatally) or pressure on the coccyx (which could become damaged). Side-lying positions may tend to put excessive pressure on one side of the pelvis rather than the other.

Penetrating Vessel

Changes in the flow of Blood are the most important at the time of delivery itself, although of course Blood needs to flow to the baby during labour, especially during each contraction. At delivery PV can be used for placental problems, excessive bleeding and to support the contraction of the blood vessels to the uterus.

The bonding aspect and connection of mother with baby during labour, how much the mother can remain aware of the baby and not just focus on the contractions and perceived pain, are aspects of PV and CV. Emotionally if the mother can remain connected with the baby, this may help support maternal and fetal relaxation.

At delivery the initial skin-to-skin contact, especially of the baby to the breast, will support the bonding and the changes in flow of the PV for the mother.

Yin and Yang Linking Wei

They are used if there is low energy and can be used if the woman is tired or Yang or Yin need to be linked.

Yang

This is a useful meridian if there is backache, especially if it involves Gall Bladder and Bladder. This is often the case in labour as it is about the shift from the Yang Water to Wood energy.

Yin

There can often be insufficient Yin energy, especially if the mother is in a stressful environment and there is pressure on her to give birth or progress in labour. This meridian can enable the mother to have space to rest, gather her energies and be nourished, in order to support the Yang energy. This is often the scenario with long labours. Some midwives will suggest epidurals in order to relax the mother and give her some 'time out'. However, work with the Yin Linking may have a similar effect.

It has a strong effect on the Heart. If there appears to be more of an emotional block to labour (such as sadness, grief, lack of joy, difficulties in the relationship between the mother and her partner, inability to shift from the prenatal bonding state to being ready to welcome the baby), then this would be a good meridian to work.

Yin and Yang Ankle Qiao

These are involved with more excess patterns. They can be used if labour is too quick or there are surges of energy followed by exhaustion. They can help with regulating the hormonal changes involved in labour and relieve structural tension, such as backache or hip pain.

Yang

They can be used if there is a fullness of Yang. Sometimes too much Yang can block labour or perhaps labour is progressing too quickly and the Yang needs to be dissipated a little. Drugs which stimulate labour, such as the oxytocic drugs used for induction, can cause too much stimulation of the uterus and so this vessel can help regulate that surge of energy.

They can also be used for the structural conditions such as backache and sciatica and hip pain.

Yin

This is used in situations of fullness of Yin. Sometimes the woman has so much Yin that the Yang energy cannot flow. She may go inside herself to the point where labour slows down. This could also be the scenario if the mother has had sedating drugs which make her go into a sluggish space. These meridians can help move the Yin energy thereby allowing the Yang energy to flow more freely.

They can also be used in cases of retention of lochia, placenta and blood stasis, fullness of the abdomen.

Baby

All Extraordinary Vessels are important during labour and in the early postnatal phase, especially if the newborn has suffered a stressful birth. With their links with the Jing and Kidney energy there is an important connection with the bones which undergo many changes during labour, the spine and skull in particular.

Conception Vessel

Yin needs to support the Yang flow of labour in order to give energy and to reduce stress. As the 'Vessel of bonding' there is a connection with the Heart. How much the mother connects or does not connect with her baby, both during labour and in the early postnatal phase, may affect both labour itself and the bonding process. The baby may sense a lack of connection and 'clutch at the mother's heart', thus slowing down or stopping labour. The baby may feel a need to stay close to the mother after birth.

There is also a connection with the Lungs and with the process of breathing. CV supports the initiation of the first breath after the Yang expulsive movement of the delivery itself. There are changes in the upper burner in the couple of days before birth in preparation for this shift. Caesarean section can affect the upper burner and the Lungs in particular, meaning that it is harder for this shift to occur and so the baby may need support. Depressive drugs given to the mother will also affect the baby, slowing down the system and bringing in too much Yin energy, making it harder for the baby to connect with the Yang energy of birth.

Governing Vessel

This regulates the Yang energy of the baby being born. It also regulates the movement of the spine and the control of the head. It embodies the movement out and down towards independence, sense of self and the expression of willpower. Too much stress will affect this and overstimulate the Yang energy, thus affecting the baby's mental emotional state.

Penetrating Vessel

This regulates the movement of Blood to the baby. If the baby is distressed, it could be due to the Heart connection with the mother or with inadequate Blood flow. Blood can be restricted due to the contractions or problems with there being a knot in the cord.

Heart-Uterus

This is closely linked with the Penetrating Vessel and relates particularly to the effects of the emotional connections between the mother and baby.

Kidney-Uterus

This is closely linked with the Jing flow and would be affected by hormonal drugs such as oxytocin which may overstimulate the hormonal changes leading to too much adrenaline, potentially causing stress to the baby.

Yin and Yang Linking Wei

These are used in cases of deficiency. This can be the case if the mother is given drugs such as pethidine which tend to suppress her system and therefore the baby's system. They are also important immediately after birth to support the baby's defensive Qi as the baby is quite vulnerable in the early weeks and months.

Yin

This can be used to support the initial breath, especially if the baby is 'flat' at birth and not breathing.

Yang

Along with the Yin Linking it can support the stimulation of the first breath if the baby needs some Yang stimulation.

Yin and Yang Ankle Qiao

These vessels embody the essence of labour for the baby: moving out into space and into form – the moment of separation from the maternal matrix.

Yin

Some babies can be sluggish in energy during labour. This can be due to the effects of drugs such as pethidine on the mother or conditions such as diabetes. After birth this vessel can be useful if the baby is lethargic due to a traumatic birth or the effects of drugs.

Yang

It can be used if there is too much Yang stimulation due to the effects of drugs. It can also be useful if the baby is getting stuck during labour for example with deep transverse arrest or shoulder dystocia. After birth it may support structural issues due to the birth such as back issues especially if forceps, ventouse or caesarean section were used. It also gives support in other structural issues, due, for example, to congenital issues such as hip dysplasia.

Girdle Vessel

If the pregnancy was stressful or if there are congenital issues or problems with any of the pelvic organs, then there may be issues here.

Movement here supports the various twists and turns down the birth canal and the opening of the hips at birth. There is a big shift at birth as the umbilical cord is attached to CV 8, a key point for the GDV. Cutting of the cord, as opposed to allowing it to stop pulsating, may influence the GDV. It will also be affected in cases of hip dysplasia and could be used to support this condition.

6.4 Changes in the 12 meridians

Mother

Water – Kidney and Bladder

This is the predominant energy of the first stage of labour as there is a shift from the energies of Kidney Yin to Kidney Yang and to Bladder.

It is important that the mother enters labour with good energy. Water can be depleted by stress and overwork which is common these days with the increased tendency for women to work later in pregnancy.

Pregnancy insomnia should also be addressed before labour if possible.

Prostaglandins and oxytocin stimulate contractions and relate to Water. Stress affects prostaglandin production as it involves the release of the adrenal hormones (catecholamines) which tend to block the release of oxytocin and endorphins. The adrenal hormones also shunt blood from the Uterus and placenta, slow down contractions and decrease oxygen to the fetus. In Chinese medicine the Kidneys relate to the adrenals. If Water does not flow, then the mother can feel like she is in a pool of stagnant water and this state is characterised by fear and trembling. It is known that *fear* is the main emotion which can block the first stage. Fear also increases the pain through the mechanism of hormones described above.

The mother needs to be in a stress-free environment to allow Water to flow and it may be this instinctive connection with water which has led to the increase in popularity of water births, or at least the use of water for pain relief during the first stage of labour. Women who have an affinity with Water will tend to find the first stage of labour easy, but may find it hard to shift to the more Yang energy of second stage. At this stage they may need to come out of water, if they have been in the pool, in order to shift the energy.

Generally it is not recommended that mothers get into the birthing pool before they are in active labour as it may slow down labour if used too early. This indicates energetically that the Water needs to shift from the Yin to the Yang phase and that too much Yin Water, as in a birthing pool, may block this shift from happening.

Kidney

- Kidney and Jing as already discussed.
- Kidney and adrenals and stress.

A long labour may weaken Kidney Yang energy which may add to the stress. It can also block the flow of fluids such as urine. A full Bladder may interfere with second stage.

Weak Kidneys may affect the Lungs. Kidney Qi needs to grasp the Lung Qi to help it descend. Shallow, fearful or inhibited breathing will adversely affect Kidney energy while deep relaxed breathing will support both Lung and Kidneys. Hypotension and hypertension can both be linked with Kidney. Wood (Liver) energy can also be affected if Water is not strong as the Water in this case will then fail to nourish the Kidneys.

Bladder

During labour there are many changes in the back, especially in the sacrum. BL30–34 points are especially important in allowing the Water energy to flow.

If the mother is lying on her back, this will interfere with the flow. Upright positions where she can move will support labour.

In the second stage a full bladder can interfere with the descent of the baby's head. In the third stage a full bladder may block the delivery of the placenta and cause excessive bleeding through blocking good uterine contraction.

Bladder can also be used for support if the mother experiences headaches or blocked sinuses. It also supports the normal functioning of the uterus.

Wood – Liver and Gall Bladder

Wood is the predominant energy for the second stage of labour. The relaxation and opening of the cervix relaxing also relates to the free flow of Wood (GB30, LV3, GB21).

As Wood types typically like to be in control, then they may find they do not like the unpredictability of labour and having a baby. They may find the first stage of labour difficult as it is about opening up and allowing energy to flow freely, like Water. Women often say they like to feel in control of labour but what they really mean by that is they are able to do what they want and make the decisions they need to make. Wood can go into over-controlling – an expression of this would be a woman who wanted to know how long labour was going to be, how many more contractions, when her baby is going to be born rather than simply staying with the energy of each contraction.

The movement of strong Wood is physically demanding and women who have been sedentary may find its power too strong. The tendency is for Wood to get stuck in the shoulders, and often during transition it is noticeable how women can clench their jaws, hold their breath and feel quite angry. A person whose Wood is flowing well tends to like the feelings of second stage and at last being able to be more active and more in control of what is going on. It is known that opening the eyes may help focus in the second stage (Simkin & Ancheta 2000: 88) and the eyes relate to Wood.

Liver

The birth process makes demands on Blood and so Liver is important first in having built up and stored sufficient Blood to support the process and then in regulating its distribution. Liver stores the Hun which is about the spiritual aspect of new life and the spirit coming in. Liver is said to rule the flow of energy in the reproductive organs, especially in the cervix, and if Liver is not flowing then it may affect the ability of the cervix to dilate.

Gall Bladder

This supports the many physical movements and adaptations which have to be made during labour. In a physiological labour, women tend to move around and this allows Wood to flow. If Wood does not flow freely then there can be tightness in the neck and jaw which can lead to tightness in the cervix and block the flow of energy down to the perineum.

Fire – Heart and Small Intestine

Fire is about providing emotional support to women in labour and allowing them to be able to express their feelings, especially if they get stuck. Feelings of connection with the baby and focus on the baby can provide a positive focus. This can involve working with the Heart-Uterus meridian.

Heart

It is important that the mother feels calm and free from anxiety. This was one of the main aspects that was emphasised by the ancients. Emotional tension and the connection between the mother and father or birth attendants can interfere with the birth process. It also supports the flow of Blood.

Small Intestine

This is about sorting the pure from the impure and is linked in with the mother being prepared emotionally to let go and birth her baby. It is an important meridian to support during times of shock, which involves sudden changes in Blood flow and sudden emotional adaptations. This is more likely the scenario if there is the need for emergency medical intervention.

There is a link with Bladder and SI can be used if there is urinary retention in labour. It is an important meridian in moving stagnation in the pelvis and can be used to help with poor circulation, including heaviness and stiffness in the hips and legs. Tightness in the neck and shoulders can be relieved by working with SI.

Supplemental Fire: Triple Heater and Heart Protector

This is about sensitivity to the environment. Often labour stops or slows down when the mother changes from being at home to being in hospital. Triple Heater is useful to work to support this adaptation and in any situation where the environment is unsupportive, whether at home or in the hospital. As it is linked with boundaries and violation of boundaries it can be used where the mother may feel cautious and hold back. It can support the mother in cases where there is medical intervention, especially instrumental/surgical deliveries such as caesarean section or ventouse/forceps.

It helps overall flows of energies, especially Kidney (and Jing) and Water energy, so it is a useful meridian for supporting the whole process. As it supports the immune system, it can be good to work if the mother is unwell.

Heart Protector

Working alongside Heart, this supports the mother's emotional connections. It is about supporting the emotional connection she feels with her support people during labour.

If the mother goes into a state of panic HC8 is especially good for calming the spirit and can often have a dramatic effect in calming strong emotions.

Metal – Lung and Large Intestine

These relate to letting go, which is what the mother is doing with her baby. It is the first stage in the separation process which will continue between mother and child until the adult offspring leaves the mother and forges his or her own independent identity. The mother herself is forming a new identify as a mother. Women may feel grief as well as joy in this process and this grief may block labour as the mother on some level does not feel ready to let go of her baby. Metal represents the basic tube of energy between the jaw and the anus: the in and out connection of birth. If it is blocked then it does not support the physical opening up which needs to happen.

Lung

This is important because of its connection with the breath. It provides the Air Qi necessary to support the process of labour which requires a lot of Qi. The out-breath provides important focus on relaxation and letting go in labour and emotionally is a good focus.

Large Intestine

This is linked with the energy of opening up and letting go. There is an interesting connection with LI4 for going into labour. Often mothers experience nausea, sometimes sickness, constipation/diarrhoea prior to going into labour or during labour itself. Large Intestine work will help these processes to be balanced and may well relieve these conditions.

Earth – Stomach and Spleen

This provides the centre of the process and governs the energy of the strong muscular contractions. If Earth is not flowing, women may feel emotionally stuck and find it difficult to get the impetus to go into labour. They may get tired. If Earth flows then women should progress easily if they are in a supportive environment and are allowed to eat as they need to. They may need to sing and make sounds.

Moving women from one environment to another, as in the transfer from home to hospital, can unsettle the Earth and may be why contractions stop. Unsettled Earth may then affect all the other elements, especially Water. Earth helps to support a grounding of unsettled energy.

Earth has a link with the muscles and the uterus at term is the biggest muscle in the body. Labour may require the use of many other muscles in the body as the mother assumes different positions. If the mother is tense and uses other muscles unnecessarily, she may tend to deplete Earth energy, and this can affect both the ability of the uterus to contract effectively and the mother's ability to have the physical strength to continue. Spleen/Earth energy is especially supported in labour by SP 6 and ST 36.

Earth energy is the energy that "digests" everything – food/drink, emotions, ideas and information. If the mother is allowed to "digest" what is happening she protects her earth energy. A bodyworker can help a mother in this process.

(Jacky Bloemraad-de Boer).

Stomach

Food Qi is an important source of energy to support labour. Some women do not want to eat but others find they need to. Some hospitals still limit food intake. It is important to support women to find out what they want because if they are not able to eat when they need they may run out of energy. If they do not feel like eating but are running out of energy, then a glucose drip may help support Stomach energy. Stomach also provides a good grounding of energy, helping the mother to feel calmer.

Spleen

This is about how the mother feels supported in labour in a tangible, mothering way. She needs Blood to flow to the baby and to her. Low Spleen energy can lead to the mother feeling tired and will often have an effect on the muscular contractions of the uterus. SP 6 is an important point for helping to strengthen a tired uterus.

I find that if a uterus 'gets tired' – which usually means that contractions slow down or stop – then SP 6 will get the contractions going again BUT it doesn't help the mother to regain strength so it should be combined with ST 36 – this works very well.

(Jacky Bloemraad-de Boer)

Baby

At birth, the meridians are activated as independently functioning in the baby with the first breath and then subsequently with the intake of food.

Bladder and Kidney

They provide a variety of cardiorespiratory and metabolic adaptations during and after labour and relate to Extraordinary Vessel energy.

Water is about change and adaptation and is particularly about the ability to cope with stressful situations. All births represent a degree of stress on some level and it can be argued that this experience of stress during birth may impact on how one experiences change and stress in other life situations.

Many of the changes around birth are due to changes in the Jing. After birth the forces of gravity start to act on the bones and joints. It is therefore crucial to work with the Extraordinary Vessels as well as Kidney and Bladder.

Bladder

Bladder, along with Governing Vessel, supports the development of the spine. It is more to do with the muscular and nerve support while GV supports the spinal column, fluid and bones. The spine undergoes many changes during the birth process and in the early days after birth. Indeed it develops greatly in the first year until the child assumes the upright position. The different organs are also working differently after birth and need to be supported by their links through the Yu (back Shu) points.

Kidney

This holds the Jing and GV 4 Kidney Yang energy: Fire of the Gate of Vitality. The Chinese felt it was important to protect this energy at birth and during the first month when the mother stayed at home. The baby would also be in a quiet environment. Kidney supports the Blood of the baby which has to make many changes immediately after birth, partly on a hormonal level, partly on a circulatory and basic composition level. Kidney also governs the bones and articulations. The newborn body goes through many changes. The bones are compressed, especially the bones of the skull and the spine. The baby may have suffered stress on the skull or back through the mode of delivery such as forceps, caesarean, or prolonged vaginal labour. A very quick birth will also affect the Kidneys as the bones, especially the skull of the baby, may have less time to adjust.

Metal – Lung and Large Intestine

This is the first separation from the maternal matrix and the baby becoming an individual. Instrumental deliveries where the separation is energetically more brutal may have more of an effect on Metal. Rather than hands being the first contact that a baby feels, instead it feels a metal implement. Furthermore modern practices have also involved separation of the mother from the baby through placing the baby in a nursery or discouraging the traditional patterns of maternal and child co-sleeping. Although some traditional practices have involved separating the mother from the child, many traditional cultures encouraged skin-to-skin contact and mother–baby contact. Progressive modern practices also encourage this.

Lung

During the last couple of days before labour begins, fetal breathing activity is reduced. At birth there are high levels of surfactant and rapid elimination of lung liquor in response to the stimulatory effects of labour.

Any problems during birth which affect fetal oxygenation or delay the onset of normal respiration – such as prolonged labour, malposition of the fetus, excessively narrow pelvic outlet, placental insufficiency, problems with the umbilical cord – can cause Qi to become trapped in the Lungs. This may lead to problems with Lung Qi in infancy and later life such as a wide variety of respiratory and allergic disorders, as well as identity issues. The old practice of slapping the baby on the back at birth would further complicate this by sending the Qi trapped in the Lungs to the Heart.

A study by Salk and others published in *The Lancet* (Salk et al 1985) suggested a link between respiratory distress for more than 1 hour at birth and an increased incidence of adolescent suicide. Lungs are the organ linked with sadness and this study fits in with the Chinese view of Heart and Lung Qi being affected at birth and setting up long-term patterns of imbalance in the organs and meridians.

After the birth, the baby's Lungs start functioning in a different way as they take in Qi with the first breath. This initiates huge energetic and physical changes. The baby becomes a separate individual, and new limits to his/her world are defined. There is space and air all around. The baby has to get used to changes in gravity. From an eastern perspective the Lungs also regulate the skin and the skin is also breathing in and interacting with the air. Most babies have some issues with their skin in the first few weeks, as they make these adaptations. There can be skin dryness, milk spots, spots and eczema, for example. The skin is activated by its massage during passage through the birth canal so that the Po-Metal is activated by the Hun: muscle of the uterus and vagina and perineum.

Large Intestine

In the hours after birth, the newborn makes the first bowel movement. This clears out the bowels from the nourishment it has received in the womb. As the infant starts to take in nourishment through the mouth and through the milk, rather than directly through the Blood, the nature of the stools changes. Large Intestine is active and changing in these early days.

Emotionally the infant has to let go of the mother, develop a new kind of attachment to her and forge a new identity. Often they may suffer from constipation or diarrhoea. This is probably not only to do with adapting to new food, but emotionally linked as well.

Fire – Heart and Small Intestine

Birth is about the baby meeting the outside world and forming relationships, both a different relationship with the mother and new relationships with others. The energy of the postnatal period is much about Fire.

The small intestine also begins to function, introducing Fire energy into the body and separating pure from impure physically as well as emotionally.

Heart

Problems at birth which affect the cardiovascular system will affect both the Heart and Lungs. Any impediment to complete oxygenation of the blood will have its primary effect on the nervous system. In addition, therefore, to the chronic Lung problems of infancy, childhood and adulthood, the effect on the Heart will cause nervousness, irritability, restless sleep and low energy in the child. These problems may continue into adulthood creating Heart issues such as a tendency to feel tired, emotionally labile, unstable, hot tempered, or even feel inexplicably anxious and nervous.

The Chinese identified two main patterns of Heart imbalance:

Heart full This is the situation where there is a delayed delivery with the head remaining inside the birth canal. People's principal complaint through life is that they are always tired, emotionally unstable, hot tempered, pulse fast, Kidney pulse usually weak. This is considered to be hard to treat.

Heart small This is where there is a delayed delivery with the head outside the birth canal. Here there is frequent unexpressed and always explained fear which creates a lifelong tension.

Small Intestine

The baby has to begin to digest food in a different way, separating the pure from the impure. It is also learning to discriminate between different types of relationships.

Supplemental Fire: Triple Heater and Heart Protector

These start functioning at birth with the first breath which represents the activation of the Triple Heater and its coordination with the Heart Protector.

The baby begins to make relationships with people other than the mother and needs its own protection and heating. It takes time for these functions to establish themselves and in the first few weeks the baby is not able to regulate these functions well. The practices of wrapping and swaddling babies indicates the need to support this protective function of the Triple Heater and Heart Protector, which can also be achieved by keeping the baby close to the mother, to give some continuity and connection to these functions. The practice of separating the baby from the mother and placing it in a nursery puts strain on these meridians and can set up an energetic pattern which can continue into adulthood of either having to overprotect themselves or disconnect from their painful emotions.

Heart Protector

This supports the infant to make emotional adaptations after birth.

Triple Heater

At birth there is also the activation of the Three burning spaces.

Earth – Spleen and Stomach

This is about coming into contact with the Earth for the first time. Earth is also about the development of muscle tone. During the birth process the baby moves around a lot, using and strengthening the muscles. With the first breath there is a big movement of the recti muscles of the abdomen (the ancestral muscle) and this is considered to activate the link with the circulation of the Jing. In the first year the baby puts on a lot of weight and so Stomach and Spleen are active.

Spleen

This changes as the baby starts to develop more muscle tone as it is exposed to the forces of gravity and the acceptance of Earth. There are also many changes in the composition of the Blood as some of the red blood cells are broken down.

Stomach

After birth the grains come into the stomach (Ling Shu) as the baby starts to take food in through the mouth. Stomach is 'opened' by the first breath. This is the link between the Pre-Heaven and Post-Heaven Jing and is possibly one of the reasons why the rectus abdominis muscle is called the ancestral muscle.

After birth, with the first intake of food through the mouth through direct contact with the mother's breast (or otherwise through a bottle), the Stomach meridian becomes activated. It is one of the most active meridians during the first year of the baby's life as the birth weight triples by the end of the first year. Much of

how the baby relates to the world in the first year is through the mouth, the sucking reflex.

Wood – Liver and Gall Bladder

The Chinese link birth with a movement of the Hun which has a link with the eyes and a connection with the outside. Energy is said to come into the body via the eyes.

There is a strong movement of the diaphragm with the first breath which is supported by Wood energy. Liver and Lung are closely connected: 1–3 a.m. is Liver time which then communicates the energy with Lung as the following organ in the cycle.

Liver

There are changes after birth for the Liver due to the fact that the greater number of red blood cells that the fetus has in the womb have to be broken down during the first few weeks. The liver has to work hard and its function may be immature – so that it may not be able to conjugate the bilirubin and jaundice may result.

There are also changes in circulation at birth, as blood which was shunted bypassing the immature fetal liver starts to be processed by it and Liver becomes more active.

As the baby starts to move then there are changes in the Liver.

Gall bladder

Physical activity; is more engaged later as the baby begins to turn from side to side and to reach.

6.5 Summary of main treatment principles for work to support the natural birth process

Support and move the Yang

In a natural birth, the mother is likely to be moving around and the Yang meridians will be easy to access. This work will include:

- Work with GV and BL and supporting the back.
- Work with the Yang Heel or Linking Vessel, depending on deficiency or excess.
- Work with Gall Bladder and Wood energies.

Support the Yin

Often it is harder to access the CV and Yin meridians on the torso if the mother is labouring naturally. However, if the mother is tired or has some intervention, then she might sit or lie down, possibly on the side, and then work here is easier. This work includes:

- Work with the Yin Heel or Linking.
- Work to support the Yin meridians, especially Liver, Spleen and Kidney.

Support the changes in Jing

Work here includes:

- Support for the Kidney and Extraordinary Vessels.
- Support for the Water energy which includes any relaxation work or encouraging the mother to labour in water.

Allow Qi to flow

Qi can potentially block anywhere but tends to block in the pelvis, lower back or jaw and shoulders. Work includes:

- Relaxation of any tense areas.
- Work on Liver and Gall Bladder.
- Work with GDV to allow flow in the pelvis is of particular relevance.

Support blood flow

This is provided by ensuring nourishment for the mother. This can be making sure she moves to allow Blood to flow but also that she eats as and when she wants to without restriction. It also includes work on:

- Spleen.
- Penetrating Vessel.

Supporting the connection between mother and baby

A lot of this work can be done by encouraging the mother to connect directly with her baby either through touch or words. It includes work with:

- Heart Uterus.
- Heart.
- Penetrating Vessel.

Supporting the energetics of the different stages of labour

First stage

- Support going with the flow.
- Water Wood meridians.
- Extraordinary Vessels.
- Flow of energy in the pelvis.

Second

- Descending movement of Wood.
- Release work into neck and shoulders.

Third

- Support of mother.
- Bonding.
- Heart, Uterus, Fire, Blood, Shen.

Fourth

- Fire Blood bonding.
- Skin-to-skin contact.

During pregnancy much focus is placed on the birth, particularly for primiparas. In reality the preparation for and recovery after birth is just as, if not more, important.

Now unable to offer care in labour, I prepare with treatment from 36 weeks gestation, and teach pain relief acupressure. Actively decreasing pain levels helps the husband/partner cope with the stress of the birth process, as well as benefiting the woman.

If you attend births it is important to be guided by the situation. Treatment is directed at symptoms as they arise; this is not a time to treat constitutional conditions, as acute changes are occurring. A birthing woman can behave outside her 'normal' personality, the quiet Yin type woman may be active and vocalise, needing firmer pressure than normally would be enjoyed, or find inner sanctum, wanting silence and not to be touched. The strongest Yang type may need soft guidance, support and encouragement. The movement from Yin to Yang can ebb and flow, changing requirements.

There is no doubt under the threat of litigation birth has become a medicalised event; however, the advances modern obstetrics offer cannot be ignored. Neither extreme of total denial of medical care or complete reliance on it is safest. I feel as a complementary medical practitioner my role is to prevent the need for intervention so far as possible, but not to impede its use if it becomes necessary.

(Lea Papworth)

I find it important to express that there is an ever changing interchange of energies BUT that the bodyworker needs to 'go with the flow' and adjust their support to each situation. I am so often surprised by how very different a client can be during her labour – a very Yin woman moving without difficulty into Yang energy and vice versa. I also believe that a bodyworker is there to facilitate the mother without judgement or a preconceived idea of how a birth should go. It may be a large adjustment due to their previous experiences, beliefs and thoughts about (natural) childbirth.

For me the most important meridians to work with have always been Spleen, Liver and Kidney with Bladder and Heart coming in at a close second. Extraordinary Vessels Yang and Yin Linking are also important. I see my work as helping the mother to make contact with her baby and her body.

I attended a birth once where the mother had been pushing for almost 2 hours (primip) and the midwife suddenly asked the mother 'Where is your baby?' The father thought she had gone nutty and the grandmother was pointing with panic in her eyes at the mother's belly as if to say 'I hope to goodness it's in that big bump we can all see?'

But the mother suddenly sat up straighter, looked at the midwife and said very clearly, 'She is so terribly far away'.

To which the midwife said, 'Would you like to call your baby then?'

The mother didn't miss a heartbeat and started singing in the most beautiful voice I have ever heard. She sang in her own words gently calling and encouraging her baby. There was an incredible change in her and within two contractions she had her baby (with a perfect APGAR) in her arms! It proves that by bringing the mother more in contact with her baby the birth ended well.

The Earth energy was most definitely involved (singing).

(Jacky Bloemraad-de Boer)

Reflective questions

Q. What would you consider to be the main differences between supporting a mother with a physiological labour and a medicalised one?

Q. Which meridians and energies do you feel are most important to support in labour?

Q. How do you feel you can best support the baby during the birth process?

References

Eyssalet, J-M., 1990. Le secret de la maison des ancêtres. Editions Trédaniel, Paris.

Kushi, M., 1979. The Book of D -In: Exercise for Physical and Spiritual Development. Japan Publications Trading Co., Tokyo.

Ling Shu Jin, 1981. Spiritual axis. People's Health Publishing House, Beijing [first published c.100 BC].

Odent, M., 1992. The Nature of Birth and Breastfeeding. Bergin and Garvey, Westport, CT.

Salk, L., Lipsitt, L.P., Sturner, W.Q., et al., 1985. Relationship of maternal and perinatal conditions to eventual adolescent suicide. Lancet 1 (8429), 624–627.

Simkin, P., Ancheta, A., 2000. Labour Progress Handbook. Blackwell Science, Oxford.

Yuen, J.C., 2005. The Eight Extraordinary Vessels. New England School of Acupuncture, Boston, MA.

Learning outcomes

- Have an overview of the main changes in energy for the mother during the first year postnatally
- Have a specific understanding of the changes in the Extraordinary Vessels and the 12 meridians for the mother
- Describe the main treatment principles for working and understand the energetics of some common patterns

Introduction

In this book we are focusing on postnatal patterns for the mother rather than the baby, although the authors work extensively with babies. In modern cultures, the health of the mother is often neglected as most of the attention is focused on the baby and whether the baby is meeting development and growth goals. In most traditional cultures, by contrast, the health of the mother in the postnatal period was considered to be of vital importance as she is continuing to nourish the baby through physically feeding with her milk as well as emotionally supporting the baby. In Japan if the baby was ill, first the doctors would look to the health and well-being of the mother. The idea in most situations was, 'Treat the mother and the baby will be well', although not in cases of severe health situations for the baby.

The modern change in focus is probably due to several factors. It is partly a reflection of the lack of value placed on the role of the mother, partly due to the fact that many women no longer breastfeed their babies, and partly due to the fact that many more ill babies are surviving because of special care, so there are more babies needing medical treatment than before.

In many traditional cultures there was an initial period of 4–8 weeks of recovery which was known as the 'lying-in' period. In the UK until recently it was respected and known as the 'confinement'. This was a time for the mother to rest and be supported. The period of full recovery was considered to be much longer and in some cultures women were advised to wait 5–7 years to have another child (Goldsmith 1984). This fits in with the idea of Jing flowing in 7-year cycles – it needs time to replenish its quality.

In traditional Chinese medicine the puerperal period is defined as the 4 months following delivery. The first month is 'small full moon' or 'Golden Month'. It was believed that any illness a mother contracted during that month would remain with her for the rest of her life. It was also believed that any existing illness a mother had could be healed. A huge emphasis was placed on healing the mother and during this time she should have plenty of rest, nutrition and support.

In traditional Japan there was an initial rest in period of 21 days (*toko age 21 nichi*) and many women still observe this. If the mother had given birth in the midwife's house she would be looked after by the midwife initially and given special foods or shiatsu for her and the baby, as needed. During the first 24 hours the mother would rest, but afterwards be moderately active in order to help restore the proper flow of Qi and Blood and accelerate the involution of the uterus. The midwife would often massage the mother's breasts or show her how to massage them, to help with milk flow and prevent mastitis. There were masseurs who specialised in breast massage before and after birth. These are now less common.

The Golden Month was time for the mother away from ordinary life, to avoid excessive stress, emotional disturbances, overwork and fatigue and be supported. It was a special time and there was a sense of family support and connection to the ancestors. The woman would abstain from bathing, washing her hair, exposing herself to cold, swimming and so on. At the end of the Golden Month there was a ritual bath containing a mixture of herbs prescribed by a traditional Chinese medicine (TCM) practitioner which would feel a positive way for the woman to enter the next phase of her life as a mother.

The remaining 3 months of the puerperium are called the 'big full moon' and the mother would continue to look after herself and be supported by the community (Zhao 2006).

Postpartum disorders are one of the four major categories of Chinese medicine. A lot is written about the various conditions, which differ from the conditions now identified. For example, there was an emphasis on how the lochia was discharging and even the idea of retained lochia (not really present in Western medicine), the openness to fever and external invasion, as well as current concerns of healing of the abdomen and breast issues.

7.1 General energy patterns for the mother

Excess and combined patterns

The postnatal period is considered a complex time. Although there is an underlying pattern of depletion there can be conditions of excess and deficiency combined with excess. Heat and sweating can build up in the body. There can be deficiency and fullness as well as stasis of Blood. There can be too much Yang energy. Different and opposite patterns can coexist. However, due to the underlying pattern of depletion, we need to be careful with dispersing and cooling techniques. In addition to all of this there is the whole emotional and physical adjustment to life with a new baby – feeding the baby, bonding, lack of sleep, fatigue and so forth.

While it is important to understand the underlying patterns we cannot be too rigid as different things can be going on in the body at the same time. We need to be aware of the complexities and work with the reality for each mother.

Different Chinese physicians would emphasise different aspects of working. Fu Qing-zhu (translation 1995) gave priority to supplementing Qi and Blood and treating other things as secondary to that. This meant he made the following recommendations:

- Do not use Qi consuming or normalising medicines. This could make stuffiness and oppression worse.
- Even though there may be damage to the Qi, do not use dispersing techniques as this may damage the Stomach's ability to take in food.

- Even though the body may be hot, do not use cold and cooling medicinals as the underlying pattern is of depleted Yin and fluids.

Another physician, Chen Liang-fang, considered that the first most common cause of problems is emptiness of Blood and consumption of Water fluids. He felt that there were three main patterns, the 'san yin':

1. Blood vacuity with stirring of Fire
2. Frenetic movement of static Blood
3. Damage due to excessive food and drink.

(Chen Liang-fang, Nu Ke Mi Jue Da Quan; quoted in Flaws 2005: 217).

Three examinations

In Chinese medicine it was considered important to ask the following three questions:

1. Is there abdominal pain? This gives indications about what is happening with the uterus and the lochia, and if there may be retention of lochia.
2. Is there constipation? This indicates the relative exhaustion of body fluids, showing if Blood and Yin are abundant or depleted.
3. Is breast milk flowing? This is linked with the intake of food and drink and indicates how much Stomach Qi has been weakened. It also indicates if there is blocked energy in the breasts.

(Maciocia 1998).

There are some typical patterns which express aspects of these energies:

- Nausea and heavy bleeding: indicates exhaustion of Penetrating Vessel.
- Sweating and fever: indicates exhaustion of Qi and Blood.
- Postnatal depression: indicates Heart Blood deficiency.

Three prohibitions

These are known as the 'San jin' (Flaws 2005). However, different physicians would have slightly different prohibitions and sometimes these would contradict each other. One set is as follows:

1. Do not cause sweating – this is because Blood and fluids share a common source and they are likely to be depleted.
2. Do not precipitate postpartum recovery – the body is sensitive.
3. Do not disinhibit urination.

It was also considered important not to raise static Blood upwards.

Depleted patterns

The force required for delivery draws upon the woman's Qi – especially her Wood and Yang Qi. The loss of blood during birth drains Blood and Yin. The expulsion of the placenta draws upon Original Qi. The huge hormonal changes during labour and the immediate postpartum draw upon the Jing. All these mean that a Deficiency of Qi, Blood, Jing and Yin are the overriding conditions of women after childbirth.

The Conception and Penetrating Vessels are depleted and the blood vessels and channels are empty and prone to invasions by external factors such as cold, heat and infection. Even if the mother had an easy birth and feels well immediately afterwards, it is still important for her to make sure that she looks after herself in the first few weeks to allow her energies to replenish themselves. Unfortunately it is common these days for women to feel pressurised to 'get back to normal' and there is little support for them to spend time with their baby. The emphasis is on getting back to work and leaving her child's care to others. If women do not get enough rest early on, they are drawing on their deeper reserves of energy, especially their Jing. Longer term they are more likely to suffer from exhaustion as well as being prone to other illness, both mental and emotional.

Depletion of Blood

We consider this separately under Blood patterns (below), as Blood is one of the most important energies to work with in the early postnatal period. Depleted Blood means that the mother is more prone to invasion by pathogenic wind.

Depletion of Qi

Sweating, fever and exhaustion are signs of depleted Qi. There will be persistent lochial discharge which is red, profuse, dilute and with no smell as the Qi fails to hold the Blood.

The most depleted area is usually the hara, the abdomen – the result of the sudden change of no longer containing the baby and the laxity of the abdominal muscles. All the meridians which pass through the abdomen, especially the Yin (Conception Vessel and Penetrating Vessel), will be depleted in energy, as will the lower back (Kidney and Governing Vessel) and the Girdle Vessel. The Girdle Vessel is particularly important because it gives support to all the other vessels. This is why women in traditional Japan would wear a wide belt 'sarashi' (girdle), to give support and bring more energy to this area.

For women who have had a Caesarean, the hara is cut through energetically and all these energy flows must be especially supported as they tend to be even more weakened.

It is important for the mother to do some gentle exercise to prevent stagnation of Qi, but not to do excessive exercise which would deplete her energy still further.

Qi will be built up also by ensuring good breathing with gentle exercise (Air) and by following a nourishing diet (Food). This means that the Lung and Stomach meridians are especially important and should not be dispersed. Qi especially needs to build up when the mother is breastfeeding.

Depletion of Jing

Kidney energy and Kidney Jing are depleted postnatally, both due to the fact that the mother nourished the baby during the pregnancy with her Jing and also because through breastfeeding she is transferring her Jing to the baby in the breast milk. Jing is required for the formation of Blood and Blood is the source of breast milk.

While Jing can never be increased it can be replenished to some extent. It is important for the mother not to be in stressful situations, especially working long hours outside the home for some time after the birth, otherwise she will draw still further on her Jing and, rather than replenish it, further deplete it. This need not necessarily be the full cycle of 7 years, but for a few years, she will need to be careful of her energy. This includes ideally spacing children at least a few years apart so Kidney energy has a chance to renew itself. Traditionally sex was avoided in the early postnatal period to allow Jing to renew and while the lochia is being discharged to prevent the counter flow of blood, similar to refraining during menstruation.

Family support may help the mother to connect in a positive way with her ancestral energy.

Food will help support the renewal of Jing as the Stomach is the link between the Pre-Heaven and the Post-Heaven Jing.

Depletion of Yin

The loss of fluids, combined with the demands made on Yin during pregnancy, may lead to there being insufficient Yin in the body, which means that the body can become too hot. If the mother is hot, it is important to avoid excessive exposure to heat, as sweating is weakening after birth. Exposure to cold is not recommended either as the Chinese considered it to be one of the main causes of postpartum problems. Cold does not allow the Yin to build up and stagnates the Blood.

Yin deficiency can be caused by overwork, Liver Qi stagnation, and expecting too much of oneself by trying to hold on to the previously ordered life which a baby throws into chaos. This can often be a cause of depression.

Blood: a key energy

There is a loss of Blood with the discharge of the placenta, the lochia and the resulting changes in the uterine lining. Furthermore a lot of the circulating Blood in pregnancy was circulating in the fetus and therefore is also lost. As the Penetrating Vessel is the Sea of Blood this channel will be depleted. Other organs especially affected are those involved with Blood production, namely Heart, Liver, Kidney and Spleen.

Depleted Blood

Signs of deep depletion include: continuous pale lochial discharge, dizziness, constipation, pale skin and tongue, restless Shen leading to sleeplessness, depression, anxiety and depressed milk supply.

As Heart governs Blood it is said that with the loss of Blood, the physical basis of the Heart, the Heart becomes restless as it has no anchor. Restless Heart energy rises, often to the head, and affects the Shen, the spirit, which it rules. This is the Chinese explanation of postnatal depression. Depression was considered linked mostly with patterns of Blood loss and its effects on the Heart.

The other main meridians connected with the Blood will also be affected – Spleen and Liver. It is important that the mother finds a balance between gentle exercise and rest to both move and restore Liver Blood. Spleen is sensitive to the food that the mother eats and therefore proper diet was considered of paramount importance.

It is considered that breast milk is a transformation of Blood, so if the mother's Blood is low, then the mother may not be able to produce enough milk. Blood is built up with diet and exercise as well as supporting the key meridians.

Stasis of Blood

As there are many changes in blood flow, the Chinese considered this to be a relatively common pattern of imbalance. Blood could remain in the uterus due to old blood or pieces of the placenta or due to retained lochia. Retention of lochia is not considered to be a condition in western medicine, but flow of Blood is considered important in Chinese medicine.

When Blood is stuck in the Uterus, the lochial discharge is dark, purplish and with clots. This can lead to emotional issues, even psychosis. There can be rib pain which would indicate a stasis of Liver Qi, or lower back pain which can indicate a stasis of Kidney Qi.

With Blood stasis, work would need to be done to move the Blood, for example by gentle stretches and working away from the Uterus. However, it is important not to do too much dispersion work as the underlying pattern is of depletion.

Heat in Blood

Heat in the Blood is indicated by heavier bleeding and the lochial discharge will be bright or dark red, often with a foul smell. The mother may feel restless mentally, have abdominal pain and dry stools. There may be infection. In this case, it is important not to use warming techniques, such as applying hot towels or the Chinese herb moxa, as these will aggravate the condition. Calming, holding but not overly cooling techniques need to be used and great care must be taken especially if there is infection. LI 11 and SP 10 clear Heat. Work with Spleen, Penetrating Vessel and Conception Vessel can also help clear Heat.

External pathogenic factors

As the channels are empty they are prone to external invasions. For this reason work with the Extraordinary Vessels is especially important as they circulate Defensive Qi (Wei Qi).

Exposure to cold and heat

The Chinese considered exposure to cold as one of the main aetiological factors of postpartum problems. However, they also considered it important to avoid excessive exposure to heat, as sweating is weakening after birth and loss of fluids may lead to further depletion of Yin.

Exposure to wind

Again due to the depletion of the channels and blood deficiency the body is prone to invasion of wind. This can lead to issues such as joint pain and wind heat invasion which causes fever.

Support for nursing and bonding

This was considered an important aspect of the Golden Month. Herbs and diet would be part of the support to build up the Blood which is the foundation of the milk. Support for the Qi was also vital and bodywork can be helpful to ensure the smooth flow of energy within the breasts.

Work could also be done to support the bonding process. The mother is considered the baby's emotional and energetic support and she herself needs to be supported so she can support the baby. There would also be specific work to support the Fire, through Heart, Ming Men and Yang Qi.

Sadly, in modern cultures, the mother often has to return to caring for other children, the household or workplace, unable to rest for her own replenishment and to bond with her baby.

Exercise and self-care

There was an emphasis on the need to rest, as lying down benefits Liver Blood and helps the body's energies restore themselves. However, a need for gentle exercise was also emphasised to prevent stagnation of Qi and Blood.

Diet

There was an emphasis on appropriate diet to support the energy patterns, especially in the building up of the depleted energies of Blood, Qi, Yin and Jing and in supporting breastfeeding. There was an awareness of the damaging effects of certain types of food to the body's weakened channels. Greasy, cold, pungent and fried foods are avoided because of the mother's weak Spleen and Stomach. Vegetables are considered beneficial because they help prevent constipation. Foods rich in protein and vitamins are important, such as pig's trotter soup and chicken soup. Brown sugar and herbs help to tonify the Qi and Blood.

Effects of medical interventions

This would not be so common in traditional China and so not much is written about this.

7.2 Changes in the Extraordinary Vessels

All the meridians which pass through the abdomen, especially the Conception Vessel and Penetrating Vessel, will be depleted in energy, as well as the lower back (Kidney and Governing Vessel) and the Girdle Vessel. This is why women wore the *sarashi* (girdle) to give support and bring more energy to this area. These days, with the increasing number of caesareans, which cut through all these vessels, and epidurals, which affect the lower back and spine, many more women experience problems with these vessels.

The pelvic floor area is also linked in with this potential pattern of weakness as the four main vessels pass through here and regulate its energy. It will have inevitably been weakened through the demands made on it during pregnancy and the stretching during a vaginal birth. If there has been an episiotomy or tearing and then stitches, then more healing needs to happen. Problems with a weak pelvic floor will express initially as stress incontinence, or haemorrhoids, or persistent general feelings of pelvic heaviness and distension. Longer-term weakness means that there is insufficient support for the pelvic organs such as the bladder and uterus, which may eventually lead to prolapse. Many women in later life suffer from weakness in the pelvic floor and it is important to do

work to encourage the building up of strength here in the immediate postnatal period.

These Vessels also circulate Defensive Qi which is important in this sensitive phase of a woman's life. They provide protection from external pathogenic factors to which the body is particularly vulnerable postnatally.

In the postnatal period, the Jing tends to depletion as it has been drawn upon during the 9 months of pregnancy and will continue to be drawn upon during the breastfeeding time. The body needs time to allow the changes in the Jing to settle. This is why that initial period of rest was considered to be so important.

The Vessels support the hormonal adjustments and the big changes in the body which happen in the early postnatal period.

The PV, CV and GV are probably the most important as they represent what Yuen calls the 'First ancestry' (Yuen 2005: 20) so are particularly relevant in establishing bonding and the early links between mother and child.

The importance of the Penetrating Vessel postnatally

Penetrating Vessel energy is perhaps the most important energy postnatally. 'Architect of creation' (Yuen 2005), it controls the breasts as well as the Blood, both of which undergo big changes. Due to its links with the Heart it helps establish bonding, supporting the mother's mental-emotional state and fostering the development of the relationship between mother and child. It provides a link between the Pre-Heaven and Post-Heaven Essence and digestion, which plays an important role postnatally both in restoring the mother's health and energy and, if she is breastfeeding, in supporting the energy of her baby.

Its main pattern in the postnatal period is likely to be one of overall depletion. However, there could be heat or coldness in the abdomen or heat or fullness in the breast.

Breasts and breastfeeding

Its pathway fans out over the breasts and chest on its way to the throat and eyes. These branches are known as the breast connecting channels. They control the major arteries which feed the breast, the axillary artery supplying the outer half and the internal mammary arteries supplying the inner half.

Breast milk is seen as a transformation of Blood, so if the Penetrating Vessel is empty, the Sea of Blood is depleted and there may not be enough milk. This is the scenario if women do not get adequate rest or nourishment – more common these days. If the Qi of the Penetrating Vessel is not flowing then the breast connecting channels will be blocked and the milk may not flow even though it is abundant.

Blood

PV helps regulate Blood deficiency, stasis and Heat and is therefore an important vessel in supporting the changes in Blood. It can be used in cases of retained or excessive lochia, supporting healing of the uterus and regulating the switch back to menstruation. It can also be used in cases of varicosities, especially of the vulva or anus. Through its links with the Heart it supports the many emotional changes and demands the mother experiences.

Newborn needs

PV meets the basic physiological needs of the newborn – the desire to be fed and to be touched. It is also about the mother being connected with her baby, both on a physical level through the breasts and through chest-to-chest, skin-to-skin contact, but also includes the Heart connection of bonding and the emotional needs of the baby.

Heart

PV is closely linked with the Heart. Some writers even consider whether the Heart Uterus meridian is a branch of the PV. Certainly this Heart/Fire Earth link expresses important qualities of PV energy. It is certainly important in supporting the huge emotional changes the mother undergoes.

Link with digestion

PV controls digestion through its link via the Stomach with Pre-Heaven and Post-Heaven Jing. It is often used in situations where there is food stasis, nausea, vomiting and diarrhoea. It also affects the baby: food intolerances in later life can often be traced back to Chong Mai energetics.

Structure: muscles and the abdomen

It is said to affect the Ancestral Muscles (Zong Jin), rectus abdominis. These need to close up both energetically and physically, to give support to the abdomen and organs. Generally abdominal energy is depleted but there can be infection or retention of Blood.

The PV affects the flow of energy to the legs through its descending branch, influencing the three Yin of leg: Liver, Spleen and Kidney. This can be useful in the early days for the prevention of thrombosis and for supporting the longer-term circulatory changes and varicose veins.

Conception Vessel and Governing Vessel

Conception Vessel and Governing Vessel continue to be important in regulating the hormonal changes of the postnatal period. They are linked with the changing energy of the abdomen and back and are especially relevant in supporting energy flow to the perineum, helping with perineal repair and recovery.

Conception Vessel

Supporting bonding

Yuen refers to it as the 'Vessel of bonding' and feels that it represents the symbiotic relationship of mother and child. It is about the mothering connection established through the front of the body as the mother holds her baby, ideally some of the time with direct skin-to-skin contact. The mother connects to her baby through the baby's mouth and eyes. This connection helps to establishing the 'maternal matrix' in time as well as place and person (Yuen 2005).

Supporting Yin and Jing

Conception Vessel helps to nourish depleted Yin and Jing and promotes the movement of body fluids, which include milk. Depletion of Yin and Jing may be linked with altered sleep patterns, especially insomnia. This is a common scenario for women suffering from sleep deprivation and interrupted sleep patterns.

Other connections

Lungs. Through its links with the Lungs it has an effect on the breathing and the movement of Qi in the upper body. Often energy is blocked here due to poor posture and feeding the baby. After a caesarean section fluid can build up on the Lungs so it is important to clear here.

Heart. The links with CV and Heart are part of the bonding process. Women instinctively hold the baby to their heart. Shen is often scattered due to changes in Blood and this can lead to depression.

Abdomen and uterus. It is linked with regulating the abdomen and uterus and so can be used: where there are haemorrhoids; in cases of vaginal or vulval pain or varicosities; where there is healing from an episiotomy; for supporting the uterus with the changes postnatally; in cases of diarrhoea with cold pain, abdominal pain, difficult urination, cold abdomen, weak rectus abdominis muscles, digestive issues and food stasis. Since weakness in the front of the body can also lead to weakness in the back it can be a useful meridian to work with cases of lower backache.

Governing Vessel

This is about 'moving forward into life' – separation from the maternal matrix (Yuen 2005). The Heart Yang of the infant develops along with the movement into the upright position. For the new mother with her first baby, this represents a further separation from her own maternal matrix, when for the first time in her life she is called upon to be the mother rather than to be mothered. GV helps her to move forward into this new identity.

For the mother, Yang energy needs to flow. The milk ejection reflex linked with oxytocin is the same energetic circuit described in the second stage of labour – and linked with Governing Vessel and Gall Bladder energy.

There are many changes in the mother's spine as her body adapts to its changing centre of gravity, coupled with the demands on the back of lifting, carrying and feeding the baby. The back will be even more affected if there has been an epidural and weakness, pain and discomfort here can last for months and years. GV is often used for occipital headaches and these tend to occur more frequently after an epidural. GV is used in all types of back problems, especially if they are centrally located.

As it influences the Brain, it is used for depression and anxiety. It helps to strengthen the Mind and the Shen as well as the Zhi of the Kidneys and willpower. It supports the Heart in helping to regulate the mental and emotional state of the Brain. It can be used where there is insomnia, feelings of fear and even of suicide, which are not that uncommon postnatally. Most women do not enact the suicidal feelings, but may experience them. Caring for a new baby often brings up issues for the mother of linking with her corporeal soul and fear of death. Working with GV can help to strengthen the mind.

Yin and Yang Linking Wei

These are important vessels to use as they tend to be used for empty conditions and the main energetics underlying the postnatal period are of deficiency.

Yin Linking

This links into the energy of the Blood and PV. It can be useful for supporting the emotional changes that the mother is experiencing, even if she is managing well with them. It is especially useful in cases where there is anxiety, insomnia and depression. It will help nourish the Heart especially when due to an empty condition. It can help to nourish the Blood.

KD 9, or 'Guest House', is a particularly powerful point as it connects Heart and Kidney energies and the mother is connecting a lot both with the acceptance of her individual destiny and the family background. Yin Linking can also be used in cases where there is backache with feelings of sadness and where there is night sweating as this is often due to Yin deficiency.

Yang Linking

It governs the exterior and a major postnatal pathology is invasion of exterior wind. It is also useful in

cases of backache especially when it involves more than one Yang channel, notably Gall Bladder and Bladder, which is also a common scenario.

Yin and Yang Ankle Qiao

These relate to the pituitary and to hormonal change. Care needs to be taken with their use as they are usually more associated with excess patterns. While there may be excess postnatally the underlying condition is more of depletion.

Yin

This is often linked with patterns involving excess Liver energy. It is a time of identity crisis due to the changes involved in becoming a mother. The mother may suffer from poor self-image, especially these days when mothering tends to be less valued by society. The mother may become lethargic and not able to care for herself or mother her child.

They are useful vessels for working with adhesions following surgery, especially in the abdomen. This means they are helpful to use after a caesarean section. Caesarean section is often accompanied by Qi stagnation in the abdomen and bloating caused by excess Yin fluids for which Yin Heel can help. They are often used even if there is no caesarean section in scenarios where there is bloating, abdominal pain, retained lochia and placenta, full conditions and Blood stasis, especially if the pain is unilateral. They are also used where there are digestive issues.

Yang

They help to absorb excess Yang from the head. They are used with mental problems such as headaches and epilepsy linked with excessive Liver Fire or Heart Fire. They can be used where there is insomnia – the eyes not closing. Insomnia can also be due to hormonal balance or simply lack of sleep due to having a newborn. Yang Heel can help balance these energies. They can be used for backache, sciatica and hip problems, all of which can be issues postnatally. They can also be used where there are urinary problems and exterior invasions of wind.

Heart-Uterus and Kidney-Uterus

Both of these vessels support the changes in the Uterus: Heart-Uterus supporting Blood and emotions, Kidney-Uterus supporting Jing.

Girdle Vessel

The Girdle Vessel continues to play its role in giving structural support to the pelvis. It has given fundamental support in the antenatal period and needs to recover from those demands. Additionally, it may have been put out of balance by excessive pressure on the pelvis experienced during labour such as with a forceps or ventouse delivery or delivery in the side-lying position putting pressure more on one side. It will have been weakened through a caesarean. It is going to have to give a lot of support as the mother takes up her daily activities, especially as the baby grows heavier, and is often put out of balance by the mother holding the baby on one hip only.

Through its link with the Zong Jin (Ancestral Sinew/rectus abdominis muscles) it will help with recovery from rectal separation. It also has links with the gluteus and paravertebrals, key muscles which support the pelvis. GDV is often used for pain in the umbilical region. Women suffering from symphysis pubis diastasis (SPD) or lower back pain are likely to benefit from GDV work.

As it binds CV and GV, then if CV and GV are empty, which they are likely to be postnatally, GDV sags.

There is often a marked pattern of imbalances between the upper and lower body postnatally. Typically there is a lack of energy in the hara combined with a fullness of energy in the upper body, neck, shoulders and breasts, particularly if the mother is breastfeeding. Work with the GDV can support these patterns.

As it links with stagnation in the lower burner and lower burner issues it is relevant to work. It can be used in situations where there is retention of lochia or as menstruation begins to be initiated. If there is a holding on or a sluggishness, which can be the scenario if the mother does not engage the muscles, then it can get stagnant. This can lead to bloating, lack of muscle tone, difficult menstruation and digestion.

It links with Liver and Gall Bladder patterns and is about control, decision-making, adaptation to the new role of mother. Again if it is sluggish there may not be this ability to move into acceptance of the new role and the emotional changes which accompany this.

7.3 Changes in the 12 meridians

Water – Kidney and Bladder

Water is about basic support systems, especially ancestral and family support. In many traditional cultures the mother would have a lot more family support, not just in the day-to-day care (mothering-earth aspects) aspects of support but drawing upon a whole body of knowledge and support in a much wider sense of the term. No wonder these days women feel isolated within a nuclear or even single-parent family unit. Where the old ancestral support is not available, society has to find new ways of providing that energetic Water support to mothers and their babies.

Kidney

Excessive physical work and overwork may weaken Kidney Yang which is needed to support postnatal recovery. Weak Kidney Yang may lead to stress and other conditions to do with the flow of fluids such as urine, urinary tract infections, cystitis and blood flow.

Weak Kidneys can affect the Lungs and so it is especially important to strengthen the Kidneys after a caesarean section. For all mothers, the need to have good Lung functioning will support the flow of energy in the chest and upper burner which may be blocked. Furthermore many women develop carpal tunnel syndrome due to the blockages in the shoulder and also the build-up of fluids which can occur if Kidney Yang is weak.

Often women have weakness in the Kidney area (L2/3) in the lower back. Strengthening here will help to support the pelvis.

Bladder

Weakness in the Bladder can be a cause of back issues, not just in the lumbar area but also in the neck, upper back and mid-back. There can be patterns of muscular weakness or tightness indicating imbalance along the Bladder. This can extend down into the back of the legs and there can be tightness or weakness in the calves.

There may be issues to do with cystitis or stress incontinence. It can also be linked with Spleen, CV and the muscle tone and energy of the perineum.

Earth – Stomach and Spleen

Earth is about the physical nourishment the mother gives to her baby and the mothering support of a mother or grandmother giving good-quality foods to the mother.

Stomach and Spleen work with the Penetrating Vessel to help build up quality reserves of milk. In modern societies more attention tends to go to the baby so that the mother may neglect herself and not eat or rest properly. Not surprisingly the breast milk then dries up. Good diet, especially Spleen nourishing foods, was considered to be of vital importance.

Stomach

Stomach influences breastfeeding as its pathway passes through the breast. Breast milk is a transformation of menstrual Blood energy which is supplemented by Post Natal Qi extracted from food by the Stomach.

If the mother is not producing enough breast milk it can be because of a depletion of her Blood energy.

As the Stomach channel passes directly through the breasts, the many physical changes in the breasts are supported by changes in the Stomach. Stomach is often used for abscesses or blockages of the breasts.

Spleen

Spleen rules the muscles and holds up the energy of the mid-line of the body. There is a link with the main areas of weak muscle: the pelvic floor may lack the strength to support the pelvic organs and lack of muscle tone in the abdomen may lead to the pelvic organs such as bladder and uterus being insufficiently supported. In the abdominal and pelvic floor areas especially there is a loss of muscle tone due to the stretching which occurred in pregnancy. Often women find it hard to accept these changes in their body shape and tone. Some women put on weight, or at least do not lose all the weight they gained in pregnancy. Due to time pressures they may find it tempting to eat empty calories and snack on biscuits and sweet food. Other women rapidly lose weight and become underweight. There may also be dampness in the hara. Spleen helps regulate damp conditions.

Spleen supports the quality of the Blood. Postnatally women may have insufficient nourishment and suffer from weakness of the Blood such as anaemia. It is also about circulation of the Blood and holding Blood in the vessels. Postnatally many women suffer from poor circulation, especially in the legs, and may suffer conditions such as varicose veins, vulval varicosities and haemorrhoids.

Fire – Heart and Small Intestine; Heart Protector and Triple Heater

Fire energy is the energy of bonding and forming a new relationship with the baby and the people around her. The mother's changing relationship with her partner is of particular importance. Initially the partner may be as excited about the newborn as the mother, but later, as the demands continue, some partners may experience feelings of jealousy.

It is also a lot about the changes in Blood which may lead to physical or emotional issues.

Heart

In Chinese terms, depression is related to the exertion and loss of Blood at birth. Since Heart houses the Mind and governs Blood, Heart-Blood becomes deficient, the Mind has no residence and it may become depressed and anxious. This may cause a state of depression, mild anxiety, insomnia and fatigue where the mother may feel unable to cope, is tearful, loses libido and feels angry. In time Blood deficiency may lead to Yin deficiency. In many women there is a mild version of this pattern. The more extreme puerperal psychosis would be seen as stagnant Blood energy harassing the Mind.

This kind of pattern can be aggravated if the relationship with the partner is unsupportive or even violent or if the birth has been particularly traumatic.

Small Intestine

This often expresses itself emotionally when the mother cannot sort pure from impure. She may become muddled about what to give to herself as nourishment and what to give to baby, or even her partner or other close family or friends. She may neglect herself in favour of others and not be receiving enough nourishment.

Shock especially affects SI so if there is trauma during the birth, the mother may experience restlessness and lack of sleep, insomnia.

Physically depleted SI can lead to Blood stagnation and poor circulation in the hips and legs. There can also be a lack of strength in the hara as it is often empty. The mother may experience pain in the ovaries. SI imbalance can express as shoulder problems and stiffness in the neck. SI can also be used for treating blockages in the breasts.

Heart Protector

This is the back-up to the Heart, so if the Heart is under strain, then the Heart Protector is likely to be involved. It is beneficial for emotional calming.

It is involved in the process of the mother bonding with her baby, and the forming of the new relationship. How much emotional support she has postnatally will affect the functioning of the Heart Protector.

The mother has been acting as the baby's Heart Protector in the womb and may find it hard to let go of this role, becoming overly protective of the baby. Of course the baby still needs to feel the protection of the mother but in a less intense way.

Triple Heater

This helps the mother adapt to her changing role and new rhythms and ways of relating to people. It is also about the adaptation to the environment: sensitivity to heat and cold. The immune system is often quite sensitive and vulnerable postnatally and women can easily become run down. It is also used for calming the spirit.

It supports the lymphatic system and its main use postnatally would be in supporting the breasts. Milk can get blocked in the ducts, creating inflammation which can lead to infection. Work to support the optimal functioning of TH and the lymphatic system will help to prevent this and even support the body to deal with issues.

The three burners are useful for supporting the distribution of energy. A typical pattern is fullness in the upper burner and emptiness in the lower burner. This will help with issues of digestion, uterine healing and recovery, and breathing.

Because of its link with Kidney energy and the Jing it is useful for supporting the depleted Kidney Qi postnatally and for supporting the process of the refocusing of Jing away from the uterus.

Wood – Liver and Gall Bladder

For Wood energy to flow, there must be some movement of the body. Posturally Liver and Gall Bladder energy in the shoulders and side of neck, tends to become quite tight. This is due mostly to the demands of holding and feeding a baby as well as sleeping awkwardly in bed at night.

Liver

Liver is an important organ in supporting changes in the blood flow postnatally. However, excessive exercise can draw too much on it. There is a need for gentle exercise combined with rest. Western views of postnatal exercise have varied over the years, but the eastern view is based on this energetic understanding. Emotional problems such as worry or anger can affect Liver energy. Liver influences the breasts and controls the nipples, so it can obstruct the flow of milk. If Liver energy is not flowing it can cause constipation, as it fails to moisten the faeces. Too many fatty foods will interfere with the ability of Liver to support digestion.

Liver also regulates the joints through the sinews, ligaments and tendons. There is often continued weakness in the ligaments due to hormonal changes. For many women it can take some time to recover. It may be that SPD is caused by the birth as well as by too much exercise in the early postnatal period. Women need to be careful not to overstretch their bodies for a while.

It affects the eyes. Often the eyes get tired or the mother may experience headaches.

Gall Bladder

This can be active due to the responsibilities of being a new mother. Tiredness and lack of sleep can manifest in the eyes.

It has close links with the Extraordinary Vessels and therefore with the hormonal system; postnatal headaches are often hormonally linked. It helps regulate bile, insulin, gastric acid distribution of nutrients. The mother's digestive system has to adapt a lot. It can be associated with neck and shoulder tightness, and headaches can be due to muscular tension along the Gall Bladder meridian.

Metal – Lung and Large Intestine

The woman has to create a new relationship with her baby and her sense of self is challenged in this post-natal period. Metal represents money and our sense of worth – a woman's capacity to earn money is usually affected while having time off to look after the baby. Furthermore, modern cultures tend to devalue women as mothers.

Lung

If the mother does not breathe deeply and relax then this will affect Lung functions. Often her posture will affect Lung energy. She may be bent over the baby while she feeds, thus blocking Lung flow. This will lead to tightness in the upper body and perhaps even a sense of tiredness and depression as the basic Air Qi does not flow freely.

Breathing is linked in with a sense of who one is and the space around one.

Large Intestine

Blood deficiency and dryness often affect the Large Intestine causing constipation, a common postnatal complaint. This may lead to haemorrhoids. Sometimes this is caused by Lung Qi failing to descend to the Large Intestine to help it in its functions.

7.4 Summary of main treatment principles

The main principle is that by supporting the mother's energy the baby will also be supported. However, it is also important to do specific work to address the needs of the mother.

The main patterns postnatally for the mother are:

Overall depletion of Blood, Jing, Yin and Qi

Rest and nourishment are the most important sources of renewal of these energies.

Work needs:

- To support the Jing. This involves work with the Kidneys and the Extraordinary Vessels.
- To support PV and the Blood (LV, HT, SP).
- To help build up the Qi. This involves all meridians but especially ST and SP as they provide the link between Pre-Heaven and Post-Heaven Jing and supply nourishment to mother and baby.

Helping to strengthen weakness in the lower back and abdominal area

Weak energy is especially noticeable in these areas, especially if there has been epidural or caesarean section.

Work here includes:

- Using holding techniques to build up energy here. Meridians especially important are:
  – CV, GV, PV, GDV, SP, KD.
- GV 4 and CV 4 are particularly important points.

Emptiness/stagnated energy in the legs

In the early postnatal period the legs are often weak and the energy may not be flowing well. There is a high risk of DVT especially after an instrumental delivery.

Work here involves:

- Moving Liver Qi especially in legs.
- Work to build up the Spleen.
- Yin and Yang Linking are also good for the legs.

External pathogenic factors

Protection and not dispersing energy is considered important.

Fullness patterns

There are areas of fullness but it is important not to overly disperse as the underlying pattern is of depletion.

Fullness in abdomen

Heat in abdomen could be a sign of infection so referral would be needed.

If there was no infection work would include:

- Holding or calming techniques.
- Working GDV to redistribute the energy.
- LI 11 clears Heat. Work with Spleen, Penetrating Vessel and Conception Vessel can help clear Heat.

Fullness/tightness in the upper back, shoulders and breasts

There is often tightness in these areas.
Work here includes:

- Work to open up the Lung to allow its energy to flow. A Collapsed Lung energy is often the cause of the tightness.
- Work to release the tightness. This is usually work in the Gall Bladder, Liver or Bladder meridians, and PV and SI.
- Position of feeding is important.

Treatment patterns by postnatal weeks

First week

- Work with the Extraordinary Vessels to support the changes in blood and hormonal flow.
- Work with the Three Burners to support the movement of energy from the Lower Burner to the Upper Burner with breastfeeding. Even if the mother is not breastfeeding, work to the Three Burners is still important.
- Work with the Uterus and CV energies to support the hara energy which feels buzzy and active as it is contracting.
- Breastfeeding: PV and ST.
- Work with the Fire energy to support the emotional changes. Heart Shen can sometimes leave. Heart connection with the baby. Fire meridians HT/HC.
- Work with Stomach/PV/CV to support Yin and nutrition.
- Do not try to inhibit dispersing Qi. It is dispersing accumulated fluid, increased urination in the early days after delivery is normal.
- Work the Lung energy – to support breathing and Upper Burner.

From 6 weeks to 6 months

- Longer-term patterns of depletion, physical and emotional may begin to become apparent.
- Emotions continue to need balancing: Heart/Heart Protector.
- Qi needs to be worked to support the postural effects of having a baby.
- GB and LV issues due to softness of ligaments and tightness of energy in shoulders and neck. Needing more physical activity.
- SP; to support demands on musculature.

From 6 months to 1 year and changes for the rest of life

- Energy more settled. Lung and link with Three Burners.
- CV/PV ST nourishment as mother, breastfeeding.
- Earth energy – mothering energy and support for musculature.
- Underlying tendencies come through more clearly now.

Many women seek treatment for 'complaints' after delivery, few see this period as a time when they need to nurture themselves. The most common complaints are poor milk production, mastitis, fatigue, particularly after the euphoria of delivering passes, depression, insomnia, shoulder back or coccyx pain. A few women present asking for general care, realising their body is depleted after the birth process.

Although certain themes are applicable when treating post partum it is important to realise each patient must be individually assessed, no one recipe fits all. Generally Qi and Blood require supplementation, dispersion is done locally and lightly.

For example, poor milk flow with soft empty breasts corresponds with Qi and blood deficiency, good diet and tonifying treatment is necessary. Stagnation of Qi produces tight swollen shiny breasts, the glands often being palpable yet milk does not flow; this requires local movement of Qi and gentle work on body points to do the same; supplementing here without moving Qi will worsen symptoms. Phlegm/damp obstructing the Qi mechanism results in swollen but soggy feeling breasts; this situation requires dietary changes and massage to move fluids, tonifying metabolism. Some gentle exercise may be beneficial in the last two cases; the first requires rest.

The concept of resting after delivery is becoming forgotten, and women quickly get back to 'normal life'. It is important to discuss a woman's expectations of herself, helping her to see the benefits of rest, good nutrition, and accepting help when it is offered. Wonder woman is only a screen goddess!

(Lea Papworth)

Reflective questions

- What are the main energies which need supporting postnatally and why?
- How can some of the eastern approaches to postnatal care be integrated into modern practices?

References and further reading

Beresford Cooke, C., 2003. Shiatsu Theory and Practice: A Comprehensive Text for the Student and Professional, second ed. Churchill Livingstone, Edinburgh.

Deadman, P., Al-Khafaji, M., Baker, K., 1998. A manual of acupuncture. J. Chin. Med. (Hove).

Flaws, B., 2005. Chinese Medical Obstetrics. Blue Poppy Press, Boulder, CO.

Fu, Q.-Z., 1995. Fu Qing-zhu's Gynecology (S.-Z. Yang, D.-W. Liu, Trans.), second ed. Blue Poppy Press, Boulder, CO.

Fu Ke Xin Fa Yao Jue, 2005. A Heart Approach to Gynecology: Essentials in Verse (S. Yu, Trans.). Paradigm Publications, Taos, NM.

Goldsmith, J., 1984. Childbirth Wisdom. Congden and Weed, New York.

Jin, Y., 1998. Handbook of Obstetrics and Gynecology in Chinese Medicine: An Integrated Approach (C. Hakim, Trans.). Eastland Press, Seattle.

Low, R.H., 1984. The Secondary Vessels of Acupuncture: A Detailed Account of their Energies, Meridians and Control Points. Thorsons, Wellingborough.

Maciocia, G., 1998. Obstetrics and Gynecology in Chinese Medicine. Churchill Livingstone, Edinburgh.

Maciocia, G., 2006. The Channels of Acupuncture: Clinical Use of the Secondary Channels and Eight Extraordinary Vessels. Elsevier, Churchill Livingstone, Edinburgh.

Rochat de la Vallée, E., 2007. Pregnancy and Gestation in Chinese Classical Texts. Monkey Press, Cambridge.

Yuen, Jeffrey, C., 2005. Channel Systems of Chinese Medicine: The Eight Extraordinary Vessels: 12–13 April 2003. New England School of Acupuncture Continuing Education Department.

Zhao, X., 2006. Traditional Chinese Medicine for Women: Reflections of the Moon on Water. Virago Press, London.

Section 2

Practical bodywork

CONTENTS

Chapter contents

Learning outcomes

- Identify appropriate assessment skills relevant to shiatsu, massage and other bodywork
- Create comprehensive health history forms relevant to the maternity period
- Describe the common postural patterns of the pre- and postnatal client
- Describe modifications required in applying orthopaedic tests for the maternity client

8.1 Assessment of the maternity client

Introduction

It is important for the therapist to make an appropriate assessment for the maternity client in order to know the most effective treatment plan and to understand the few cases where work would not be appropriate. Many therapists use the SOAP charting procedure (Thompson 2002) – formulating Subjective (S) (client perceptions) Objective (O) (therapists findings) Assessment (A) into the (Treatment) Plan (P). The maternity assessment will include understanding the relevance of existing assessment skills and awareness of any modifications to the assessment which need to be made.

Assessment procedure

Depending on their training and skill set, the bodyworker will have variations in emphasis in their intake/assessment. Common components include:

Observation/visual assessment

Visual assessment should begin with the first moment of contact. This may begin before the client has even crossed the doorway into the therapy room. How is the client carrying herself in her pregnancy? How is she holding the newborn? How does she approach the therapist, both in her demeanour and her mobility? What does her face express?

Some therapists prefer to keep the visual assessment informal and simply observe the client's posture while others conduct a more formal postural assessment including use of a plumb-line and specific orthopaedic tests. Another option is to observe clients while they are carrying out any suggested exercises.

It is important to understand the common postural patterning of the maternity client in order to guide and inform specific tests. This understanding will also inform the therapist regarding the appropriateness of exercises.

In Chinese medicine this aspect of the assessment is called *Bo shin* and includes observation of the colour of the skin and the tongue. In pregnancy there is a greater circulating blood volume, the core body temperature is higher and there are various changes in the skin. Understanding thoroughly how the body changes will influence this aspect of the assessment and the therapist's ability to determine effective ways of treatment.

Listening and questioning

Filling in the health history form forms a significant part of this aspect of assessment. The form which is used for the non-maternity client may well be inappropriate both in its inclusion and exclusion of certain questions. Understanding the potential emotional as well as physical changes of the maternity period will help guide the therapist in determining appropriate questions to ask in order to elicit relevant information.

In Chinese medicine these are two distinct assessment categories. *Bun shin* is the listening aspect which includes listening to the type of sound and tone of the voice and *how* the client is talking rather than specifically *what* they are saying. It also includes the use of smell, as specific body odours relate to expressions of different organ energies.

The second assessment category is *Mon-shin* – questioning which would include more specific information gathered verbally from the client.

Touch/palpation

This may occur as part of the postural assessment and during specific orthopaedic tests. For some therapists it may include pulse or Hara (abdomen) and back energy assessment. However, the client is also being continually assessed during the treatment. As the therapist touches the tissues of muscle, ligaments, and the joints of the body, as well as contacting lymph and the pulses, and different types of energy, their work is constantly being informed. Again, understanding how the body changes will affect the understanding of this information. The Chinese referred to this aspect of assessment as: *Setsu shin*.

The maternity health history form: modifications

For most therapists, the form that is used for non-maternity clients is incomplete with respect to obtaining comprehensive information. For example on many forms pregnancy is listed as a 'condition' or even a 'caution' or 'contraindication' for bodywork. Furthermore, common case history questions are not specific enough to elicit the kind of information which is needed in order to work safely and effectively with this population group.

Taking a good health history provides the basis for assessment and treatment decisions. However, sensitivity is needed in eliciting appropriate information. Asking open questions may be the most non-invasive way to receive information. For example, it may be inappropriate to ask directly if the client has had a previous miscarriage (spontaneous abortion) but by asking if they have had previous pregnancies the possibility is opened up for the client to share information about any pregnancy losses she has experienced. It may not seem appropriate to ask direct questions

about the woman's partner, since she may not be in a relationship, but the therapist can ask whether the woman has people who can provide support to her.

The therapist should be aware that some questions may be construed as invasive or irrelevant for the client. The ability to connect with a new client and good communication skills are essential when asking potentially challenging questions. Ensure clients are able to refrain from responding if they so choose. The therapist may also need to explain why they are asking specific questions and their relevance to the session. The client's right to privacy as well as confidentiality must be underscored.

As each bodyworker has different needs for their health history form, we have focused on general items that the therapist might consider including with their own form. These items are in addition to the information which is gathered with non-maternity clients. General information gathered for any client such as previous health history issues, injuries or medical conditions, lifestyle factors, and goals of the treatment are obviously also relevant for the maternity client.

Common abbreviations in clinical notes

In some countries the woman may carry her clinical care notes from her primary care provider. She may willingly share this information with her therapist. Common abbreviations used in clinical notes are:

Para 0 – no previous birth

Para 1 or 2 – 1 or 2 previous births

Para 2 + 1 – 2 previous births plus a miscarriage before 28 weeks

LMP – last menstrual period

EDC/EDB/EDD – expected date of confinement/birth/delivery

Alb – albumin in urine (protein). This may be a sign of pre-eclampsia

Hb – haemoglobin. If less than 10.5 considered anaemic

Hct – haematocrit: percentage of red blood cells. If less than 32% considered anaemic

Fe – iron

BP – blood pressure

FHT/R – fetal heart tones/rate

H/NH – usually refers to heart tones

Fundus – top of uterus

Cx – cervix

PP – presenting part of fetus

Vx/Vtx – vertex (head down)

Ceph – cephalic

Long L – longitudinal lie (fetus lying parallel to mother's spine)

LOA – left occiput anterior

LOP – left occiput posterior

LOT – left occiput transverse

ROA – right occiput anterior

ROP – right occiput posterior

ROT – right occiput transverse

RSA – right sacrum anterior; the most common breech presentation

Eng/E – engaged

T – term

The areas covered below may be included on the case history form or asked as additional questions.

Pregnancy history

- **Menstrual history**. A longer menstrual cycle may indicate a tendency for a longer pregnancy, a shorter cycle a shorter pregnancy; a history of heavy bleeding may indicate a tendency to bleed.
- **History of previous pregnancies, length of gestation, any complications**. This provides a foundation for possible issues or conditions which may be relevant for care in the current pregnancy.
- **Was the pregnancy planned?** This may elicit information about whether the pregnancy involved assisted reproduction.
- **Gestational age/EDB**. This is needed so the therapist knows what to expect in terms of possible symptoms, as well as positional and technique adaptations.
- **Any issues in the current pregnancy history to date**. This will help highlight key issues such as nausea, backache, fatigue, stress, etc.
- **History of vaginal bleeding**. This may or may not mean that bodywork is contraindicated depending when the bleeding commenced, how heavy it is, whether it is resolved, and so on. The cause of any bleeding in pregnancy should be assessed by the primary care provider before the therapist proceeds to do any treatments. Current bleeding would, in most cases, be a contraindication to bodywork (Box 8.1).
- **Abdominal pain**. This will determine whether abdominal care will be included in the treatment – is the client suffering from overstretched skin, ligamentous discomfort, or experiencing more serious issues such as premature labour, placental issues or blood pressure problems (HELLP)? (See Box 9.2 p. 254.)
- **Problems with urination**. Frequency or burning could indicate a urinary tract infection. Lack of urination may indicate a more serious complication which would require immediate referral.

Box 8.1 Bleeding in maternity care

Active uterine bleeding: immediate referral; no bodywork

Any case of active uterine bleeding needs immediate medical attention. If the bleeding has settled, a detailed health history needs to be taken to establish the cause, if known, in order to determine appropriate work. Possible causes of bleeding are:

First trimester

- Implantation bleeding; if mild not necessarily an issue once settled.
- Threatened abortion/miscarriage. Once this has settled, if the fetus is still alive, then work may continue.
- Ectopic pregnancy or hydatidiform mole: immediate referral if active bleeding and once diagnosed the woman would receive appropriate medical treatment. Work can then be done to support the recovery process.
- Cervical lesions: once these have been assessed and there is no bleeding then work may continue.
- Vaginitis: again work may continue once the bleeding has settled.

Second and third trimesters

- Placenta praevia; may be from mild to severe; if no bleeding can work with modifications (see high-risk chapter)
- Placental abruption: may only present with mild bleeding, but is always a potential emergency, particularly if the pregnant woman shows signs of shock and a hard uterus.

Labour

- Placental detachment.

Postnatally

- Retained placenta.
- Placental issues.
- Infection.

Exception

Where there is bleeding but the woman knows she is miscarrying and that the fetus has died, and wants support in that process then it is her choice to receive bodywork.

- **Groin pain or discomfort**. Could indicate possible PGI/SPD.
- **Blood pressure: current and previous history**. Some therapists take the BP at the beginning and/ or ending of the treatment. If not, the therapist needs to know when blood pressure was last taken,

and whether it was within normal limits. Blood pressure is an important indicator of health in the maternity period.

- **Varicose veins, leg cramping or pain, sensory loss (numbness).** These kind of issues are fairly common and it is important to identify them in order to establish appropriate work to the legs.
- **Clotting issues/suspected DVT. This is potentially an emergency situation and needs to be screened for.** It is rare in healthy pregnant clients.
- **Date of last visit to primary care provider.** This will ensure that the client is receiving regular antenatal care, and inform the therapist of the type of care received whether midwife, obstetrician, or family physician.
- **Position of baby (from week 28) if known.** If it is not known then the therapist may feel it is appropriate to encourage the woman to be aware of her baby, ask if she is feeling movements, and perhaps elicit a discussion about how she feels about her pregnancy, her baby, birth, and so on.
- **History of previous labours.** This can indicate problems or anxieties which may affect the client in her current pregnancy. It can also provide useful information for the therapist who offers birth preparation work or who attends births.
- **Birth plans for this labour.** This is more appropriate to ask during the last trimester, unless it is relevant earlier. It opens the possibility of talking about bodywork as an option during the birthing process and potentially as a means of pain relief.
- **History of the previous postnatal period.** This is important to establish if there were any problems with postpartum depression, or issues adapting to motherhood or breastfeeding in order that preventative type of work may be done.
- **Family information,** e.g. how many other children, family support. This gives an idea of the kind of demands made on the client, for example if she is well supported, single or with partner and so on.
- **Available support.** This elicits further information about family set-up but also emphasises the need for support in pregnancy.

Labour support form

If a therapist is attending their client's birth, there will be additional information that will need to be obtained both in advance of the birth and during the birthing process. Note taking during the delivery would be in alignment with the requirements of the therapist's scope of practice. A post-birth debriefing session may also be included as part of client care.

Questions/information to be gathered include:

What are your hopes for this delivery?

Are there specific reasons for why you want a doula/birth support person for your birth?

What are your beliefs about birth? What sort of births did your mother/sister/close family members have? What was your own birth like? (This information gathers the kind of beliefs, conscious and unconscious, the woman may have about birth and also memories/imprinting of her own birth.)

Birth record:

Gestational age at delivery (in weeks)

Time labour contractions began

Time labour contractions were 5 mins apart

Dilatation/effacement/station when admitted to hospital if applicable

Spontaneous rupture of membranes? Yes/ No

If Yes, what time?

Place of rupture (home, hospital, car, other)

Dilatation, if known, at time of rupture

Colour of the amniotic fluid? Was meconium present? Yes/No Light/Moderate/Thick

What was the approximate length of first stage (0–10 cm)?

How did the mother feel during first stage? What kind of support did you offer? Bodywork given. Effect.

Second stage (bearing down)?

How did the mother feel during second stage? Positions. What kind of support did you offer? Bodywork given. Effect.

What was the approximate time/length of third stage (delivery of placenta)? Were there any third stage complications?

If yes, please explain

How were the mother and baby? Any support given?

Was the mother breastfeeding? Who helped her establish breastfeeding?

Any other issues before you left? Bodywork given? Further emotional support?

Time doula arrived. Time doula departed. Total time doula in attendance.

Debriefing visit:

How did the mother feel after the birth? Any issues? Was any postnatal work done? How did the therapist spend time with the mother after the birth?

Date of first postnatal visit.

Postnatal work

Pregnancy questions

If the therapist is seeing the client for the first time in the postnatal period, then relevant information about the pregnancy and birth history as well as previous pregnancies/births should be obtained. This includes questions about stress, fatigue, and family/friend support.

- **What kind of labour?**

If the therapist attended the birth this will have been recorded in detail (as above). If the therapist did not attend the birth, then they will need to find out what happened during the birth, both physically and emotionally, in order to inform the postnatal approach.

- **How many weeks postnatal?**

This is important in order to know what to expect in terms of types of conditions and cautions.

- **How are they recovering postnatally?**

This includes both emotional and physical aspects of recovery.

- **Breastfeeding/feeding issues?**

If the mother is breastfeeding, she may need lymphatic work and breast massage or another treatment modality. If she does not wish to have treatment directly from the therapist, she could be shown some self-care modalities.

- **Baby.**

How is the baby? Any health issues or concerns related to the baby? If the therapist is trained in baby massage, some simple techniques can be shown. Regardless, if the baby is with the mother, it is usually helpful to try to include the baby in the session, perhaps by letting the baby lie beside the mother, encouraging the mother to tend to her baby's needs, cuddling, feeding or changing her baby. Postpartum care on the floor can be effective in allowing more space for mother/baby bonding.

- **Any specific pain in the perineal or groin area?**

This is important to screen for possible PGI/SPD. As this could be caused by the birthing process itself, it is worth repeating as a postpartum question.

- **Incisions: healing of caesarean section and episiotomy scars.**

This is vital to know in order to establish appropriate postnatal work.

- **Temperature/fever/discharge of lochia issues.**

Cautions/contraindications/modifications

One of the aims of questioning is to establish if there are any situations where the client would need to be referred or if there are any cases where bodywork needs to be modified (Boxes 8.2, 8.3, 8.4).

Box 8.2 Urgent referral in pregnancy

Urgent referral: no bodywork should be carried out until medical diagnosis is made. Women need to be referred *immediately* to their primary care provider.

- Severe continuous unexplained abdominal pain (many causes – see box 9.2 p. 254–255).
- Current uterine bleeding (many causes – see box 8.1 p. 183).
- Loss of amniotic fluid prior to 37 weeks and/or strong contractions; pre-term labour.
- Inability to urinate; UTI with possible bladder complication.
- Severe facial oedema; possible PET.
- Oedema which is visibly increasing and which does not respond to elevation or mobilisations; possible PET, hypertension or kidney issues.
- Severe headache, blurry vision, flashing lights; possible PET.
- Symptoms of shock in woman: pale face, mental confusion, dizziness; possible placental separation or DIC.
- Lack of fetal movement which the woman feels is of concern; possible still-birth or fetal issues.
- Severe vomiting; T1 possible hyperemesis, hydatidiform mole. T2 and 3 premature labour.
- Signs of severe depression or psychosis.
- Suspected thrombosis.

Box 8.3 Signs of eclampsia/toxaemia (PET)

Eclampsia may be a medical emergency. It occurs in the second or third trimesters as it is dependent on there being a placenta.

It may be fine to work with a pre-eclampsic woman with modifications (see high-risk chapter) but if it starts to develop into eclampsia then it is becoming a medical emergency and needs immediate medical referral. The therapist needs to be clear that all the following are possible signs:

- Severe frontal headaches.
- Visual disturbances, e.g. blurry vision, flashing lights.
- Swelling of face; severe including swelling of eyelids.
- Epigastric pain/pain in upper right upper quadrant of abdomen (HELPP syndrome).
- Generalised oedema, more than just some oedema in the legs and arms. It would be experienced throughout the leg and not just in the extremities.
- Severe abdominal pain.
- General malaise, agitation, nausea.

Testimonial: do not be afraid to refer if you have concerns

I am usually able to work out if a mum has cholestasis from the feet and the abdomen and I have had four cases of this where it has been dismissed by the medical professionals, but I have insisted that the women leave my session and go straight to the hospital for a blood test. It has always proved positive. One women said that her reflexology session saved her life. On arrival at the hospital, the doctor was so shocked at the results of her liver function test that he ordered an immediate caesarean section. Hospital protocols have been changed as a result of this. He said if she had left it for another day then it would have been fatal for her.

(Catherine Tugnait, UK Maternity Reflexologist and Reflexologist Therapist)

Modifications to treatments

In order to understand how treatments should proceed, a clear understanding of the physiological changes occurring in the maternity period is crucial.

If the client is presenting with more pathological conditions, then often work can be done but with modifications. These types of conditions are outlined in the high-risk section. Conditions warranting early referral to primary caregiver but where the therapist may be able to work are outlined in Box 8.5.

Postural assessment

This is key to assessment. It should include some assessment from anterior, lateral and posterior view of the body. It must include an understanding of the physical structures such as joints and muscles as well as how the meridian pathways may be distorted through decompensated posture. The therapist may wish to palpate the bony landmarks of the body. The woman's posture will show significant movement to change in the areas of most flexibility. Physiotherapy studies (Polden & Mantle 1990) suggest that the increase in kyphosis and lordotic sways in the spine will be exaggerated as the pregnancy progresses.

Usually assessment is made from assessment in the standing posture; considering the anterior, lateral and posterior view. However, in pregnancy alignment may also be assessed while the client is sitting or while she is on all fours.

While the client is sitting (for example on the ball) it can be helpful to notice how the legs support the sitting posture and any alterations in position. The hips will be externally rotated increasingly as the fetus grows in size. While the client is on all fours (for example resting over the ball) assessment can be made of lumbar lordosis and supportiveness of the abdominal muscles. Observation can be made of the shoulders and neck and which way the client places the head.

Assessment can be made of the comfort of the knees in this position and any knee issues may become apparent.

Typical posture of pregnancy

Postural habits pre-pregnancy tend to be exaggerated. The typical posture in later pregnancy is caused by:

- Hyperlordosis. The increasing weight of the abdomen, accompanied by lengthening of the muscle and some weakening of muscle tone, increases anterior pelvic tilt, especially when accompanied by a lack of postural awareness. The increasing weight causes additional work load on the lower vertebrae, lower erectae spinae and transversospinalis groups. The muscles respond to this lengthening by contracting and tightening. This means that lordosis of the lower back is increased.
- Other muscles which tend to be involved in this pattern are:
  - *Weak or inhibited (hypotonic)* – rectus abdominis, transverse abdominus, external and internal obliques, pelvic floor.
  - *Short and tight (hypertonic)* – gluteus maximus and minimus, hip flexors (psoas major and iliacus), rectus femoris, tensor fascia lata (TFL), quadratus lumborum, lumbar erector spinae, iliotibial band as they engage to stabilise the lower back.
- The knee joints tend to be slightly hyperextended. The ankle joints tend to be slightly plantarflexed. There can also be a narrowing of the intervertebral discs and foramen, leading to possible nerve root irritation.
- Sometimes the woman responds to this by bringing the weight back onto the heels to compensate for the forward pull of her body.
- Weight of the baby. Factors here include the weight of the baby and also softening of pelvic joints, external rotation of the hips and compression of the lumbosacral area. The weight of the fetus in the pelvis, combined with the hormonally induced softening of the pelvis, causes a widening of the hips and external rotation.
- This relative pelvic instability may also lead to sacroiliac (SI) joint instability or sacral misalignment. The weight of the fetus may also put pressure on the sacroiliac and sciatic nerves, causing sciatica.
- If the baby is lying in the posterior position, its pressure is likely to be more uncomfortable.

The pelvic floor muscles contract and the uterine tilt is increased anteriorly which perpetuates the postural fatigue of the skeletal muscles with prolonged upright postures and increases the likelihood of uterine muscle contraction.

(Averille Morgan, personal communication, 2008)

Effects on the rest of the body

The neck and shoulders may express patterns of compensation in response to the changes in the pelvis. Typical patterns here can be grinding of the jaw and temporomandibular joint (TMJ) issues and excessive tension in the neck and shoulders:

This is due to the cranial membranes being strained via the sacral attachment. If, for instance, the sacral drag is a result of pelvic muscular or ligament weakness then the spinal membranes are also straining from their interspinal attachments and cranial base attachments. The resultant inferior drag can manifest as throat, sinus and jaw contraction.

(Averille Morgan, personal communication, 2008)

The pelvic position and weight will affect the legs, positions and joints. The gastrocnemius and soleus tend to be hypertonic in addition to the tensor fascia latae and rectus femoris. The adductors tend to be hypotonic. Often there can be a collapsing of the inner arches of the feet (pes planus).

The changing weight necessitates adaptations to changes in the centre of gravity via stretch or contraction of skeletal muscles and disproportionate loading on viscera or fascial structures, eg uterus and mesenteries. Balance may become an issue for pregnant women.

Hyperkyphosis

The increasing weight of the breasts contributes to the postural imbalance in the maternity period. They tend to pull down on the front of the upper body meaning that hyperkyphosis may be an issue. The lungs and front of the body – rib cage and intercostals, diaphragm – tend to become compressed with the result that breathing may become more laboured and there may be thoracic outlet syndrome issues:

With increased anterior fascial strains of the thorax, the thoracic inlet tension increases. This area is important for lymphatic drainage via the lymphatic ducts. Improved respiration using the abdominal diaphragm will encourage the thoracic inlet to reciprocally pump and aid spinal circulation and drainage, gradually improving postural compensation mechanisms.

(Averille Morgan, personal communication, 2008)

Typical patterns

- Short and tight (hypertonic). Sternocleidomastoids, upper trapezius, suboccipitals, levator scapulae, scalenes, pectoralis major and minor, subclavius, serratus anterior, anterior intercostals, splenii, supraspinatus, infraspinatus, teres minor.

- Weak or inhibited (hypotonic). Rhomboids, middle trapezius, thoracic erector spinae, suprahyoids, infrahyoids, longus capitis, longus cervicis.

Energy patterns

- Collapsed Lung energy; Kyo patterns more common.
- Wood energy, especially Gall Bladder around the shoulder blade is tight/Kyo sometimes even though the muscles may be weak.
- There can be a narrowing of the intervertebral discs and foramen, leading to possible nerve root irritation.

Individual variations

The 'typical' presentation of pregnancy will vary (Fig. 8.1). Individual assessment will be needed to determine which of the muscle patterns is present for each client. This is particularly necessary relative to pre-existing musculoskeletal issues. For example if the pelvis is already in lordosis this pattern will be exaggerated. If the pelvis is rotated or higher on one side this will add variation to the basic pattern.

If the client has pre-existing imbalances in their legs, this will affect the pelvic alignment. Shortened or lengthened quads/hamstrings affect the pull on the pelvis and the ASIS and sacrum may be out of alignment.

The focus of postural alignment in pregnancy is primarily to correct excessive anterior pelvic tilting. This includes exercises and techniques which lengthen the lower back, helping to aid posterior tilting of the pelvis to a more neutral position and shortening the abdominal muscles as well as opening the chest and lungs.

Passive movements and joint mobilisations are especially helpful as the fetus tends to create compression in areas of the mother's body, especially in the pelvis and ribs. Where the fetus is pushing on the maternal pelvis, ligaments and muscles will stretch and at times, strain. Care needs to be taken to monitor the stability of the pubic bone, as PGI becomes a possibility and would result in avoiding movements which could aggravate the symphysis pubis.

Energy patterns: postural

- The postural changes will in turn have an effect on the meridians of the body which will affect the various energies. The main energy that is weakened is the energy of the Kidneys, due to their role in storing the Jing which is sent to the baby and their relationship to the Extraordinary Vessels.

This is the energetic root of the lordosis pattern. It would be aggravated by weakness in the lower Bladder area.

- Changes in the pressure on the discs reflect patterns of the Governing Vessel. Blocked energy in the back also reflects blockages in energy of the three burners. The lower burner is considered to be 'blocked' by the fetus which in turn affects the middle burner and upper burner energy.
- These postural changes would affect the Yin meridian of the front of the body. There is a tendency for weaker energy in the Yin meridians, especially CV and KD, PV.
- The Yin meridians of the legs are often weaker – SP, LV, KD. The Yang meridians of the legs often compensate by contracting.
- Due to the weakness of the Kidney there is often excess energy blocked in the neck and shoulders, particularly in the Wood meridians of Gall Bladder and Liver.
- All of these patterns need to be assessed individually.

Typical posture postnatally (Fig. 8.2)

Weakness in the pelvis

The muscles which have been weakened due to the demands of pregnancy (abdominals and pelvic floor), if not appropriately strengthened, may remain potential areas of weakness for the rest of the woman's life. In the initial postnatal period, the pelvis tends to be even less stable than during pregnancy, due to the pressures of the fetus descending and the forces of opening out in labour and the resulting weakness in the musculature and ligaments. It takes time for the muscles and ligaments to strengthen. Some women continue to have lower back and pelvic issues into the postpartum and beyond. These type of issues will tend to be aggravated by the additional weakness in the abdominal wall caused by a caesarean.

Women may have PGI issues, especially PGI, caused by strain placed on the pubic bone during labour through either prolonged straining in second stage in a squatting position or lying in lithotomy for extended periods straining.

Postnatally women often have tight psoas muscles as these work to support the pelvis.

One-sided patterns due to carrying infant on one hip

Weakness in the pelvis can be further exacerbated by poor posture postnatally. Many mothers carry their infant on one hip, especially as the baby gains weight in the weeks and months post delivery. This creates

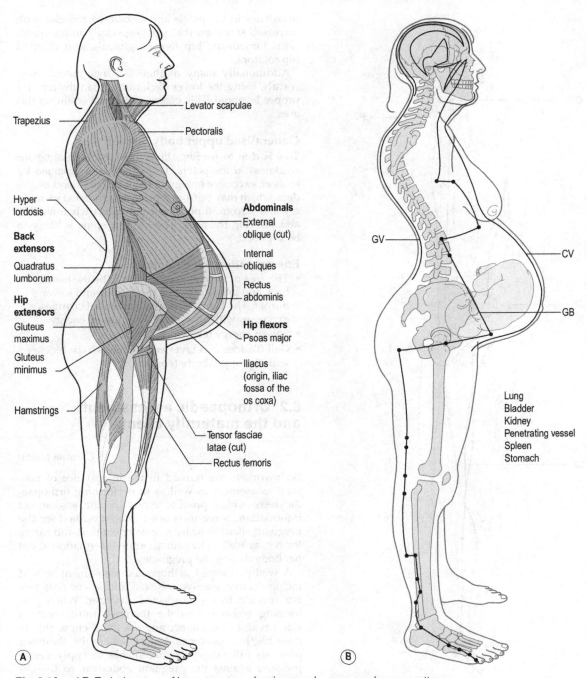

Trapezius

Levator scapulae

Pectoralis

Hyper
lordosis

Abdominals

External
oblique (cut)

**Back
extensors**

Quadratus
lumborum

Internal
obliques

Rectus
abdominis

**Hip
extensors**

Hip flexors

Gluteus
maximus

Psoas major

Gluteus
minimus

Iliacus
(origin, iliac
fossa of the
os coxa)

Hamstrings

Tensor fasciae
latae (cut)

Rectus femoris

Ⓐ

GV

CV

GB

Lung
Bladder
Kidney
Penetrating vessel
Spleen
Stomach

Ⓑ

Fig. 8.1A and **B** Typical posture of late pregnancy, showing muscle groups and energy patterns.

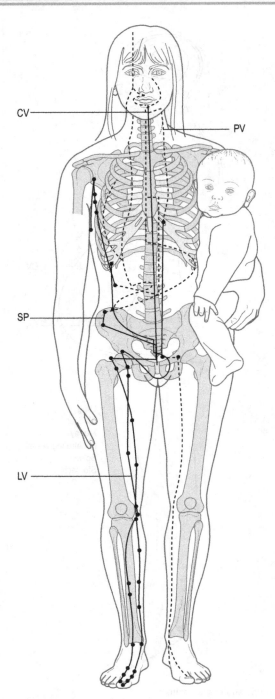

CV —

PV —

SP —

LV —

Fig. 8.2 Areas weakened through pregnancy and strains placed on the body through caring for young children, showing muscle groups and energy patterns.

imbalance in the pelvis and associated muscles with increased strain on that side, especially in the quadratus lumborum, hip flexors, gluteals, and external hip rotators.

Additionally many mothers lift their infant awkwardly, using the lower back rather than the legs for proper leverage. This places additional strain on this area.

Generalised upper body tension

This is due to feeding, lifting and compensating for weakness in the pelvis. This can be accompanied by tension/excessive energy in the head, neck and shoulders, which may be from tension accumulated in delivery and also from poor postural habits when feeding and carrying the baby. The thoracic spine is likely to be kyphotic.

Energy patterns: postnatally

- The area of weakness continues to be the lower back and pelvis which is the Kidney and lower burner. The Hara itself, after the initial changes, expresses with an overall weakness of energy.
- Spleen energy tends to be weak.
- Gall Bladder and Liver energy tends to be blocked; with the upper body tensions.

8.2 Orthopaedic assessment and the maternity client

Caroline Martin

Bodyworkers are trained in the importance of postural assessment as well as in performing orthopaedic tests which provide more specific assessment information. Some tests need to be modified for the pregnant client in order to ensure comfort and safety for her, as well as to gain accurate information about her body during the pregnancy.

A well-performed orthopaedic assessment should include active, passive, resisted and *special tests* that are specific to the suspected disorder. When performing resisted tests the therapist must create a safe amount of resistance and ask the client to slowly meet his/her resistance. In tests where the abdomen prevents full range it is acceptable to apply gentle pressure against the pregnant abdomen, to the client's comfort level.

Together all the tests will help better determine what muscles, tendons, joints or nerves are involved and/or affected. These tests are very important in making a differential diagnosis because minor disorders can mimic very serious problems. A proper orthopaedic assessment can mean the difference between a minor inconvenience and a fatal medical condition.

The bodyworker's role is not to diagnose medical conditions, but to play an important part in referring the client back to her primary healthcare provider for further assessment when it is thought necessary. Whether or not the questions lead to any conclusive assessment, it is still necessary for the therapist to refer the client to the MD with all negative and positive findings documented.

Below is a list of some physical disorders that have similar symptoms but very different diagnoses and which the therapist may encounter with the maternity client:

1. Low back pain caused by tight/strained low back muscles is similar to that caused by kidney problems. This is important because kidney issues may be a factor in pregnant clients. Findings from a back assessment may show that the client has tenderness with certain active ranges of motion (AROM) but if the resisted tests are negative then this suggests there is no muscle involvement. If the passive tests are also negative then this suggests it is not ligament or joint related either. At this point it is important to run through the low back special tests including myotomes and dermatomes, and if these are all negative then the therapist should consider involvement of the kidneys. The therapist can ask questions regarding colour of urine, frequency of urination as well as any signs of burning and unusual odour. The therapist should then refer the client to the appropriate healthcare professional who in turn should do the necessary urine tests to determine if there is any urinary tract or kidney involvement.

2. Thoracic outlet syndrome (TOS) that presents with left-sided weakness may actually be the signs and symptoms of a mild stroke. It is therefore imperative that the therapist can properly test for TOS.

3. Carpal tunnel syndrome (CTS) needs to be assessed to determine if it is being caused by tightness of the fascia/muscles/tendons due to excessive swelling in the wrists or whether active trigger points in the neck/shoulder muscles are the cause. The therapist must also consider blood pressure (BP) in addition to swelling. They must determine if the onset of swelling is sudden, dramatic, in the face as well as the arms and legs, and be aware of the additional symptoms as listed in the BP section 1.4 p. 20. The client may

be suffering from pre-eclampsia which needs immediate medical attention.

4. Shoulder pain is often caused by tight neck, shoulder, chest, upper back muscles or may sometimes be due to a rotator cuff bursitis/ tendonitis/strain. But shoulder pain that has a sudden onset and is isolated to the left side, and that may or may not show other symptoms of a heart attack, must be properly assessed – referral to a physician may be wiser than a shiatsu/massage treatment.

5. Pain in a client's leg may be caused by tight, fatigued or cramping calf muscles which are very common during pregnancy. However, these symptoms may actually be due to a deep vein thrombosis (DVT), so it is important to know the difference.

6. Low back pain that exhibits symptoms of a tight iliopsoas muscle is identical to pain caused by an aortic aneurysm. This is an extremely rare complication, especially in pregnancy, so the therapist is unlikely to encounter it. However, any attempt to release an iliopsoas could rupture an aneurysm, and the misdiagnosed client would likely die on the massage table. Although an MRI would be needed to diagnose an aortic aneurysm, an orthopaedic assessment can determine the involvement of the iliopsoas.

Having the training and ability to assess a client orthopaedically ensures an accurate clinical impression and improves quality of care for the client. The knowledge of the individual bodyworker in regards to orthopaedic tests may vary from country to country and there are specific books that discuss orthopaedic testing in great length. We have included tests which cover the main areas of the body most likely to be affected by maternity changes.

Orthopaedic testing and positioning

Generally, near the end of the first trimester, the expectant client will find the prone position too uncomfortable during orthopaedic testing. The therapist will need to adjust and modify their assessment techniques specifically when the pelvic/hip joints are involved. From the middle of the second trimester she is likely to find supine less comfortable. In the postnatal period, prone and supine become testing options once more, although care needs to be taken with clients after surgery, that there is no pain experienced in different positions due to incision discomfort.

Table 8.1 lists the typical joints assessed actively, passively and with restriction. It notes their movements and approximate normal ranges of motion (ROM). For

Table 8.1 Joints with their movements and approximate normal ranges of motion (ROM)

Cervical spine	Thoracic spine	Lumbar spine
Flexion – 45°	Flexion – 30–40°	Flexion – 80°
Extension – 45°	Extension – 20–30°	Extension – 20–30°
L/R sideflexion – 45°	L/R sideflexion – 20–25°	L/R sideflexion – 35°
L/R spinal rotation – 60°	L/R spinal rotation – 35°	L/R spinal rotation – 45°
Hip	**Knee**	**Ankle**
Flexion – 120°	Flexion – 135°	Plantarflexion – 30–50°
Extension – 30°	Extension – 0–10°	Dorsiflexion – 20°
External rotation – 60°	External rotation – 40°	Eversion – 10°
Internal rotation – 40°	Internal rotation – 30°	Inversion – 20°
Abduction – 45°		
Adduction – 30°		
Shoulder	**Elbow**	**Wrist**
Flexion – 180°	Flexion – 140–150°	Flexion – 80–90°
Extension – 45–60°	Extension – 0–5°	Extension – 70–90°
Abduction – 180°	Pronation – 80–90°	Ulnar deviation – 40°
Adduction – 45°		
External rotation – 90°	Supination – 90°	Radial deviation – 30°
Internal rotation – 90°		
Horizontal abduction – 45°		
Horizontal adduction – 135°		
External rotation with 90 degrees elbow flexion		
Internal rotation with 90 degrees elbow flexion		

the most part these tests can be done in a seated, semi-reclined or standing position. Often a seated position will be the least compromising, most comfortable, and safest for the maternity client. If supine is the only option, avoid keeping the client in this position for any longer than she is comfortable and be alert to any signs or symptoms of supine hypotension. The values in italic font are the orthopaedic tests that are usually performed prone or supine and positional modifications will be discussed later in this chapter.

Modifying basic orthopaedic tests for the maternity client

Before discussing maternity positional modifications during an orthopaedic pelvic assessment, it is important to ensure the therapist remembers the minor modifications for other joint assessments.

When testing the cervical spine have the client seated to avoid loss of balance. The therapist will need to support the client at the hips when performing the

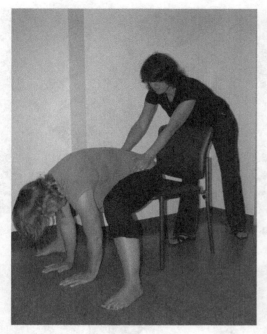

Fig. 8.3 Forward lumbar flexion.

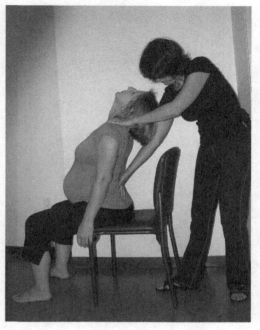

Fig. 8.4 Therapist spotting active lumbar extension.

active range of motion for the thoracic spine while having the client in a standing position. Resisted ranges of motion of the thoracic spine can be done with the client seated.

Active, passive and resisted tests of the shoulder, elbow and wrist can also be achieved with the client in a seated position whereas the knee and ankle assessments can be completed successfully with the client either semi-reclining or seated.

Always test the uninjured side first to determine the client's normal ranges and rule out the joints above and below the chief complaint site to ensure there are no other complications. Give a full explanation and, where necessary, a demonstration of the testing movements prior to performing the test.

Pelvic assessments of the maternity client

When assessing pelvic disorders a gait analysis and postural assessment should be done first. The therapist should note any strained walking gait such as a 'waddle' or limp and use a plumb line for a proper postural assessment to determine the degree of increased kyphosis or lumbar lordosis.

Following the gait and posture analysis a full hip *and* lumbar assessment must be completed as both regions affect pelvic movement. For example, when

the lumbar region is flexed forward a problem with the articulation of the ilia on the sacrum could be detected, just as hip tests can uncover lesions at the sacroiliac joint. The therapist must be aware of any imbalanced movement which could expose hyper- or hypomobility.

Forward lumbar flexion can be performed safely and effectively, even in the later stages of the third trimester, by having the woman seated with her feet firmly on the floor and her legs spread apart enough to accompany her growing belly (Fig. 8.3). As noted in Table 8.1, the hip is tested in six different ranges of motion and the lumbar in four, two bilaterally. Special tests are performed after a full hip and lumbar assessment is completed, followed by palpation. The special tests for the pelvis are discussed later in this chapter.

In assessing the pelvis the therapist must initially test the client in her active range to see if any limitations exist. It is important not to physically stress the client and therefore the therapist needs to avoid having the client switch back and forth from standing, to seated, to semi-reclined and so on. All the active and resisted ranges of motion of the lumbar assessment can be done in the seated position; therefore it is more efficient to test this region first (Fig. 8.4). Due to the increased laxity of ligaments and weight of the perinatal client passive testing can sometimes be awkward and the results

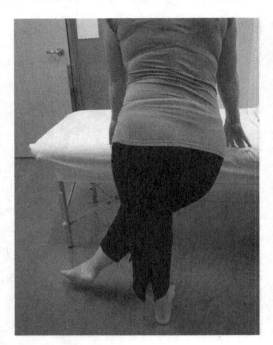

Fig. 8.5 Active hip adduction.

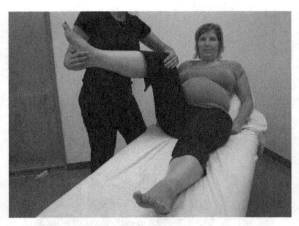

Fig. 8.6 Passive hip internal rotation.

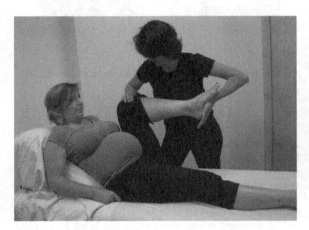

Fig. 8.7 Passive hip flexion.

inconclusive. Therefore it is best to place a gentle overpressure at the end of each active range of motion as long as the client exhibits normal and pain-free ranges. A normal overpressure end-feel should be a 'tissue stretch' sensation for all ranges of the lumbar spine. During the active testing phases in the seated position always stand within a safe close range of the client to assist her should she lose her balance.

For the hip assessment all tests that can be done standing should be performed first as the rest will be done with the client semi-reclined. These are: active extension, abduction, adduction, then passive and resisted extension. Position the client beside the therapy table so she can utilise it for support then direct her to extend her leg backwards, out to the side and then across the body. At this stage it is best to test the passive and resisted actions of the client's hip while she is still standing (Figs 8.5 and 8.6). When applying resistance always have the client just meet your resistance and hold the test for 5–15 seconds (Fig. 8.8A).

Next position the client semi-reclining. The most logical order of testing in this position is hip flexion, internal rotation, and external rotation actively, passively then resisted. Finish off with passive and resisted abduction and adduction. For active flexion direct the client to bring her knee toward her chest. Have her relax and repeat the movement passively (Fig. 8.7) then with resistance (Fig. 8.8). Again, the expanding abdomen will determine the amount of range enabled.

For external and internal rotation have the client turn her foot inwards and outwards while the hip and knee are at 90° of flexion. Next perform the passive and resisted tests of these ranges and then move onto testing abduction and adduction. When performing abduction stabilise the opposite side at the pelvis and thigh. For adduction assist the client by lifting the opposing leg. Resisted adduction can be done with the client semi-reclining, while resisted abduction is most effective with the client side-lying (Fig. 8.9).

Throughout the tests note any decreased ranges of motion, abnormal end-feels and pain or discomfort.

Special testing and modifications for common maternity conditions

There are a number of *special tests* that can be performed to help determine what anatomical structures are involved in a condition. Listed below are

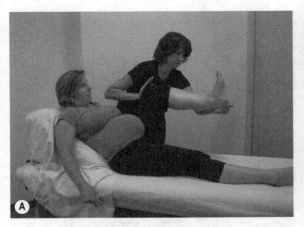

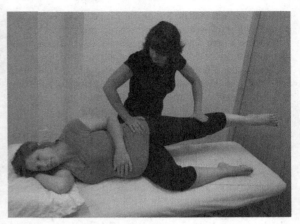

Fig. 8.9 Resisted hip abduction.

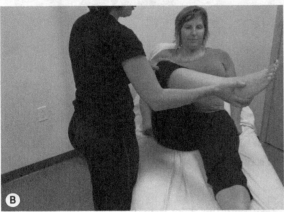

Fig. 8.8A and B Resisted hip flexion. (A) Passive external rotation and (B) resisted internal rotation.

just a few examples of common and effective tests. It is highly recommended that therapists should get further training with instructors who are skilled in teaching orthopaedic special tests and assessments if they have not covered this skill in their professional bodywork training.

Compression syndrome tests

Wright's test

Objective: Test for thoracic outlet syndrome (TOS) due to tightness in the pectoralis minor muscle.

Test: With the client seated palpate her radial pulse and then hyperabduct the client's arm so her hand is brought over her head. Instruct her to take a breath and note if her pulse dissipates. If there is no change have her rotate or extend her head and neck as this may also create a positive test result.

Results: Positive if pulse dissipates or she experiences tingling and numbness in the upper limb.

Adson's manoeuvre

Objective: Test for TOS related to compression of the brachial plexus caused by tight anterior scalenes.

Test: Locate the radial pulse, have client rotate her head *toward* the test shoulder. Next ask her to extend her head back while the therapist passively externally rotates and extends the client's shoulder. Ask the client to take a deep breath and hold it for approximately 15 seconds.

Positive sign: If the pulse fades or disappears.

Travell's manoeuvre

Objective: Test for TOS related to compression of the brachial plexus caused by tight middle scalenes.

Test: Locate the radial pulse, have client rotate her head *away from* the test shoulder. Next ask her to extend her head back while the therapist passively externally rotates and extends the client's shoulder. Ask the client to take a deep breath and hold it for approximately 15 seconds.

Positive sign: If the pulse fades or disappears.

Phalen's test

Objective: Tests for carpal tunnel syndrome (CTS) caused by pressure on the median nerve.

Test: The therapist fully flexes the client's wrists bilaterally and places them so the posterior aspects of the client's hands are touching. Gently compress the wrists together for approximately 60 seconds.

Positive sign: Tingling in the first to third digits and the lateral half of the fourth digit.

Straight leg raising (SLR) test

Objective: Tests for disc-related compression disorders.

Test: Position the client in semi-reclined. With the client's leg straight the therapist internally rotates, slightly adducts and flexes the leg at the hip; discomfort in the posterior leg indicates the hamstrings are tight.

Positive sign: Pain within 40–90° is indicative of a disc-related condition and/or tension on the lumbosacral nerve roots between L4 and L5. If both legs are lifted passively and pain is felt prior to 30° then this is suggestive of an SI joint dysfunction.

Valsalva's test

Objective: Tests for compression to a spinal nerve due to a herniated disc/tumour/osteophyte.

Test: With the client seated, ask her to take a deep breath and hold it for approximately 15 seconds. At the same time instruct the client to moderately bear down as if emptying her bowels.

Positive sign: Localised pain at site of compression which may radiate downwards. This indicates a possible disc-related disorder.

Note: Avoid this test if the client is beyond 36 weeks or has had any signs or symptoms of early delivery.

Slump test

Objective: Tests for compression/impingement of the dura and/or spinal nerves.

Test: The client is seated, with feet on the floor and legs slightly open. Ask the client to slump so that the spine flexes forward and the shoulders drop toward the floor. At the same time the therapist holds the client's chin and head up. If there is no reproduction of symptoms then the therapist flexes the client's neck forward. If there is still no reproduction of symptoms, passively extend the client's knee and if this does not recreate any symptoms, dorsiflex the foot. Perform test bilaterally (as in Fig. 8.3).

Positive sign: Pain along the spine or symptoms of sciatica. The pain is usually felt at the site of the lesion.

Hip/sacroiliac joint

Kemp's test

Objective: Tests for facet or SI joint dysfunction and/or a nerve root lesion due to a herniated disc.

Test: With the client standing the therapist positions him- or herself behind her. The client must extend the spine while laterally flexing and rotating to the affected side. At the same time the therapist controls the movement by holding the client's shoulder while directing the client to reach towards the back of the opposite knee. Gentle overpressure is applied in extension while the client side-flexes and rotates to the side of pain. Movement continues until limit of range or until symptoms are produced.

Positive sign: If symptoms are reproduced.

Patrick's/Faber test

Objective: Tests for SI joint dysfunction or a tight piriformis muscle.

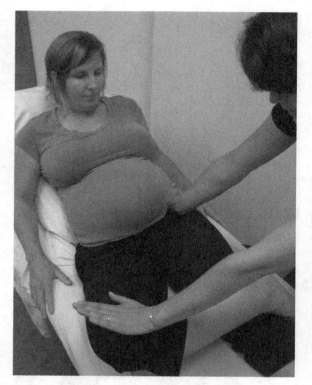

Fig. 8.10 Patrick's/Faber test.

Test: With the client seated, the therapist places the client's leg so that the foot of the test leg is on top of the opposing knee. This places the hip so it is flexed, abducted and externally rotated. The therapist must stabilise the client by placing one hand on the anterior superior iliac spine (ASIS) of the non-test leg and gently push the test leg down towards the table (Fig. 8.10).

Positive sign: If the leg remains above the non-test leg or if the client feels pain in the hip or SI joint.

Transerverse anterior stress test/sacroiliac joint 'gap' test

Objective: Tests the stability of the anterior ligaments of the SI joints.

Test: Facing the client, who is semi-reclined, the therapist places his/her left hand on the inside aspect of the client's left ASIS and the right hand on the right ASIS. Gently apply cross-armed pressure outwards. Normally the direction of pressure is also downwards but this is difficult to do later in the pregnancy. However, the unidirectional position is still quite successful during pregnancy.

Positive test: If the client feels unilateral discomfort/pain in the SI joint or gluteal region.

Transverse posterior stress test/sacroiliac joint 'squish' test

Objective: Tests for stability of the posterior ligaments of the SI joints.

Test: Facing the client, who is semi-reclined, the therapist places his/her right hand on the outside aspect of the client's left ASIS and the left hand on the right ASIS. Gently apply pressure downwards and inwards.

Positive test: If the client feels discomfort/pain in the SI joints or gluteal region.

Trendelenberg test

Objective: Tests for weakness of gluteus medius or hip instability on the stance side.

Test: Standing behind the client the therapist places his/her hands with the fingers on the ASIS and thumbs on the SI joints. Next ask the client to stand on one leg and observe whether the iliac crest of the non-stance side drops, stays level or rises. Repeat test on the other side.

Positive test: If the pelvis drops on the non-stance side then this displays weakness of gluteus medius in the *stance* side.

Lower leg
Homan's sign

Objective: Tests for deep vein thrombosis.

Test: First note if the client has palpable tenderness, increased warmth, decreased pedal pulse and/or swelling in the calf region. Then, with the client's knee in extension, passively dorsiflex the ankle.

Positive sign: Sharp pain in the calf with passive dorsiflexion and tenderness with palpation of the calf.

Note: In the absence of a positive sign, DVT may still be present, therefore this is an inconclusive test.

Other tests relevant to the maternity period
Rectus abdominis separation (Fig. 8.11)

Test: Get the client to lie in the supine position if possible, otherwise minimal semi-recumbent. Let her place her legs over a bolster and allow the lumbar curve to flatten. As she breathes out, get her to curl forward and flex her head, neck and shoulders. The therapist can then place four fingers 1 cm below the navel and feel the connective tissue between the two medial borders of the recti muscles. If more than 2.5 fingers fit into the gap then the muscle is considered separated. Repeat this test for the musculature 1 cm above the navel.

Energy assessment tools: shiatsu

Hara assessment

Some therapists use Hara assessment as a prime focus. However, Hara assessment is not as accurate in pregnancy, particularly after the middle of the second

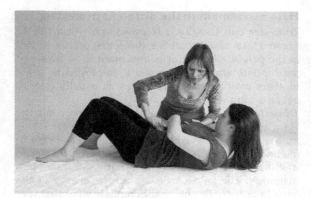

Fig. 8.11 Rectus abdominis muscle separation check.

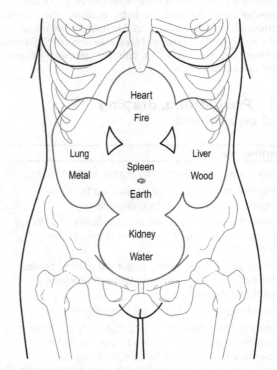

Fig. 8.12 Five element Hara assessment.

trimester. The therapist will need to include back energy assessment (Yu points and organ zones) and rely on other assessment tools.

A modified version of Hara assessment can be carried out using five elements rather than a full organ/meridian (12 area) assessment (Fig. 8.12).

The therapist needs to learn to focus on the assessment areas of the mother while almost ignoring the baby. This becomes increasingly difficult as the pregnancy progresses.

Hara assessment in the different trimesters

Trimester one Usually it is possible to do a full 12 organ Hara assessment, as the fetus/uterus is still in the pelvis, although it is important to be aware of appropriate amount of pressure employed as some mothers may be very sensitive. It is usually easy to get an accurate picture.

Trimester two The fetus begins to move more into the Hara and is at the level of the navel by 23 weeks. This means that the lower Hara diagnostic areas begin to include within them the energy of the fetus. However, it still may be possible to do a fairly accurate Hara diagnosis. The key is to focus on the energy of the fetus in order to be able to differentiate what that specific energy feels like and then shift the focus to the energy of the mother and see what can be picked up.

Trimester three By now the baby is filling the whole abdominal and Hara area, and it is usually not possible to do an accurate 12 organ Hara assessment. Reliance is placed more on the five element assessment and other assessment tools.

8.3 Positioning, draping and equipment

Learning outcomes

After reading this section the reader will be able to:

- Position the client on the floor or the table, depending on their working preference.
- State the advantages and disadvantages of different positioning choices for different stages of the maternity period.
- Make an informed choice about the optimal position for a client during different stages of pregnancy, birth and the postpartum.
- Monitor client comfort level(s) and objective signs.
- Identify client-centred factors that guide positioning choices and show understanding of the fact that clients may not always be able to clearly identify issues regarding maximal comfort, for example with supine hypotension.
- Move the client into and out of different positions and modify or change positions to alleviate discomfort.
- Negotiate draping for the client securely and in a boundary-conscious way when treating her whole body in the side-lying and forward leaning positions.
- Describe which techniques and areas of the body are most suitable to work with in different positions.
- Decide upon the type of equipment they will need for their individual practice.

Introduction

Bodyworkers have differing position and equipment needs for their maternity clients. These depend on whether they work on the floor or on the table, with the client clothed or not clothed, and the types of techniques they use. Current literature on maternity bodywork does not tend to reflect this diverse reality. There are various considerations for each therapist in choosing both the optimal position for a client, how to position them safely and how long to work in each position. Each position has its advantages and disadvantages which we outline. We also give some indications, based on research and our clinical and teaching practice, of how to use each position, including relevant equipment and draping needs. However, ultimately each therapist is responsible for determining the optimal position for each of their own clients.

Equipment

There are many diverse pillows and tables marketed for the bodyworker and their clients. Equipment designed for maternity work ranges from the 'pregnancy beanbag' to the 'pregnancy massage table' to the 'body cushion' and breastfeeding pillows. For the therapist developing their maternity practice the array can be both daunting and costly, especially when the therapist may be unsure which position is the most effective to work. Pregnant women need additional support, but when starting in practice begin with a few simple things such as pillows of varying sizes and a 'physio' (Swiss or gym) ball in order to determine what works best, both from the therapist's and the client's point of view. Equipment can be built up gradually as an understanding of different positions is developed. Specialist systems are not necessary in order to work effectively.

Pillows and support

It is useful to have a range of different shapes and sizes of cushions/pillows. Include square and rectangular-shaped cushions and experiment with rolls and bolsters of different sizes. A helpful addition is to have some cushions which mould to the shape of the woman, especially for breast or abdominal support, such as traditional Japanese buckwheat husk pillows. These give good support and retain their shape, and may be preferable to fillers such as large polystyrene beads and kapok which tend to become compressed with time, thereby losing their shape and support. However, there are newer pillows on the market which are filled with smaller polystyrene beads which tend to mould even more than the traditional pillows without becoming compressed.

Another pillow to consider, which tends to be a little more expensive, is a breastfeeding 'sausage' cushion. This is typically a long roll, or a full-length cushion, which can be placed under the breasts, abdomen and legs when the woman is lying in the side position. This pillow may limit access to the front of the client's body, but it offers good support while working on the back, legs and arms. Other useful cushions include V-shaped breastfeeding pillows, which offer support for the neck and shoulder/chest, but which may also be used between the legs. A triangular wedge is an excellent option in offering effective support in the semi-reclining position if the therapist does not have a massage table with a reclining back. This wedge usually needs building up with other regular pillows to ensure the correct angle and support.

Working on the floor or on a table

Massage therapists tend to work on tables while shiatsu practitioners tend to work more on the floor. Offering the option of floor or table work is an example of being able to provide additional positioning options for the client, but considerations must be made to ensure the therapist is comfortable and utilising their own body effectively and without strain.

It is not difficult to learn to use either option effectively. The majority of strokes and positional guidelines are identical – it is the therapist's body which is positioned differently. If the therapist wants to work with an unfamiliar option further training is recommended to ensure that good body mechanics are maintained.

Working on the floor

Working on a mat on the floor offers the advantage of having space for the therapist to move the woman easily between different positions, without worrying about her falling off the table. The client also has more space in which to lie. Additionally it is an effective position, especially during the last trimester, for helping the woman get used to positions she may use in labour such as leaning over a ball. In the postnatal period it can mean that the woman can lie next to her baby with more space than the table affords. For the mobile therapist, a mat is often lighter and easier to carry than a table.

There are several issues to consider for the therapist who is not used to working on the floor. It can be more draughty and cold than working on a table. For most pregnant women this will not be an issue, as their core body temperature is higher, but it is vital to ensure that the room is warm enough. Also ensure that there is sufficient padding, both for the client and for the therapist's knees. The traditional Japanese method is to have a futon, a cotton mattress, on the floor. This needs to be wide enough to fit both therapist and client. A double size usually works well.

Working on the floor raises issues such as being in closer physical proximity to the client. The therapist needs to be especially careful draping during massage using oils and to respect the client's boundaries. It tends to feel overly invasive to be positioned at the front of the client when working on her head or abdomen, although work to the legs may be acceptable from the front. The majority of the techniques tend to be performed with the therapist positioned at the back of the client's body.

Table issues

The main criteria in table selection is to get a well-made table, which is as wide as possible, in order to provide a sense of security for the pregnant woman's growing body, especially in the side-lying position. This is also relevant if the woman brings the newborn with her postnatally. The table tends to be set at a lower height than when working with clients who may be worked on exclusively in prone or supine. In the side position the superior aspect of the woman's body is higher than in prone or supine. Furthermore, different areas of the client's body are at different heights. The therapist needs to be able to adjust their height at different stages of the treatment. It can help the therapist to have a ball on which to sit while working the spine or head and to have a small stool to rest their foot on for the extra height with arm elevation. If the therapist can afford it, or works in a clinic where there is one, a hydraulic table provides an excellent way of adjusting the height during the treatment itself in order to work different parts of the woman's body.

As prone positioning tends to be considered a less safe positioning option and is not recommended for extensive use in pregnancy, it is unwise to invest in a costly 'pregnancy table' which has a hole cut out in which to place the woman in a prone position. Depending on the client and the type of technique, prone may be appropriate, but in this case, pillowing is usually sufficient.

Working with a chair

Another positioning option is to use a forward leaning massage chair, such as an on-site chair. These vary considerably in their design. The therapist will need to ensure that there is enough space for the pregnant client's abdomen and ideally it should have facilities for adapting the position. Depending on how the legs can be positioned, the chair may or may not be suitable for positioning women with pelvic girdle dysfunction (PGD) or symphysis pubis instability (SPI).

Working with an exercise ball

An exercise ball offers a further positioning option for some clients. The client can sit on it and lean over the table with pillow support, or it can be placed on the floor on a mat or futon so that the client can lean over in the all fours position.

Draping issues

Many therapists use a large single sheet for draping, although some favour towels. In pregnancy the sheet tends to be the most effective form of draping and its use is outlined in more detail under the side and forward leaning positioning sections (below). A single sheet covers the whole body easily, even in the side position where different areas of the client's body are at varying heights. Being light and less bulky than a towel, a sheet is easy to position and re-position, especially when moving or mobilising the limbs. Another advantage of the sheet is that if there are areas the woman is less certain of being worked, especially the abdomen, breasts or buttocks, then initial work can be performed through the sheet. As the client often feels warmer in pregnancy, a sheet may be more comfortable for them than towels or blankets.

Selecting the optimal position for maternity treatment

This can be seen as one of the most creative aspects of working with maternity clients. The position a woman is comfortable in can vary from week to week and the needs of different women also vary significantly. The therapist needs to be adaptable so that they can respond to the changing shape and weight of the woman's pregnant body and meet the varying postnatal recovery needs. Some women like to stay in one or two positions during most of their session, while others need to change position more frequently. The more skill the therapist has in offering different position possibilities for their clients, the more likely it is that the client's comfort needs are met, while the therapist is able to access different areas of the body. The woman's safety must always be the first priority, but comfort must not be neglected. The therapist may find that they suddenly have to change what they are doing, as the woman needs to change her position. Therapists also need to be aware of their own comfort when working in less familiar positions.

There have been to date, in bodywork literature, confusing guidelines on the use of different positions. Obstetric texts and guidelines are not especially detailed on the use of different positions apart from guidelines for exercise. In this chapter we review the advantages and disadvantages of different positions and explore some of the myths which have grown up in the bodywork world around positions to help each therapist make the most informed decision on the most appropriate positioning options for their individual clients.

The only hard facts are the following:

Fact 1. *Supine hypotension (SHS) may be an issue for some women from 16 weeks (see relevant parts in pregnancy theory chapter).*

Fact 2. *If the woman shows signs of suffering from SHS then the way to correct it is to adopt the left lateral position to take pressure off the inferior vena cava.*

Myths

Some of the myths are as follows:

Myth 1. *It is safe to position a pregnant woman in prone with appropriate pillows.* There is no research on the disadvantages of prone positioning as it is not a position which is utilised as part of obstetric or midwifery care. This raises implications for bodyworkers as to how safe it is to position a pregnant woman in a prone position, especially as it is not a position that pregnant women would themselves naturally assume. In considering these issues we conclude, for the reasons outlined under prone (section 8.4 p. 202), that it is a position to be utilised as little as possible during pregnancy.

Myth 2. *Forward leaning positions rotate a fetus into the anterior position from posterior both during the third trimester and in labour.* While this is accepted 'fact' among many midwives, doulas and childbirth educators, it is not clearly substantiated by research.

Myth 3. *The right lateral position should be avoided.* Varying reasons are given for this: it puts undue pressure on the inferior vena cava, encourages right-sided positioning of the fetus, which is less optimal, and impedes placental flow. There is in fact no evidence to validate any of these claims and it does not make sense in terms of body mechanics for a pregnant woman to lie exclusively on one side.

The different position options

The following are common positions that can be used during maternity work, with suggestions for when these positions are most suitable.

1. Prone: most often used for back and neck and for posterior leg massage.
2. Supine: used when massaging arms, legs, abdomen, head, face, neck and shoulders.

3. Semi-lying/or semi-reclining is a useful alterative in maternity work to the fully supine position and can be used when the client is not comfortable supine.

4. Side-lying: used to massage the back, arms, legs, head, neck and shoulders, and abdomen.

5. Forward-leaning: using a bodywork chair with special adaptation for the pregnant abdomen: using pillowing, such as a beanbag or wedges, designed to support the anterior torso and head, neck and shoulders of the pregnant woman or using a birthing ball. This is used for the abdomen, back, neck and shoulders and legs.

6. Sitting; more upright on the ball or chair. This can be used for the neck, head, face and shoulders, arms, abdomen.

Factors affecting positioning choices

It is the responsibility of the therapist to be able to work confidently in the position which is the safest and most effective for the client. Factors affecting the position chosen include:

- Case history information given by the client.
- General health status.
- Health status related to this pregnancy as well as previous pregnancies, including general health and obstetrical history.
- History of musculoskeletal well-being, areas of stress, tension, injury, pain, muscle strain, and/or any overuse or repetitive strain issues.
- Stage of pregnancy, birth or postnatal.
- Client comfort.
- Therapist preference for floor or table.
- Type of technique the therapist will be utilising.

Case history information and health status of the client

This information must always be considered. For example, a client with PGI will need alterations for the side-lying position. A client presenting with a recent caesarean section incision or scar may have difficulty lying in prone or side for the first week or two.

Stage of pregnancy

First trimester The majority of pregnant women in their first trimester (up to 13 weeks gestational age) can lie in prone or supine with comfort and safety as the uterus is still a pelvic organ. In the first trimester breast sensitivity/tenderness or nausea/vomiting may interfere with the client finding comfort in the prone position. The side position can also be an effective option. Forward leaning tends to be less included due to nausea and client sensitivity.

As the pregnancy progresses into the second trimester (14–26 weeks gestational age), and the gravid (pregnant) uterus expands, alterations to positioning must be made for safety and comfort reasons. This is the time when side-lying, semi-reclining, forward leaning and sitting tend to be more appropriate than prone or supine.

Stages of labour

During labour the woman will not be lying prone or fully supine. Side-lying, semi-reclining and forward leaning are all potential options depending on progress of labour and comfort of the woman. Other positions may also be effective such as standing, including leaning forwards and rocking, or standing in more of a squatting position. These additional positions are discussed in more detail in the labour sections (theory and practical) and in the aftercare sections.

Postnatal stages

After birth, the woman may once again lie safely, and usually comfortably, in both prone and supine. She may want to continue using side-lying and sitting positions. Forward leaning may be less appropriate, especially in the early stages, due to pressure on the abdomen, especially after a caesarean section, and issues of client comfort.

Therapist preference and client comfort

While it is important that the therapist feels comfortable working, they should not utilise any position for their own comfort if it is not safe for the client. It is the therapist's responsibility to learn to work with their client in a variety of positions so they can select the most appropriate for each client. We have had reports of pregnant women being told to lie face down in advanced stages of pregnancy because the therapist was not comfortable providing therapy in a side-lying position! We have also had reports from clients who have been placed fully supine for extended periods and have felt dizzy but not informed their therapist because they thought therapists knew what they were doing.

Many women remain in the position they are placed in by the therapist, even if they feel slightly uncomfortable as 'pleasing the therapist' may override their natural instincts. Before beginning any treatment, the client must clearly understand that if they are feeling discomfort in any position they should inform the therapist immediately so that the position can be altered. It may be helpful to ask the client what position they sleep in as this will give some indication of how comfortable they are in the different positions. This client involvement will help to establish a dialogue for effective care and increase the woman's self-awareness.

Cautions for all positions in maternity bodywork

- **Pelvic girdle dysfunction, PGI issues.** If the woman is suffering from PGI or SPL issues, care must be taken in all positions that the bones are not destabilised, either bilaterally or unilaterally.
- **Abdominal comfort.** In all positions care needs to be taken to ensure that the abdomen of the pregnant client is comfortable and not being compressed. Postnatally abdominal comfort is also an issue, particularly for women who have had a caesarean section.
- **Breasts.** Some women have leakage of colostrum or milk during pregnancy and postnatally. Place towels between the breasts and table/floor/ cushions and follow body fluid control guidelines.

8.4 Prone, supine, semi-reclining, side-lying

The prone position

Advantages

- Easy access to structures of the back and posterior of legs.
- Allows maximum use of the therapist's weight for increased depth of pressure.
- With a face cradle the prone position helps the client maintain symmetrical alignment of upper back, shoulders, and neck which provides effective care and assessment in the event of musculoskeletal issues in these areas.
- Client preference: clients who are stomach sleepers may have difficulty resting in other positions due to their preference in sleeping face down. Clients may feel familiar with this position from bodywork received prior to pregnancy.
- The gentle pressure experienced on the abdomen postnatally may support the abdomen and aid postnatal recovery.

Disadvantages

- During the second and third trimesters, as the uterus and baby expand, downward pressure from lying prone creates added stress on the client's body.

- The increased lordotic curve of the pregnant client along with the anterior shift in gravity due to the expanding pregnant belly may create musculoskeletal issues related to the areas of the lower lumbar, gluteal and leg regions. Additional pillows may need to be placed under the shins to minimise lordosis.
- Pressure may be increased on the uterine ligaments.
- The downward weight of the pregnant woman can increase challenges to the uterosacral ligament which helps to stabilise the uterus in relation to the sacrum in the pelvis. This could also potentially manifest as increased sacral discomfort.
- Challenges to SI joint stability may occur in this position. This may increase aggravation to an already irritated SI joint.
- The breasts may feel uncomfortable, even with pillowing, and the woman may feel breathless due to pressure in this area.
- The weight of the therapist as they apply pressure to the lower back area in conjunction with the factors mentioned above present an increased downward force or load on musculature which may already be challenged by the growing pregnant belly.

Considerations in prone

In pregnancy

First trimester. Prone positioning is an option for treatment although the woman may require extra pillowing under the breasts for breast comfort and under the calves to reduce lordosis.

Second and third trimesters. Some bodyworkers do use cushioning systems or tables which allow the pregnant abdomen to rest prone in a hollowed structure during the second and third trimesters. There is insufficient evidence on the safety of prone for bodywork and it seems wise to limit or avoid prone positioning in these trimesters. Some therapists, such as osteopaths or chiropractors, use pillowed prone for specific techniques of limited duration with feedback from the client.

The individual therapist who wishes to treat a pregnant client prone must be responsible to determine the professional safety of their clients, and to express this in their informed consent with the client. When working prone, care needs to be taken with ascertaining depth of pressure in the lumbar and sacral area because this excessive pressure will put strain on the uterine ligaments and excessively pull on the lower back. Deeper work on the upper back is also likely to be uncomfortable because of tenderness of the breasts.

In labour
This is not a position which supports labour and is therefore not utilised.

Postnatally
As in the first trimester, with cushions for the breasts and to reduce lordosis. Care must be taken with those clients who have had a caesarean section to ensure that it does not increase strain on the incision.

The supine position

Advantages
- This position facilitates the possibility for the therapist to work evenly both sides of the body at the same time and is a familiar working position.
- It is an effective position for passive mobilisations of the hips and pelvis and checking pelvic alignment.
- It is especially effective for neck and face work.
- It can be a balanced position for doing breathing and visualisation work.

Disadvantages
- From 16 weeks onwards supine hypotension may be an issue for some women.
- *It increases pressure on the lower back and sacrum.* At any stage some women experience discomfort in these areas. As the fetus increases in size during pregnancy additional stress may be created so often it is not comfortable for the woman to lie supine even with pillows under the knees.
- *Position of the baby.* With the woman supine, the fetal back tends to move towards her back – it assumes the posterior position and has less space. Extended periods of supine, particularly if not balanced by forward leaning, are generally not encouraged during the last trimester as the fetus is settling into position.

Considerations for use
First trimester
Supine can be used if the client is comfortable.

Second and third trimesters
Limit the use of supine and replace it with semi-reclining where possible. If the woman expresses a desire for supine work, the therapist needs to be responsible for ensuring the safety of the client. This means being alert for signs of possible SHS and then immediately repositioning to the left side (SOGC/CSEP 2003).

In labour
Semi-reclining is preferable to full supine because of the additional demands of labour.

Postnatally
Supine can be recommenced although care still needs to be taken with lower back issues. Pillowing under the knees is usually needed to reduce the lordotic curve and ease positional low back discomfort.

Semi-reclining

Advantages
- It has the benefits of the fully supine but is usually much more comfortable for the woman from the second trimester if she is adequately supported.
- It eliminates the concern over SHS issues.

Disadvantages
- *Pressure on the lower back and sacrum.* The increasing size of the baby may cause stress on the bones of the pelvis, although less than fully supine, so that it is important to check that the woman is comfortable in this area and place additional towels if necessary.
- *Position of the baby.* As with fully supine, the fetus tends to move into the OP position. It is therefore important to combine bodywork in supine with bodywork in either side or forward leaning to balance out these effects.
- More suitable on table or when client not moving as can be a little more fussy to move the client and the wedge may move more on the floor.

Considerations for use
- **In all maternity periods**: *Mayes' Midwifery* demonstrates utilisation of the 45° wedge (Fig. 8.13) as valuable for both exercise and relaxation practices (Henderson & Macdonald 2004: 388). Specific to the client receiving bodywork, care should be taken to ensure the woman's posture is not slumped as they lie into the wedge. It is often necessary to place an additional three pillows on top of the wedge to increase comfort. This increases the angle of incline to closer to 60°. As well, the sacrum and lower lumbar region need to be well supported. For some clients with pain in this area, a rolled up towel can be added for lumbar support. The client's neck and head should also be supported so the neck is not in a hyperextended position.
- With adequate support, the client usually feels very comfortable in this position, even if she has low back issues.

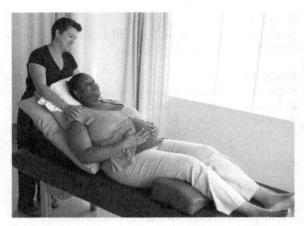

Fig. 8.13 Client lying semi-reclining with wedge cushion.

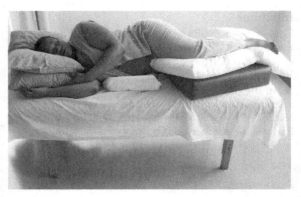

Fig. 8.14 Client in the side-lying position on a table. Cushions under the neck need to be placed at a height that ensures that the neck is in line with the spine. Usually there is a cushion between the breasts or under the upper arm to keep the weight off the lower shoulder and give space in the breast area. If desired, a cushion may be placed under the abdomen to give support. A cushion under the superior leg takes pressure off the abdomen and reduces lateral torsion of the lower back.

- It is particularly effective for work on the face, including sinus draining techniques.
- Since it encourages anterior fetal positioning balance semi-reclining work with work in other positions, especially forward leaning ones.

Side-lying

Advantages

- It is a comfortable and familiar resting position for most women during their pregnancy and many women sleep on their side.
- It is an excellent position for supporting labour.
- It is a position in which many women breastfeed their baby postnatally.
- Left lateral minimises pressure on the inferior vena cava and is used if woman is suffering from supine hypotension.
- Left lateral maximises renal plasma flow.
- There is no pressure on the lower back.
- Virtually the whole body can be treated in this position, except the lateral superior aspect of the inferior leg, inferior hip and side of body, the inferior side of the face and neck.

Disadvantages

- Sometimes, discomfort can occur on the weight-bearing joints, particularly the shoulders and hips, as a result of lying on the side and with the increased weight gain during pregnancy. Appropriate pillowing can reduce these issues considerably.
- The asymmetry of spinal, hip and shoulder positioning and weight-bearing may make

assessment while working more challenging for the therapist.
- Relative contraindications include right leg pitting oedema, right pulmonary dysfunction (e.g. chronic asthma or bronchitis affecting the right lung), venous return insufficiency (e.g. liver congestion or tricuspid valve insufficiency).

Considerations for use

When to use it

With appropriate support and feedback from the client it can be safely used at all stages of pregnancy, birth and the postnatal period. Side-lying should present no increased risk of harm in the majority of pregnant clients unless they disclose particular issues related to lying in this position.

Correct positioning (Fig. 8.14)

Although the side-lying position is essentially beneficial, this is only if the client is appropriately positioned. Key factors to be aware of are:

- *Correct alignment of spine.* Care needs to be taken to ensure that the spine is not in hyperlordosis and that it is in alignment. The neck needs to be supported so that it is on the same level as the rest of the spine. The hips and pelvis need to be aligned with the spine.
- *Musculoskeletal issues relating to shoulder.* The body needs to be aligned, or supported with pillows so that there is not excessive weight placed on

the inferior shoulder as this may cause nerve/circulatory impediment expressed as discomfort, tingling or numbness in the arm. This usually means placing a pillow between the client's breasts on which to place her superior arm. This alleviates pressure on the inferior arm, keeps an openness in the chest and may also provide some support for the thoracic and waist area.

- *Correct alignment of the hip and knee to avoid possible pressure on the uterus.* The knee of the superior leg needs to be positioned alongside the body so that is not placing undue pressure on the uterus and there is no internal rotation of the hips and misalignment of the lower back, and the gluteals and piriformis are relaxed. The exact placement varies for different women:
  - for most women place the inferior leg in extension and bend the superior leg over pillows. The pillow needs to be long enough so that the ankle, foot and knee are all on it to ensure comfort of the knee and to keep the hip aligned. How near to the abdomen the knee is placed, and therefore how flexed the leg is, depends on how much space is required by the abdomen and in creating correct alignment of the lower back.
  - if the woman prefers to have the knees and legs together then a pillow may be carefully placed between the knees to prevent pressure on the abdomen and promote correct alignment of the back.
- *PGI/SPL positioning.* If the woman is suffering from PGI, then care must be taken to position the legs together (knees and inner thighs together) with only a small towel for padding between them.
- *Right side-lying issues.* If the woman is higher risk and there are issues with placental, renal or plasma flow, then left side-lying may be encouraged more than, although not to the exclusion of, right side-lying. Encourage if oedema issues (Monga 1999).
- *Abdominal support.* Some women appreciate a small pillow or baby wedge under the abdomen to relieve pressure. This may also help to minimise any forward twisting of the torso.

Women who have particular difficulty getting comfortable in bed or on the massage table may find an egg-carton mattress helpful for alleviating discomfort. This is utilised in some hospitals for clients on prolonged bed rest.

How to work and techniques which can be performed

It makes sense, if the woman is comfortable, to assess what is going to be worked with the woman lying on one side and complete that work before turning her on to the other side. In terms of assessing which side to begin with there are various factors to consider:

1. *One-sided musculoskeletal issues*: different therapists work differently, but assess which side will be addressed first, the weakened side or compensating side.
2. *Lymphatic work*: if lymphatic techniques to address oedema in the legs are to be utilised, then the left terminal node will need to be stimulated prior to commencing work on the legs. This means that prior bodywork will be concluded with the client lying on their right side.
3. *Comfort of the woman*: the woman may feel more comfortable on one side than the other. Depending on the nature of the work, the therapist may want to begin with either the more or less comfortable side.

Consider that the client may need to change position during work on one side. It may mean that the client may need to be turned a second time to complete work on the first side.

In terms of techniques which can be used, the whole of the client's body can be worked from a combination of work to both the left and right sides. Not everything worked on one side need necessarily be repeated on the second side although the therapist may choose to do so. Some work can only be done on the superior side (side of neck, shoulder, upper arm, side torso, lateral aspect of upper leg), and so if these areas need to be worked on both sides of the body, they will need to be worked from both the left and right sides. Some work can be done from either side (abdomen, back, medial aspects of both legs). The therapist may choose to do them from each side or only from one side, depending on the nature of the issue and the way in which it is being addressed. For example, if there are issues with the back, then it makes sense to work it from both sides as forces of gravity and pressures on the back will be acting differently on both sides. However, if there are no particular issues then more work may be done on the back from one side than the other.

Although some therapists may not be used to working in the side-lying position, it offers an effective way of working with any client, even a non-pregnant one. Many of the techniques described in the practical section are described in the side-lying position. Initially it may feel a little awkward if the therapist is only used to working from prone and supine as different parts of the client's body are at different heights and it may shift while being worked. It is important therefore to keep checking on correct body alignment Some areas can be accessed more effectively from the side position than from prone or supine, namely the shoulder and the gluteal area. The other possibility which side-lying opens up is the direct connection between the front and the back. Holding the abdomen and lower back together is an effective way of connecting with those areas simultaneously and can be used for both energy-based and physical techniques. For example, placing a hand on the lower back while performing effleurage with the other hand on the abdomen can help the woman feel more secure with the abdominal work. Making a link with CV and GV meridians can help the therapist balance the Yin and Yang aspects simultaneously. This two-handed connection is also an effective way of making contact with the fetus from front and back, as it is essentially being held between the therapist's hands.

The arms, shoulder, neck and face

Side-lying is an effective way of working on the shoulder and the chest and exploring the movements of the shoulder girdle of the superior side. It is an excellent position in which to access the scapula for release. Work can be done on the side of the neck, taking care to work at the appropriate depth for the client.

Full range of movement and many different positions for working the superior arm are offered and because of this, it may be a more complete and effective way of working on the arm than supine or prone.

It is not so good for the face as only half the face can be worked from one side.

The legs

It is possible, through appropriate positioning, to work all aspects of the superior leg and all aspects of the inferior leg apart from the lateral aspect of the upper leg. It may feel somewhat disjointed initially to be working mainly on the medial side of the inferior leg rather than being able to work the whole leg effectively from one position. However, provided basic principles of treatment and flow of technique application are ensured, the client will not experience it as disjointed. The upper leg can be mobilised effectively and all aspects may be worked.

The abdomen

Side-lying is not necessarily the position of choice for working the abdomen in the first trimester or postnatally as it may be harder to access than in supine. However, as the abdomen starts to grow, side-lying offers an effective option for work. The side position also offers the possibilities of the connections between the lower back and abdomen, as previously stated.

The back

While side-lying might not appear to be a position of choice for work on the back because the pressure between the two sides may be slightly uneven, work can be effective. For most women, work is usually effective for both sides of the erector spinae, even if work to latissimus dorsi and quadratus lumborum may be less specific on the inferior side. The whole of the sacrum can usually be accessed, although depending on the type of techniques used, the symmetry of a forward leaning position may be optimal for some of the work. However, it is an excellent position for working the gluteals and piriformis of the superior side as the muscles tend to be relaxed and more accessible than with the client prone or forward leaning.

Moving from one area of the body to another

One of the main issues for the therapist, when beginning to work in the side position, is how to ensure a sense of continuity and flow. Long sweeping effleurage strokes can sweep down the back, over the hip and gluteals and down into the legs and include the abdomen. Depending on draping boundaries as outlined in the therapist's scope of practice, some of these may need to be through the sheet. Another possibility is to transition simply by placing a hand on one area and then moving to another area. For example, after work has been completed to the back a hand can be placed on the hip prior to beginning work on the leg. This helps to give a sense of continuity and flow. Another possibility of linking is to use passive movements; these are very effective for relaxing limbs and joints and improving blood flow. These include movements of the arms such as shoulder rotations, hand and arm stretches, leg stretching and rotations, both single and double leg, and foot and ankle rotations and movements. All of these are explained in the practical section.

Turning from one side to the other

On a table

Women who are comfortable rolling on to their back and who have no pelvic instability issues may simply roll to the other side through supine. The therapist should stand on the side they are rolling towards so that the client feels secure and can place their back along the edge of the table. Another option can be to get the woman to roll from her side onto all fours. Work could be done in the forward leaning position (see that position for ideas), usually supporting the client with pillows, before she lies on her other side. Changing position via all fours is a good option for women with PGI as, especially if they keep the supporting towel between their knees, it will ensure stability of the pelvis. Another option can be to get the woman to sit up, swing her legs over the side of the table and then lie down on her other side.

On the floor

As on the table, the client could roll on to her back or go through all fours. On the floor the woman could lean over the ball while the therapist does some work. It is also possible for the therapist to turn the woman by bringing her into supine, using movement of the client's superior leg and shoulder. If the woman is comfortable in supine, the therapist could do some passive movements of both legs before using the other leg and shoulder to turn the client to the other side.

Draping

Side-lying draping can make some bodyworkers and students nervous. With sufficient practice, this can become a quick and easy activity. In some countries draping is more regulated than in others and if standards of practice are not followed then the therapist could face misconduct charges and loss of practice privileges. It is important to ensure that the breasts are covered and that the groin and perineal areas are covered. A very secure draping procedure for groin coverage is outlined below.

Secure side-lying draping

Courtesy of Lisa Ivany,
Atlantic College of Therapeutic Massage

(see also massagetherapy.com)

Have the client covered with a large sheet.

Place pillows under client's head for support.

Place another pillow under her arm for comfort and stability.

Straighten top hip and knee.

Flex bottom hip and knee.

Secure the top sheet at the hip level.

Take the back corner of the top sheet and bring it over the top leg, making sure the sheet undrapes to above the knee.

Bring the same corner underneath the top leg to create a fan which will be used to cover the gluteals.

Bring the top sheet upwards to undrape the greater trochanter and posterior superior iliac spine.

Move the fan under the top sheet and pull the top sheet securely against the gluteals.

Holding the sheets in place, ask the client to flex her top hip and knee and extend the lower hip and knee.

Readjust the draping and securely tuck the top sheet under the lower gluteal area.

Place pillows under the flexed knee for client comfort.

Undraping protocol

Remove pillows from under the knee.

Ask client to extend top hip and knee and flex lower hip and knee.

Untuck top part of sheet and pull it and the fan section down over the gluteals.

Take the bottom part of the sheet and bring it back over the leg.

Another version

Simply pull the lower corner of the sheet from over the inferior leg and pull it up between the two legs, letting the corner rest in front of the client's body. Alternatively pull the upper corner from the front of the body down between the client legs.

For the breasts, especially if arm and shoulder mobilisations are going to be performed, it can be helpful to have a small hand towel to drape over the breasts so that as the arm is moved, the breasts remain covered.

8.5 Forward leaning and sitting (Figs. 8.15–8.17)

Forward leaning

This relates to all forward leaning positions such as:

- Sitting on a stool or ball leaning over a table.
- Sitting in an orthopaedic back care or massage chair leaning forward.
- Kneeling on a table over pillows or the back of the table.
- Kneeling on the floor leaning over a ball or cushion.
- Kneeling forward briefly on hands and knees.

Advantages

- A good position for spinal and pelvic assessment as the body is symmetrically aligned.
- *Supporting optimal fetal positioning*: this may help to encourage cephalic anterior positioning of the baby during the third trimester. It helps to create space in the 'functional maternal cavity' (Averille Morgan, personal communication, 2008) by relaxing the abdomen and ligaments. This

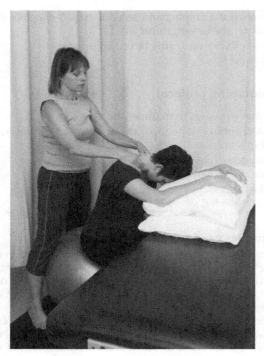

Fig. 8.15 Sitting on a ball and leaning over a table. Cushions on the table provide comfort for the neck and shoulders.

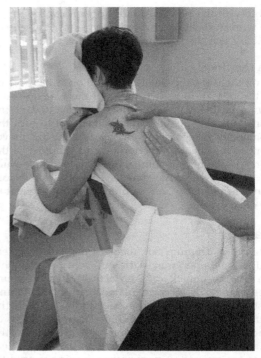

Fig. 8.16 Sitting in an orthopaedic back care or massage chair leaning forward. The chair must be well supported with pillows on the seat and in front.

may help the baby to move, especially from a less optimal position such as breech, oblique or transverse.

- *Relief of pressure on the lower back*: this position tends to offer the most effective relief to the lower back by taking the weight of the baby away from it. If the woman is suffering from sciatica or lower back problems, often simply placing her in the forward leaning position is enough to ease and potentially resolve the problem.

- *Preparation for labour position*: this is an effective position for supporting the physiological process of labour, so it is helpful to encourage the woman to feel comfortable in it. It can also be used to teach labour support techniques to the partner or labour support provider/doula.

- *Relief from pressures on the pelvis during the treatment*: it is a good transition position between work on the two sides. It offers some time when there is no pressure on the hips and pelvis and circulation is facilitated in the pelvic area. The client can even be encouraged to rock and move her pelvis to provide additional relief and movement before lying on the second side.

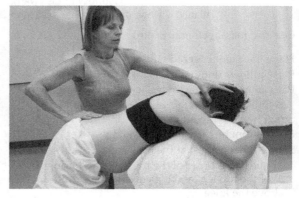

Fig. 8.17 Kneeling on the floor leaning over a ball. The woman should not sit back with knees apart if she has symphysis pubis instability (SPI). Support is needed for breasts and knees, the abdomen should not lean directly over the ball, and only the areas of the back which are supported should be worked on deeply.

- *Good working position for women with PGI/SPI*: if the woman is suffering from PGI, she can rest in this position quite safely. It is a good position to encourage her to become more aware of her abdominal and pelvic floor muscles. Her knees do not need necessarily to be completely together, although they must not be further apart than hip width. It offers an option for working the medial side of the leg with this client group; this would not be possible in the side position as women need to keep their knees adducted in side-lying.

- *Possibility for deep sacral work*: it offers the possibility for effective deep sacral work and is a valuable position for this type of work in the third trimester. Pressure on the sacrum does not involve compression of the uterus or ligaments, as it would in prone. Deep sacral work is often the type of work that the woman enjoys during labour.
- *Possibility for abdominal relaxation and work*: this position can be effective for work which involves the baby. As the abdominal muscles are engaged but also relaxed, it is an effective way of working the abdomen. It also offers the possibility of working symmetrically around the abdomen as the whole abdomen can be accessed more readily than from the side position.
- *Comfort for the woman*: once the woman has tried out this position, she often finds it the most comfortable position to be in during her last trimester. She can even move and rock her hips and change position if she needs to if she is using the ball.

Disadvantages

- Some knee issues may become aggravated in the all fours version.
- If there is excessive separation of the rectus abdominis muscles (more than four finger widths) it may place too much strain on the abdomen.
- If there are issues with caesarean section incisions/scars it may create too much downward pressure.
- For women suffering from nausea or blocked sinuses it may not be very comfortable due to the forward movement.

Considerations for using forward leaning

It tends to be used during:

- **Second and third trimester**. It tends to be used more in the second and especially the third trimester as the fetus grows in size and puts more pressure on the sacrum, and during the third trimester as the fetus begins to settle into the position for labour.
- **Labour**. It can be used extensively for birth preparation and work during labour itself.

It is less used during:

- **First trimester**. It is less used here because it may aggravate nausea and sinus congestion. Furthermore there is no pressure from the fetus on the sacrum or abdomen to relieve through the position nor are the deep sacral and abdominal techniques indicated. Due to the subtle changes going on in the pelvis and uterus, if the woman is not used to this position she is less likely to feel comfortable.
- **Early postnatal period**. It is less used because there is no longer the weight of the fetus to relieve. Further, the relative weakness of the pelvic area and abdomen post birth and potential caesarean section issues tend to indicate less use of a position where these muscles are engaged. The types of techniques utilised are less likely to include deeper techniques on opening the sacrum and pelvic area and it is not likely to be a restful position for the woman.

How to ensure correct positioning

It is only a safe and effective position if the following key factors are observed:

Care not to aggravate carpal tunnel syndrome

Care must be taken not to position the woman in such a way that she is taking her body weight on her wrists. She needs to ensure that she is leaning on her forearms over the ball, beanbag or pillows or when resting without support.

Care that the back does not go into hyperlordosis

Care must be taken to ensure that the back does not go into hyperlordosis because the weight of the baby could put too much downward pressure on the lumbar vertabrae. Encourage the woman to move around a little to find the best position, especially over the ball. For some women this may involve leaning more over the ball, while for others it could involve sitting back on the heels.

Using a ball

A ball is often a good way to support this position as it is soft. It will need to be the correct size, usually about 65 cm but it could be slightly larger or smaller depending on the woman. Ensure that the ball is not too inflated but has a little give. It will be slightly less deflated than when used in the gym but it must not be too deflated or it will give too much. The ball needs to be used on the floor. Place a towel over the ball to make it more comfortable. Extra pillows may also be placed on top of the ball. Place a soft cushion in front of the ball to stop it rolling, or buy a ball with sand already in it, which stabilises it.

The woman should not sit back with knees apart if she has PGI.

Support is needed for breasts and knees, the abdomen is not leaning directly over the ball and only areas of the back which are supported can be worked on deeply.

How to work and techniques which can be performed

This position often becomes the favourite for many women in the last trimester, as it creates so much relief for the lower back and space for the baby. It is a very versatile position and can have many different versions. If the woman is not comfortable with one version, she is often comfortable with another. It tends to be used for only part of the treatment, unlike the side which could potentially be used for the whole treatment.

It can be used at the beginning of the treatment. Some therapists, even if they work with oils, encourage the woman to lean fully clothed over the ball and do some exercises. They then do some bodywork through the clothes before the woman undresses and lies down on the table or the floor. Other therapists like to use it as a transition between the two sides or as a position with which to end the treatment.

Some women may only be comfortable for a few minutes, while others may be comfortable for up to half an hour, although probably no longer. When it is used in labour, women will be moving around much more than during a treatment and will tend to have short breaks from it by standing up or walking around.

It is an effective position for:

- Deep work on the sacrum: but it depends on the support for the rest of the back how deeply you can work other areas of the back. Any areas where the back does not have support need to be worked quite lightly.
- Working the neck and the top of the shoulders.
- Working the abdomen.
- Working the posterior aspects of the whole of both legs and the medial aspects of both upper legs.
- Working the lower arm and hand.

Depending on how the woman is supported it may or may not be effective for working the proximal aspect of the arms and back of the shoulder.

It is not such an effective position in which to work the anterior of the legs, chest or face.

Draping

A large towel is draped over the upper body. This can either be tucked around the woman or is draped to reach the table or the floor. A large sheet can then be placed over the towel and draped over the rest of the body. When the therapist wants to work the upper back they can tuck the sheet at the level of the woman's hips and fold the towel to the top of her upper back, allowing the draping to come down to the floor. When they want to work the abdomen, they can reposition the towel. When they want to work the legs they can tuck the sheet to the front of the body.

Sitting

Issues related to sitting position

This is similar to what has been described above in forward leaning but the woman is sitting in a more upright position, either on the floor or on a chair or ball, rather than forward leaning.

Advantages

- Good position for accessing neck and shoulders.
- Good position for accessing face.
- Can work the abdomen and back.
- If sitting on ball can move around a little and get relief from hip tension/congestion.

Cautions

- PGI/SPI – legs should never be more than hip width apart.
- If on static surface such as floor or chair, as opposed to the ball, pay attention to comfort of the pelvis.

Considerations for use

When to use

As this position does not include the forward leaning component, then it may be used in the first trimester and postnatally. From the second and third trimesters of pregnancy, due to fetal pressures and position, ensure that the ball is the right height, so that the client's knees are slightly lower than her hips.

Often in the maternity period a ball is used rather than a massage chair as it can provide a softer surface for the sacrum and coccyx and, depending on the type of chair, it may offer more possibilities for position alteration.

Types of strokes possible in this position

It may be an effective position for working the face and neck and upper part of shoulder in late pregnancy. Work can also be done for the back and especially the sacrum. Abdominal work and arm mobilisations can be performed. It is not so effective for work with the legs.

A final word

Each therapist has a different way of working and each woman presents with different needs. The possibilities of utilising the different positions as part of maternity work have many variations and we encourage each therapist to explore fully the options and limitations of each position in order to create effective options for their clients. One of the most important aspects rather than rigidly work with only one or two positions is to use a range of positions during bodywork and to encourage the client to continue to use them herself. This will both help with her comfort and encourage optimal fetal positioning and labour preparation.

Fetal rotation anterior can be promoted by maternal positions which generate a co-ordinated softening and support of the fetal presenting part. So it makes sense that women move through various postures, particularly from 36 weeks on, to support the co-ordinated muscular and ligamentous softening. Standing forward flexion movements are best if co-ordinated with flexed knees, externally rotated hips and relaxed abdominal muscles. Forward flexion over the bed with knees bent and lower back softened into the lumbar lordosis improves the synchronised movements of the abdominal diaphragm and pelvic floor muscles, and with a broad pelvic brim the anterior occiput presentation will be enhanced.

(Averille Morgan, personal communication, 2008)

As I work with both shiatsu and massage, and some of my clients come to me for a mix of the two, I tend to work more on the floor. Further, for 12 years I taught antenatal and postnatal exercise classes in Bristol and so I was used to working with clients moving around. I was also influenced, as many of us were at the time in the early 1990s, by the work of Jean Sutton and optimal fetal positioning. It made sense to me and still does, although I am always careful not to be overly rigid in focusing on the negative aspects of babies in the OP position, but on the positive aspects of the forward leaning position as a counter to the sedentary positions which many of my clients were in for large parts of the day due to their work. Certainly from my own practice I have observed from incorporating forward leaning into daily life and activity as well as into my bodywork treatments, women have reported a number of benefits. These include decreased back pain, more comfort in the pelvis, more confidence in their bodies, more awareness of their baby, not just physically but emotionally, empowerment in the process of labour and, for the most part, much more enjoyable labours than previous ones. I think this is an example of something which may not have an RCT to validate it yet, but makes sense in terms of both anatomy and 'common sense'.

For the majority of my third trimester clients I will begin with a section over the ball. Then they often want to lie down

on their side. Of course, if they are not comfortable on the ball, or just want to lie on their side, I don't rigidly include the ball as part of the session. If they are comfortable lying supine briefly, I may do a few gentle mobilisations as a transition movement between the sides, or I may do some more ball work, or I may simply get them to roll to the other side themselves, dependent on their needs and presenting issues. Again with supine positioning, I find that clients are very clear if it is a suitable position for them or not. Most women are not comfortable for most of the third trimester supine, but some are. Most clients I find are comfortable for the majority of the second trimester and so I do tend to use it then. I never work with them for very long – never more than 10 minutes and usually only 5 – always monitor their responses and actually tend to do more gentle mobilisations and stretches, so they are not statically supine.

With my postnatal clients, I tend to use the side-lying position if they bring their newborn with them as that way they can feed the baby or rest next to them and I can still continue with the work. I am often surprised how many women find it difficult to relax while they are feeding and so my work may include specific relaxation focus while they are feeding. I am always open to new possibilities and encourage my clients to show me how they feel comfortable. I have lots of different size cushions and feel it is worth spending the time to ensure that they are comfortable before I start working with them.

Positioning is one of the aspects I enjoy about my maternity work. I never quite know what I am going to do, or how the client is going to feel each week, and I truly have to be present in each moment with her.

(Suzanne Yates)

8.6 Definitions of techniques included in bodywork sections

A basic description of common techniques used is included in this section to help inform the reader about technique applications for the various maternity issues and stages. For further clarification on these strokes, in depth practical training should be undertaken alongside additional reading. (See the further reading and references section.)

Effleurage (Swedish massage), saka (shiatsu)

Swedish massage

Effleurage comes from the French verb *'effleurer'*, to stroke. Some authors refer to it as stroking or gliding (Cassar 1999, Loving 1999, Tappan & Benjamin 1998) while others describe stroking and effleurage as two different manipulations (Hollis 1998, Rattray & Ludwig 2000).

It can be varied in terms of: *pressure* (superficial to deep) and *direction* (longitudinal or transverse to the muscle fibres).

Longitudinal and superficial strokes are often used at the beginning of the treatment to spread oil, warm up the tissue, as an introductory technique of connection, and to make an initial assessment through palpation. These strokes tend to be performed with a wide palm and cover a broad area.

More pressure is generally applied with the long upward stroke toward the heart (when treating a limb) and a lighter pressure on the return stroke (Andrade & Clifford 2001, Beard & Wood 1964, Kellog 1895, Palmer 1912). This is in part due to a belief among some authors that structural damage may occur to the valves within the veins if effleurage is applied in a centrifugal direction (Tappan & Benjamin 1998). However, there is no evidence to substantiate this claim and it is generally considered safe to stroke down a limb with pressure which is comfortable for the client.

To apply deeper effleurage strokes, more pressure is applied, such as reinforcing the contact by putting one hand on top of the other, using fists or forearms, or using one's body weight to increase the strength of the technique while maintaining a broad contact.

These strokes should be applied repeatedly and rhythmically as this is an important aspect of the application. The therapist proceeds systematically across the specific part of the body, concentrating on any areas which feel harder, tighter or more tense.

The primary effects of these strokes are to promote circulation and identify areas of tension within the soft tissue.

Transverse superficial strokes. Transverse strokes are applied with a focus to loosen and separate muscle fibres by working across them.

With legs, transverse strokes can be applied by grasping around the belly of a muscle and drawing the tissues towards the thumb.

Longitudinal and transverse deep strokes. Smaller points of the hand can be used such as the pad of the thumb, fingers or elbow to focus the pressure deeper into the tissue. They are effective for working on deep lesions and should be performed slowly.

- Transverse strokes will stretch the connective tissue between the muscle fibres.
- Longitudinal strokes will stretch and realign the muscles.

These strokes stimulate local circulation.

Shiatsu

Stroking – saka – is performed usually in the direction of classical energy meridian flow. Faster and more superficial strokes are considered to be more sedating (for areas of where there is more or excess energy). Slower and deeper strokes are considered to be more tonifiying (for areas of less or depleted energy).

Petrissage/kneading (Swedish massage) – kenbiki (shiatsu)
Swedish massage

Petrissage comes from the French verb '*petrir*', to knead. One or both hands work in a smooth rhythmical way to grasp, squeeze, compress and lift the tissue. As one hand releases its grip, the other takes up a grip adjacent to it. It is much like kneading dough (Salvo 2003).

Petrissage may stimulate local circulation, loosens and softens tissue, and has a warming effect. It may be useful in situations of muscle contracture or soft tissue adhesions (Liston 1995). If the muscle tissue is tense due to minor injury or fatigue it may be uncomfortable, so effleurage should be applied before attempting petrissage in order to help prepare the tissue for this more intense application.

Squeezing

This can be done through the clothing or the sheet, or directly on the tissue.

Shiatsu

Usually used with more of a focus on releasing areas of contracted muscular tension. It is also used to release 'Jitsu' full areas.

Friction
Swedish massage

The term *friction* comes from the Latin '*fricto*', meaning 'to rub'. This is the deepest technique and is targeted at specific areas of soft tissue injury, such as scar tissue and adhesions. It is a specific, repetitive, non-gliding technique where superficial tissues are moved over the underlying structures.

The digit or elbow is used in a similar way to deep effleurage, but greater pressure is applied. It is applied more lightly initially until sufficient depth has been achieved to locate adhesions, after which deeper frictions are applied. A rotation or short rocking movement can be included.

The depth at which the friction is applied can change, with an angle of 90° being the deepest. Sensitivity is needed to get maximum pressure without causing pain. Frictions are powerful and can create inflammation or tissue damage if used too forcibly. They should never be used in acute conditions.

Usually, before applying friction the area is warmed up and prepared with effleurage or static holding. After an area has been treated with deep friction it is stretched either with superficial or deep longitudinal strokes and/or with passive functional stretches and/or hydrotherapy applications.

Frictions can improve mobility, increase local blood flow and decrease pain (Tuchtan & Stelfox 2005).

Shiatsu

Digit or elbow pressure is sometimes used with rocking as preparation or release for the more typical holding pressures of shiatsu work. Typically used in Jitsu areas.

Other

Friction is often used in neuromuscular (NM) techniques.

Percussion/tapotement

Tapotement is derived from the French verb '*tapoter*', to tap. This is a firm, repetitive, rhythmical striking manipulation of the superficial and deep tissues followed by a quick rebound. Percussion techniques use alternate hand striking which is performed using a loose wrist.

There are different types of tapotement techniques. They are (in order of strength, from deepest to lightest):

- Pummelling/beating: this is carried out with palmar surface of loosely held fists.
- Shearing: this is not strictly a percussion technique but involves rapid movement and has similar effect. The belly of the muscle is grasped with the hands close together. The open hand makes a sudden thrust, pulling tissues away, while the other pulls them back.
- Cupping: the hands form a cup so that a pocket of air is trapped against the skin as the hand strikes. This creates a deep but soft percussion effect and should make a hollow sound.
- Hacking: the ulnar border of the hand is used with the wrist held loosely. This can be light or slightly deeper.
- Plucking/pincement: this is also a light and springy technique where the superficial tissues are picked up between the thumb and first two fingers. The fingers and thumb glide over the tissue until they come together. It is rapid, gentle, and rhythmic.
- Tapping: this is the lightest tapotement technique and is applied with slightly bent fingers, allowing the fingertips to tap the tissue. It can be used on delicate and sensitive areas of the body.

All these techniques are stimulating and are less appropriate if relaxation is considered the primary goal. They can be used to awaken a client at the end of the treatment. They may help with some nerve conditions such as multiple sclerosis, and can help stimulate muscles and nerves after a period of immobilisation.

When applied slowly and lightly they may be more relaxing and can be used to release muscle spasm. They are locally contraindicated during early stages of injury repair as it may further damage the tissue or affect the formation of scar tissue (De Domenico & Wood 1997).

Rocking and shaking

In *rocking* a firm and gentle pressure is applied to any part of the body which is then rocked. The therapist should tune into the rocking rhythm which feels appropriate to the client, which may be slow or fast in nature. Slower rocking can bring about a deep sense of relaxation. It can be a good way of starting or finishing the treatment and can be used at the same time as deep friction to encourage relaxation.

A more vigorous *shaking* can be carried out on one limb by grasping at the ankle or wrist and raising the limb along with applying mild traction. The whole limb can be shaken with varying degree of vigour. It can relax muscles and help to mobilise joints.

Breathing

More information on specific breathing in the maternity period is given in the aftercare section 12.2 p. 340. Breathing is an important technique for increasing relaxation.

Lymph drainage techniques

These techniques are light in pressure and are applied just below the surface level of the skin and superficial to the veins. The pressure is applied in one direction only, towards the lymph nodes. The stroke tempo is slow. There are specific sequences that have been developed for each area of the body. It can be taught as a complete therapeutic system in itself but bodyworkers can work to address movement of lymph by applying knowledge of the basic principles.

Static pressure and holds

These techniques include golgi tendon release, origin and insertion, myofascial trigger point release, pressure points, energy holds. They are one of the main technique applications which characterise the shiatsu approach. Pressure is applied at tsubos (points) along meridians.

Holds can be performed lightly or deeply with a goal to relax, to make contact, or to integrate work.

Stretches/passive movements/ joint mobilisations

These include shaking, rocking, tractioning, rhythmic mobilisations, recoil, joint play, muscle energy and counterstrain. They can be used with a focus on mobilising joints, stretching and working muscles, and allowing energy to flow through meridians.

Fasical techniques and soft tissue release

Soft tissue release is in fact a hybrid of techniques including:

- Friction and stretching.
- Pressure techniques.
- Skin rolling, crossed hands, fascial stretch, fascial spreading, cutting, torquing.
- Stretches and mobilisations.
- Strain/counterstrain.
- Connective tissue massage and manipulation.
- Neuromuscular therapy.
- Visceral manipulation.
- Craniosacral therapy.
- Myofascial – pressure at the level of the fascia.

Neuromuscular technique (NMT)

This is an extension of deep friction and pressure techniques (Schneider et al 1988). In trauma there is an increase in local muscle tension around the damaged area due to a response in the peripheral nervous system as part of the initial healing process. However, if this continues for a period of time, the nervous system becomes used to holding this degree of tension and accepts it as 'normal'. This can remain even if the initial trauma has recovered.

The aim of this work is to consciously focus the client's mind on relaxing into the pain. The nervous system suppresses its normal reflex. After a period of time (up to 90 seconds) the tension in the local tissues releases and the pain diminishes as relaxation occurs.

Muscle energy techniques (MET)

This is a collective name for a variety of techniques that stretch, strengthen or break down fibrous adhesions. It is one in which the patient's own effort and movement, rather than that of the therapist, provides the primary focus. It works well on muscles that are excessively tight, but cannot be used to achieve hyperflexibility. It involves using the period of relaxation following isometric contraction to increase the passive stretch in tissues.

8.7 Eastern bodywork concepts

While still retaining an awareness of achieving muscular relaxation, a connection can be made with other energies in the body. Some of these relate to physical organs but they can relate to thoughts and feelings, as well as the more 'spiritual' aspects of a person. This can be an important element to bring to work maternity, as not only is the mother going through

quite profound physical and emotional changes, but work is being done with two people, the baby as well as the mother. It may enhance the work to include an energetic as well as physical awareness of the baby and to encourage the mother and the father to relate to the baby, emotionally as well as physically, if this seems appropriate.

This type of approach can be included before, after or at the same time as applying more muscular-focused techniques.

How is energy felt?

More and more massage therapists who have not specifically studied shiatsu may have some training in a variety of modalities that primarily address an energy-based approach such as reiki, craniosacral work, polarity, touch for health, kinesiology and 'spiritual healing'. Individual therapists relate to energy in a variety of ways. Some 'see' energy, even as specifically being able to see meridian pathways or specific visual images. Others 'feel' sensations which may be hard to describe. Other therapists intuit emotions.

Typical sensations experienced when working with energy include sensing:

- Hot/cold.
- Movement/waves.
- Tingling/buzzing.
- Physical feelings of sinking into or being pushed away.

One of the main concepts used in shiatsu and other eastern traditions is the idea of 'excessive' and 'deficient' or 'depleted' energy patterns.

Key concepts of working in shiatsu: full and empty energy patterns

The underlying idea is that there is one energy in the body which can become blocked, so that in some places there can be too much and in other areas too little. The aim of bodywork is to facilitate the flow of energy. These concepts are all relative as the flow of energy is ever-changing and never static and varies according to age, stage of life, time of day, season and so on. This energy moves in pathways known as 'meridians' and powerful points along these pathways are called 'tsubos'.

Kyo/Jitsu (Table 8.2)

In terms of feeling the energy of the meridians or tsubos it can be either 'Kyo' or 'Jitsu'. These concepts are similar to Yin and Yang, but refer to unhealthy expressions of energy:

Table 8.2 Comparison between characteristics of Kyo and Jitsu

Kyo	Jitsu
Empty	Full
Expansion	Contraction
Loose	Tight
Deep	Surface
Slow	Fast
Cold	Hot
Yielding	Resisting
Weak	Strong
Soft	Hard
Depleted	Energetic
Receptive	Repellent
Drawing in	Pushing away

Table 8.3 Ways of working with Kyo and Jitsu – tonification and dispersion

Tonifying techniques for Kyo	Sedating/ dispersing techniques for Jitsu
Hold for longer – generally more emphasis on holding techniques	Hold for less – generally more emphasis on movement and stretches
Use soft parts of your body, e.g. palm	Use sharper parts of your body, e.g. elbow
Use slow stroking techniques	Use faster stroking techniques
Work more slowly	Work more quickly
Work with aim to bring energy towards	Work with aim of moving energy away

- Kyo is the condition of *depleted energy*, which is more *hypo*.
- Jitsu is the condition of *excess energy*, which is more *hyper*.

This can be illustrated by thinking of a round ball representing a healthy person. Now think of a distorted ball with indentations and protrusions marring its circumference. The indentations which are hollow and below the surface are the areas of Kyo. The protrusions are Jitsu. It is easier usually to spot the Jitsu areas because they project from the surface, but it is much more difficult to find the Kyo areas which are the cause of the problem, as they are more hidden. This condition of distortion is relative to the healing power and constitution of each individual.

The techniques used to normalise Jitsu points are called *sedation* and those to normalise Kyo areas, *tonification*. In shiatsu often the Kyo is tonified before the Jitsu is sedated. With sedation the Jitsu area is stimulated with short, sharp, fast strokes and possibly stretches, and the protrusion will normalise. The hollow areas of Kyo require patiently holding shiatsu, using long, slow, soft strokes. This takes more time because warmth must reach deep inside to nurture, strengthen and normalise the area. By building up the Kyo areas first, the Jitsu areas often soften before doing any work directly on them. This expresses the idea that all energy is interconnected – working on any area in the body has an effect on the whole of the rest of the body.

Work to balance Kyo and Jitsu
See Table 8.3.

Other key principles of shiatsu
Two-handed technique
One of the key features of working with shiatsu, which is slightly different from working with massage, is the technique of working with two hands following the Kyo-Jitsu principle. One hand is assuming the supportive or Yin role and the other hand the active or Yang role. By working with these two different energies at the same time, we can promote balance in the body. The supportive or Yin hand is important as it provides the penetrating support needed to prepare the body for treatment. Without this connection, the manipulation with the hand in motion (Yang) tends to remain superficial and often painful.

Perpendicular pressure
The way that pressure is given is by using different parts of the body, most commonly the palm of the hand, but also thumbs, elbows and knees. The pressure comes from the whole weight of the body being behind the part that is actually touching the body. In shiatsu, as in massage, the body weight needs to be applied through moving the abdomen and keeping the shoulders and arms relaxed. If this is not done, then the therapist may get sore thumbs and wrists and become easily tired. The pressure does not feel as comforting or penetrating for the client. The abdomen is known as the Hara and is seen as the energetic centre of the body. The person giving the shiatsu

ideally should be as relaxed as the person receiving because their own energy is flowing well.

Be relaxed

One of the most important principles is that there is an inter-relationship between the giver and the receiver. The way that the therapist feels when giving shiatsu can be transmitted to the client. If the therapist is feeling tense and uncomfortable, the work they do is often experienced by the client in a similar way. If the therapist is holding their breath, so too may the client. If the therapist's energy is not flowing, then the client's energy may not flow so well.

Another aspect of being relaxed is that, in essence, shiatsu is about 'doing nothing'. This expresses the idea that no effort should be involved, rather it is simply connecting with the client's energy and allowing change to happen. Sometimes this happens easily, sometimes not as easily, but it is the client's energy which ultimately decides to change. The therapist cannot make change happen. In doing shiatsu the therapist is merely acting as a facilitator of change within the client's energy field. Nothing is 'done to the client' as such. In this sense it is different from pharmacological treatments, for example. Shiatsu is about working with the energy which is there and in this sense is very safe, as change is limited to what the body can produce and process.

Work from the Hara

Shiatsu has its roots in the eastern traditions of bodywork, which means that it shares similarities with eastern martial arts. The emphasis in all of these, such as tai chi, chi qung and karate, is that the centre of the body, the centre of being, is the Hara. The Hara covers the area from above the pubic bone, round the side of the body, defined by the anterior iliac spines, to under the rib cage. In some traditions there is a more specific focus on points. An important point is CV4, three thumb-widths below the navel, sometimes known as the Tan Dian.

The way to cultivate awareness of coming from the Hara is by breathing exercises and by movements which encourage the body to move from here. The out-breath is the Yin breath – the breath of letting go, the breath of relaxation. Modern cultures tend to emphasise the in-breath – the Yang aspect of the breath. The in-breath is about taking on new things, drawing things towards us. It is helpful to emphasise the out-breath as this is the aspect of the breath most of us find more difficult to connect with.

When working with shiatsu, it is important to be aware of the breathing of the client. Often simply placing a hand on someone else and being aware of their out-breath helps them relax and is shiatsu at its simplest level. The Japanese called this 'te ate', which literally means putting a hand on the pain to heal and

it is a term often used in nursing practice. An experienced therapist can tune in to the best place on the body to place the hand, how long to hold it there and how much pressure to give.

Summary of basic principles for energy work

- Be relaxed while doing shiatsu.
- Centre attention on the Hara (abdomen) and work from here.
- Work with penetrating perpendicular pressure not physical pressure.
- Work to balance Kyo and Jitsu – empty and full patterns.
- Use two hands – mother hand, working hand principle.
- Work with continuity and flow.

8.8 The selection of the base; oil/lotions/wax and the use of essential oils in maternity care; aromatherapy

With contributions from Fiona Mazurka and Jan Caruana, and from Rhiannon Harris (aromatherapy)

Learning outcomes

- To be able to describe the types of oils/lotions which are appropriate to use with the maternity client
- To be able to discuss the issues relating to aromatherapy

Working through the clothes or using oils

While there seems to have developed a convention for massage to use oil and shiatsu to work through the clothes, this does not have to be adhered to. Although many shiatsu schools in the east and west teach shiatsu through the clothes, some schools do use oils. Shiatsu derived from *tuina* and *ampuku*, which often use oil-based techniques. Many massage techniques can be done through the sheet or even clothes. Apart from deeper kneading and long gliding effleurage, most strokes adapt well. In labour work some women want to keep their clothes on and it is useful for therapists to be versatile in their approach.

Use of oils and lotions

Key issues in selection of oils/lotions for the base

The selection of the bodywork medium varies considerably from country to country. In some countries wax is used, often beeswax, and in other countries oils, sometimes nut-based. In other countries, the use of creams and lotions has taken over from oils to address potential allergy issues. Some of these lotions are made of natural products. It is important to select lotions which are not made of mineral oils as these petroleum-based products are not beneficial for the skin and may deplete it of vitamin D. It is also important to select lotions which do not contain perfumes.

With the increasing incidence and awareness of potential nut allergies, many therapists have changed to non-nut-based mediums, especially in some countries. In these countries, sunflower, canola, jojoba or apricot oil are suggested as alternatives. This seems a shame since many of the nut oils have beneficial qualities. Jan Kusmirek (2002) lists five nut oils in his top 12 vegetable oils: hazelnut, kukui, macadamia, sweet almond and walnut. He suggests using walnut for general massage mixed with 30% sweet almond and 20% hazelnut. Research on the use of nut oils is not conclusive and allergies are usually more linked to peanuts; however, some therapists may prefer not to use nut oils.

It is possible that the allergy may be caused by the processing of the nut oil. Many therapists use inexpensive oils which are often highly processed. As the oil penetrates the skin then it makes sense to use the best-quality and least-processed oils, keeping to principles such as organic, cold pressed and virgin where possible. Always patch test a small amount on the inside of the client's wrist for 24 hours to rule out any allergic reactions.

Oils which many therapists do find helpful in the maternity period to nourish the changing skin are wheatgerm oil or evening primrose oil, which are high in vitamin E content and can be mixed in a ratio of 1:3 with another vegetable base oil. Wheatgerm oil is rich in essential fatty acids and has the highest content of vitamin E of any of the plant oils, and so will be effective in nourishing the skin and helping protect against stretch marks. Rosehip seed oil has become popular over the last few years for the prevention and treatment of stretch marks, and for its wound-healing abilities (and wrinkle prevention). It has high levels of the essential fatty acids including omega 3 and 6, as well as vitamin C and, unusually for a plant, vitamin A. Wheatgerm and rosehip seed oils can be combined. Another oil almost as rich in vitamin E as wheatgerm oil, with less of an odour, is soya bean oil.

Other therapists find that beeswaxes are a good medium to use, especially if working on the floor, as there is no risk of spillage. Often the beeswax is mixed with olive oil or arnica or vitamin E as in the Tui basic blend which is often used in Australia and New Zealand. Butters such as cocoa butter (*Theobroma cacao*), which is a vegetable butter extracted from the cocoa bean, and shea butter (*Vitellaria paradoxa*) which is a fat extracted from the fruit of this tree, are both solid in texture and very moisturising and emollient (protective). They both have a long history of use in cosmetics and can be applied directly to the skin and they will melt at skin temperature. Coconut oil is another wonderful product that in its organic cold pressed state is solid at room temperature but will melt as it is applied to the skin. It is also rich in essential fatty acids.

All these oils may help minimise stretch marks on the abdomen, although remember that stretch marks are the result of over-stretching of the skin and ultimately dependent on the woman's weight gain as well as her basic skin structure, which is genetically determined. It is therefore important not to claim that these oils 'will reduce stretch marks'. The woman may also want to use them to nourish the skin of the perineum to help it stretch during the birth.

In labour, it is best to keep to the same oils used during pregnancy. Postnatally in Japan, white sesame oil was used for shiatsu on the breasts, which was done directly on the skin.

For perineal massage

Any of the above oils can be used to massage the tissues of the perineum but it is probably best to use a rich oil that penetrates the skin a little more slowly such as wheatgerm. Jojoba seed oil (*Simmondsia chinensis*) can also be used. This oil differs from other plant oils in that it is a wax that is harvested from the seeds. It has been used to replace whale oil (since that was banned) as it is an oil that most closely resembles human sebum.

For healing perineal tears and episiotomies

A sitz bath of salt water can be done twice a day, followed by an application of calendula-infused oil. Oils rich in vitamin E and essential fatty acids can also be used.

For healing caesarean scars

As above, calendula-infused oil will help the area heal at a much more rapid rate. After the stitches have dissolved and the area is healing nicely, continue to use oils and butters to feed and nourish the tissue to help the scar tissue heal well.

The primary role of aromatherapy in maternity care

Rhiannon Harris

Without doubt, the main role of aromatherapy in maternity care provision is that of stress reduction, with its multiple benefits to both mother and child. Other advantages, such as helping the mother to physically adapt to her pregnant state and dealing with minor problems as they arise, are secondary to stress management with essential oils.

Any measure that helps reduce anxiety levels will have a positive impact on both mother and child. Aromatherapy excels in the domain of stress management; however, its inclusion in maternity care requires specialised training in the safe and effective use of essential oils. This overview highlights key areas and is provided only as general guidance to the massage practitioner wishing to further their studies and extend their practice.

The anxiety-reducing and mood-enhancing benefits of essential oils cannot be emphasised too much. The most effective results are found when the person:

- Likes the fragrance of the essential oils used.
- Participates in their application/administration.
- Has a positive expectation as to their anticipated effects.

In general, for reduction of anxiety and mood enhancement, low doses of essential oils via inhalation are the most effective interventions. As a woman's sense of smell generally becomes more acute during pregnancy, the traditional practice of using lower doses of essential oils in aromatherapy treatments for the pregnant woman (e.g. 0.5–1% concentration in general bodywork treatments) appears well justified.

Aromatherapy provides anxiety-reducing benefits from preconception, through the antenatal period and into the postnatal period.

Aromatherapy in preconception care

Even before conception the stress-reducing effects of aromatherapy have an important contribution to make since preconception stress and anxiety are established factors for some women who have difficulty conceiving. It is thus increasingly common to find preconception care advice and support including stress management techniques such as aromatherapy along with other lifestyle and nutritional measures to optimise the chances of conception (Williams 2005).

Some aromatherapists suggest that the ideal essential oils and extracts to use at this time are those that are derived from plants that produce their volatiles primarily for the purposes of sexual reproduction. This includes, for example, the use of floral essential oils and extracts such as *Rosa damsacena* (rose), *Cananga odorata* (ylang ylang), *Jasminum officinale* (jasmine), *Citrus aurantium* ssp. *aurantium* (flos.) (neroli) and *Lavandula angustifolia* (lavender). Incidentally, these are the same essential oils also classically used in traditional aromatherapy for anxiety and stress management.

Antenatal stress

Working with the woman throughout her pregnancy can provide immense support and benefit. To be able to aromatically accompany the mother-to-be as her body changes and adapts offers real benefit to the mother in terms of stress management as well as promoting a healthy pregnancy and a healthy child (Bastard & Tiran 2006). The various physiological and hormonal changes, coupled with anticipation, fear and concern for the baby's health, often lead to peaks of anxiety at different stages in pregnancy and these factors can be further exacerbated by sleep disturbance and fatigue. Thus the support provided with the use of relevant essential oils goes much further than providing a 'pleasantly fragrant gestation'; by helping reduce maternal stress, aromatherapy also contributes to promoting positive health of both mother and child.

Anxiety reduction during labour

Using the fragrance of essential oils to assist with reduction of anxiety during labour is probably the most established benefit of aromatherapy in maternity care. This is further enhanced if the therapist is able to work prenatally with the woman; in this way, she can help establish a powerful odour-associated relaxation response that then can be re-evoked during the labour process. The advantage of using odour as a cue for relaxation in this way is its speed of action (i.e. immediate). Linked closely with reduction of anxiety comes a welcome reduction in pain perception.

In the largest observational study thus far conducted on aromatherapy during labour (Burns et al 2000), observing more than 8000 mothers over an 8 year period, reduction of anxiety and fear were the most significant benefits reported. *Lavandula angustifolia* (lavender) and *Boswellia carterii* (frankincense) essential oils were the most commonly used for this purpose.

Anxiety levels during labour can significantly impact the health and well-being of both mother and baby (Burns 2005). Some aromatherapy benefits consequent on anxiety reduction to mother and baby during labour and immediately postpartum might include:

- Reduced incidence of epidural anaesthesia.
- Reduced use of opioid medication.
- Greater control over the labour process.
- Greater control over pain, more able to mobilise.
- Greater partner participation/involvement.
- Reduced incidence of mechanical interventions.
- Promotion of endogenous oxytocin through relaxation and pain relief.

- Optimum placental oxygenation.
- Successful establishment of breastfeeding.
- A more alert baby, able to suckle.

(Burns 2005, Burns et al 2000, Fanner 2005, Simkin & Bolding 2004)

Essential oils commonly employed by midwives and aromatherapists during labour include:

Lavandula angustifolia (lavender)
Boswellia carterii (frankincense)
Citrus bergamia (bergamot)
Citrus paradisii (grapefruit)
Citrus limon (lemon)
Mentha spicata (spearmint)
Cananga odorata (ylang ylang)
Salvia sclarea (clary sage)
Mentha × piperita (peppermint)
Citrus reticulata (mandarin)
Rosa centifolia (rose absolute)
Rosa damascena (rose otto)
Jasminum grandiflorum/officinale (jasmine absolute)
Eucalyptus globulus (eucalyptus)
Rosmarinus officinalis (rosemary)
Chamaemelum nobile (Roman chamomile)
Origanum majorana (sweet marjoram).

(Fanner 2005; Burns et al 2000, 2007)

Postnatal depression/postpartum psychosis

Helping the woman make a successful positive transition into motherhood is another area where aromatherapy is increasingly used. Postpartum mood changes are commonly reported and can persist for extended periods, affecting the mother's self-esteem and her ability to interact with her baby. Although there are few reported studies in this area, aromatherapists are working in different countries with women suffering with postpartum depression and postpartum psychosis, usually in conjunction with touch therapies and essential oils in dilute doses. Aromatherapy provided in this way has been shown to help improve physical and mental well-being (by reducing anxiety, fatigue and physical tension) as well as improve the mother's feelings towards her baby and thereby facilitate mother–baby interaction and bonding (Antoniak 2008, Imura et al 2006, Meyer 2005).

In a recent report (Meyer 2005), essential oils preferred by women with postpartum depression included:

- *Boswellia carterii* (frankincense)
- *Cananga odorata* (ylang ylang)
- *Citrus bergamia* (bergamot)

- *Citrus limon* (lemon)
- *Citrus sinensis* (sweet orange)
- *Lavandula angustifolia* (lavender)
- *Pelargonium graveolens* (geranium)
- *Pogostemon cablin* (patchouli)
- *Rosa damascena* (rose)
- *Santalum album* (sandalwood).

Essential oil safety in pregnancy

Apart from deliberate or accidental poisonings following ingestion, there have been no reported cases of serious problems arising from the use of essential oils in pregnancy (such as premature labour, spontaneous abortion, fetal abnormality, etc.). Yet it is normal to be concerned about potential risk and there are numerous opinions and 'safe/unsafe lists' expressed in the literature. Indeed, some authors ask if essential oil hazards in pregnancy constitute an 'accident waiting to happen' (Tiran 1996).

In our opinion, any advice concerning aromatherapy and the pregnant woman needs to be based upon the following:

- Awareness of the changes that occur during pregnancy.
- Respect for the developing fetus.
- Access to the limited information available concerning essential oil pharmacodynamics and pharmacokinetics.
- Understanding of essential oils, their chemistry and their possible hazards.

There is now ample evidence that essential oils do penetrate the body after application, irrespective of which route is used. Medical practitioners and herbalists alike exercise caution with drug administration and remedies during pregnancy. Thus a degree of caution is also warranted with essential oils. However, the risk of serious harm occurring to either the mother or baby from the appropriate use of essential oils is considered negligible, particularly when the oral, rectal and vaginal routes of administration are excluded.

There are three main risk factors concerning essential oil hazard:

1. *The amount/dose absorbed*. Toxicity is always dose-dependent and can be acute or chronic. In maternity care, it is normal practice to use lower doses of essential oils as compared to doses for a non-pregnant woman. Usual doses for general bodywork in pregnancy include essential oils at 0.5–1% concentration, diluted in a suitable medium (fixed oil, cream, etc.). If there is an acute or localised physical problem, then normal doses apply (2–5%).

2. *The route of administration used.* The oral, rectal and vaginal routes carry a greater risk of toxicity than skin application and inhalation of essential oils. It is extremely unusual to use essential oil via these more hazardous routes during pregnancy unless prescribed by a medical practitioner. There have been a number of reports of toxicity to both mother and fetus during pregnancy due to the accidental and deliberate ingestion of essential oils (Anderson et al 1996, Weiss & Catalano 1973).

3. *The potential toxicity of essential oil components/ their metabolites.* Oils containing high amounts of phenols, toxic ketones and phenylpropanoids carry a greater risk in general and thus their use during pregnancy is unusual unless there is specific indication. Certain components such as the ester sabinyl acetate (found in *Juniperus sabina* (savin) and *Salvia lavandulaefolia* (Spanish sage) essential oils for example) are considered potentially abortifacient and inhibitors of implantation and are also therefore avoided (Pages et al 1996).

Some compounds have the potential to be transformed into potentially toxic intermediary metabolites before they are fully metabolised and cleared from the body. This is reportedly the case for the main ingredient in *Mentha pulegium* (pennyroyal) essential oil where the main component (pulegone) is possibly less toxic than its intermediary metabolite, menthofuran. Due to repeated attempts to cause abortion by deliberate ingestion of extracts of pennyroyal, including its essential oil, the pharmacokinetics of pulegone have been examined in both animals and humans (Anderson et al 1996).

Risk to the fetus: essential oils and the placental barrier

The permeability of the placenta is reduced for polar water-soluble substances and also most microbes but it is readily permeable to lipid-soluble drugs with only a limited amount of metabolism of drugs at the level of the placenta itself. This means that a small proportion of essential oil components that reach the mother's blood in their unchanged state are likely to also reach the baby. It is for this reason that aromatherapists exercise caution in their:

- Selection of essential oils (i.e. those that have low risk of toxicity).
- Route of administration (limited to external and inhalation).
- Dose (low, usually half that of a non-pregnant person or less).

Many therapists avoid the use of essential oils and herbal remedies during the first trimester. This is often implemented more as a safeguard against uncertainty and doubt concerning responsibility if the woman was to miscarry during that period than as a protection against fetal malformation or potential abortifacient risk.

Symptom management with essential oils

There are a wide range of symptoms during pregnancy that frequently cause discomfort and distress. Many respond well to essential oils and aromatherapeutic interventions and these may offer significant support and relief. The most commonly reported symptoms and complaints that generally respond well to aromatherapy interventions are listed below. To address these issues, the massage practitioner requires adequate aromatherapy training:

- Altered body image
- Back pain
- Breast tenderness
- Breathlessness
- Fatigue
- Haemorrhoids
- Headaches and dizziness
- Heartburn and indigestion
- Leg cramps
- Mood swings
- Nausea and vomiting
- Nasal congestion
- Nosebleeds and bleeding gums
- Numbness and tingling in the arms and legs
- Stretch marks
- Sciatica and hip pain
- Skin changes
- Sleep disorders
- Swollen ankles.

The role of related products

In many cases, symptoms encountered during pregnancy can be effectively addressed without essential oils by the judicious use of hydrolats and/or vegetable fixed or infused oils. This is particularly the case when addressing symptoms that are skin-related, including, for example:

- Reducing the appearance of stretch marks.
- Addressing skin changes such as itching and skin dryness.
- Relieving the tightness of swollen ankles.
- Soothing cracked nipples.

- Reducing breast engorgement.
- Preparing the perineum with perineal massage.
- Accelerating tissue repair following surgical interventions (Lavanga et al 2001).

If essential oils are added, their fragrance further enhances the aesthetic appeal of the product and thus encourages its regular use. However, in many cases, essential oils are not required, thus further reducing the potential 'chemical burden' to the mother and fetus.

Breastfeeding and essential oils

Mothers often ask if there is a chance that essential oils may adversely affect the nursing baby. Ito and Lee (2003) acknowledge there is much confusion concerning the issue of potential breast milk contaminants and the therapist is also presented with conflicting advice in the literature.

While there is no existing direct evidence concerning essential oil accumulation in breast milk, it should be assumed that if essential oils are ingested or applied directly to the breast, some components will enter breast milk due to their lipophilicity and low molecular weight. However, if essential oil components enter the systemic circulation via body massage, the amount absorbed is likely to be very low and thus the risk is considered negligible.

In general, advice to nursing mothers is that they avoid ingestion of essential oils and application of essential oils directly to the breast and continue receiving the benefits of general aromatherapy massage treatments once the baby is over a month old. Avoidance of essential oils in the immediate postnatal period is linked to the potential conflict of essential olfactory cues (Davis & Porter 1991, Porter & Winberg 1999), such as the mother's own odour, as well as minimising overexposure to chemicals at this early age when the baby's own detoxification/metabolic processes are not yet fully mature and their skin permeation dynamics lead to increased risk of toxicity (Alcorn & McNamara 2003, Harpin & Rutter 1983, Hoeger & Enzmann 2002).

General guidelines for aromatherapy in maternity care

- Always recommend that the mother-to-be seeks advice from a professional aromatherapist before using essential oils at home, particularly if she has poor health and/or a poor obstetric history.
- We advise that essential oils are avoided during the first trimester unless carefully supervised by a trained aromatherapist/midwife.

- If essential oils are to be used at any stage during pregnancy, the dose/concentrations administered are traditionally lower than for a non-pregnant person.
- Regular application of undiluted essential oils is not advised on any part of the body.
- Oral, rectal and vaginal uses of essential oils are inappropriate in pregnancy unless medically prescribed.
- The regular, daily use of essential oils via different routes is not advised.
- The choice of essential oils used should be limited to those with a low history of toxicity.
- There is no accepted, authoritative list of oils that are safe or unsafe to use as all information is based upon common sense as opposed to proven hazards during pregnancy.
- Hydrolats, fixed oils and infused oils can often substitute essential oil use.
- Unless an essential oil is applied directly to the breast, the levels of components in the breast milk are likely to be extremely low.
- If breastfeeding, only use essential oils with a confirmed lack of toxicity and avoid application to the breast itself.
- Consider using related products such as infused and fixed oils and hydrolats. These are extremely versatile agents in pregnancy care and carry negligible risk.
- Pregnant women or new mothers should avoid continuous exposure to fragrances (synthetic or essential oil based).

References and further reading

Alcorn, J., McNamara, P.J., 2003. Pharmacokinetics in the newborn. Adv. Drug Deliv. Rev. 55 (5), 667–686.

Anderson, I.B., Mullen, W.H., Meeker, J.E., et al., 1996. Pennyroyal toxicity: measurement of toxic metabolite levels in two cases and review of the literature. Ann. Intern. Med. 124 (8), 726–734.

Andrade, C., Clifford, P., 2001. Outcome Based Massage. Lippincott Williams and Wilkins, Philadelphia.

Antoniak, P., 2008. Essential oil therapy with a client experiencing post-partum psychosis: a case study. Int. J. Clin. Aromather. 5 (1) in press.

Bastard, J., Tiran, D., 2006. Aromatherapy and massage for antenatal anxiety: its effect on the fetus. Complement. Ther. Clin. Pract. 12 (1), 48–54.

Beard, G., Wood, E.C., 1964. Massage Principles and Techniques. WB Saunders, Philadelphia.

BeFit-Mom, 2009. Prenatal and postpartum fitness and exercise. Supine hypotensive disorder during pregnancy. Available at: <www.befitmom.com> (accessed 02.04.09.).

Burns, E., 2005. Aromatherapy in childbirth: helpful for mother – what about baby? Int. J. Clin. Aromather. 2 (2), 36–38.

Burns, E., Blamey, C., Ersser, S.J., et al., 2000. The use of aromatherapy in intrapartum midwifery practice: an observational study. Complement. Ther. Nurs. Midwifery 6 (1), 33–34.

Burns, E., Zobbi, V., Panzeri, D., et al., 2007. Aromatherapy in childbirth: a pilot randomised controlled trial. Br. J. Obstet. Gynaecol. 114 (7), 838–844.

Cash, M., 1996. Sport and Remedial Massage Therapy. Ebury Press, London.

Cassar, M., 1999. Handbook of Massage Therapy: a Complete Guide for the Student and Professional Massage Therapist. Butterworth Heinemann, Oxford.

College of Massage Therapists of Ontario, 1999. Code of ethics standards of practice, 12 June 1999 (Note that the CMTO Standards of Practice 12 lists specific modifications for the birthing client.). Available at: <cmto.com/pdfs/99june.pdf>.

Davis, L.B., Porter, R.H., 1991. Persistent effects of early odour exposure on human neonates. Chem. Senses 16, 169–174.

De Domenico, G., Wood, E.C., 1997. Beard's Massage, fourth ed. WB Saunders, Philadelphia.

Fanner, F., 2005. The use of aromatherapy for pain management through labour. Int. J. Clin. Aromather. 2 (1), 10–14.

Fraser, D.M., Cooper, M.A., 2003. Myles' Textbook for Midwives, fourteenth ed. Churchill Livingstone, Edinburgh.

Harpin, V.A., Rutter, N., 1983. Barrier properties of the newborn infant's skin. J. Pediatr. 102, 419–425.

Henderson, C., Macdonald, S., 2004. Mayes' Midwifery: A Textbook for Midwives, thirteenth ed. Ballière Tindall, London, p 386.

Hoeger, P.H., Enzmann, C.C., 2002. Skin physiology of the neonate and young infant: a prospective study of functional skin parameters during early infancy. Paediatr. Dermatol. 19 (3), 256–262.

Hollis, M., 1998. Massage for Therapists, second ed. Blackwell Science, Oxford.

Imura, M., Misao, H., Ushijima, H., 2006. The psychological effects of aromatherapy-massage in healthy postpartum mothers. J. Midwifery Womens Health 51 (2), e21–e27.

Ito, S., Lee, A., 2003. Drug excretion into breast milk: overview. Adv. Drug Deliv. Rev. 55 (5), 617–627.

Kellog, J.H., 1895. The Art of Massage: Its Physiological Effects and Therapeutic Applications. Modern Medicine Publishing, Battle Creek, Michigan.

Kendall, F., McCreary, E.K., Provance, P.G., et al., 2005. Muscles: Testing and Function with Posture and Pain, fifth ed. Lippincott Williams and Wilkins, Baltimore.

Knuppel, R., Drukker, J., 1993. High-Risk Pregnancy: A Team Approach, second ed. WB Saunders, Philadelphia.

Kusmirek, J., 2002. Liquid Sunshine: Vegetable Oils for Aromatherapy. Floramicus, Somerset.

Lavanga, S.M., Secci, D., Chimenti, P., et al., 2001. Efficacy of *Hypericum* and calendula oils in the epithelial reconstruction of surgical wounds in childbirth with caesarean section. Il Farmaco 56 (5–7), 451–453.

Liston, C., 1995. Sports physiotherapy applied science and practice. In: Zuluaga, M. Australian Physiotherapy Association Sports Physiotherapy. Churchill Livingstone, Melbourne.

Littleton, L.Y., Engebretson, J.C., 2002. Maternal, Neonatal and Women's Health Nursing. Delmar, Thomson Learning, Albany, NY.

Loving, J., 1999. Massage Therapy: Theory and Practice. Appleton and Lange, Stamford, CT.

Magee, D.J., 2008. Orthopedic Physical Assessment, fifth ed. Saunders, Philadelphia.

Meyer, M., 2005. Aromatherapy in a Melbourne baby unit. Int. J. Clin. Aromather. 2 (1), 33.

Monga, M., 1999. Maternal cardiovascular and renal adaptation to pregnancy. In: Creasy, R.K., Resnick, R. (Eds.) Maternal Fetal Medicine, fourth ed. WB Saunders, Philadelphia.

Pages, N., Fournier, G., Baduel, C., et al., 1996. Sabinyl acetate the main component of Juniperus sabina L'Herit essential oil is responsible for anti-implantation effect. Phytother. Res. 10 (7), 438–440.

Palmer, M.D., 1912. Lessons on Massage, fourth ed. Baillière Tindall and Cox, London.

Parenthood.com, 2009. Sleeping positions while pregnant (why is sleeping on the left side so often recommended?). Available at: <Parenthood.com> (accessed 20.04.09.).

Polden, M., Mantle, J., 1990. Physiotherapy in Obstetrics and Gynaecology. Butterworth Heinemann, Oxford.

Porter, R.H., Winberg, J., 1999. Unique salience of maternal breast odors for newborn infants. Neurosci. Biobehav. Rev. 23, 439–449.

Rattray, F., Ludwig, L., 2000. Clinical Massage Therapy. Talus, Ontario.

Salvo, S.G., 2003. Massage Therapy: Principles and Practice, second ed. WB Saunders, St Louis.

Schneider, W., Dvorak, J., Dvorak, V., et al., 1988. Manual Medicine Therapy. Thieme, New York.

Simkin, P., Bolding, A., 2004. Update on nonpharmacologic approaches to relieve labor pain and prevent suffering. J. Midwifery Womens Health 49 (6), 489–504, 555, 556.

SOGC/CSEP Clinical Practice Guideline, 2003. Exercise in pregnancy and the postpartum period. No. 129, June 2003. Society of Obstetricians and Gynaecologists of Canada.

Tappan, F., Benjamin, P.J., 1998. Tappan's Handbook of Healing Massage Techniques: Classic Holistic and Emerging Methods. Appleton and Lange, Stamford, CT.

Thompson, D.L., 2002. Hands Heal: Communication Documentation and Insurance Billing for Manual Therapists, second ed. Lippincott Williams and Wilkins, Baltimore.

Tiran, D., 1996. Aromatherapy in midwifery: benefits and risks. Complement. Ther. Nurs. Midwifery 2 (4), 88–92.

Tuchtan, C.V., Stelfox, D., 2005. Foundations of Massage. Churchill Livingstone Elsevier, Australia.

Weiss, J., Catalano, P., 1973. Camphorated oil intoxication during pregnancy. Pediatrics 52 (5), 713–714.

Williams, W., 2005. Preconception care and aromatherapy in pregnancy. Int. J. Clin. Aromather. 2 (1), 15–19.

World Health Organization, 2003. Pre-operative procedures. Available at: <http://www.who.int/reproductive-health/impac/Clinical_Principles/Operative_care_C47_C55html>.

Yates, S., 2003. Shiatsu for Midwives. Books for Midwives, Oxford.

CHAPTER **9**

Chapter contents

See theory section

For more information on:

Eastern and western theory

See Chapter 15

For more information on:

Professional issues

See Chapter 14

For more information on:

Higher-risk clients

Learning outcomes

- Describe the benefits of bodywork in pregnancy
- Outline different approaches and considerations for each of the three trimesters of pregnancy
- Describe special issues relating to pregnancy including miscarriage and working during tests
- Outline cautions and contraindications
- Evaluate different techniques and their suitability through pregnancy
- Approach each area of the body, understanding the changes and considerations on how to work

9.1 Overview and key themes

Introduction

Pregnancy can be a very happy and positive time for mothers – an expression of a woman's health and creativity. Pregnancy is not an 'illness' as it is sometimes presented. Women will not necessarily experience any 'problems' and some women even feel healthier than at other times in their lives.

However, each woman responds very differently to the major physical and emotional changes of pregnancy. To some extent this response will be based on her pre-existing emotional and physical state. It will also be based on her life situation: her family situation and support, financial and housing situation, work, cultural situation and so on. Every woman experiences pregnancy differently, and even the same woman may experience different pregnancies quite differently. The key to working with pregnant women is to be adaptable and versatile. Some women may feel extremely well during their pregnancy and able to maintain a high degree of physical activity. Other women may develop health concerns or feel debilitated, even to the point of having to restrict their usual daily activities.

Pregnancy places demands on the body. For some women, these demands seem to 'wake up' their body and improve functioning of many different systems, on both an emotional and physical level. For other women, pregnancy may exacerbate weaknesses in her bodily system(s), whether on a musculoskeletal, circulatory, respiratory or emotional level.

Many women suffer from what are called the 'minor ailments' of pregnancy. Most of these respond well to work with massage, shiatsu and other forms of bodywork. These are the easier and rewarding realities to work with and the practitioner beginning to work with pregnant mothers can feel fairly comfortable working with this group of mothers. Practitioners need to build a sound knowledge of what the common realities are for pregnant women, both physically and emotionally, and understand the best approach to help ease these discomforts. Some issues such as symphysis pubis problems (PGI), will require good knowledge not only of relevant bodywork techniques but also of aftercare, as the condition can be aggravated without appropriate self-care.

Sometimes women suffer more serious illness during pregnancy. This may be due to an underlying condition, such as a respiratory or heart problem, or it may be pregnancy-induced, for example pre-eclampsia or gestational diabetes. Some of these conditions can be supported through appropriate bodywork. However, they raise more issues and are best left for the more experienced practitioner to work with at their discretion. If the therapist works with this group of mothers, there needs to be clear collaboration with the primary maternity caregivers. The therapist may need to work within the hospital setting. Guidelines to these 'higher-risk' conditions are given in Chapter 14, and there is some exploration of relevant professional issues in Chapter 15.

The therapist also needs to be aware that while for most women pregnancy is ultimately a joyful time, it can be unpredictable. It is a time which may include working with issues such as loss, bereavement, depression and grief. Many pregnancies fail in the first trimester, but pregnancy loss may occur at any stage of pregnancy, including during labour and the first few weeks post-delivery. It may be that the baby survives but has minor or severe medical issues or physical or mental disabilities. This means that the therapist needs to know how best to support women through potentially challenging times. This involves examining their personal qualities and being aware of what they can offer, as well as ensuring that they have an appropriate support structure, both professional and personal.

The role of the pregnancy bodywork therapist is to support the mother in the unfolding emotional and physical journey upon which she has embarked – whether joyful and easy or challenging.

Benefits of bodywork in pregnancy

For the woman

1. Offers complementary support to medical care for the physical changes experienced through the pregnancy, for example bodywork for headaches rather than medication, strategies for working with common complaints such as oedema, varicose veins, musculoskeletal tension.
2. Relaxation helps support the woman emotionally and physically.
3. Helps to enhance the positive aspects of pregnancy, and the woman's connection with the baby and with her changing body and emotions.
4. Offers a time (1–1½ hours) when the woman can voice concerns or fears which may not be overt and some degree of emotional or practical support may be offered.
5. Provides continuity of care. The bodyworker may have been working with the woman before the pregnancy, can work with her throughout the pregnancy, may be at the birth and then continue to work with her postnatally.
6. Appropriate self-care strategies can be an integral part of the bodywork:
   - breathing and relaxation techniques can support the woman to relax and tune into her body, baby and feelings
   - exercises can be shown which can support the physical changes of pregnancy and be useful for birth preparation, e.g. stretches to alleviate leg cramps, forward leaning to relieve backache and encourage fetal positioning
   - postural awareness can be encouraged so that the physical changes can be better integrated
   - the partner and other children can be involved in learning massage techniques and other self-care strategies. This will help encourage communication between the couple and family and facilitate prenatal bonding with the baby.
7. The partner can also receive bodywork and be supported in their role.

For the baby

1. A calm, relaxed environment is likely to benefit the baby as well as the mother.
2. Encourages mother/baby connection/bonding.
3. May help encourage optimal fetal positioning.

Testimonial

I had the pleasure of Suzanne working with me during my third pregnancy. She came recommended by my midwife and I was also aware of her through my involvement with natural childbirth groups. I had enjoyed the benefits of shiatsu in my two previous pregnancies and was looking forward to the relief that I knew it could bring.

Early in pregnancy I had a tendency to develop sciatic pain and lower back issues as I have a moderate scoliosis. This presents in a very 'tension'-like pain and Suzanne worked hard on releasing the muscles and allowing more movement into the area. After each session I felt as if I had regained some level of flexibility which was hugely appreciated! As I also suffer from symphysis pubis issues, the whole lower back/pelvic area becomes a worry for me as I get larger, and this is where I felt most in need of the physical release Suzanne provided.

For the first time I also visited a chiropractor in conjunction with the shiatsu massage. I do feel that the combination was hugely beneficial, although the main benefit I received from shiatsu (and Suzanne) as my pregnancy progressed was emotional. My second child was born by caesarean section which had, in addition to my heavily medicalised and painful first birth, severely dented my confidence in terms of birthing. As committed as I was to having a natural home birth, there were many fears and tensions that Suzanne worked through with me.

In addition this pregnancy was not easy for other reasons – I developed gallstones which affected my sleep badly and increased my neurotic belief that my body was useless! Combined with weeks of prodromal labour I was physically very tired and worn out at points but always felt calmer and stronger after seeing Suzanne. She truly healed me physically and mentally and the birth of my daughter was all that I had hoped for.

Key themes

Working to help the woman connect with her changing body

The therapist needs to clearly understand the many changes which are happening on many levels for the woman, physical and emotional, in order to support the woman effectively.

Working with awareness of the baby (embryo/fetus)

It is important to remember that the work involves at least two people – the woman and the baby (or babies). The therapist needs to be aware of how the baby develops in utero and what senses are developed at any given time. For example, the baby will be aware of touch from 7 weeks old. It makes sense to include the baby in the therapeutic relationship, rather than simply as a by-product of working with the mother. Sensitivity is also required in the awareness of the relationship between woman and baby. In the first trimester, the woman may be unsure about what she feels about her baby, even if the pregnancy is planned. She will be aware of the high rate of miscarriage and this, combined with not being able to feel her baby move, may increase her feelings of insecurity. However, some women are tuned into their baby even at this stage and the therapist needs to be aware of that reality. By the second trimester, the woman will be feeling her baby move (from about 16 weeks) and will tend to be more settled in her response to the pregnancy as well as feeling more confident of the pregnancy continuing. This relationship with her baby will deepen through the third trimester.

If possible, and appropriate, in all trimesters it may be helpful to make a direct connection with the baby, ideally early on in the session (perhaps through touch or, if more appropriate, through breathing and visualisation), and encourage the woman to be involved with this. For the baby, bodywork may offer a positive experience of touch and communication. This relationship to touch may support not only the pregnancy but also the birth experience and the postnatal period.

For the woman, including the baby in the treatment offers an opportunity to spend time bonding and communicating with her baby. At the first session, the therapist may not feel that it is appropriate to make a connection with the baby right at the beginning. It is important to ask both woman and baby 'permission' to touch the abdomen before making a direct connection with the baby. This 'permission' can be asked verbally or more energetically (tuning in). Women usually enjoy this work, experiencing it as extremely beneficial and calming. During the third trimester, techniques may be performed which may be able to help with the optimal positioning of the baby.

Core body temperature

In all trimesters care needs to be taken in terms of monitoring the woman's body temperature. Normal core temperature is between 36.2 and 37.6°C (97–100°F) and it is 0.5°C (0.3°F) higher during pregnancy (36.7–38.1°C). There are no really clear guidelines on how high the woman's temperature can rise before it poses a risk to the baby but 38.9°C (102°F) may be the upper limit. It is for this reason that women are generally advised not to use saunas, hot tubs or tanning booths during pregnancy, although some Finnish studies were done on the use of saunas which showed no adverse effects. It makes sense for the therapist to be sensitive to the woman's temperature and to recognise that the room may need to be cooler than for non-pregnant clients. Care must be taken when using hot packs, moxibustion or any heat-based techniques. Electric heating pads have not been shown to cause harm. Infrared lights should not be used, not only because of heat considerations but also because of hormonally induced sensitivity of the skin. Sensible guidance seems to be to use heat applications *with care* in the extremities and to avoid their use in the pelvic area.

Be aware of higher circulating blood volume and relative softness of connective tissue

See Ch. 1.

9.2 Specific considerations for each trimester

First trimester

In this trimester there are hormonal adjustments and there may be anxieties about the well-being of the baby and about being pregnant; it is a time of change and instability, both emotional and physical. Even if the pregnancy is planned there may be worries around miscarriage and the health of the baby, and concerns about the reality of a new baby becoming part of the family. It raises questions such as: How is my life going to be after the baby is born? Will I be working? Will I have enough money and support? Will I need to move house? If unplanned, then serious life and death issues are brought to the fore: Do I want this baby or not?

Many women are concerned about bonding with their baby, or acknowledging their pregnancy because of these factors. The newly pregnant woman may be worried about activities she engaged in before knowing she was pregnant, such as alcohol use, and may be nervous about doing any activity which could potentially be harmful in any way. Due to lack of information and myths perpetuating outdated information, she may be unsure about the safety of bodywork and exercise. The inexperienced therapist may also feel quite tentative about working with clients at this time.

The general guidance is for the woman to continue with her normal day-to-day activities as long as she feels comfortable doing so, rather than stopping activities. There is recent research suggesting that moderate exercise and certainly reducing stress levels may be the most beneficial ways of supporting this first trimester (Latka et al 1999). By extension this tends to indicate that bodywork may also be beneficial, and certainly there is no research to show that bodywork

is harmful. Bodywork is often no more vigorous than many of the day-to-day activities the woman may ordinarily be engaged with such as walking to work, exercising in the gym, continuing to engage in sexual activities, running around after toddlers or carrying heavy shopping.

Many women feel that they need to conceal the fact that they are pregnant because of the risk of miscarriage and considerations such as job security or family pressures. This may lead to increased stress, particularly as it is difficult to ask for sympathy or time off when they may be feeling unwell. The therapist may be one of the few people who knows that the woman is pregnant and she may appreciate the space to be able to express her doubts and insecurities.

There are no obvious outward signs of being pregnant yet physically and emotionally this can be a difficult trimester. Many women feel incredibly tired due to the huge hormonal changes and adaptations their bodies are going through and may in addition feel sick or nauseous. They may be increasingly sensitive to food, alcohol, cigarette smoke and other smells. Their breasts may feel heavy and they may experience headaches, nasal congestion, hoarseness and coughs. There are initial changes in the chest and breathing patterns which bodywork can support.

Diastolic blood pressure falls in early pregnancy. This means that the woman may feel faint or dizzy and care needs to be taken when getting on or off the table or when performing exercises. At this stage she is not likely to suffer from varicose veins and other related problems. Lymphatic system changes begin but there is no oedema of the extremities.

The woman will probably not be seeing a primary healthcare provider unless she has a pre-existing medical condition or has gone through an assisted conception. Conventional maternity care begins more at the end of this trimester when the risk of miscarriage decreases. While it is important to be aware of any potential complications and referral issues, it is often beneficial for clients to receive bodywork in the first trimester, especially if they have been receiving bodywork prior to becoming pregnant. Support can be offered for the huge emotional and physical changes the woman is undergoing.

Bodywork

Essentially most practitioners would agree that, if the implantation is strong and the developing cells are healthy, it would be difficult to do anything which could cause harm. Therapists would have to work with inappropriately strong techniques to cause an increase in risk. Some women do not even realise that they are pregnant and may have already been seeing their therapist without harm.

The approach will be determined by how familiar the woman is with bodywork. If she is a pre-existing client, depending on how she is feeling, the approach need not necessarily be changed dramatically. If it is the first time she has experienced massage, then the therapist will need to be more communicative and cautious in approach, as with any first-time client.

It is important to remember that some women do not feel tired or sick in the first trimester and may still be keeping to a fairly similar exercise/lifestyle regimen as they did before they were pregnant. (Remember the young gymnasts of the Eastern bloc countries who were competing in the Olympics in their first trimester.) More active clients may still enjoy vigorous work, so this can be offered provided there is good communication and feedback. However, as the woman's and baby's systems are in such a rapid phase of change and adaptation, physically vigorous work may be uncomfortable and inappropriate for some clients. This may be the case for those clients who have a history of miscarriage or IVF treatments or clients who are depleted due to the demands of a stressful job or caring for other young children. In these cases a gentle relaxing approach may be more appropriate. Often energy-based work can be particularly beneficial, especially if the client is suffering from nausea and sickness.

When working extensively with women in the first trimester, it is likely that some clients may experience miscarriage. The therapist needs to be aware of these issues and how to support the client during this difficult time.

It is generally considered inadvisable to use physically strong strokes/techniques around the pelvis/abdominal areas as there are many nerve, circulatory and lymphatic links between the abdominal organs (e.g. bladder, intestines) and the uterus and the sacral nerves which supply the uterus. It is thought that stimulation of the abdomen and sacrum may trigger stimulation of the uterus. Certainly there are many internal changes occurring in this area: the embryo/fetus is still developing all its major organ systems and there are daily changes in the structures and 'energies' (eastern view). As well, the pelvis is beginning to 'soften' due to the effects of relaxin and progesterone. However, there is currently no clear definition as to what would constitute 'over-stimulation'. Women are not restricted from eating food which may irritate the GI, the sacrum is stimulated while sitting and moving around, and the physical reactivity of the body with sexual activity will most likely be far more 'stimulating' than the application of bodywork techniques. The uterus is still a pelvic organ in this trimester and it only begins to rise above the pubic bone at the end of the first trimester, so work with the abdomen does not involve directly working over the uterus. Indeed, many women instinctively rub their abdomen when feeling nauseous. However, some women may be sensitive to abdominal touch and may not be comfortable with bodywork in this region.

If the woman is comfortable with the idea, gentle, energetic holding or touch relaxation to the abdomen can be a wonderful element of care and may provide a calming, reassuring connection between the client and her baby, as well as between therapist and client. If appropriate, the therapist can begin to focus the woman's attention on her early connection with the baby. Some women find this challenging as they cannot yet feel the baby and they may not want to connect because of the higher risk of miscarriage. This choice needs to be respected, even if the therapist's own belief may be that connecting and accepting the pregnancy offers the first stage in being able to let go if the pregnancy fails.

Work can be done to the legs and feet. This can be more vigorous or more gentle, depending on the client's needs. It can include energy work down the legs and holding the feet to ground the energy.

The upper body can be treated with fewer cautions. Although the eastern view is that the chest is linked to the pelvis, direct work here will not be too stimulating. It can be worked more vigorously, although bear in mind the relative softness of the tissue. Particular attention to the cervical and thoracic areas may be needed, especially if the woman spends considerable time in an office where she is using a computer and/or telephone, driving a car, or spends time in more static positions in her daily activities. Particular care must be taken when working around the diaphragm and intercostal spaces due to the increased sensitivity of breast tissue. Gentle stretches to open the chest may be encouraged, but be aware that women may feel vulnerable in the first trimester and this type of work may not be appropriate.

Energy work may be beneficial in terms of addressing nausea.

In terms of bodywork position, work can be done as for the non-pregnant client. Both supine and prone positioning can be used if comfortable. The client may not need any additional cushions/pillows, apart from possibly additional support for the breasts which may feel sensitive, sore or heavy.

A key element of care at this stage is to include work with breathing and visualisations to help with relaxation. This can be included as part of the bodywork itself or done as a self-care exercise before or after the session.

The main focus of first trimester work is to support the multitude of changes which the woman is undergoing. Stress reduction and acceptance of the changes is a key part of this. First trimester work lays the foundation for the rest of the pregnancy.

Bodywork cautions

- Passive joint mobilisations and techniques such as rocking and shaking may aggravate nausea.
- Levels of relaxin are at their highest in the first trimester and so body tissue in the pelvis may be more lax than usual. Care needs to be taken with stronger strokes and pressure in this area. Gentle hip stretches and passive movements may be appropriate but it depends on the client.
- Manual lymphatic work for the legs and arms is generally not advised. Firstly, it is considered inadvisable to encourage the elimination of toxins this may stimulate, particularly in the inguinal area. Secondly, it is not indicated: if a woman is suffering from oedema in the first trimester then this would be not be considered a 'normal' response to pregnancy and referral for medical diagnosis would be required. Some gentle lymph work on the neck and face may help with sinus congestion, but again it is important not to over-stimulate toxic release.
- Heavy tapotement is not advised because:
  - there are high levels of relaxin in the first trimester
  - it is considered less advisable to stimulate the body at this stage, as so many changes are occurring, especially at the level of increasing blood volume
  - this type of action may not be rhythmically soothing for the woman or the developing baby.
- Care and awareness of the lower back and sacral area is important due to the changes taking place in this area. Techniques which are more physical in nature tend to be less advised. Lower back pain which is not muscularly related needs to be taken seriously as it may indicate miscarriage or infection.
- It is important to avoid stimulation of any of the labour focus shiatsu/reflex points/zones as this stage is the least stable and they may trigger threatened miscarriage.
- Be alert to and refer any bleeding as this is a sign of potential miscarriage.
- For referral issues see Box 8.2 (p. 185) and Box 8.5 (p. 188).

Aftercare

- It is helpful to begin to introduce postural awareness exercises if the woman is open to this, before the weight of the baby becomes an issue.

- It is not a good idea to begin dramatically new or intense exercise regimes in the first trimester, but introducing some simple, gentle exercises, such as breathing or pelvic floor exercises may be helpful. For someone who is already exercising, provided they feel comfortable continuing and are not overly tired, they can continue and modify as they feel appropriate. The main guideline for intensity is to listen to the body. For some women this may mean continuing with fairly vigorous exercise. For someone who was not exercising and who feels quite tired and nauseous this may mean minimal exercise.
- It needs to be taken into consideration that the levels of relaxin are high and therefore tissues in the pelvic area are relatively softer and more unstable, although there are not the additional issues to do with increased weight in the pelvis.
- If the client is doing no exercise then consider introducing at least some work with the breath. This will help to relax the client, as the first trimester may be a stressful time. Introducing breathing awareness early on will also mean that the client has plenty of time to practise techniques for connecting with her baby and labour, which will hopefully become life-long methods of coping with stress.
- Pelvic floor exercises are important to do during this trimester, especially if the woman has not been doing them routinely prior to pregnancy.
- If the woman has been doing supine abdominal exercises it is advisable to continue them if possible as usually at some stage of the pregnancy she will not be comfortable lying supine. It is important to check that she is doing them correctly, as often women do not, especially making sure that she is breathing correctly, not jerking or bouncing, and is drawing the abdominal muscles in and not allowing them to bulge. It would tend to be less advisable to do versions which include leaning back over a ball, although modified curl ups would be appropriate to continue. It is a shame that many women feel that they have to stop doing their abdominal exercises as soon as they are pregnant, when in fact they could have continued and gained an extra 3 months of value from performing them.
- During this trimester there can be neck and shoulder tension so it is usually of benefit to show some stretches for these areas.
- The more vigorous exercises, especially those where some pressure is put on the pelvic floor, such as the standing squat and squat, are best left to be introduced in the second trimester when the pregnancy is more established, unless the woman is already doing them and feels fine with continuing.

- The partner may not want to become too involved with bodywork support until the pregnancy is more settled. However, if s/he is interested, then there are some effective techniques for helping with nausea and aiding relaxation and connection which may be shown.

<hr>

Summary box – first trimester

- There are potentially many benefits of bodywork in the first trimester: reduction of stress, increased relaxation, alleviation of early pregnancy symptoms, encouragement of early pre-natal bonding, supporting self-awareness, encouraging good breathing and promoting well-being.
- The therapist needs to be aware of the huge changes that are occurring for both woman and baby. The women may be more sensitive to touch and so gentler versions of all techniques may be requested. As so many changes are occurring and the woman may not feel well, she may want to come for weekly or even daily sessions for support and relief of symptoms.
- The therapist needs to include an awareness of pre-existing postural and energy patterns as well as treating current symptoms.
- The therapist needs to be aware of their client's fatigue, energy level, and nausea if present, and adapt techniques accordingly. Energy work may be best for nausea and for supporting the neuroendocrine changes. Relaxation-style work is often most appropriate.
- The upper body may have increased tension – headaches can be common during pregnancy. Many women are working at desks. Upper body work is often indicated.
- Most therapists agree that only gentle work is applied to the pelvic area. This includes both the abdominal and lower back regions. This is erring on the side of caution and it is up to the therapist, with the client, to decide on appropriate work in this region.
- No heavy tapotement techniques should be used as the tissue is softening/elastic and tends to be a less soothing rhythm, especially if the woman is feeling nauseous.
- Stretches for pregnant clients should be slow and gentle rather than vigorous and prolonged because of relative joint laxity.
- Most commonly used bodywork positioning is supine and prone. Breast tenderness may indicate position alteration, e.g. increased support in prone or offering the side-lying position for comfort.
- Avoid stimulation of labour focus shiatsu points and reflex zones on the foot.

- The therapist needs to be aware of the emotional aspects of the pregnancy – the therapist may be one of the few people who know the mother is pregnant and therefore one of the few able to offer support if the woman miscarries.
- Breathing and visualisation techniques are excellent options at this time, and help the woman become more comfortable with their usage during the remainder of pregnancy, the upcoming birth process and as life skills for being a parent.
- Exercise routines can be suggested in conjunction with the health status and current activity levels comfortable for the client. It may be appropriate to reduce intensity of sessions if the client is used to high-performance vigour. This stage of pregnancy is not considered the time to undertake new exercise regimens. However, for women unused to exercise simple shoulder and neck releases as well as pelvic floor exercise are examples of effective home care exercises.

Second trimester

This is a time to process and adapt with more ease: the golden time. Generally it is an easier time, both physically and emotionally. The woman's energy is usually more stable and she tends to feel less tired. She is often 'blooming' and begins to feel more of a connection with her baby. Around 16 weeks the woman may first notice her baby's movements. With a first pregnancy she may not be aware of the baby's movements until around 19 weeks. In most traditional cultures, it was only when the woman felt the signs of the baby moving that pregnancy was considered established. It was referred to as 'quickening'.

The woman has decided whether or not she wants the baby and probably begun to tell other people, but she is not yet carrying as much weight as she will in the third trimester. Morning sickness usually settles from around 12–16 weeks and the rate of miscarriage drops. By the end of this trimester the baby may survive if born – as early as 23 weeks fetuses are 'viable' although the baby will need to be in an intensive care unit.

However, it is important to remember that for some women this 'easy' time does not occur. Some women suffer with nausea and morning sickness throughout pregnancy. They may feel even worse as they are waiting for an 'easy' time which never comes. Issues related to body perception may also create a lack of ease, especially if eating disorders or self-esteem issues become triggered due to the changing pregnant body. Some women enjoy their changing shape whereas others try to hide the fact they are pregnant and feel uncomfortable with the weight gain.

This trimester is essentially a time of transition between the major hormonally driven changes of the first trimester and the major physical changes, largely due to the increased weight of the baby, of the third trimester. Some of the feelings of the first trimester may continue into the early part of the second trimester, and some of the changes of the third trimester may begin in the second trimester. There is usually a noticeable point during this trimester when the woman finds she needs to begin to slow down once more. If she does not her body may send her warning signals, such as stitches or cramping if she is over-exerting herself, or heartburn/indigestion if she eats too much at a time or too late at night. If she is able to slow down, listen to her body and adapt, she can enter the third trimester feeling well, unless of course complications develop.

Bodywork

Much of the work in the second trimester is about encouraging good postural awareness to prepare the body for the increased physical demands of the third trimester. Key areas to focus on in this regard are the back and abdomen.

Since the major organ systems are formed, the rate of miscarriage/stillbirth is much lower and the pregnancy is considered more 'stable' from about weeks 16–18. This is the time to begin to include stronger physical work around the sacrum and pelvic areas, depending on the level of comfort of the client. Abdominal work can begin to be deeper, depending on the woman's preference, although strokes must always be careful not to pull on already extended muscles and ligaments.

Physical work around the neck and shoulders continues to be beneficial and is often indicated.

Many of the conditions of the third trimester can begin in the second trimester, so it may be relevant to address any body systems which begin to show signs of strain such as the lymphatic, circulatory, musculoskeletal and digestive systems. Be alert to the possibility of PGI or sacro-iliac (SI) problems developing.

Energy work can be continued, aimed at supporting specific energy changes for the client.

Although many women still feel comfortable for short periods lying on their backs, in the therapeutic context, it is best to provide the majority of care in the side-lying position. In the second trimester typical prone work is not advised.

Bodywork cautions

- Continue to be aware of not over-stimulating labour focus points and reflex zones.
- Begin to watch for signs of symphysis pubis and pelvic girdle instability (PGI) and adjust bodywork and self-care suggestions accordingly.

- Refer any bleeding to primary care provider to establish its cause.
- Be aware that the woman may begin to develop pre-eclampsia (signs include raised blood pressure, protein in the urine, oedema – see theory and Box 8.3 (p. 185)) and it is important to recognise oedema related to pre-eclampsia as in this case lymphatic work would be avoided.
- Be aware that although relaxin levels are not as high as in the first trimester, the tissue is still softer than normal and therefore heavy tapotement strokes are best avoided.
- **Referral issues see Box 8.3 (p. 185) and Box 8.5 (p. 186).**

Aftercare
Lifestyle and exercise

This is the time to encourage the woman to take up exercise as she can begin to prepare herself for the increased physical demands of the third trimester and help to prevent some of the problems which otherwise might develop, particularly musculoskeletal issues such as backaches, cramps or circulatory issues such as varicose veins or heartburn, constipation and indigestion. As she continues and the weight of the baby increases, she will be working harder by doing the same exercises.

Since many of the minor ailments of pregnancy are caused by poor posture, postural awareness exercises are particularly important to include. This includes breath awareness and pelvic tilting as well as spine lengthening. Abdominal exercises can be safely begun, if the woman had not been doing them in the first trimester. These would probably be all fours exercises. Pelvic floor exercises should also be initiated or continued.

Some of the stronger exercises can now be introduced such as squatting and the standing squat, as appropriate, paying attention to any cautions.

The partner may want to become involved, especially now that the baby's movements can be felt. S/he will not feel so wary and it is lovely to introduce abdominal work to support the partner's connection with the baby. Partners can also learn techniques to ease neck and shoulder tension and other ailments.

The woman may well want to begin to attend some antenatal yoga or exercise classes, take up swimming or some regular aerobic exercise such as walking.

Summary box – second trimester

- For many women, this is the 'easiest' (blooming) phase of the pregnancy and she may not need as frequent sessions as in the first trimester. Often woman choose to come every 2–3 weeks, if they have no particular issues.

- Benefits of work in the second trimester include: supporting the mother to continue looking after her body in this easier phase of pregnancy; helping to prevent conditions developing; encouraging good body posture and awareness; supporting prenatal bonding and involving the partner.
- This is a time of transition between first and third trimesters – symptoms of the first trimester may persist, while symptoms of the third trimester may develop.
- Side-lying positioning should begin, although supine with support may be used in the early phase for brief amounts of time.
- Be aware of increased musculoskeletal issues such as lower back pain, sacroiliac (SI) dysfunction, SPD and pelvic instability (PGI). Other issues such as oedema and varicosities may become more pronounced.
- Postural changes will become more evident.
- Stronger/deeper/more specific strokes may be appropriate depending on the physical realities of the woman.
- Deep tapotement such as pounding and hacking are still best avoided.
- The therapist and woman/partner can work more with the abdomen and the connection to the baby (see abdomen section).
- Lymphatic work may be indicated towards the latter end of this trimester.
- Be aware of pre-eclampsia from week 24. Work may need to be modified (see higher risk, Ch. 14).
- This is the time to encourage the woman to take up exercise, especially focusing on postural awareness and the abdomen and pelvic floor.
- The partner may begin to want to be more involved, especially as they will begin to be able to feel the baby.

Third trimester

In this trimester there are structural effects due to the growing baby. The focus is on birth and motherhood. Although many women may continue to feel wonderful throughout the third trimester, this is the most physically demanding phase of pregnancy. Usually by the end of this trimester, most women feel some degree of tiredness. Many of the issues of this trimester are caused by the increasing weight of the baby and the effects that this has on the woman's body. Good posture can make an enormous difference to how the woman feels.

By this trimester, postural imbalances which may have begun in the second trimester have become more marked and the typical pregnancy posture presents (see

Fig. 8.1A and B, p. 189). Bodywork to balance this and to increase postural awareness is usually beneficial.

The third trimester is the time when the baby begins to settle into the position for birth and so work can be done to encourage optimal fetal positioning.

The woman may suffer from circulatory problems in arms and legs such as varicose veins, oedema, carpal tunnel syndrome. Due to compression of internal organs the woman may suffer from constipation or indigestion. Gestational diabetes may develop. Appropriate exercise, dietary advice and self-care strategies can go a long way to help minimise the discomfort of these conditions.

The therapist needs to be alert to the fact that more serious problems may develop in this trimester such as hypertension, pre-eclampsia or obstetric cholestasis. The placenta could present with issues such as abruption as it detaches, or it can begin to function less efficiently as the pregnancy progresses.

The woman may be waking more frequently during the night, either due to the need to urinate or to physical discomfort, particularly in the hips and shoulders. This may lead to her feeling increasingly tired. Women currently are working increasingly longer in their pregnancies with many working until weeks 34–36 or even week 40. This can add increased stress, especially if they have other children. They may not have time to focus on preparing for birth either emotionally or physically. Their bodywork sessions may offer the only time that the woman focuses on herself and her baby. It is therefore important not only to address the physical issues but also to support the client in processing her emotions.

Emotionally the woman focuses more on the impending birth and may be feeling anxious about how she will cope. She may be more motivated to practise birth positions and breathing for labour and her partner may want to become more involved.

During the last few weeks the woman needs to be supported both physically and emotionally, to begin the process of letting go of being pregnant and preparing to birth her baby and journey to the next stage of being a new mother.

First-time mothers tend to focus almost exclusively on the birth, and it is helpful to encourage them to begin to look beyond motherhood. Some women are concerned about the responsibility of being a mother. Second-time mothers may express concerns about life with an additional child and sibling rivalry or issues such as sleeping, breastfeeding, postnatal depression, particularly if they had difficulties previously.

Bodywork issues

Work in this trimester is focused on giving the woman and baby more physical space. The woman's internal organs are compressed because of the growing baby and stresses are placed on the spine and abdominal muscles. Bodywork can be done in these areas. The ribs may be feeling the pressure of the baby and feel bruised (rib flare), which may also restrict breathing. Gentle diaphragm release work and work for the intercostals may help. Later as the baby engages, there may be pressure down in the pelvis and the client may benefit from hip stretches, provided there are no symphysis pubis issues.

Stretching movements are especially beneficial during this phase of pregnancy as the increasing size of the baby tends to block the flow of blood, lymph, and energy. Pregnancy can be a time to improve flexibility, both through exercise and massage, but it must be done with awareness. Side stretches can help open up the ribs. Elevations and passive movements of the arms and legs will help to improve circulation and the flow of lymph.

Care needs to be taken with regard to the increasing softening of connective tissue which may lead to pelvic instability.

The client may be experiencing sinus congestion and work to support lymph flow in the neck as well as opening up the chest and clearing the sinuses can be helpful.

Energy work can support the woman in making the shift from the state of pregnancy to birth – supporting both the emotional and the hormonal changes.

Side-lying positioning continues in the third trimester, and it may be worth considering if the woman may feel more comfortable lying on the floor. Forward leaning work can be included.

Knowing the basic position of the baby can help prepare the woman for her birthing process, and may help inform the therapist of the best positioning for implementing the treatment.

Bodywork cautions

- By the third trimester, most women are not comfortable lying on their back, even for short periods. Be aware of supine hypotension (SHS).
- Mobile joints especially SI, symphysis pubis (watch out for (PGI).
- Be aware of the signs of pre-term labour.
- Be alert to the realities of pre-eclampsia, obstetrical cholestasis, gestational diabetes, placental issues.
- **Referal issues see Box 8.3 (p. 185) and Box 8.5 (p. 186).**

Aftercare

The main focus in this trimester is on preparing for birth and beyond. It is helpful for the client to continue as much as possible with the exercises she has been doing in the second trimester, although she will probably find at some point that she is no longer comfortable doing exercise in the supine position. She may also find that she needs to slow down a little and exercise less. It can be helpful to remind her that even if she does not exercise as much, she may still be working as hard because the baby is increasing in size. What often happens during this trimester is that the woman has days when she has more energy and days when she is more tired. These ups and downs are normal and the woman needs to be encouraged to listen to her body and adapt her daily exercise to what she feels like doing on that day.

The focus is on practising positions which will be useful during the birth. It is a good idea, if the partner has not already been involved with the exercises up to this point, to begin to practice with the woman. Massage from the partner may add to the woman's comfort in the latter stages of her pregnancy. Sessions involving the partner are an excellent way to help the couple learn how to work together for the common goal of the birth of their baby. This may help communication and facilitate confidence and self-esteem in both individuals, supporting the transition of forming a new relationship as a family.

A focus while doing the exercises is to be aware of the baby's position and to focus on those exercises which support the baby to be in the optimal position.

Bear increased joint laxity in mind when suggesting exercises and movements to do or to avoid. In the case of symphysis pubis laxity (for more information see theory, p. 28–30, and aftercare, p. 348), appropriate exercise and postural modifications will need to be shown.

Summary box – third trimester

- This is the time when many of the ailments of pregnancy become more obvious and the woman may need more frequent sessions again.
- Be aware of positioning to prevent supine hypotension and to support optimal fetal positioning.
- The woman may be more restless and need to change position more frequently.
- Be aware of the increased laxity of the ligaments and joints when utilising stroke applications, mobilisations, etc.
- Observe for oedema, varicose veins, carpal tunnel, rib flare.
- Be aware of the possible onset of systemic issues such as pre-eclampsia, gestational diabetes.
- Allow for bathroom breaks, and consider hydration/nutritional elements.
- Include work to support optimal fetal positioning and connect with the baby.

- Include self-care strategies for optimal birth readiness, e.g. cat stretch, on all fours with pelvic rocking and breathing/visualisations.
- Include the partner in strategies to help prepare the couple for labour and include work where possible as preparation for the postnatal period. This will help support both individuals physically and psychologically.

9.3 How to support women who are going through difficulties

Difficult test results

- This is likely to be during the late first trimester and early second trimester depending on the tests.
- Be clear of the type of tests and if it is an assessment of maternal or fetal health.
- Estabish if the result is a risk factor or diagnosis of condition.
- Consider what the woman's options are.
- If the woman has to make a decision then the focus of the bodywork is to encourage the mother to be able to tune into her own feelings about what feels the right choice for her and the baby from a place of relaxation. The aim is not for the bodyworker to impose a particular viewpoint. Respect the woman's choice.
- If a decision has already been made then the bodyworker can still help to support the woman to relax into what she has chosen and to find a place of relaxation.
- Depending on the woman and the situation, it may or may not be appropriate to include work on connecting with the baby.

Working with miscarriage/loss

- Miscarriage or loss may occur at any stage of pregnancy. It is most common in the first trimester and much less common after that. Refer to eastern and western theory section for more information and causes and patterns.
- Working with women suffering loss may trigger feelings for the therapist, so it is important to be clear about boundaries.

Working with a pregnant woman who has a history of miscarriage

Previous miscarriage may affect a woman's experience of the current pregnancy. Women who have undergone fertility treatments may have had a history of miscarriage.

Often the client may not feel relaxed until she has got beyond the stage at which she miscarried in a previous pregnancy. She usually feels quite anxious about doing exercise or having bodywork as she may be worried that this may cause a miscarriage. It is helpful to reassure her that exercise is now being shown to have a possible protective, rather than harmful effect and this is likely to be true for bodywork. The therapist should not make definite claims that bodywork may help prevent miscarriage although they can reassure the client that at the very least bodywork will not cause harm, and may indeed be able to support the pregnancy by promoting relaxation and supporting key energies such as Jing, Blood.

Establish the cause for previous miscarriage if known. If there is no known cause then it is likely to be a one-off cause and genetically based; therefore work to support Jing (Kidney) is likely to be appropriate. If the cause remains an issue, e.g. uterine issues (Extraordinary Vessels), incompetent cervix (Spleen), sticky blood (Penetrating Vessel), support these energies.

Type of work

- As the woman might be anxious, energy-based or relaxation techniques rather than more physically challenging work may be more appropriate.
- The woman is likely to be extremely sensitive to work around the abdomen. She is probably wary of bonding with a baby she is afraid she might lose, and the approach will need to be extremely sensitive. Working with breathing and visualisations can be supportive. The woman can visualise letting go of her feelings of fear and anxiety and simply come to being in her body. For some women, feeling connected with the baby may be helpful. She can visualise, if she feels she can and wants to, the baby growing in the womb and being held there. She can visualise her body nourishing her baby.
- Abdominal energy work and holds may be supportive, depending on the woman.
- Energy work: support the Jing, Kidney, Extraordinary Vessels. Chong mai if there are issues related to Blood conditions.

Supporting women during and after miscarriage

Women often feel guilty that maybe there was something that they could have done to prevent the miscarriage. It is helpful to reassure them that in fact most miscarriages are the body's healthy response to letting go of a baby which is not developing properly.

For the woman, whatever the stage of pregnancy, it is a process of grieving for her baby and it can be helpful for the therapist first to acknowledge that process of grief rather than try to negate it. It may also be helpful to encourage the woman to find the most appropriate way to grieve. Some women like to have some kind of funeral ceremony for their baby, even though it may be a simple lighting of a candle and saying goodbye. Some women like to bury their baby, or what remains, under a tree or in a special place. Some women even carry blood from their baby around with them. Other women may find these kinds of ideas distasteful and need to be encouraged to find what works for them.

Often, if a woman has had a previous termination, feelings of guilt may rise to the surface. She may feel in some way she is being 'punished' for what she did before. In this case it may be helpful for her to grieve for the previous baby as well as the current one, so that she can let go and move on.

During a miscarriage

This is similar to work for birth preparation, but of course includes awareness of the grieving process. Support includes:

- Supporting the woman to 'birth' the dead baby.
- Lung is useful to support the grief process and letting go.

I worked on a friend with reflexology and shiatsu points to help her with a missed abortion. She was close to needing surgery to remove a fetus that had died a few weeks earlier, but her body and mind would just not let go of it. After a very emotional session of reflexology for the both of us, the baby miscarried that night. Her whole family were grateful for being able to ease her pain and avoid medical intervention.

(Catherine Tugnait, maternity reflexologist and massage therapist, UK)

After a miscarriage

Often bodywork is extremely helpful for helping women get in touch with their feelings of grief and to give them the space to feel what they need to do from a space of relaxation and stillness, rather than anxiety and guilt. One of the most crucial parts can be simply creating a space in which the mother can acknowledge her 'lost' baby – whatever age the baby was when s/he died.

Work is similar in approach to the postpartum period, depending on how long after the miscarriage the therapist sees the woman. The aim is to help restore the woman's energies and support the grieving process.

Case study

Suzanne

Client B's baby had died some weeks prior to our session and she had come to me because she did not want to have a dilatation and curettage (D&C) and wanted to try to see if bodywork could help her miscarry naturally. I had not seen her for bodywork before but she knew I specialised in maternity work. I was careful not to guarantee any outcome but agreed to support her in whatever process she was going through. She was very distressed. On taking the case history, I discovered that, mixed up with the feelings of distress over this miscarriage, were feelings of guilt over an abortion she had undergone many years previously. She was feeling that maybe somehow she was being punished for getting rid of her previous baby. She was effectively grieving the loss of two babies. I did a combination of massage and shiatsu work, focusing on the 'labour focus' points and doing some deep work around the sacrum. I also did a lot of connecting work with her abdomen and the baby. We talked a lot about the baby she was still carrying and she felt that she wanted to create some kind of ceremony. We then spoke about including her previous baby in the ceremony. She came back a week later, after she had miscarried naturally, the day after receiving the treatment, to help her with the recovery. She was feeling much better and felt that she had been able to let go of her previous feelings of guilt. She had involved her partner in the ceremonies. She was feeling ready to move on. Some years later I worked with her again; she was expecting another child and the pregnancy was going well at this time.

How to support women with pelvic girdle and symphysis pubis instability (PGI/SPI)

This is often weakness in the symphysis pubis, possibly combined with weakness of the sacroiliac joint. The main aims of treatment are:

1. To avoid strain and mobilisation of the symphysis pubis and sacroiliac joint. This is achieved by taking care to position the client as much as possible with the knees together. If wanting to work the adductors and inner leg, then it is preferable to position the client in forward leaning or sitting, rather than the side, and to minimise the distance between the legs. Care needs to be taken when the client moves in and out of different positions.

2. To strengthen areas of weakness.

   Abdominals (transverse and oblique) (meridians: CV, ST, KD, PV) and pelvic floor meridians (CV/GV/GDV, pelvic floor energy holds)

   CV/GV hold to bring energy to the perineum

   Weak adductors (Yin leg meridians: SP, LV, KD)

   Girdle Vessel and Conception Vessel, give support to the pelvis

   Points, especially CV 2, to strengthen the symphysis pubis CV

   Spleen to support the weakened muscles

   Liver and Gall Bladder support the ligaments

   CV 2 to benefit symphysis pubis

3. To give some release to contracted/overcompensating areas.

   Contracted gluteals and piriformis and iliotibial band (meridians: GB and BL)

   Sacral work: BL and GV balance spine

In releasing these contracted muscles/energies without having done sufficient compensatory work for the weakened muscles/energy areas, pelvic instability may tend to be aggravated. A good rule of thumb is to do a little less than seems appropriate and monitor the effects of any release on the stability of the pubic bone.

Other patterns

There may also be other patterns which need to be addressed:

- Tight quadriceps or hamstrings may also relate to symphysis pubis weakness.
- Leg imbalance; one shorter than the other will contribute to pelvic instability.
- Pelvic misalignment; ligaments, SI, piriformis.
- Feet; fallen arches may also contribute.

9.4 Overview of practical techniques

Different types of techniques and their suitability at different stages of pregnancy

The usual precautions apply for all these techniques, for example fever, infection, DVT and so on. There are some further specific cautions in pregnancy which are outlined in assessment (section 8.1 and 8.2 p. 181–198) and under specific areas of the body.

Specific areas more sensitive to issues in pregnancy include:

- Breasts
- Abdomen
- Legs.

Summary of maternal changes in pregnancy with most implication for bodyworkers

- Effects of progesterone and relaxin relaxing connective tissue, smooth muscle and ligaments, especially in the pelvis.
- Increased blood flow and changes in composition of blood.
- Increased likelihood of oedema.
- Increasing size of the fetus and weight gain.

Higher circulating blood volume and changes in composition and circulation of blood

There is limited research on the effects of bodywork on blood circulation but certainly it is wise to take the increased blood volume into account. This means that techniques which encourage vigorous movement of blood such as heavy tapotement and vigorous petrissage tend to be used less. Overall stroke application also tends to be a little slower. Of course, this is all relative and depends on the overall health status of the client. It is more likely to be an issue in cases with underlying pathologies in addition to the normal circulatory changes of pregnancy. This would include women suffering from hypertension, kidney or heart issues and placental issues.

There are changes in clotting factors but for most healthy women this would not lead to an increase in DVT.

Relative softness of tissue

This will be more of an issue for women who were hypermobile before pregnancy as the joints will become even more mobile. For other women, this increased flexibility can offer a positive possibility for postural, muscular and soft tissue change and re-education which can remain postnatally. In the muscles, there will still be patterns of hyper- and hypotonicity. However, the hypertonic areas will tend to respond a little more quickly and release a little more rapidly. This means that often less physical release is needed than with the same client prior to pregnancy. Strokes, stretches and mobilisations tend to be performed at a slightly slower pace, with good support. It is important not to do jerky or ballistic-type movements because of the increased risk of over-stretching (as advised in the RCOG guidelines on exercise in pregnancy, RCOG 2006). Qualifications as to depth of pressure, mobilisations and resisted techniques must, however, bear in mind the general health and fitness level of the pregnant woman as well as her underlying, genetically determined, softness of tissue.

Issues of oedema and increased fluids

As there is more oedema, there is likely to be more of an issue with extra fluids and therefore work to support lymphatic and venous return is often indicated. If there is oedema then the tissue will be more sensitive to stronger physical type techniques.

Effleurage (Swedish massage), saka (shiatsu)

These types of techniques are generally suitable at all stages of pregnancy as they can be varied in depth from gentle to deep and in speed from slow or vigorous depending on the client's needs. They can be used to facilitate circulation, either lymph, blood or energy. They can be calming strokes if the client is tense or anxious. In the first trimester if the client is feeling sensitive to touch, then the lighter nature of these strokes may be more beneficial than deeper strokes.

Cautions

There may be certain areas of the body, where care may need to be taken at different stages: notably legs with varicose veins and oedema, abdominal and breast work if the woman does not feel comfortable with it. These are outlined in more detail under specific sections of the body.

Kneading/petrissage/frictions (Swedish massage), kenbiki (shiatsu)

This type of work is generally beneficial at all stages of pregnancy. As pregnancy progresses and certain muscle groups and meridians may become more contracted, petrissage techniques offer increasingly valuable modalities. Deeper petrissage in areas of tense and contracted muscles can be particularly effective. This is often indicated for the gluteals, trapezius (GB) upper thighs (TFL and iliotibial band, quadriceps and hamstrings) (ST, BL, GB), and calves (BL), especially in later pregnancy.

Cautions

- As there is greater circulating blood volume, care needs to be taken to monitor increased blood flow for client comfort, but it is not usually an issue of concern.
- Due to relative softness of tissue, kneading may have a slightly slower rhythm than with

a non-pregnant client, but the rhythm depends on the actual softness of the tissue for each client.
- More care needs to be taken in the first trimester due to the changes in the body and because the client may be feeling both tired and anxious. Women usually appreciate work in the neck and shoulders but they may be more cautious when consenting to gluteal or low back work. Work in these areas does not increase harm to the client if it is done with sensitivity to her needs, her health situation and the state of her soft tissues. Additional respect must be exercised in working with women who have a history of miscarriage.
- During the first trimester most women would probably not appreciate kneading to the abdomen. However, if it is not a first pregnancy, the tissue may well be quite stretched and the uterus is not in the abdomen, so no harm would be caused if the client would appreciate some gentle or moderate kneading.
- Basic gentle strokes of petrissage, such as reinforced palmar kneading, may be appropriate in the second and third trimesters, provided that they are gently or moderately applied, respect the changes in the underlying structures (uterus, baby and other abdominal organs) and do not add any further stretch into the lengthened abdominal muscles.

Percussion/tapotement

Light tapotement strokes may be beneficial in stimulating the terminal lymph nodes and thymus. This work is often indicated throughout pregnancy due to the increased incidence of sinus congestion. It is particularly indicated in the second and third trimesters due to the increased likelihood of oedema in the limbs. Moderate tapotement may be beneficial in certain areas depending on the client's tissue and presenting issues. The client's response to tapotement must be paramount.

Cautions

The stimulating nature of these techniques means that strong tapotement is generally a less suitable technique in pregnancy. There are two main reasons:

1. The softening of the tissue means it springs back more readily and can more easily be overstretched. Pregnant women are advised to minimise ballistic-type movement in exercise.
2. The rhythm of tapotement may feel unsettling for the pregnant client, and potentially also the baby.

Rocking and shaking

Once the pregnancy is more settled, from 16 weeks onwards, some gentle rocking, in tune with the woman's and baby's rhythms, is often appropriate. It depends very much on the client. These techniques can be beneficial for releasing tension and the rhythm can feel calming.

Cautions

- Generally not advisable in the first trimester due to the fact that many women feel sick or nauseous. Rocking is likely to aggravate feelings of sickness.
- More vigorous rocking and shaking would be less advisable throughout pregnancy because:
  - relative softness of the tissue
  - it is likely to feel unsettling for the client and potentially her baby.

Breathing

Breathing can be used as a primary form of stress reduction and to promote relaxation in pregnancy; it can also be encouraged as a tool to help prepare the woman for her birth.

Pregnant mothers breathe more from the diaphragm than non-pregnant mothers, and they also need more air. It is helpful to encourage women to learn to breathe more deeply and to breathe into the abdomen, where they may feel blocked due to the pressure of the fetus. If the client is breathing her body is going to function more optimally.

Breathing is a useful tool to support self-help visualisation techniques. Appropriate breathing is important when undertaking abdominal and pelvic floor exercises.

Lymph drainage techniques

In all trimesters work to support the terminal nodes and the neck, along with sinus draining, may be of benefit in aiding the sinus congestion which pregnant women often experience.

In the second and third trimesters stimulating the main lymph nodes and doing manual lymph drainage work for the arms and legs is beneficial for reducing oedema and for alleviating carpal tunnel syndrome.

Cautions

See lymph section (p. 274).

Static pressure and static holds including soft tissue release and neuromuscular technique (NMT)

These are generally suitable for all trimesters and are often enjoyed by pregnant women, who appreciate the calming yet deep nature of the techniques. The techniques are particularly effective in the sacral area, gluteals and upper leg in later pregnancy due to the demands placed on the body by the growing baby.

Cautions

Avoid:

- Specific 'labour focus' points until 37 weeks.
- Significant pressure over the abdomen in the first trimester.
- Pressure on the uterine fundus at any time.
- Pressure over varicose veins.
- Strong sacral pressure in the first trimester.
- Any pressure which would cause pulling on the uterine ligaments.

More specific information on these situations is given under the relevant practical sections.

Stretches/passive movements/joint mobilisations

These types of techniques are beneficial at all stages when performed in a gentle rhythmic manner with good support to the joints. It is important to perform the mobilisations with more support and a little more slowly than usual and not to use any bouncing, ballistic-type movements due to the relative softness of tissue and laxity of joints. Rocking movements (as outlined above) would tend to be smooth and relatively slow.

Stretches and especially the use of limb elevation are often beneficial, especially in late pregnancy, as many of the issues are caused by restricted circulation due to the fetus in the pelvis and the increased weight of the breasts.

During the first trimester, women who remain well and physically active may experience the benefit of muscle tension release from stretches.

Cautions

Strokes involving movement, especially in the pelvic area, may be less suitable or need to be modified in the first trimester. This is because a primary focus is to support the physical and energetic formation of the fetus and a 'gathering' rather than 'opening' approach is preferred. This is especially true if the client has a history of miscarriage or is feeling nauseous.

In all trimesters particular attention should be paid to the relative laxity of joints, especially the joints of the pelvis (sacroiliac and symphysis pubis). While most women will present with no particular issues, caution to ensure that joints are not overstressed, overextended or injured should occur at all times. This means that movements need to be performed a little more slowly than usual and the movement should never be overextended. Stronger resistance techniques may be best avoided in order not to overextend the client and because the body is undergoing so much change it may be hard for the client to gauge how much resistance is appropriate. Gentle resistance or overpressure at the end of each active range of motion is acceptable as long as the client exhibits normal and pain-free ranges of movement. A normal overpressure end-feel should be a 'tissue stretch' sensation. When performing any stretches or mobilisations, make sure that the joints are supported, especially the knees when lowering the legs.

Fascial techniques and soft tissue release

During pregnancy the fascia is affected in many ways with the physical changes which are occurring. For this reason, fascial techniques can be excellent modalities in helping ease discomforts in the musculoskeletal system.

Cautions
Local area cautions apply.

9.5 Approaches and techniques for different areas of the body

The main postural patterns of pregnancy are described under 'assessment' (see Chapter 8). Specific areas of the body are described in the sections below (9.6–9.11).

9.6 Head, face, neck and shoulders

Appropriate work to these areas may be of benefit throughout pregnancy and there are few cautions beyond those considered for any client. It is an area which is often tense, due in large part to our modern sedentary lifestyle of sitting at desks, working at computers, and driving cars.

In pregnancy these issues tend to be exacerbated. Most women continue to do their normal desk work through most of their pregnancy. Because of all the emotional and physical changes they are undergoing they may be under more stress, and these areas are likely to be even more tense than normal.

There is often hyperkyphotic pattening. Work to the neck and shoulders may relieve some of these patterns as well as increasing postural awareness leading to its improvement. These patterns may be the cause of headaches, thoracic outlet, de Quervain or carpal tunnel syndrome, difficulties with breathing and tightness in the chest and costal border area.

Clients may enjoy work on the face, especially if they are feeling anxious. It can be a soothing way to finish the treatment. Face massage may help relieve headaches during pregnancy, many of which are posturally or hormonally related.

Women often experience nasal congestion along with a tendency to develop colds and nasal tract infections due to hormonal changes and the lowered immunity of pregnancy. They are not able to take medications for these conditions. These changes also mean that fluids tend to drain less effectively and sinus draining techniques can be effective. Nosebleeds may also occur. The therapist needs to remember that the tissues are relatively softer. Work can be beneficial all the way through pregnancy from the first trimester when the client may experience hormonally related headaches.

Energy wise the Gall Bladder and Bladder tend to be contracted and Lungs weakened. PV and CV may be congested.

Types of techniques

The style of technique would not necessarily be that different than with non-pregnant clients. The therapist can use stretches and passive movements, although they need to be aware of the potential nausea of the first trimester.

Working positions

The semi-reclining position is the preferred position for facial work as it affords good symmetry and access to all areas. However, if the client is not comfortable, then the side position or sitting on a ball can be used. The side position is not so easy to work the sinuses as only one side can be accessed at a time; however, work can still be done if it is the only position available.

Side-lying is an excellent position in which to work the lateral aspects of the neck and the shoulder girdle area and is often the preferred position for the therapist working these areas, even in non-pregnant clients. Work can be done with the therapist positioned in the front, back or superior aspect of the client's body. It offers an excellent position for thorough mobilisation of the shoulder joint. Techniques need to be applied bilaterally.

Leaning over a physio ball can also offer effective positioning for accessing the shoulders.

Cautions

No direct stimulation of GB 21 on the top of the trapezius until 37 weeks (or earlier if induction indicated). Work to this point only needs to be avoided by using stimulation with deep specific downward pressure. General petrissage over the point is not a concern for potential labour stimulation.

Technique suggestions for the lateral aspect of the neck and shoulder work in the side-lying position

We have suggested these techniques in the side position, as many therapists are not so confident when working in the side position. For all the following techniques, the client can be either on a floor or a table. For techniques applied in the side-lying position, the therapist and client may find them most effective when the therapist is positioned on the side of the client's back rather than at their front. Any technique which is done without consideration of the special needs of the client may feel invasive, particularly in pregnancy or when in proximity to the abdominal or breast area.

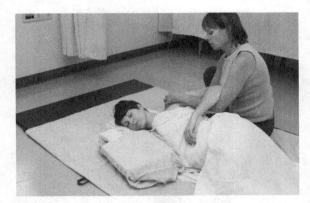

Fig. 9.1 Shoulder stretches side-lying.

Shoulder and neck stretches in side-lying position

Benefits

An excellent way to reduce tension in the shoulder and open up the chest.

The technique

Kneel or stand beside the client's back at the level of their shoulder. Take hold of their upper arm, linking both hands around their shoulder, so that the fingers are on top of the shoulder (Fig. 9.1).

Lean back so that the neck and shoulder are extended. Repeat this movement several times until the area relaxes. This is an excellent passive movement which lengthens the muscles (scalenes, trapezius, SCM) and meridians (GB, TH).

From this position the therapist can also perform some shoulder rotations and explore the range of movement of the shoulder joint. More detailed work of the meridians and muscles in the shoulder can also be undertaken.

Work for the neck and head (Fig. 9.2)

Keep the hand which is nearest to the client's body on the shoulder, applying slight pressure. Place the hand or forearm which is furthest from her body on the side of her head. Lean between the two hands to extend the top of the shoulder.

Effleurage down the side of their neck using hands or forearm. This is good for warming up the muscles and meridians here. Palming can also be used along the side of their head.

The therapist can use pressure techniques along these muscles or meridians. Thumb pressure, knuckle pressure, palm or forearm pressure can be applied.

Neck stretch

From the same position as above, use the hand which is nearest to the client's body to continue supporting

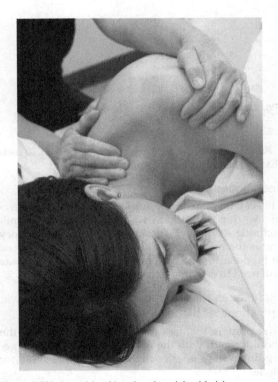

Fig. 9.2 Work to side of head and neck in side-lying.

and applying gentle extension to the shoulder. Rest the forearm of the other arm along the side of the neck, with the palm facing up. Gently slide and roll the forearm along the side of the neck up to the base of the occiput. Gently nudge the occiput with the forearm, just below the elbow, to give the neck an extra stretch (Fig. 9.3).

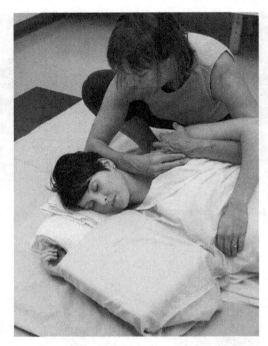

Fig. 9.3 Forearm stretch to side of neck in side-lying.

Repeat this procedure several times, until it feels that the head/neck have sufficiently relaxed.

Techniques for the face

This can be done in the supine position and is effective work postnatally as well as in pregnancy. Semi-reclining work can be done for the face in pregnancy and is the preferred working position. If work needs to be done for the face from the side, first one side will need to be worked, then the other.

Techniques for the upper back and shoulder blade

First prepare the area by keeping one hand on the shoulder and, with the other, palming or effleuraging down the upper back and around the shoulder blade.

Scapula stretch

This is a familiar stretch which can be effectively performed in the side (Fig. 9.4). Place the fingers of the hand which was palming under the medial border of the scapula. Use the other hand to retract the shoulder while applying pressure with the fingers or thumb under the scapula border. Work all around the border of the scapula. Repeat the pressures until the scapula feels released.

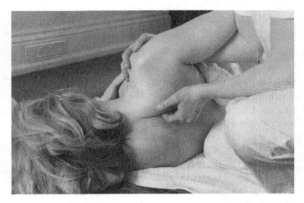

Fig. 9.4 Scapula release side.

The thumb or fingers can be applied along the border while elevating the scapula.

If the client's shoulder is sufficiently flexible, their shoulder can be more fully retracted and the arm placed against the back, as in the scapula release in the prone position. This may be a more effective way with some clients to perform the technique.

In any of these positions, work can be done systematically around the shoulder joint, and surrounding tissues. It can be useful to hold the attachments of a muscle, while working with finger effleurage and friction or vibration into the belly, or insertion of the muscle. This increases the stretch of the fibres, but remember to work slowly, in case the stretch reflex is stimulated. In this basic working position many of the neck and shoulder muscles and points can be worked such as teres, rotator cuff muscles, Yang and Yin Heel and SI work (Fig. 9.5). Pressures can also be applied to acupoints directly on the scapula or around the medial or superior borders can be worked (e.g. SI, TH, GB).

Trapezius release

The trapezius is a common site of chronic tension and hypertonicity. To perform the release in the side position there are two options:

Option 1 (Fig. 9.6) This is a technique which is often performed prone which can be effectively done in the side position. Work around the neck and shoulders with effleurage and petrissage to prepare the tissue to facilitate relaxation of the muscle. Place the hands on top of each other with the fingers moulding over the top of the clavicle at the insertions. Using body weight, gently, slowly and firmly apply pressure into the muscle while sliding the hands over the top of the clavicle and following the trapezius round into the back. Just over the superior border of the scapula it feels as though the muscle is gathering up. Keep

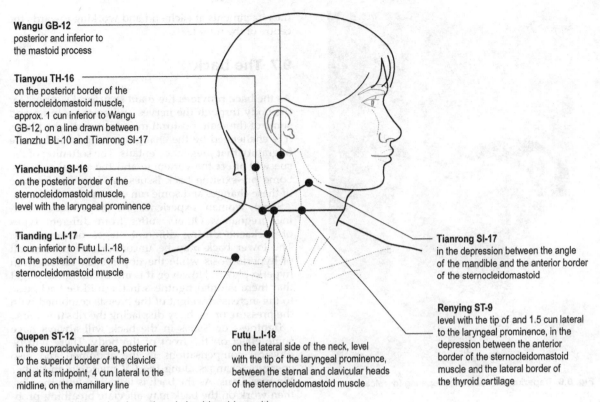

Wangu GB-12
posterior and inferior to
the mastoid process

Tianyou TH-16
on the posterior border of the
sternocleidomastoid muscle,
approx. 1 cun inferior to Wangu
GB-12, on a line drawn between
Tianzhu BL-10 and Tianrong SI-17

Yianchuang SI-16
on the posterior border of the
sternocleidomastoid muscle,
level with the laryngeal prominence

Tianding L.I-17
1 cun inferior to Futu L.I.-18,
on the posterior border of the
sternocleidomastoid muscle

Quepen ST-12
in the supraclavicular area, posterior
to the superior border of the clavicle
and at its midpoint, 4 cun lateral to the
midline, on the mamillary line

Futu L.I-18
on the lateral side of the neck, level
with the tip of the laryngeal prominence,
between the sternal and clavicular heads
of the sternocleidomastoid muscle

Tianrong SI-17
in the depression between the angle
of the mandible and the anterior border
of the sternocleidomastoid

Renying ST-9
level with the tip of and 1.5 cun lateral
to the laryngeal prominence, in the
depression between the anterior
border of the sternocleidomastoid
muscle and the lateral border of
the thyroid cartilage

Fig. 9.5 Meridian points in neck and shoulder side position.

applying pressure and the muscle will eventually start to release, feeling as though it is trickling through the fingers. Repeat again at least once, or more, as necessary.

Option 2 With your client on their side again, prepare the muscles of the upper trapezius with effleurage and kneading techniques. Feel along the upper margin of the muscle with the thumbs and note any areas of contraction. There may be a particular area of heat, or thickening, or hardness. Place the thumb into one of these areas and use firm but gentle pressure to release the point. A combination of holding into the point for some seconds, feeling how deeply and how long to hold, and then releasing and then repeating several times can provide effective release. Vibration can also be used into the muscle.

Rhomboids and levator scapulae

Working with the attachments This technique can be used on shorter muscle groups. It is not so effective for longer muscles as the distance between the attachments is greater. It is effective for these two muscle groups which are often contracted in pregnancy, as they are for many clients, due to modern sedentary and often desk-bound lifestyles.

Muscle testing can help ascertain whether the muscle is contracted (hypertonic) or lengthened (hypotonic). With hyperkyphosis the rhomboids may be lengthened rather than shortened, although due to underlying tension patterns there may be a degree of contraction. Assessment can be verified through palpation with general massage techniques such as effleurage and some passive movements of the shoulders. This will also prepare the tissue for deeper work and help rule out any injuries.

Work can then become focused around the attachments of the chosen muscle groups with techniques such as petrissage and friction. As this is done, palpation can reveal restrictions or hypotonicity in the muscle. In areas of hypotonicity, work can be done, such as with pressure techniques or gentle movement of the muscles, to build up strength.

If the muscle is hypertonic, use the thumb to stabilise a point along the attachment and stretch along the

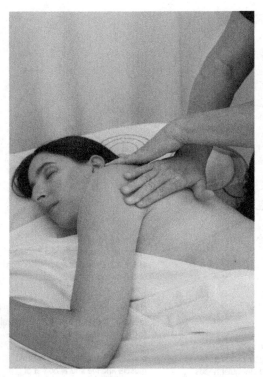

Fig. 9.6 Trapezius release side; preparing for release.

fibres of the muscle with the thumb or fingers of the other hand to the attachment at the other end of the muscle with the aim of slowly lengthening the muscle. For example, with contracted rhomboids, hold a point against the spine between T1 and T5 and stretch towards the scapula. For the levator scapula, hold with one thumb against the vertebrae (C1–C4) and stretch with the forearm or fingers/thumb along to the superior medial border of the scapula. Pressure should be applied to maximum depth of comfort for the client. If restrictions or points of tension are palpated in the belly of the muscle then these can be released with appropriate techniques, such as thumb or knuckle static pressures, or vibrations or frictions.

Once this work has been completed, use scapula stretches and shoulder rotations to help the muscle get used to being in the lengthened state.

If the muscle is weakened or lengthened, as the rhomboids may be in hyperkyphosis, then work around the attachments, including deeper work into the belly of the muscle, but without the stretch. Passive movements can then be included to help strengthen the muscle – with the rhomboids external rotations of the shoulder, with levator scapula upward rotation. Work can also be done using pressure from the attachments at each end and working towards the centre of the muscle.

9.7 The back

As the back provides the main structural support for the body through the nerves and spinal column and some of the main postural muscles are attached here, it is challenged by the changes in weight and centre of gravity that pregnancy entails. The softening of tissue will affect the vertebrae and the spinal muscles. Some pre-existing back issues can improve because of these changes and some can worsen.

Some women experience no back issues during pregnancy. Others suffer from different types of backache during different stages of pregnancy. The lower back may be uncomfortable as a result of hyperlordosis while the upper back suffers from hyperkyphosis. However, it is important not to forget that there is often tightness in the middle back, due to the increased weight of the breasts combined with the pressure of the baby displacing the ribs upwards.

Tightness or issues in the back will always have some effect on the front of the body. There will be physical compensations in the abdomen and also energetic changes along the CV meridian and other Yin meridians. As the back is linked in with the ribs, then work on the back may alleviate breathing problems. Tightness around T7 often correlates to tightness in the area just below the sternum. Releasing T7 may help alleviate heartburn.

The back responds well to bodywork in pregnancy and a main benefit of work is to increase postural awareness. It is vital therefore that appropriate postural exercises are shown alongside the hands-on work.

The initial focus of work to the back is to correct the pelvic tilt. This will involve work to lengthen and strengthen the lower back muscles (combined with abdominal strengthening work).

Deeper techniques to the lower back have often caused concern for therapists anxious that release here may affect the uterus, especially sacral work, because of the connections of the sacral nerves to the uterus. This has not been shown to be the case and indeed deep work to the sacrum and lower back becomes increasingly indicated with weight gain through the pregnancy. Deeper work in the pelvic area is generally not advised in the first trimester, but from around 18–20 weeks the depth of strokes can be increased according to the comfort of the client. Work can be done which includes deeper work to piriformis, and gluteals which are often hypertonic and sacrum. This can often release lower back pain, due to compression of sacral iliac nerve by tight muscles in this area.

First trimester work is helpful to gain an accurate picture of underlying energy and structural patterns pre-pregnancy. Deeper work on muscles such as the piriformis and quadratus lumborum is not so indicated in first trimester due to their proximity to the uterus which is undergoing significant changes, and potential pulling on the tendons combined with potential increased sensitivity and protectiveness of the woman. A gentler approach to this area is usually advised, especially during the first 8 weeks.

Postural assessment is best carried out standing before the treatment commences as much of the back work in pregnancy will be performed in the side position.

Type of strokes

The back torso can be worked with most of the strokes and techniques which are normally used with non-pregnant clients. A key focus of the work is often to utilise strokes which lengthen the lumbar spine, thus reducing anterior pelvic tilt. Alongside this, work will need to be done to address abdominal weakness.

The main issue is that if the side position is used there may be some asymmetry between stroke application and muscle response between the two sides, as the back is resting on the floor/table on one side only. This can make it more challenging to access the degree of release on the inferior side. It is therefore important to have the client lie on both sides to provide a thorough therapeutic approach to both sides of the back.

If the all fours position is used, then it is important to ensure that pressure is comfortable for the client with stroke application over the upper back, as the breasts may be compressed through the client resting over the ball or cushions. Lighter strokes also need to be utilised for the lumbar area which is less supported in this position: it is important not to increase lumbar lordosis or place stress on the vertebrae (Fig. 9.7).

Working positions

The side position is one of the main positions in which to fully work the back. The main focus of work is related to the spinal column and attachments such as the erector spinae bilaterally as well as the lateral muscles of both sides, though with an emphasis on the muscles that are on the superior side of the spine. The side resting on the table/floor will be worked more effectively when the client lies on her other side.

The forward leaning position provides a more accurate picture of postural patterns although work in the lumbar and upper back area is usually not as deep as in the side, due to ensuring breast comfort and the fact that the lumbar area is unsupported. In the forward leaning position, much of the therapist's work is already done; pressure

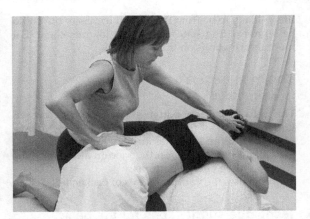

Fig. 9.7 All fours work to the back showing sacral and head hold. Note that upper back and lumbar areas should receive light pressure for breast comfort and due to the lumbar spine being unsupported.

has been taken off the lower back, the abdominals are engaged and the pelvis can begin to realign. It is useful to encourage the client to use forward leaning regularly to ease sacral tension and sciatica.

Prone positioning, even with body or pregnancy cushions, is not an ideal position to do any deeper work on the back and is not recommended by the authors for women during the second or third trimesters of pregnancy (see positioning issues).

Cautions

Deep cross fibre release work to the quadratus lumborum in the side-lying position which involves work towards the spine is less advised as this will tend to pull laterally on the abdominal wall and may feel uncomfortable as well as potentially pulling on the uterus and its supporting ligaments. However, work from the spine towards the lateral side of the body across the fibres is acceptable. Work can also include effleurage and stretching in the direction of the muscle fibres, which are often contracted (hypertonic), or static holds to release muscle tension to help to increase muscular relaxation.

The sacral and lower back area tends to be worked gently in the first trimester, because of the high relaxin levels which support the many internal changes (uterine, embryological) occurring in this area. As the pregnancy progresses and the weight of the baby increases strain on the sacrum, and the supporting musculature tends to be more contracted, it can be worked more specifically/vigorously. Attention must be paid to the balance between the sacrum/SI joints and the symphysis pubis. Problems may arise with pelvic instability; in a first pregnancy this is likely to be from the second trimester but could be a pre-existing state with a multiparous client. For more informations on this see p. 236.

Common patterns of the back in pregnancy

The three common patterns have been discussed under assessment (p. 187). These are: hyperkyphosis, hyperlordosis and the pressure caused by the increasing weight of the baby on the sacrum along with the corresponding energy patterns.

Box 9.1 lists the various causes of backache.

Technique suggestions for the back in the lateral and forward leaning positions (Figs 9.8–9.11)

We have selected techniques in the side position and the forward leaning position which are less familiar for the therapist.

Work with the erector spinae and bladder meridian in the back from the side position

To work the erector spinae, deeper techniques are often indicated such as: circling pressures, friction, transverse frictions, muscle stripping and stretching along the muscle fibres. These integrate well with shiatsu work to the Bladder meridian. Do work both sides, even if a slightly different pressure is utilised on each side.

Often, due to hyperlordosis, it may be more beneficial to use a stronger downward stroke in the lumbar area to encourage correction of anterior pelvic tilt. The upper back may benefit more from sweeping outward strokes which integrate with the arms.

With energy work, the Yang meridians tend to be worked downwards. The Bladder meridian lies in the centre of the erector spinae, with a second branch 1½ thumb-widths lateral to the first. A relaxing and connecting technique to work to balance Bladder is to place the palm of one hand in the lumbar area and with the other palm, palm down the erector spinae from the thoracics to the sacral area. Begin by palming to the side of the spine which is superior but also palm down the lower side of the spine. Ensure the hand position is comfortable in this less familiar position and that the wrists do not hyperextend.

- The therapist can do this work from the top of the head, working down; this is beneficial for strokes which lengthen the back (Fig. 9.9).

Box 9.1 Possible causes of backache

Immediate referral

- Suspected pre-term labour.

Referral after bodywork

- Kidney issues, unless the therapist feels they are urgent. These can be distinguished from musculoskeletal issues as they are not usually relieved with client change in position or activity.

Issues bodywork can support

- Musculoskeletal issues.
- Issues relating to the sacrum and uterus.
- Sacroiliac pain.
- Pelvic girdle instability.
- Discogenic issues.

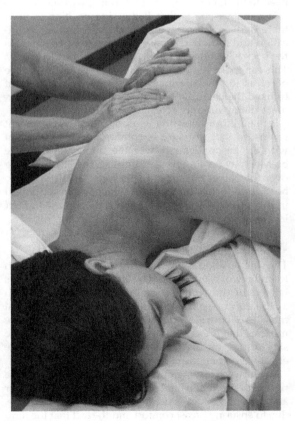

Fig. 9.8 Work on back: therapist facing back.

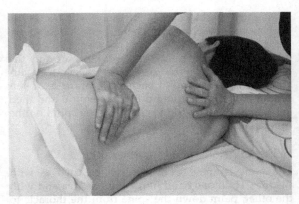

Fig. 9.9 Work on back: therapist at head and working down to hips.

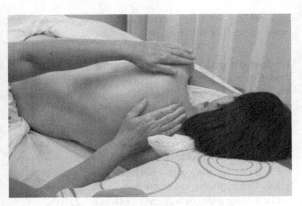

Fig. 9.11 Work on back: at hips up into shoulder.

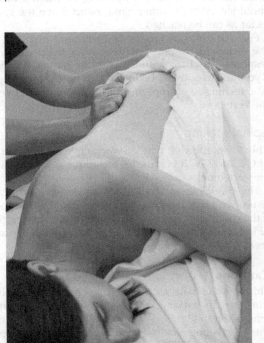

Fig. 9.10 Work on back: therapist facing back and working hips.

- They can work from the hips; this is beneficial for work which includes the shoulders (Fig. 9.10).
- They can face directly on to the back; this is beneficial for work which is more specific to the erector spinae and Bladder (Figs 9.8 and 9.10).

Important points on bladder line

The following three points are particularly important in pregnancy:

- Jinggong (*Palace of the Essence*) – coincides with BL52. It is on the outer Bladder line, three thumb-widths lateral to the space between L2 and L3. This is an important point to strengthen the Kidneys although more on a physical level than the deeper Kidney tonification level of its neighbouring points BL 23 (at the same level but medial to BL 52 in the erector spinae). It is indicated for regulating urination and for oedema. It is used in the treatment of pain that spreads widely to the muscles of the lumbar region.
- BL51 *Vitals gate* – 3 cun (or thumbwidths) lateral to the midline. Lateral to BL 22, back transporting point of Triple Heater. The Qi of TH is essential for proper movement and transportation of Qi in all physiological processes. Its action extends up to chest and downwards to Bladder and uterus. Used in postpartum abdominal pain, breast lumps and breast pain. It is therefore also useful postnatally.
- BL 53 *Bladder's Vitals* – 3 *cun* lateral to midline, level with spinous process of second sacral vertebra. Its action affects the abdomen, bladder, uterus and genitals.

Direct work with the spine (Governing Vessel) – in the side position

In Swedish massage therapists are wary of working directly with the spine. However, some work to the vertebrae is often indicated in pregnancy, especially with an energy focus as opposed to a physical focus.

In working with the vertebrae the scope of practice must always be adhered to.

Important points on the GV line and their actions

The GV points lie between the spinous processes of the vertebrae. Some important ones in pregnancy are:

- GV 2 *Transporting point of lower back* – junction of sacrum and coccyx. Can be used in chronic sacral backache from Kidney Yang deficiency.
- GV 3 *Lumbar Yang gate* – between L4/5 (iliac crest L4). Strengthens lower back.
- GV 4 *Ming Men: gate of life* – between L2/3 (navel level). This is the most powerful point for strengthening Kidney Yang and all Yang energies in general. It tonifies and warms the fire of the Gate of Vitality. It strengthens original Qi (related to pre-Heaven Qi) and therefore is indicated for chronic weakness on a physical and mental level. It strengthens the lower back which is often slightly weakened in pregnancy due to the focus of sending energy to the fetus. It eliminates cold from the uterus and intestine. It can be used for abdominal pain and infertility.
- GV 9 – below T7 (level to inferior angle of scapula, at the bottom tip of the shoulder blade T7/8). This regulates the Liver and Gall Bladder. It affects the chest and abdomen and is used when there is stagnation of Qi in the middle burner, which is often the case in pregnancy.
- GV 11 – below T5 – same level as BL 15 (5/6 T)-Heart Yu. Its action extends to the Heart; and there are many emotional and Blood changes in pregnancy.
- GV 12 below T3 – same level as BL 13 (3/4 T)-Lung Yu. It tonifies the Lungs; as the body needs more air in pregnancy, this is an important point.

It is advisable to first do some work with the erector spinae/Bladder before doing work on the spine itself. This will help to identify if there are any local problems with any of the vertebrae, as this is often reflected in these muscles. If there are local issues then direct work would be avoided in those areas. By relaxing the muscles, the structures of the spine can be felt more easily.

Effleurage down the GV/spine

When commencing work with the spine, begin with the lighter strokes to identify any potential spinal issues. Begin making contact with GV with light effleurage strokes down the spine, using the fingertips. If this is comfortable for the client, stroke depth can be slightly increased. The pressure will not be as deep as with the erector spinae, as bone and joints are being worked with, rather than muscles.

Next some firmer fingertip stroking around the vertebrae can be introduced. This can be as a circling movement around each vertebra or as a spiralling movement, going down in a spiral and then starting back at the top to complete the spiral on the other side.

Spine/GV holding and connecting

The same palming technique can be used as with Bladder. Hold one hand in the lumbar area and with the other, palm down the spine from the thoracic to lumbar areas. An alternative position for the mother hand can be to have it supporting on the top of the shoulder. With the other hand, palm down the spine as far as can be reached.

Feel for areas of tension, either more physical, in the vertebrae, or more energetic. Vary the pressure in response to what is felt beneath the hands. Balance, Kyo and Jitsu areas. Follow this with the more specific technique of applying thumb pressure between the vertebrae.

Spinal rocking

This is an effective way of working with the energy of CV and GV. It is a useful technique for mobilising the vertebrae.

The mobilisation should not be done if there are issues with the vertebrae and should be discontinued if the client feels any pain or discomfort. When beginning the rocking, start gently, in order to identify any areas which will not respond well.

Cautions

This is not usually such a good technique for the first trimester. Its rocking motion may be unsettling at a time when the body is in a state of change and if the client is feeling sick, will tend to aggravate the feelings of nausea. Furthermore, at this stage, the spine is not yet experiencing the increased loads of later pregnancy and so it is less indicated.

The technique (Fig. 9.12)

The first three steps can be done with one hand around the shoulder (the hand closest to the client's body), as in the shoulder stretch (Figs 9.1 and 9.4):

1. Use the free hand to spiral with gentle pressures around the spinous processes in a figure of eight-type movement (as in Effleurage down the GV/Spine).
2. Hold each side of the spinous process.

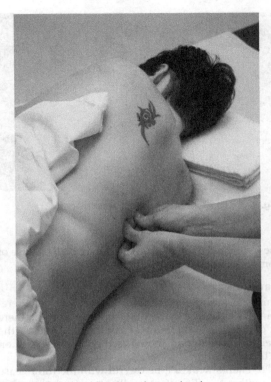

Fig. 9.12 Spinal mobilisation using two hands.

There are several hand positions which may work:

   (i) Fingers and thumb holding each side of the vertebrae.

   (ii) Knuckles.

3. **Mobilise the vertebrae.** There are three rocking movements that can be performed:

   (i) From side to side (i.e. medial to lateral across the spine) which in the side position translates to up and down (from the inferior side of the spine to the superior). This is the hardest movement to do, as it is working against gravity on the upward part of the movement. It often works better to do it as two separate movements: first lift the inferior aspect of the spine away from the table/floor and then push down on the superior aspect of the spine.

   (ii) From head to toe (i.e. superior to inferior).

   (iii) In and out (i.e. from posterior to anterior – from the back to the front).

See which direction the vertebrae most easily move in – do not force them. Only one or two of the movements may feel easy and there may be resistance in the others. The movements which feel easy may change in different parts of the spine.

These three steps can then be repeated with the therapist facing the body, holding the vertebrae with both hands and rocking them.

The three different movements can be performed. Make sure that the hands are positioned close together so that only small segments of vertebrae are worked at a time (Fig. 9.12).

Sacral work

This can often be worked quite deeply and usually more deeply as the pregnancy progresses. Deeper pressures must always be assessed according to the comfort of each client and should never cause pain or discomfort. They need to be worked up to gradually. The sacrum is one of the key areas where women appreciate strong work during labour and the techniques are described on p. 302–305. The same type of work can be used during pregnancy in the second and third trimester, although it is usually lighter earlier on, becoming deeper as the pregnancy and labour progress.

Deep sacral work can be done in the side-lying position, but is often most effective in a forward leaning position as the sacrum can be accessed evenly on both sides and the weight of the gravid uterus is taken off it. This work should not be done with the client prone, as it is likely to cause too much pressure to be placed on the uterus/baby and it would not be comfortable for the client.

Stretches for the back and side

These stretches are especially beneficial in the second and third trimesters when the woman is beginning to feel the physical challenges from the weight of the growing baby. However, if the woman is physically active and wants some work to the side of the body in the first trimester, they are not contraindicated.

Side stretch (Figs 9.13, 9.14)

This stretch is beneficial for lengthening the side of the body. It works on stretching out the quadratus lumborum, latissimus dorsi and serratus posterior. It also opens up the ribs, intercostals, oblique muscles and, to some degree, the iliopsoas. It releases tension locally in the hip and the shoulder. It releases the energy of the meridians of the Gall Bladder, Triple Heater, Small Intestine, Yin and Yang Linking Vessel. After this stretch, more specific work can be done into these muscles and meridians using the web of the hands or thumb pressure.

Face the client, with the body placed midway between her hip and shoulder. Cross the hands, placing one hand just below the axilla on the side and the other hand on the hip. Leaning the body weight,

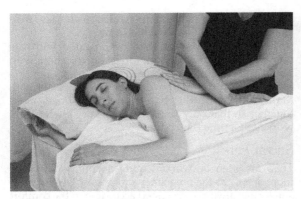

Fig. 9.13 Side stretch with palms.

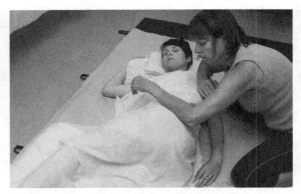

Fig. 9.15 Hip and shoulder stretch simultaneously.

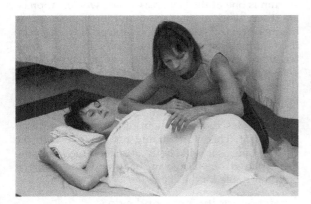

Fig. 9.14 Side stretch with forearms.

apply hand pressure in a lateral application to stretch the tissue away from itself, thus stretching the lateral fascia and the muscles (Fig. 9.13).

This stretch can also be done using forearms, in which case the arms are not crossed and pressure can be applied by laterally rolling out the forearms (Fig. 9.14).

With both versions, it is important that the majority of the pressure is applied parallel to the side of the body and not straight down into the hips and the shoulder. Downwards pressure would simply compress the hip and the shoulder and not achieve the goal of a longitudinal stretch.

A stretch can also be performed for the hip and the shoulder at the same time (Fig. 9.15).

Piriformis release

Benefits

This technique is often indicated in the second and third trimesters. A contracted piriformis is part of the hyperlordotic patterning and may be the cause of compression on the sciatic nerve.

Cautions

This is a significant soft tissue release which is therefore less indicated in the first trimester. Further, there is not the same amount of contraction due to the weight of the gravid uterus as there will be later on in the pregnancy.

For clients with SPI, be careful with the full release as, without sufficient strengthening work for other muscle groups (e.g. abdominals and lower back), it may destabilise the pelvis further.

The technique

Orthopaedic tests can be performed to assess the side of the more contracted piriformis. Other clinical observations of the hips (e.g. observing the external rotation of the feet) and palpation can also be included.

This technique is often more effective with the client in the side position, as opposed to prone or forward leaning, as the gluteals are in neutral and it is easy to access the piriformis. Begin by warming up the tissue. This can be done either through the clothes or sheet, if the client prefers, or directly on the skin with lotion or oil. Begin with effleurage and then apply deeper petrissage and frictions to the gluteals. When the gluteals are more relaxed, palpate and apply deeper pressure to access the belly of the piriformis. Palpate into the buttock between the sacrum and the top of the femur. The most tender point here will be the release point mid-muscle.

Keeping the thumb in the belly of the piriformis, place the other thumb resting along the side of the sacrum, stabilising the origin. Now give gentle pressure into the release point for a few seconds as the client breathes out. The exact amount of time and pressure will be determined by how much the muscle

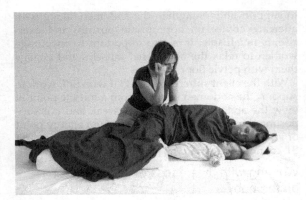

Fig. 9.16 Piriformis release elbow side.

relaxes. Once the muscle has relaxed maximally, gradually release out of the muscle. This may need to be repeated several times in order to achieve maximal relaxation. Between each time, effleurage can help the muscles relax, ready for the next release.

If more pressure is needed then the elbow or fist can be used rather than the thumb (Fig. 9.16). Place the elbow with the forearm at a 90° or greater angle to the upper arm. Wrap the other hand around the elbow to stop it slipping off the muscle. Gradually raise the forearm to increase the pressure in the elbow and hold with pressure.

Repeat this several times, and wait for release (heat, tingling, softening).

Palpate the piriformis on the client's other side to assess for muscle tension or contraction. Perform the technique bilaterally if indicated.

This area may need repetitive treatments as it frequently contracts due to pregnancy posture.

9.8 Chest/abdomen and front of body: changes and working principles

The abdomen

Since this area, like the back, undergoes major change in pregnancy, knowing how to work it safely and effectively is important. Many myths exist regarding bodywork in this area. It is not uncommon to find massage texts advising against touching the abdomen not just during the first trimester but throughout the pregnancy. These precautions seem to be based on a vague fear of causing harm to the client or fetus rather than a sound therapeutic rationale.

The abdomen needs to be approached with respect, sensitivity and a clear understanding of what is occurring with each specific week of the pregnancy. There are certain cautions regarding types of strokes and times when it would be less advisable to use certain types of strokes. However, there is no reason why the abdomen should not be massaged if sound treatment protocols are followed. Indeed in many traditional cultures (Davis-Floyd 1999, Kitzinger 2000, Priya 1992) abdominal massage in pregnancy was and still is a key part of care. It often includes fairly vigorous work, especially if the aim is to help with good fetal positioning. For many women self-abdominal massage is an instinctive and intuitive way of connecting with their changing body and baby (Verney 2002). In modern cultures, the primary care provider will palpate the abdomen at various stages throughout the pregnancy. Initially this is to feel fundal height and assess fetal growth; in the last trimester it is also to assess fetal position. This type of palpation involves deep, and at times uncomfortably deep, pressures, with no increased harm to the baby.

Of course, the therapist always needs to respect how the client feels about someone else touching her pregnant abdomen. Even if women are massaging their own abdomen, they may need time to trust the therapist to work on it. For women who are wary of massaging their own abdomen, it is usually best to encourage them to do so before the therapist starts to work on it. The therapist can also encourage partners to massage the abdomen and teach them some simple strokes. As the woman gains in confidence with touch, strokes can gradually be included. Initially a light touch through a sheet, perhaps focusing with the woman's breathing pattern or even working through her hands, may be sufficient. Gradually more vigorous strokes can be utilised and work directly on the skin with oil can be commenced. A woman's relationship to her abdomen can change substantially during pregnancy – often women who normally would not enjoy abdominal work love it. Touch and subtle communication can support a woman's awareness of her changing body. However, if she does not want abdominal work, that choice needs to be respected.

Key principles for working on the pregnant abdomen

First trimester work

More caution should be exercised with abdominal massage in the first trimester while the uterus is accommodating for implantation and development of the placenta. Deep physical work with the abdomen is less indicated. This is not necessarily because it will cause harm. Indeed the uterus is still a pelvic organ in the first trimester and is well protected. Rather, it is because the woman will probably feel quite protective of this area as a result of the significant emotional and physical changes she is experiencing.

Musculoskeletal and structural changes

Through the pregnancy there are many changes going on in the abdominal area, from a muscular and also an internal organ point of view. In terms of muscles, the abdominal muscles are being stretched by the growing baby. By the second trimester the uterus is rising into the abdomen and by the end of the third trimester it is under the ribs. The rectus abdominis muscles lengthen and separate. The transverse muscle of the abdomen and the obliques are pulled laterally. It is important not to put further stretch into already stretched muscle groups. This means that all the work on the abdominal muscles tends to utilise the stronger stroke towards the midline, to support the stretched recti, oblique and transverse muscles. When working between the ribs and the pubic bone, emphasise the stroke to shorten longitudinally as opposed to lengthening, as there are many of the attachments for the abdominal and pelvic floor muscles here.

Deeper abdominal muscles such as the iliopsoas can not be worked directly as they lie inferior to the baby but they may be indirectly accessed through stretches.

In terms of the uterus itself, techniques must not be performed which pull on the ligaments, especially the broad and round ligaments. This means that the angles of pressure need to be in the direction of holding the uterus and therefore involve pressure from the abdomen towards the centre of the body, with the hand cupping around the form of the uterus so that there is no pull on the skin. Further, there should be no techniques which apply pressure directly down on to the top of the uterus (the fundus) as this may stimulate contractions.

The therapist needs to be aware of the size and location of the uterus and the baby so that work, including depth of pressure and sensitive contact, can be appropriate and comfortable for the client.

In terms of the digestive system, the stroke should be performed in a clockwise direction to support the movement of the intestines. The intestines lie behind the baby by the third trimester and they cannot be accessed directly but, none the less, their direction of flow should be respected.

Balance is vital between the abdomen and back. Often back hypertonicity is an attempt to balance the pregnant abdomen, and this may accentuate previous weakness in the musculature, ligaments or structural alignment of the lower back. The weakened abdominal muscles may contribute to hyperlordosis. Work to support and strengthen the abdomen, along with aftercare advice on appropriate posture and exercise, is invaluable. It is also important to encourage women to relax the abdominal muscles and engage them with pelvic floor exercises.

With the client suffering from PGI with SPI, work to support the abdomen is vital. From a muscle point of view the abdominal muscles are weak and not supporting the joints of the pelvis. From an energy point of view the core meridians of the PV and the CV and ST are not supporting the joints.

Working with awareness of stroke effect on the baby

It can be helpful to encourage the woman to make contact with her baby as much as is appropriate, even in the first trimester when it is more at the level of an energy connection. The therapist can also try to tune into the energy of the baby, with permission of the client. As the baby grows in size, then a more physical connection can begin and the strokes of the abdomen can become firmer. The baby is well protected by the amniotic fluid, the walls of the uterus and muscles of the abdomen and yet is often responsive to touch and may even move towards the hands of the therapist. The woman usually begins to feel excited about including the baby in the work from 16 weeks when she can feel a response and the risk of potential miscarriage is much reduced. Some women do not want to connect with their baby until around this time. However, other women like to connect on a more intuitive level with their baby before.

As the baby gets bigger, hand contact needs to be moulded to the shape of the baby so that there is no pull on its body. Some pressure can be applied with the woman's breathing and responding to her comfort levels. Pressure should be applied at 90° to the body and aimed towards the woman's back so as not to pull on the tissue.

In terms of fetal position, which is a factor in the last trimester, bodywork may involve stroking down one side of the abdomen in the reverse direction to that which supports the digestive system, for example in order to encourage the head to move to the pelvis.

Work with the baby tends to be intuitive. Apart from being aware of the fetus's position and physical response, the therapist may 'tune in' to the baby. Different babies respond differently to touch. Some may be alert and aware and their movements can be playful. Other babies are still and appear to be relaxed or sleeping.

Energy work on the abdomen

Hara assessment and work to specific points may become more challenging as the pregnancy progresses.

In the first trimester it is more like working on a non-pregnant abdomen, although being sensitive to the woman and how she feels to the touch. However, as the baby takes up more of the abdomen its energy can tend to dominate and the therapist needs to be able to differentiate between maternal and fetal energies. Sometimes the baby will be so active and communicative that it is not possible to ignore it, while at other times the woman's energy will be clearer.

Points below the umbilicus tend not to be used by acupuncturists in pregnancy and points above the umbilicus only in the first 3 months. The rationale behind this is to prevent potential problems being caused by insertion of the needle. However, this does not necessarily make sense as the uterus does not reach the level of the navel until around 22 + weeks and the depth of insertion is unlikely to be so deep as to penetrate into the uterus. In bodywork, as the pressure can be varied, this caution does not apply.

Conception Vessel brings energy to the centre; Spleen in legs brings energy up and supports muscle and organs; Kidney and Kidney-Uterus support deep energy and help with fatigue; Penetrating Vessel balances Blood energy; Heart-Uterus balances Blood energy, is emotionally calming for the baby and helps the mother's connection with baby. Girdle Vessel can support ligaments, joints and deep abdominal muscles as well as helping balance energy from front to back. CV3–5 and Uterus points all help with abdominal pain.

Energy work in the different trimesters

First trimester

Deep ampuku style techniques would generally not be appropriate due to the huge changes in the area. Deeper point work can be included depending on the mother's preference. Although physically the baby is tiny, it is growing so rapidly it is often possible to pick up on its energy. This tends to be experienced as buzzing and active.

Second and third trimesters

As the woman can feel her the baby move, work needs to include an awareness of the two energies. Deeper work may be more appropriate, although with any physical techniques the guidelines outlined in the musculoskeletal section need to be adhered to.

Summary of principles of working on the pregnant abdomen

- If the pregnant client presents with any unexplained severe abdominal pain or discomfort,

always refer first to her primary care provider for assessment prior to commencing bodywork.
- Lighter work on the abdomen, even simply holding techniques, is usually more appropriate in the first trimester. Work can become more physical, depending on the client's preference and state of health, as the pregnancy progresses.
- Include awareness of stroke effect on the baby.

Musculoskeletal principles

- Emphasise the stroke towards the midline from the hips.
- Emphasise the stroke shortening between the pubic bone and the ribs – work longitudinally towards the navel (i.e. strokes from pubic bone to navel and from ribs to navel, not stretching out from the navel).
- Work in a clockwise direction to support the digestive system.
- Support the uterus and its ligaments in terms of stroke and pressure direction and do not overstretch tissues which are experiencing stretching.
- Effleurage, flat-handed techniques and even gentle kneadings or superficial fascial techniques may be utilised. Deeper strokes such as vigorous or strong kneading, frictions and tapotement should never be used. 'Gentle but firm' may be a guideline for depth of pressure which is similar to that used on the newborn with baby massage.

Benefits of abdominal work

- The increasing size of the uterus places pressure on the abdominal organs, such as stomach, liver, intestines and in working the abdomen these strains may be alleviated.
- The connection with the baby can be important for prenatal bonding and relaxation and may help support the baby getting into an optimal position for birth.
- Work can be done to help keep some tone and strength in the abdominal muscles, especially the rectus abdominis muscles.
- The skin may benefit from the application of oil due to the stretching which occurs. While stretch marks are primarily determined by weight gain and the elasticity of the skin, oil will help nourish the skin and may help alleviate some of the discomfort experienced through the stretching.
- Lymphatic work can help reduce fluid retention which may be experienced in the abdomen in the second and third trimesters.

Types of techniques

These have been largely outlined in the principles. See also section 9.9.

Working positions

- In the first trimester work can usually be done supine.
- From the second trimester work is usually done in the side position.
- From the third trimester forward leaning can be included, which may help the baby settle in the anterior position as well as creating more space both for the baby and for the abdominal organs.

Cautions

- It is important at all times to make sure that no techniques create strain for the uterus or its ligaments or for the abdominal muscles.
- Techniques such as direct work with the psoas and ileocaecal valve work are too deep for any stage of pregnancy. They become suitable in the later stages of the postnatal period and are outlined there.
- If there is ever any concern about the integrity of the placenta, particularly if there has been a history of bleeding which may indicate possible placental abruption, even once the client has been given the all clear, work to the abdomen should be limited to light, even off the body energy work and encouraging the client to connect with her breath. This is because any pressure, even stroking, could potentially cause the placenta to detach.
- If there is any pain when working over the abdomen, then the work should be discontinued.

Pain needs to be identified as to its source. If the therapist has any concern that the pain is not musculoskeletal then they need to refer the client immediately to their primary caregiver.

- It is not uncommon during the last few weeks of pregnancy for the client and therapist to feel the uterus contracting. This could be the early Braxton Hicks contractions or even, if working past 38 weeks, early labour contractions. The client will probably not want any work done to the abdomen other than gentle holding while the contraction is present. However, once the contraction has ended, after a couple of minutes, then work appropriate to that stage of pregnancy can resume.
- If the uterus presents as hard, like in a contraction, but the contraction does not fade after a couple of minutes work should be stopped and the woman referred to her primary care provider. This could indicate placental problems (such as retroplacental clots). Be aware, however, that the uterus does feel quite firm at the end of pregnancy, so do not unduly worry the client. Retroplacental clots are quite rare.
- Oligohydramnios and polyhydramnios (too little or too much amniotic fluid) are potential cautions as they may indicate pathologies. This diagnosis will need to be made by the primary care provider. It is a tricky diagnosis to make and in many cases does not necessarily indicate any problems. If there is no underlying pathology then some gentle abdominal work may be considered although more at an energy/connection level rather than a physical level.

Causes of abdominal pain in pregnancy are outlined in Box 9.2.

Box 9.2 Abdominal pain in pregnancy

There are many types of abdominal discomfort which women may experience during pregnancy. Most are not dangerous, but some may be the signs of serious conditions which need immediate medical referral. It is important for the therapist to understand the types of abdominal pain. If in doubt, it is best to err on the side of caution, referring the client to their primary care provider, and not treating until medically clear. This should be done without unduly alarming the client.

Severe continuous abdominal pain: emergency referral

Causes include:

- *Ectopic/tubal pregnancy – first trimester.* When the tube ruptures there will be severe intraperitoneal haemorrhage and the women will experience

intense abdominal pain. There may also be referred shoulder tip pain on lying down as blood tracks up to the diaphragm. The woman will appear pale, shocked and nauseous and may collapse. This is an acute surgical emergency and requires immediate treatment.

- *Acute appendicitis – any time.* This is the most common cause of emergency non-pregnancy-related issues during pregnancy.
- *Gallbladder issues: suspected gallstones cholelithiasis.* This is the second most common cause for emergency non-pregnancy related issues during pregnancy.
- *Threatened abortion (miscarriage).* Lower abdominal pain which will probably extend to the lower back.

- *Placental issues: placental abruption, placenta praevia.* A hardened uterus which does not soften as would be expected with Braxton Hicks may indicate placental problems. There may also be bleeding (see p. 378).
- *Perforation of a duodenal ulcer.*
- *Acute pancreatitis.*
- *Retroverted uterus.* Abdominal pain with inability to urinate: can be a sign of a retroverted uterus which has become fixed. Referral is required as the bladder needs to be drained, after which the uterus usually corrects position.
- *Hydatiform mole.* Abdominal pain accompanied by sickness.
- *HELLP syndrome.* Deviation of PET, pain in upper right quadrant of abdomen – this may be the only symptom.

Moderate abdominal pain

If the therapist and client feel that there is no imminent danger and the client would benefit from bodywork prior to visiting their primary care giver the treatment may continue, although any physical work to the abdomen would be avoided. If both client and therapist are uncomfortable with continuing then referral should be immediate. It may be hard to decide the best course of action and the individual therapist must decide based on their skill level and knowledge of the client. Moderate abdominal pain in the absence of other serious symptoms would tend to represent milder conditions in the less acute stage as listed below. However there are two cases of emergency referral.

- *Suspected tubal pregnancy.* Although this may present with moderate to mild abdominal pain, if the woman describes vaginal bleeding, especially following intercourse, this is an emergency referral issue.
- *Preterm labour.* If this is suspected then immediate referral is required.

- *Urinary tract infection.* If it is suspected but the woman is able to urinate and does not have other symptoms such as fever, bodywork may continue, but immediate referral after treatment is important.
- *Gallbladder disease (cholecystitis or billiary colic).* If there is no current pain but the therapist suspects it may be an issue then bodywork may continue but immediate referral is important.
- *Fibroids and cysts.* Work can proceed as per the comfort of the client but if undiagnosed fibroids or

cysts are suspected, refer back to primary caregiver for further diagnosis and monitoring.
- *Moderate aches around previous caesarean incision.* This can indicate weakness with the scar so holding/energy techniques only should be employed and the client referred back to the primary healthcare provider for further advice and support. If the client is concerned then immediate referral.

Mild, physiological 'normal' kinds of pain

Provided basic principles of abdominal work are followed and the woman is comfortable, there should be no immediate referral issues. It is helpful if the client mentions the symptoms to her primary care provider but bodywork should be able to continue using appropriate techniques as per the comfort of the client.

- *Stretching of uterine ligaments:*
  - Broad: low, sharp abdominal pain which is often on one side or the other, especially in first trimester; second trimester pain usually less but increases again in third trimester and may be referred to the groin and back.
  - Round: one-sided diagonal pain from top of uterus to groin; can often be a brief stabbing pain or longer dull ache, usually beginning from the second trimester.
  - Uterosacral ligaments: could be cause of aching in the sacrum, especially in the third trimester.

- *Pressure from the fetus.* Fetus kicking, engaging, pushing.
- *Stretching of the abdominal wall.* Stretching feeling, dragging, heavy feelings in the muscle.
- *Braxton Hicks contractions.* Provided these are intermittent, irregular and not strong, with no backache or breaking of water then work may proceed.
- *Stretching under ribs.*
- *Ribflare.*
- *Mild aches around previous caesarean incision.* This can indicate weakness with the scar so holding/energy techniques only should be employed and the client referred back to the primary healthcare provider for further advice and support.
- *Symphysis pubis pain.*
- *Pain around the pubic bone.*
- *Heartburn and constipation.*

The chest and breasts

This is an area where many changes occur. Like the abdomen, it is an area in which many therapists are wary of working and may indeed have been told not to work. This relates to a lack of knowledge and understanding of the profound therapeutic benefits of breast massage. Many pregnant women experience tenderness, discomfort or breast pain which is a result of the normal changes of the body. Women are often unaware that breast massage is an option for promoting healthy breast tissue and easing some of these discomforts. Explanations of how bodywork

Dialogue: Cindy and Suzanne

Suzanne

As both a shiatsu practitioner and massage therapist, I have always loved working with pregnant women's abdomens. I remember from my own first pregnancy, in 1990, I had some wonderful massages from a colleague but she never did much work on the abdomen. I had to go home and work on it myself and get my partner to massage it too. I found it a lovely way of communicating with my babies and I think it is something very instinctive that women do when they are pregnant. Provided I trusted the person who was working with me, I was quite comfortable with having my abdomen touched. I had quite a lot of shiatsu also during my pregnancies, and found I really did enjoy the pressure work.

Of course everyone is different, and some women are going to enjoy work on the abdomen more than others. However, in my experience, I find that once I do start working with the abdomen, my clients generally love it.

I always feel very privileged when mothers in the first trimester feel comfortable enough with my touch to let me connect with their abdomens. There is such a buzz of energy. I do not think I have ever felt drawn to doing deep work, but with some women I simply hold gently and connect, with others I might work in a few different areas, connecting both with the energy of the baby and with Hara diagnostic areas. Sometimes when I work with women who are used to bodywork, they are quite happy for some gentle effleurage with oil.

Later, the energy of the baby becomes clear and the mums usually love someone else communicating with their baby. The baby often responds, either by going to sleep or by kicking and becoming playful. It really

does feel like working with two people. Sometimes I get a clear sense of the baby in the womb, but I am always careful not to feed back too literally what I have felt. Usually it has been positive but sometimes I have had babies who have been breech or I have picked up on feelings of unease or discomfort: I do not talk about those kind of things with the mother unless she initiates the conversation. It could just be 'my stuff' and even if it is not, I feel it is important to encourage the client to communicate directly with her baby, rather than through me.

I also feel that abdominal work is a great opportunity for the partner to connect with their baby in a very tangible way from the second trimester.

Cindy

Many therapists feel nervous about working on the abdomen of their pregnant clients, but like Suzanne, I present this option in an open and enthusiastic way. Like most aspects of bodywork, if the therapist is confident and knowledgeable, the client is much more likely to feel at ease with their treatment choices. A full explanation of how abdominal massage is done, including a comparison of the difference in pressure utilised by the therapist relative to that used by the obstetrician or midwife, listing the indications for abdominal massage and an openness to accept whatever decision the client makes, often increases the client's willingness to try out this abdominal work. For many women it can also be considered baby's first 'therapeutic massage' – an idea that often delights many women! It is an excellent first opportunity for the mother to experience nurturing touch with the baby growing inside her.

can benefit the pregnant woman can be given and then it is the decision of the client whether she wishes to try this option as part of her treatment.

Towards the end of the pregnancy, breast work can be done which will support the physical changes in the tissues and help prepare the woman's body for breastfeeding.

Thankfully, pioneering work by registered Canadian massage therapists Debra Curties, Pam Hammond and Pam Firth have resulted in educational workshops throughout North America that have now widely been integrated in the curriculum of North American massage therapy colleges and postgraduate training. For more information about the therapeutic benefits of breast massage, see Curties (1999).

Testimonial

During both my pregnancies, I felt both soreness and congestion in my breasts. I found breast massage to be very relaxing and appreciated having it included in my pregnancy treatments. I found that I got instant relief from both the soreness and the feeling of congestion. I feel my overall breast health was improved. I also feel more connected to this very important part of my body. I continue to receive breast massage as part of my routine massage therapy care post delivery. I feel that regular breast massage can benefit all women at all times, and that there are very specific indications for it during pregnancy due to the hormonal and physiological changes that occur. Breast massage is something that is easy for a massage therapist to teach to a client for self-care purposes in addition to including breast massage in treatment sessions. Once women understand the structure and function of the breast and lymphatic system, learn how easy it is to do on themselves, they really appreciate having this knowledge. My clients report that breast massage helps improve their general breast health. I see breast massage as a way to improve both drainage and tissue health in the breast area.

Canadian Massage Therapist

From the first trimester there are significant changes in the breasts, and for many women, heaviness in the breasts is one of the first signs of being pregnant. They are often quite sensitive and gentle bodywork may be appropriate.

As the pregnancy progresses, the breasts become fuller and heavier and pull down, contributing to shortening in the pectoral region. These changes may also restrict breathing, especially if accompanied by poor posture. The fetus pushing up towards the ribs in the last trimester can cause the woman to feel bruising and discomfort along the lower costal margin (commonly known as 'rib flare'). Clients often appreciate work here to open up the chest and diaphragm, to encourage deeper breathing patterns and create the feeling of more space.

Tightness in the upper back and shoulders will tend to aggravate tension and discomfort in the breasts, so work often needs to be done to address concerns in those areas too.

If the woman is considering breastfeeding, then work with the breasts can form part of her preparation, and may increase comfort on both an emotional and physical level. Work can also be done to support the lymphatic changes and help to prevent mastitis.

Types of techniques

- Work can be done with different types of stretches to release tensions and tightness in both the energies and muscles of the chest and breast area.
- Direct and indirect work can be done in the rib and intercostal areas. These techniques will tend to be less deep than with the non-pregnant client, due to the changes in the tissue and the expansion and pressures on the rib cage.

- If the client is not comfortable with direct work on the breasts, then work can be done around the breast tissue. Direct work on the breasts can be done either directly on the skin with oil or over the sheet. The client can also be shown techniques which she can do herself. This can help prepare both physically and psychologically for breastfeeding.
- Be aware of the possibility that colostrum could leak from the areola during the session. The therapist needs to treat colostrum as any other bodily fluid, exercising universal standards of infection control. When treating any lactating woman directly on the breast, this would mean wearing gloves during this aspect of the treatment.
- Lymphatic style work in the breast area can often be effective, comfortable and supportive.

Working positions

Work on the breasts is often done more towards the end of the pregnancy and side-lying and semi-reclining are usually the most appropriate positions at this stage. Both positions are effective for accessing and treating the breasts and including shoulder and pectoral work. Side-lying, with the therapist positioned behind the client's body, may feel less threatening if the client is shy or new to this aspect of treating her body.

Cautions

Women need clear explanations from the therapist about the benefits of breast work. Work should not be carried out on the breasts, especially directly on the skin, without first obtaining the client's consent. Clear instruction and informed consent is crucial. There may be gender issues and the client may feel less comfortable with a male therapist doing breast massage.

9.9 Chest/abdomen and front of body: techniques

These techniques are grouped together as some involve working with both the abdomen and breast. The client may find it more acceptable if the breasts are linked in with other work on the front of the body.

Abdominal pressures/holds/strokes/kidney/uterus

Benefits

This is a simple and non-invasive technique to begin to make a connection with the client, her abdomen and baby. It can be done through the sheet if the client is not sure about whether she wants to have direct work on the skin with oil/lotion. It can also be done after some oil/lotion has been applied to the abdomen.

Cautions

Since this is a technique which can be light in nature, it does not have many cautions attached to it. However, if there is any concern regarding work with the abdomen per se, then appropriate cautions should be respected. Feedback from the client is always essential.

The technique (Figs 9.17, 9.18)

The client can either be side-lying, semi-reclining or sitting. She could also be leaning forward over a ball.

To start or finish this work, off the body connecting work can be done. This can be helpful if the client is unsure about whether she wants work directly on her abdomen. Place one hand a few centimetres above the navel and the other hand under the spine directly underneath the upper hand. Imagine energy travelling from one hand to the other. Spend a couple of minutes or so in this position until a 'warming' or 'expanding' sensation is felt between the hands. A connection may also be felt with the baby. After this, work can be continued on the abdomen or the work to the abdomen can be concluded by slowly removing the hands.

Place one hand on the abdomen and slide the other hand under the lower back. The location on the lower back can be where the therapist feels most appropriate in the lumbosacral area. If the client is forward leaning then the hand on the lower back needs to be on the sacrum. Spend some time allowing the hands to rest and tuning into the client's breathing pattern. If the client is breathing shallowly, she can be coached through some deeper abdominal breathing. Visualisations, if appropriate, may be included. This holding may also be focused on the Kidney/Uterus connection; this involves having one hand over one of the kidneys and the other over the uterus.

Once the woman is used to the touch and she is breathing deeply, work can be commenced with utilising some pressure. Apply pressure with both hands, 'sandwiching' them together with the client's out-breath. Assess how much pressure is comfortable and appropriate. Try to tune in to the baby in the womb, as well as the woman. Firm pressure, if applied sensitively and gradually, is usually preferable to a pressure which is too light or tentative. As the woman breathes in release some of the pressure, but still remain in contact. Repeat this several times. As the client relaxes more, the pressure may become a little deeper.

At this point, some single hand effleurage strokes can be included. This can be done with or without oil. Keep the hand on the lower back and work with clockwise effleurage strokes. Mould the hand which is effleuraging to the shape of the client's body. Tune in to the client's response. Be aware of how the baby responds to the touch.

Keeping the hand on the lower back, move the hand on the abdomen in a clockwise direction, coming to rest a few centimetres from its original position. Repeat the work, before moving the hand on the abdomen again. Continue this until the hand is back at the starting point. Work can then be commenced for a second time, with a closer or wider circle away from the navel. The hand on the back remains in the same position. The pressure on different areas of the abdomen will probably be different as it depends on what is felt between the hands. For example, when

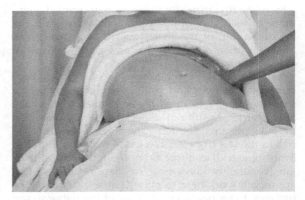

Fig. 9.17 Work on abdomen: pressure/stroking with one hand on abdomen and one hand on lower back, semi-reclining.

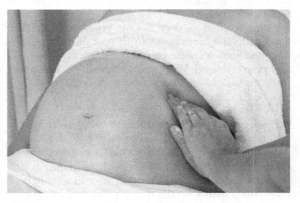

Fig. 9.18 Applying some pressure to the abdomen, semi-reclining.

working over the fetal spine, the pressure is likely to be deeper. When working over an area of the uterus where there is not much of the baby's body, the pressure will probably be lighter. By repeating the pressures, sensitivity to these differences will increase. If unsure of pressure, elicit feedback from the client. It should feel comfortable at all times.

Abdominal muscle gathering technique/Girdle Vessel and connecting with the baby

This helps to support the lengthened obliques, transverse and rectus abdominis muscles. It also provides a passive lateral stretch to the erector spinae. Women report an easing of back tension along with a sensation of warmth in the abdomen which they tend to experience as a feeling of more support from their abdominal muscles. They especially like the pressure on the midline and often say that they feel like they have 'been put back together' again. The baby may also respond to this stroke. It can be linked with more specific work to the Girdle Vessel by including the GDV points and holding.

Semi-reclining

This can be done with or without oil but is an effective technique to incorporate with abdominal massage using oil/lotion for treatment application (Fig. 9.19).

Begin by holding both hands together under the back at the level of the lumbar vertebrae. Tune in to the woman's breathing. Start with a fairly light stroking to gradually draw the two hands together towards the midline of the abdomen, focusing on gathering from the lower erector spinae and drawing the obliques and transverse towards the midline. As the hands come over the recti muscles, the tissue

will feel firmer due to the bulkiness of these muscles and the pressure may become a little firmer. This can be repeated a few times and each time a little more pressure can be applied as appropriate. Hold the hands one on top of the other, with the lower hand fingers facing the clavicle and the upper hand at 90° to the lower, together over the midline. As the client breathes out, a little firmer pressure may be applied at a 90° angle down into the midline.

Side (Fig. 9.20)

Stand or kneel behind the client's body facing her back in the same position. Place both hands side by side covering the side of the abdomen closest to the floor/table. Hold the hands here and tune in to the woman's breathing. Some gentle abdominal rocking could also be included, with the rocking movement being initiated in the therapist's body. Draw both hands towards the midline and rest them on the midline. Do not continue the stretch beyond the midline, otherwise the muscles on the side superior to the table will be pulled laterally, away from the midline. Repeat this a few times. Each time the gathering may become a little deeper, depending on the comfort of the client.

The same technique can be repeated on the superior side of the client's body. This time the pressure needs to be lighter, especially until the tissue of the rectus is reached. This is because this area is not protected by the bones of the rib cage or hips and if strong pressure is used, there is likely to be excessive pull on the abdominal tissue including the uterine ligaments, which are quite vulnerable in this position.

Begin with both hands on the side of the spine away from the floor/table. Pressure around the erector spinae can be firmer but as the hips are reached then less pressure should be applied. Continue gathering towards the midline and as the lateral border of

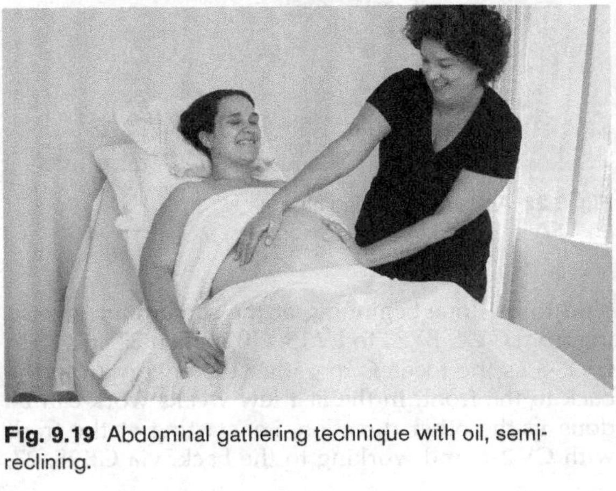

Fig. 9.19 Abdominal gathering technique with oil, semi-reclining.

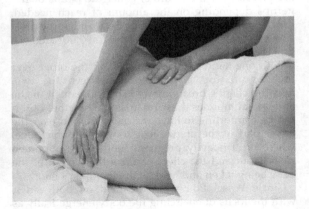

Fig. 9.20 Side abdominal gathering.

the recti muscles is felt, a little more pressure may be applied.

Finally, finish by drawing the two sides together at the same time using one hand to work each side. This is achieved by starting with one hand on the side of the abdomen inferior to the table as in the first part of the technique, while at the same time placing the other hand around the back and doing the second part of the technique. Finish with both hands holding over the midline and apply some gentle pressures towards the spine. This may seem slightly awkward initially as the hand on the far side can be firmer but has less distance to travel, and the hand starting on the upper side of the body has to be less firm but has further to travel. With practice this can feel like a continuous, flowing movement.

Working the Girdle Vessel can also be done, although technically it may feel a little more uneven for the therapist as the belt can not be accessed so easily physically all the way around.

Place one hand under the side of the client's body which is resting on the couch/floor, ideally cupping around the space between the ribs and the pelvis. If this is not comfortable place this hand over the centre, along the CV line.

With the other hand work the Girdle Vessel points of the upper side of the body, beginning with GV 4 and moving out to BL 23, LV 13, GB 26, 27 and 28, coming round to the CV in the midline. Try to feel the connection around as much as possible.

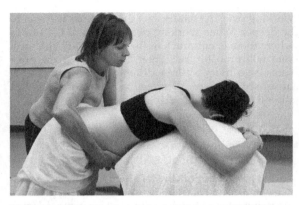

Fig. 9.21 Forward leaning abdominal gathering, GDV all fours.

Forward leaning (Figs 9.21, 9.22)

This can be done with the stroke beginning at the sacrum and gathering together at the front of the abdomen. The therapist will need to stand or kneel behind the client and place their hands on the sacrum. Both hands can move from the sacrum to the front at the same time, or one hand at a time. Once both hands are placed over the midline, either the palms or fingertips depending on the amount of reach needed, the therapist can lean their body back and apply pressure from the abdomen to the spine, at a 90° angle so that there is no pull on the tissue.

With one hand over the uterus and the other over the sacrum, feel a connection between the two. Feel the client's breathing and the movement of the abdominal muscles drawing in as she breathes out. It can be comforting to have the hand cupped over the lower part of the uterus, just above the pubic bone, where on a heavily pregnant mother the abdomen rounds out and the client can feel the weight of the baby being taken and held by the therapist's hands.

Girdle Vessel Points can be held on both sides, with the focus of encircling the body energetically as well as physically. For most of pregnancy work will

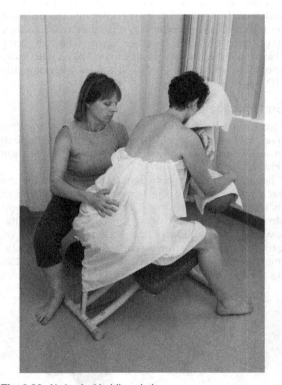

Fig. 9.22 Abdominal holding chair.

tend to be done beginning at the sacrum and working from GV 4, BL 23 to LV 13, GB 26 then 27 and 28 to CV 2–8 as the focus is to gather the energy from the back to the front. In the last few weeks work can be done in the other direction, i.e. starting at the front with CV 2–8 and working to the back, via GB 28, 27,

LV 13, BL 23 and finishing with GV 4, with a focus on 'opening up' the Girdle.

Work for the Penetrating Vessel – main meridian pathway, chest and sacrum

Benefits

PV can be useful to work at all stages of pregnancy, although it is particularly indicated in the first trimester, because of the changes it undergoes. At any time PV work can be useful to ensure a good flow of Blood and Jing to the fetus and is especially useful in cases where the fetus may not be developing properly/well (e.g. concerns over growth). In this case a clear understanding of the implications and an awareness of any potential issues which might contraindicate stronger abdominal pressure is required, but work with more of an energy rather than physical focus is likely to be beneficial.

PV work in the torso

Work with the Penetrating Vessel will help with the flow of energy along the front of the body. It can often get blocked at the level of the clavicle and the pubic bone, because the flow of energy tends to change as it passes through the bones and joints. Physically many muscles have attachments in these areas and work here will also impact on the muscles. The clavicle is often involved when there are difficulties with breathing fully and with respiratory/immune conditions. The pubic bone is often involved with problems of energy flow into the pelvis, which includes conditions such as pelvic girdle instability (PGI).

PV breast work

Techniques affecting the connecting pathway in the chest help in preparation for breastfeeding and for the woman to feel more relaxed about her changing breasts.

Semi-reclining position

If the client is uncomfortable with work directly on her breasts, then it can be done through the sheets.

The therapist needs to be standing or kneeling facing directly over the client's body. Place one hand over the clavicle and the other hand over or just above the pubic bone. Make sure that it is the ulnar edge of the hand over the upper border of the pubic bone so that the rest of the hand is covering the lower abdomen and is not below the pubic bone.

Feel for a rhythm of connection and also how much pressure feels appropriate. Respond to the rhythm of the body. Sometimes it feels appropriate to continue with a stabilising hold. At other times it feels more appropriate to include some gentle rocking during

the second or third trimester when the client is not experiencing nausea.

Get a sense of where there is more energy (Kyo-Jitsu) and begin working where there is less energy. This could be at the level of the pubic bone or clavicle. Generally in pregnancy there will be more energy in the pubic bone area, and this is where the energy needs to be supported to flow. Work is usually done from the clavicle down to the pubic bone, keeping the hand over the pubic bone.

Pathway of PV in torso

Keeping the mother hand over the lower abdomen, use the other hand to work down the PV. Begin by palming down over the PV pathway and then repeat by using more specific thumb pressure. The PV pathway is two thumb-widths from midline to bottom of ribs and then narrows to ½ *cun* from the midline on the abdomen. When using the thumb, place the rest of the hand so that it is comfortable and gives support to the thumb. Around the breast area it is often better to use fingers rather than the palm for support to reduce the amount of pressure applied.

Some therapists prefer to work the whole of one side of the PV in this way and then repeat on the other side, rather than work the two sides at the same time, because the mother hand can remain in contact with the uterus/baby. However, if specific points of Kyo and Jitsu are felt, then two points can be held, either on one side or on two different sides. This will mean moving the mother hand away from its position over the uterus.

There are also the PV connecting channels which run horizontally from the main pathways towards and into the breasts. With consent from the client to work on the breasts, the therapist can try to feel these energetic pathways.

Pathway of PV in sacral area

Benefits

This work can be beneficial for balancing the sacrum both structurally and energetically. It may help with PGI issues and to support caesarean scars from previous pregnancies. It may also help in healing structures after birth.

This work is usually done through the sheet, because of the closeness to the coccyx and pubic bone.

Ask the client to lift up their pelvis so that one hand can be slid underneath. The middle finger should rest lightly over the body of the coccyx (or as close as the client is comfortable with) and the sacrum is cupped in the palm. The other hand lies with the ulnar edge along the top of the pubic bone so that the fingers point to the side of the body (Fig. 9.23A).

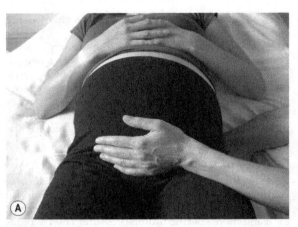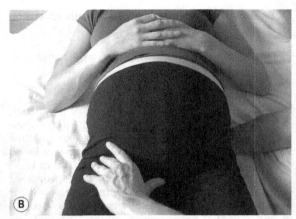

Fig. 9.23 Sacral hold working PV points above the pubic bone. A, cupping with ulnar hold: forearm resting on thigh; B, thumb pressure.

Feel the energy connection between the two and respond accordingly to balance Kyo and Jitsu. Some gentle rocking may feel appropriate, although not in the first trimester or at any time if the client is experiencing nausea.

Specific points can be worked with the hand on the pubic bone. Thumb pressure can be applied to the point on the centre of the upper border of the symphysis pubis (CV 2) (Fig. 9.23B). If the client has PGI this is likely to be sensitive and so pressure will need to be very light or even off the body. Pressure can also be applied to KI 11 (half a thumb-width each side) and ST 30 (two thumb-widths each side).

While working, the forearm of the working hand may be placed so that it is resting on the client's thigh. This can add a grounding quality to work. Energetically it is providing a connection with the Stomach meridian which links with the PV through ST 30. Clients often find this connection reassuring. It may also provide a 'distraction' so that they are not so focused on the potentially more sensitive area of the pubic bone. This position allows the therapist's arm to be more fully relaxed.

Point actions

ST 30 'Rushing Qi' – regulates Qi in the lower burner, the Penetrating Vessel and subdues 'running piglet Qi' (the rebellious movement of Qi upwards along the PV which is a common scenario in the first trimester).

KD 11 'Pubic bone' – regulates the lower burner.

Side position

PV can also be worked from the side position. There are two options for this:

Option 1

Face the client's head with the hip of the side nearest their body placed alongside the client's hip. The mother hand is placed on the client's lower back and the working hand makes contact with the abdomen. The abdomen can be worked with the palm of the hand or the thumb or fingertips. The breast area may be more problematic as the client's breasts may be in the way.

Option 2

This can provide an easier way for accessing the PV in the breast area. Face the client's back as in the hip/shoulder rock. Place one forearm over the hip with the palm over the abdomen. Place the other forearm over the pectorals with the fingers or the ulnar side of the hand over the midline (CV) or 2 *cun* lateral (PV). Lean back to apply a slight stretch between the forearms which opens up the PV (Fig. 9.24). This gives easier access to the front of the body. Some gentle rocking may feel appropriate.

The upper part of the pathway can be worked with the ulnar side or fingers of the upper hand while keeping the lower hand over the abdomen. The ulnar side of the hand is generally more appropriate over the breasts as it tends to feel less invasive. However, depending on the size of the breasts, it may be more appropriate to work with the fingertips, rather than the side of the hand. If the breasts tend to fall over the hand, then simply lean back further to move the breast tissue away. How far down the PV work can continue will depend on the size of the breasts and length of the mother's torso. When the upper hand can no longer make a good connection with the PV, place it back over the pectorals so that it becomes the mother hand and carry on working down PV with the hand which

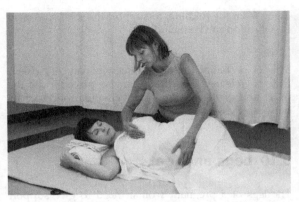

Fig. 9.24 Working the PV in side facing the back and using forearms to open out body.

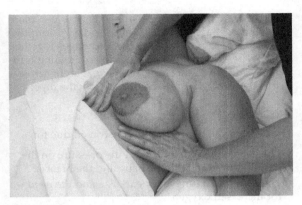

Fig. 9.25 Working the breast in semi-reclining.

was over the abdomen. It may be more comfortable for the client to receive palming over the lower part of the pathway as it passes through the abdomen; however, if the client is comfortable the work can be repeated using thumb pressures. Use the fingers of the hands to cup the abdomen, while working with the thumb.

Of course this position and type of work may not feel appropriate to all women because of its intimacy. This is where the sheet can be a useful tool for massage therapists, instead of working directly on the skin with oil.

Direct work for the breasts (Figs 9.25, 9.26)

Direct work can be done. It should never be overly strong and depends on client feedback. It is usually done more to the end of pregnancy and can include gentle stroking, palming and cupping. Lymphatic strokes over the breasts can also be included. This is described in the postnatal chapter (p. 324 and 333–335).

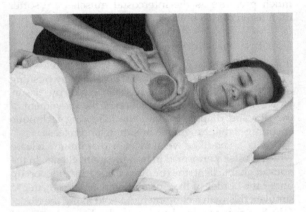

Fig. 9.26 Work to the breast from the side.

Pelvic floor work

For most bodyworkers, apart from some osteopaths and chiropractors, direct work with the pelvic floor is outside their scope of practice. However, this muscle group is significantly challenged in pregnancy and does need attention to ensure optimal immediate and long-term function. A holding technique is outlined in the postnatal section which offers a way of supporting the muscle and energy flow without directly applying touch. It can also be used during labour.

Heart Uterus

This simple technique is a great one to show parents to use themselves. It is usually a calming technique as it is connecting the energy of the Heart, with its role of regulating all the emotions, with the Uterus, where the baby is. It provides a lovely emotional connecting focus for the client with her baby.

Place one hand over the physical organ of heart and the other over the physical organ of uterus. Feel which is more Kyo (empty) and which is more Jitsu (full).

In pregnancy although the Uterus may feel more full, this is how the energy needs to be. The emphasis on work in pregnancy is therefore to allow the energy of the Heart to support and nourish the Uterus. To do this, keep one hand over the uterus and with the other hand move it a few centimetres closely to the hand over the uterus. Hold the hands over the two new connections for a few of the woman's breaths. When good connection is felt, move the upper hand a few more centimetres closer to the hand over the uterus. Hold it there for a few breaths. Keep repeating this until the two hands are together over the uterus.

Try to get a sense of the quality of the connection – a good connection often feels like a nice firm rope, coiled around and strong. Sometimes, however, it feels like the rope is more frayed and the energy is not held between the two organs. In this case use more gathering techniques. This work is fairly intuitive and is focused on drawing the frayed edges together. This can be done with either stroking or holding techniques. Sometimes the 'rope' feels like it is cut across – in this case work needs to be done to join the rope.

Rib, diaphragm and intercostal work

The rib area can become quite constricted due to:

- The expansion of the ribs and the pressure on the diaphragm from both the baby and the breasts.
- The increase in lung and heart size and the need for increased oxygen.

Techniques to release constrictions are often indicated, but care needs to be taken not to apply too much pressure as the intercostal muscles are softer than usual due to hormonal changes.

Diaphragm release and Lung release

It is not advisable to do strong diaphragm release in pregnancy because of the pressure of the baby pushing under the ribs and the relative softness of the tissue. However, there is often restriction in the movement of the ribs and diaphragm and the following technique encourages diaphragmatic breathing and release.

This is a modified version of a diaphragm release which is often performed in non-pregnant clients. In the non-pregnant client, the thumbs or fingers can scoop up under the border of the ribs. In pregnancy it is better to simulate this with a cupping hand hold along the ribs.

To begin, place one hand over the lower border of the front ribs, on one side, cupping them along the diaphragm. Place the other hand under the back ribs. As the client breathes out, sandwich the two hands together so that the hand under the front cups the edge of the ribs. As the client breathes in, release the pressure.

For the Lung release, move the hand which was under the back to line up under the clavicle so that the middle finger rests over the LU1 point. The other hand remains cupping the lower front ribs. As the mother breathes out, apply pressure to the hands; as she breathes in, release the pressure. This moves the diaphragm but links it with an energetic Lung release.

The other side can be released when the client has turned over.

Intercostal release

The intercostals have to support the additional weight in pregnancy due to increased fluids and breast tissue. Gentle release work is appropriate. It is often most effective when performed directly over the skin with oil, as there can be some glide. The movement here is

away from the midline, to support the release. A gentle vibration can be included.

Side

This is probably the most effective way of achieving the release. One hand can be placed over the other and gentle springing movement applied across between the intercostals with gentle pressure. Repeat several times.

9.10 Legs and feet

The legs of a pregnant woman need to give support to the pelvis due to the increasing weight gain. Key postural muscles such as the quadriceps femoris, iliotibial band, tensor fasciae latae and hamstrings are often hypertonic as they compensate for the additional weight, potential weakness in the pelvis and lower back and changes in the gait. GB and BL may be contracted. The calves are also often hypertonic and these patterns may contribute to leg cramps. The adductor group and Yin meridians may tend more towards hypotonicity and often need to be strengthened. Further, the growing baby tends to interfere with the circulation of blood and lymph in the legs as well as the flow of energy.

Bodywork to support all muscles, lymph, blood and energy is of great benefit – especially when it includes some mobilisations, to stretch overworked muscles and get energy flowing in meridians. Work in positions where the limb is elevated will support venous and lymphatic return and meridian flow. Work needs to respect the general tissue changes which occur in pregnancy and the effects of oedema which is common. The legs may feel heavy by the end of pregnancy, especially in hot weather, and most women appreciate work to their legs.

The knees and ankles are more prone to injury due to increased ligament laxity coupled with the increased weight load. The plantar arch muscles of the inner feet may collapse if footwear which restricts, overflexes or rotates the foot during late pregnancy is worn, such as high heels or flat, unsupportive shoes such as flip flops or Wellington boots. There may be oedema of the ankles, feet and toes which can cause discomfort and decreased motility. Foot work can have far-reaching effects for the pregnant client and is often much appreciated.

Lymphatic and circulatory systems: oedema and varicose veins

It is common for women to have oedema in the legs, especially the lower part of the limb and the ankles and feet, in later pregnancy. This is due to the increased fluid volume, combined with the softening of tissue and increased weight of the abdomen blocking the flow of lymph in the inguinal nodes and the legs. This type of oedema is worse at the end of the day, especially if the woman has been standing on her feet, and responds to leg elevations. It is better after a night's sleep and worse in hot weather. When there are no other symptoms, especially no increase in blood pressure or proteinuria, this onset of oedema is not the result of pre-eclampsia. Manual lymphatic techniques are particularly effective as they help clear lymph nodes and support the flow of lymph. Energy wise it responds to work with Spleen, which helps to transform and transport fluids, as well as Kidney, which supports fluid.

Many women develop varicose veins along with oedema, for the same reasons. Later in pregnancy the weight of the fetus compresses the pelvic veins as well as affecting venous return to the legs. Women who stand for long periods of time without regular movement during the day may aggravate the development of varicose veins.

Most varicose veins are superficial and non-pathological and respond well to appropriate bodywork. Care needs to be taken to monitor that there is no development of more serious issues such as phlebitis or blood clot formation (e.g. DVT/thrombosis).

Leg cramps

Leg cramps can be common in the second and third trimesters due to increased weight, circulation changes and calcium and phosphorus mechanism. Cramps usually occur in the calves. Bodywork to stretch and relax the muscles of the legs, especially the calves, and improve circulation, is often beneficial. Work with the Bladder meridian, especially BL57, which is locally indicated to relieve cramps.

Exercise is important, especially stretching and mobilising the legs. Women need to be reminded not to plantarflex their feet which is a natural stretch response during rest or sleep or when awakening. The impact of several intense onsets of leg cramps is usually enough to emphasise the importance of keeping the feet in a neutral or dorsiflexed position!

Dietary attention may also be important because calf cramps can be linked to the calcium, phosphorus mechanism including a lack of magnesium, salt, and vitamin C. Eating foods rich in these minerals and vitamins may be of help. Many primary care providers recommend a prenatal vitamin.

Restless legs syndrome (RLS)

Restless legs syndrome (RLS) is fairly common and may be experienced by as many as 1 in 10 women. It usually involves legs which feel restless and may suddenly feel twitchy and jumpy when resting. Like many other leg issues, it is due to the increased weight and circulation but it also seems to have a hereditary link, as it runs in families. Energetically this is linked with Kidney and Extraordinary Vessel energy. It also seems to be linked with low blood sugar as it is more common in diabetics and hypoglycaemics. This would be linked with Spleen energy. It seems to be worsened by coffee (which affects Kidney energy) and alcohol (which affects Liver energy).

All of the above indicate that the problem is with the Yin energy of the legs and these meridians are in the medial aspect of the legs. This means that work to release any blockages in these meridians and work to improve circulation, especially to the medial aspect of the legs, is indicated. Exercise and stretches to the legs, both while massaging and also for the mother to do herself, is indicated.

Types of techniques

Bodywork needs to respect the fact that for all women the tissue is relatively softer. If there is oedema it will also be more stretched, and so deep pressure would not be comfortable. However, there are no major adaptations to work with legs in pregnancy. If there are no varicose veins or oedema, phlebitis or DVT and the woman is carrying out normal activities, then the pressure and depth of stroke can be to the comfort of the client and muscle work and energy work can proceed according to the client's needs. Due to the musculoskeletal structure, as with all clients, the deeper work will be to the lateral and dorsal aspect of the legs more than the medial aspect.

Working positions

In order to support flows of energy and blood and lymph to the leg, elevated positions are often indicated. For these, the client could be side-lying with the therapist supporting the leg in an elevated position. Alternatively, the client could sit, possibly on a ball, and rest her legs on a chair.

The client may also appreciate leg work while she is on all fours. She could have deep work to the dorsal aspect of the legs. This is also an effective position in which to work the medial aspect of the upper leg, especially the adductors, which is safe to use if the woman has PGI.

Cautions

Varicose veins, DVT and phlebitis

Many therapists are concerned whether bodywork on the pregnant woman's leg will increase circulation in the area and might exacerbate any potential risk. Some authors (Osborne-Sheets 1998, Stillerman 2008) have indicated that deep work to the medial aspect of the legs is not advisable at all in pregnancy due to the slightly increased risk of DVT in pregnancy. However, even light work would potentially dislodge a DVT so treating all women as though they are at risk would actually mean that all women could have no bodywork. This is nonsensical – especially when bodywork is likely to reduce the risk of DVT forming.

In the second and third trimesters especially, and even in the first trimester, especially for subsequent pregnancies, the therapist must note the presence of varicose veins, and should monitor for issues such as phlebitis or the possible onset of blood clots – thrombus formation. If varicose veins do appear, it is wise to remind the client to tell her physician or midwife, and some explanation of the issues related to circulation in the legs may be warranted by the therapist. It is important to communicate the concerns without being alarmist. If varicose veins do exist, the degree of severity is important to note. This includes appearance, texture, temperature, level of discomfort/pain and location. Local work directly over varicose veins, even those which are considered to be only in the superficial category, should be avoided, but general work to the legs and around the area may be very beneficial in helping promote healthy circulation.

In the event that phlebitis or thrombus is suspected or present, it is important to seek attention from the primary care provider. Signs that this may be the case include one-sided oedema or heat, inflammation or pain or a positive Homan's sign. However it is important to recognise that a thrombosis can be present in the absence of these signs.

If thrombosis is suspected then immediate referral to the primary care provider is essential as even getting on and off the floor or table could potentially dislodge a thrombus. Once the clot has been treated and the situation has stabilised, then work may be resumed, as long as the woman is under continuous supervision by her primary care provider. In this instance work would always need to be more physically gentle to the legs as the client would be on blood-thinning drugs which means there is more risk of bruising. Energetically there would be some weakness to the Spleen and possibly Liver meridians.

Oedema

It is important to be clear that the oedema is lymphostatic (the 'normal' type due to increased volume of fluid and poor circulation) and not lymphodynamic (linked with pre-eclampsia or other systemic failures) in order to decide on the most appropriate treatment.

Dialogue

Suzanne

There are differing opinions on how to work or not work with thrombosis and whether to treat all pregnant women as potentially at risk of thrombosis. From my point of view thrombosis is potentially a risk, but if I was really going to treat all pregnant women as though there were at risk from a DVT I would actually not be giving them any bodywork at all. We could argue that anything could potentially dislodge a thrombosis. In fact, if I did suspect that one of my clients had a thrombosis, I would not do any bodywork but would send them straight to hospital.

If they were put on blood-thinning drugs and the thrombi then broke down, and provided they were receiving regular medical check ups, I would be quite happy to work with them again. If they were still taking blood-thinning drugs to manage their condition, then I would focus more on energy techniques and light work to the legs because of the increased risk of bruising.

I would argue that bodywork is of benefit in preventing the build of thrombosis and varicose veins in the first place. I would always be a little more cautious of working with women who have been on bed rest but I think if we take a clear case history and screen for possible risk factors, and they are doing regular exercise, I would not assume that they are at risk.

I suppose my bottom line is I see pregnancy as essentially a time of health and my job as being to support that process of health. Of course there can be problems and I would support a woman who has health issues as appropriate, but I see one of my main tasks as being to work in the preventative arena.

Cindy

Existing massage therapy textbooks advise against doing any bodywork on the legs of a client who has been put on bed rest during her pregnancy. The first question for the therapist to consider is why that client is on bed rest. Then the therapist must ask the extent of the bed rest. Can the client get up to go to the bathroom, walk around the room or home for limited amounts of time? What other activities has she been told to abstain from or to do?

One of the most common exercises prescribed to women on bed rest by physiotherapists is plantarflexion/dorsiflexion of the foot. If the reader tries this repetitively, they will understand that this is a fairly significant pumping action which creates strong contractions in the lower leg muscles.

If one compares this to gentle massage or shiatsu techniques, the question arises about the possibility of increased risk of releasing blood clots with a woman who is already stimulating her leg muscles in a fairly intense way.

As well, women may be given the blood-thinning drugs such as Fragmin or heparin prophylactically. This is significantly different than actively treating a client who has been diagnosed with an actual blood clot.

If the therapist and/or client has any concern regarding bodywork increasing risk of harm to the client, then it is best to focus on relaxing work to areas not involved, for example gentle massage to the head, neck and shoulder area might be most effective.

That said, therapists may consider the active care strategies given for clients who have had a knee replacement or a caesarean section where gentle mobility and/or ambulation is encouraged as soon as possible in order to prevent the formation of blood clots. To consider leg massage prohibited for any or all pregnant bed rest clients who are free of contraindications or circulatory pathologies such as blood clots seems to be fear based rather than related to existing evidence-based practice.

Reflex and acupuncture points – labour focus points

Several of the 'Labour focus points' are around the legs and ankle – LV 3, BL 60, SP 6 – and these tend to be avoided until 37 weeks.

The reflex points for the uterus, ovaries and fallopian tubes are around the ankle. There is differing opinion on how safe and appropriate it is to work these areas. Some therapists advocate avoiding the ankle area totally but this is like saying avoid the uterus/abdomen totally. The health of the client and the type of approach are the most important factors. Avoid deep stimulating work and approach the uterus zones on the ankle using the same principles as for the abdomen.

First trimester

During the first trimester the passive movements of the legs and hips may or may not be comfortable; it depends on the client's health status and their level of physical activity. If the client is feeling weak and nauseous and has a history of miscarriage, they may feel

---

> **Testimonial: one view of working the uterus reflexes**
>
> *Catherine Tugnait, UK maternity massage and reflexologist*
>
> *I always work the uterus reflex in every treatment in every trimester. I just work it differently depending on need. In the first trimester I do lots of gentle linking balancing work. Often I am able to palpate the reflexion of the baby's heartbeat and I connect this with the mother's heart reflex. I link the energy I feel from the uterus with the mother's kidney reflex which is K1 in shiatsu. I build in some visualisation for the mother to imagine her baby in utero, even if it is only weeks old.*
>
> *In the second trimester I work the uterus reflex to balance, strengthen and tone it, though still quite gently, for example thumb walks. When women get close to dates, I do drainage work and endocrine balancing to get them ready for labour. I also link the mind, the solar plexus and the uterus to encourage positive thinking about the birth. I am able to palpate the reflexion of the baby on the feet and so can very accurately tell what position the baby is in and how engaged its head is. I can also feel the position of the cervix reflex and ascertain how ripe it is. I link this with GB 34 on the knee to stimulate the cervix into action. Some women can actually feel sensations in their cervix while I am doing this which shows how powerful it must be. The endocrine reflexes also give good clues to how close labour is to starting. I also build in linking work with SP 6 when priming labour.*
>
> *Once the woman is post dates then I work very deeply into the priming points if the mum's energy allows me to. You get a feel for what is the right level for each individual mum and I never work beyond comfortable tolerance levels. I have on a few occasions been able to work out that the baby has its head deflexed and is malpresented, much to the amazement of the midwives when told by the mum that their reflexologist thinks this may be the case. It has been accurate in all three cases.*

that this work is too stimulating because of 'opening effect' for the hips and pelvic area at this time when there are significant changes in the uterus and energy wise, the body is gathering energy. If the client has a history of SPI then these movements would also not be indicated.

However, if the client is already doing a lot of sport or other exercise which is working this area and the body is used to this type of movement, then she may benefit from the release work offered by gentle mobilisations.

The manual lymphatic techniques for the legs are not used in this trimester as they are potentially too detoxifying and if the woman is presenting with oedema this is not a normal symptom of this stage of pregnancy. This means the therapist needs to refer back to the primary care giver.

Deeper work to the lateral aspect of the upper leg is often indicated.

Be aware that rocking movements may aggravate nausea.

Deeper work on abductors (pectineus, sartorius, gracilis) which are attached to the pubic bone may be too strong because of the changes in the ligaments and muscles of the abdomen and pelvis.

PGI/SPI cautions

If PGI is present, then it is important to minimise movement of the pubic bone. It can be helpful to imagine that the legs are glued together at the knees or the client is wearing a tight mini skirt. This means that no mobilisations can be performed. When the client is lying in the side, the lower leg may be moved to rest on a cushion in order to work the lateral aspect, provided the knees are kept together. Great care needs to be taken when getting the client to change position, especially when moving from one side to the other. It is usually best for the client to move through all fours.

Sometimes it can be helpful to get the client to sit or lean over a ball. In this position some work can be done to the medial aspect of the leg, as long as the knees are kept fairly close together.

9.11 Legs and feet: techniques

The main issues when working the legs are not so much a whole new range of specific techniques, but rather adapting current techniques to the side, all fours or sitting positions as well as including work with mobilisations and elevation.

Hip rotations/leg rotations and stretches and working with the leg in the elevated position

Benefits

- These movements are beneficial for supporting lymph and blood circulation, meridian energy and working muscles and joints. They can be good

to include with the lymphatic work and both the inguinal and spinal nodes can be stimulated.

- The semi-reclining position is used more in the second trimester with the side position being favoured from late second into third trimester.
- An elevated position offers an additional option for working the upper leg, which can support release of oedema and take pressure off the abdomen. Lymphatic work can be done in this position.

Cautions

- These movements should not be done if the client is suffering from PGI/SPI.
- If the client has a high-risk obstetric history and is in hospital, then these techniques would tend not to be performed, as they may be potentially over-stimulating.
- If the client is higher risk but not in hospital, then these techniques may possibly be performed if deemed appropriate, but slowly, gently and in a relaxing, rather than stimulating, manner.

Semi-reclining position (Figs 9.27, 9.28)

Table version

Bend one of the client's legs at the knee. Support the knee/leg with hands around the knee and do some gentle rotations of the leg to work the hip and upper leg. Explore the full range of movement. There are three basic positions:

1. The knee can be eased into the abdomen, taking care not to put too much pressure on the abdomen. This is good for releasing the lumbar vertebrae.
2. The knee can be externally rotated to the side. This stretches the adductor group and Yin meridians of the leg.
3. The knee can be taken internally rotated towards the other leg. This stretches the iliotibial band, and Yang meridians of the leg.

The leg can be worked in any of these three basic positions. Care needs to be taken to give adequate support to the leg.

The work can be repeated on the other side.

Floor version

The same three movements with one leg can be performed from the floor and the therapist can also do direct work to the leg in each of these positions. Movement 1 can be done with both legs simultaneously.

Keeping this can usually be done for the client with PGI as the knees are being kept together, but

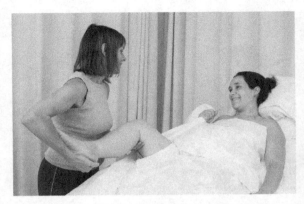

Fig. 9.27 Semi-reclining movements of the legs: externally rotated.

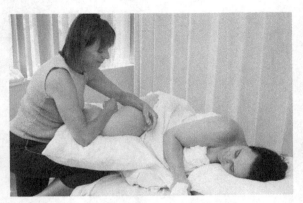

Fig. 9.29 Working leg in side on table: upper leg.

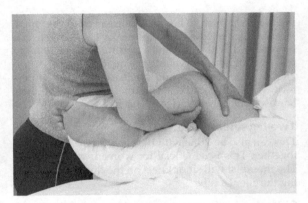

Fig. 9.28 Semi-reclining movements of the legs: working on the leg.

care must be taken that there is no discomfort in the pubic joint.

Side position

From the side position, mobilisation work is focused on the upper leg. No mobilisation work can be done if the client is suffering from PGD/SPD as the knees need to be kept together.

Draping

If working with massage, the sheet needs to be well tucked in between the legs.

Table version (Fig. 9.29)

The therapist stands in front of the client. The therapist supports the ankle and knee of the client's leg. The therapist then moves her own body forward and backwards, flexing the client's hips and pumping the inguinal nodes. Gentle rotational movements can

also be performed. The therapist can also work with the leg in the elevated position. In this case, she will probably need to rest her knee on the table to give support or support the leg against her body, using a cushion as appropriate. Work will tend to be more for the lateral aspect of the leg (IT band, GB) as it is harder to work the medial aspect of the leg in this position.

Floor version (Fig. 9.30)

The easiest position for the therapist is to step over the client's lower leg, pick up the client's upper leg and support it over their own leg. Make sure that the client's leg is only lifted as high as it is comfortable. The knee needs to either be supported on the therapist's leg or the therapist uses their arm resting on their own leg to support the client's knee. If the knee is unsupported it will tend to rotate, causing the gluteus and piriformis muscles to contract in order to give support to the hip. The therapist may want to place one hand over the gluteus to check this is not happening. This may feel comfortable and supportive to the client.

From this position, the therapist can move their body back and forth in order to create a pumping movement for the leg. This is useful for stimulating the lymph nodes and supporting pelvic circulation as well as releasing muscular tension. Rotational movements can also be done for the leg by using the arm.

The leg can be worked in this elevated position. For the upper aspect of the leg, work can be done to both the medial and lateral sides of the leg. The therapist will probably need to support the leg at the knee and work with the other hand or forearm.

For the lower aspect of the leg, the therapist will need to rotate their hips so as to face more towards the leg. If this feels uncomfortable, then they may step back over the client's inferior leg and place their

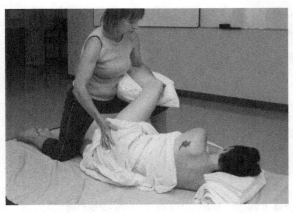

Fig. 9.30 Floor side-lying: work to leg in elevated position, showing therapist body and hand positions.

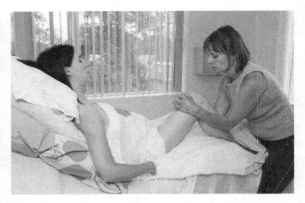

Fig. 9.31 Table semi-reclining: double leg quadriceps/hip release with therapist hands showing work to the legs.

elevated leg on the other leg in a kneeling position. Work can be done to the medial and lateral aspect of the lower leg.

If the therapist is not comfortable, they can lift the client's leg onto a small ball (45 cm) and rest it there. Again the ball must not be too big and the knee must be well supported over the ball so it does not rotate causing pulling on the hips and contraction of the gluteus muscles and piriformis.

Quadriceps (Stomach) and hamstrings (Bladder) release work

Benefits

Releases for these muscle/meridian groups are safe to do in pregnancy and often indicated. Tight quadriceps or hamstrings can affect both the pelvis and the spine. They are often involved in musculoskeletal issues in the low back, and may relate to symphysis pubis discomfort.

Cautions

Do not work with the legs apart in SPI/PGI cases.

Quadriceps
Semi-reclining
This release can be performed on one leg or both legs simultaneously.

One leg release
The therapist stands or sits on the table or floor. The client's knee is flexed and her foot is placed on the floor or table. The therapist stabilises the foot and knee with their own hand (table) or foot (floor).

The therapist places their hands on top of the quadriceps muscle and gently leans back, allowing the

muscle to stretch. This also releases into the hips. It may also release into the neck. This stretch can be repeated with the hands in different positions to release different areas along the quadriceps.

From this same position a release can also be performed on the calves. The therapist moves their hands to the calves and leans back.

Two leg release (Fig. 9.31)
This can also be done with the client's two legs placed together. This is beneficial for women with SPI/PGI. The therapist will sit or kneel on the floor or table facing the client's hips.

Side

This can only be performed for the superior leg. The superior leg is bent at the knee and the foot is brought into the gluteus muscles. The therapist leans back, giving good support to the leg. This cannot be done for women with SPI/PGI.

Bladder work/posterior leg muscles

This work can effectively be done in the side position, a forward leaning position or with the client sitting on a ball or chair.

Benefits

Bladder is good for general relaxation of the legs, for working the muscles in the centre of the back of the leg (hamstrings, gastrocnemius, soleus) and relieves leg cramps, as well as urinary problems and water retention (oedema).

Side-lying

This work can be done on either leg. With the upper leg, it can be done with the leg either on the floor or table or in the elevated position (Fig. 9.30) with the

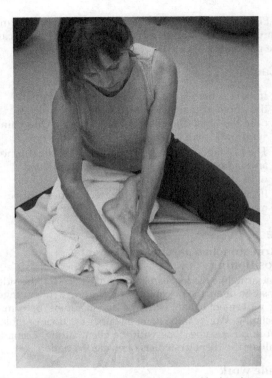

Fig. 9.32 Floor side, lower leg calf release with elevation.

lower leg, the calf can be elevated over the thigh, or cushion, to work (Fig. 9.32).

Forward leaning version or sitting on a ball or chair (Fig. 9.33)

The client needs to be leaning forward in such a way that there is access to the back of the legs.

Place one hand on the sacrum and with the centre of the palm of the other hand, apply pressure down the back of the leg. At the knee move the hand which was on the sacrum to the back of the knee and repeat going down the back of the leg. With the lower leg, it is a less familiar position for most therapists but work can be effective: it simply takes a little getting used to the fact that the hands are not pushing down on the same plane when working in the lower leg.

Work can also be done on the foot, resting the foot over the therapist's thigh.

Bodywork for varicose veins/legs

Bodywork is recommended for this condition, as it relieves oedema, improves the condition of the smooth muscles, and increases venous outflow.

Energy work to support varicose veins includes work for the Spleen and if there is oedema also include Bladder meridians.

Goals of treatment

Goals are threefold:

- To decrease oedema (for an additional approach see manual lymphatic techniques).
- To support venous return from the lower extremities; this is achieved by raking effleurage, leg elevations and mobilisations.
- To support the smooth muscles in order to normalise venous function; this is achieved by local massage or energy work on the muscles of the legs.

Two simple techniques aid this work: continuous effleurage and continuous vibration. The area of application will depend on the severity of the condition and there is never any direct work over the varicose vein.

It is helpful to combine it with hydrotherapy (e.g. cool cloths and foot baths) and to teach the client appropriate self-care.

Continuous effleurage and vibrations

Work in the sacroiliac area using strokes such as raking or flat hand effleurage. After a period of 3–5 minutes, move to the thigh with raking effleurage strokes only. Raking effleurage is of support where there are varicose veins because the fingers, held in a rake-like fashion, can fit between the varicosities, and thus avoid any pressure on the vein itself.

By working rhythmically with the strokes of raking effleurage and light shaking vibration (with the hand still maintaining the rake-like position), oedema should visibly start to decrease, and the client should report a feeling of lightness or tingling in the calf or toes, as well as in the thigh.

After a while work can be done on the calf in the same way as on the thigh.

The effleurage and vibration strokes run only in the direction of the venous flow, i.e. towards the heart. The work is concluded with some long strokes all the way up the leg. If there is still some oedema present, then proceed to the more specific lymph strokes (see section 9.12, p. 273).

In terms of frequency of treatment, daily or every second day treatments for approximately 2 weeks gain the best outcome. This is where it can be helpful to show the partner simple self-help techniques which can be used at home.

Hands/arms

Physically the arm is often tense due to the sedentary lifestyle combined with poor posture. Repetitive movements from working at a keyboard, or professions such as hairdressing can create or aggravate conditions such as carpal tunnel (inflammation or

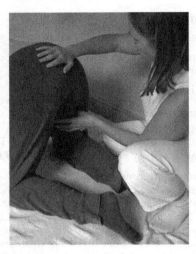

Fig. 9.33 Work to Bladder/hamstrings with client on all fours.

compression of the medial nerve), thoracic outlet syndrome, de Quervain syndrome (inflammation of the radial nerve resulting in thenar pain) brachial nerve plexus irritations or rotator cuff strain.

There is often oedema in the arms and hands due to the increased fluids and potentially impaired circulation caused by poor posture. This may cause compression of the median nerve and create or aggravate carpal tunnel syndrome.

Energy wise, the arms represent the emotional aspects of energy and the Heart and Heart Protector together regulate all emotions. Slow holding work can often be calming for the emotional changes which the woman is likely to be experiencing during pregnancy. Even when working on a more physical level, it is recognised that problems with shoulders and arms, especially conditions like frozen shoulder, can often be due to emotional causes as well as physical ones.

Opening up and releasing tension patterns in the arms will also support breathing techniques and work to support the lungs, as well as releasing tension in the chest and upper back.

Types of techniques

As with the leg, there are not many new techniques but the approach is more about getting used to working in different positions and including mobilisations and elevations.

Working position

Work can be done effectively in the side position, although only the superior arm can be worked with mobilisations and elevations.

Sitting positions can offer alternatives. Both arms can be accessed and so mobilisations of both arms can be performed.

Cautions

- If there is nerve damage, which may happen in the upper arm around the brachial nerve plexus, or in the wrist due to carpal tunnel or de Quervain syndrome, then local work is inadvisable.
- The LI4 labour focus point lies between the thumb and index finger and should not be stimulated until around 37 weeks.
- If there is oedema, then lighter techniques will be more suitable.

Techniques

Arm stretches/passive movements/positioning

The arm, like the leg, can be mobilised. In fact, the side position offers the possibility of including a fuller range of movements than with the client supine or semi-reclining. Work can be done on either the floor or table. Work can also be done with the client sitting. Using a ball for the client to sit on is often a good option.

Side work

For all these positions, the therapist stands or sits by the client's upper arm with their body at the back of the client. The hand furthest from the client's body is placed on the top of the client's shoulder and the other hand supports the arm at the elbow with the forearm and the hand holding at the wrist.

Three stretches can be done from this position. These also offer different positions for working the arm. With all of these ensure that the elbow is supported and that there is no strain on the shoulder girdle.

1. Extend the arm as far as it will go behind and in a line with the head. In order to do this the therapist will need to shift their body position to be a little more at the head of the client. This stretches the Heart and Small Intestine meridians and the muscles of the inside arm. The stretch can be extended by the therapist swapping their supporting arm and placing it on the client's hip. Do ensure that the hand is on the bone, as it would be too much pressure on the muscles and ligaments above the hip (Fig. 9.34).
2. Extend the client's arm up at 90° to the side of their body and, using a small cushion to avoid the client resting directly on the body, rest it against the cushion. This stretches the Heart Protector and Triple Heater meridians and the muscles of the inside and outside arm (Fig. 9.35).

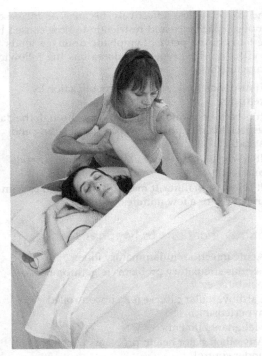

Fig. 9.34 Side position work to arm; arm in Heart Small Intestine stretch with side stretch.

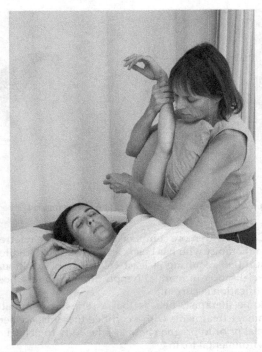

Fig. 9.35 Side position work to arm; arm in Heart Protector stretch.

3. Externally rotate the shoulder and allow the arm to abduct and the shoulder to retract, as far as it will go. Give support with the leg (floor) or arm (table) as needed. This stretches the Lung and Large Intestine meridians and muscles of the medial arm and shoulder. The pectorals are also stretched in this position.
4. Rest the arm along the side of the client's body. Some wrist movements and stretches can be done from this position. Work can be done for the lateral aspect of the arm and it is especially effective for the deltoids, brachialis and extensor group.

Lymph pumping technique
Benefits
This is beneficial, not only for releasing muscles of the upper arm and shoulder, but also for stimulating the axillary nodes, which will help with oedema.

The technique (Fig. 9.36)
Stand or sit by the arm. The arm can either be flexed or extended depending on what is most comfortable for therapist and client.

Holding the arm with relaxed hands, the therapist uses their own upwards and downwards body movement to pump the arm vertically up and down.

9.12 Lymphatic work

Written in consultation with Pam Hammond

This section is written for therapists who do not have in-depth training in lymphatic drainage and is directed towards working with oedema secondary to healthy pregnancies without underlying health issues or pregnancy-related complications. It is not a prerequisite to have done manual lymphatic drainage courses in order to apply some lymphatic principles to enhance the work. These basic techniques can be very effective in relieving the pain and discomfort associated with pregnancy-related oedema.

It is important before treating any oedema to determine the cause in order to ascertain if it is within the scope of practice. If there is any suspicion that there are underlying causes the client should be referred to their primary care provider for an accurate diagnosis.

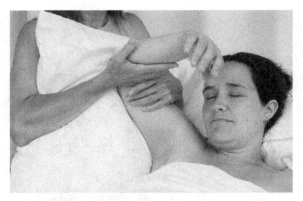

Fig. 9.36 Side position lymph pump; arm either extended or bent.

Clients with more complex oedema may be referred to a therapist who has been certified by an accredited institution requiring at least 160 hours of additional specialisation in manual lymph drainage and whose certification is current.

Some therapists believe that a series of lymphatic drainage treatments with a certified therapist are beneficial prior to pregnancy to aid the body to get rid of environmental toxins.

Complex oedema is referred to as lymphodynamic oedema. This means that the amount of fluid to be disposed of has increased and there is too much fluid for the transport capacity to drain. An example of this in pregnancy is oedema related to pre-eclampsia, when the kidney, liver or heart are starting to function less optimally and, with eclampsia, may begin to fail. It can also be the case with hypertensive disorders or other kidney, heart or liver conditions. In this case lymphatic drainage is not effective or recommended. This type of oedema presents with the following characteristics:

- It does not respond to elevation.
- It tends to be constant throughout the day.
- It is present through the whole limb, rather than more pronounced at the extremities, and may present in the face and even the eyelids.
- It has a harder crystalline feel. It is often called 'pitting oedema'. This can be hard for the therapist to distinguish initially as in pregnancy even lymphostatic oedema can indent a little due to the increased fluids.

The type of oedema which can be worked with in pregnancy is known as lymphostatic oedema. This is when the amount of lymph fluid that has to be disposed of is normal (in pregnancy there is more, but this is normal not pathological) but the transport capacity of the lymphatic vessels is compromised or exhausted. In pregnancy the lymphatic vessels tend to drain less effectively because of increased venous capacitance and restriction to flow caused by the fetus in the pelvis. Lymphatic drainage tends to be effective. This type of oedema has the following characteristics:

- It responds to elevation and mobilisation by reducing.
- It is better on waking and worsens through the day, especially after prolonged periods of sitting and standing.
- It is worse in the extremities of the limbs (hands and feet).
- It is less crystalline. It may still indent and remain indented for a few minutes.

Contraindications to lymphatic work

- Acute infection/inflammatory illness.
- Serious circulatory problems (e.g. thrombosis, phlebitis, etc.)
- Cardiovascular disease (e.g. uncontrolled hypertension).
- Malignant ailments.
- Any other major health problems which are not under control.

Precautions or relative contraindications

- Lymphodynamic oedemas of the heart, liver and kidney.
- Thryoid problems (hyper- or hypothyroid). Lymphatic drainage on the neck and sternum could possibly alter blood hormone ratio and stimulate the thyroid.
- Bronchial asthma or allergies; drain when the symptoms are in remission.
- Abdominal surgery.
- First trimester of pregnancy: some believe that it may over-stimulate the release of toxins at a time when the body is in a state of transition. Furthermore if there is oedema in the first trimester this is likely to be linked to a pathology and is not suitable to work.

Lymphatic work

In terms of when to include the lymphatic work in the treatment, it is best to do it at the end, when all the other work has been done. It can be done as a section at the end or it can be done as a completing stroke for the arm or the leg. This is because the other work will already have supported the lymphatic and circulatory systems, and work around the neck and the abdomen can be included as part of this, finishing with the lighter lymphatic strokes. Further, it is much easier to do lymph drainage without oil. Excess oil can be removed with the sheet before commencing. Some people believe that if deeper strokes are done after lymphatic work they will negatively impact on the lymphatic work by causing the vessels to be compressed again. Although this is unproven it makes sense to finish with a lighter stroke.

Lymph work for the client feels rather different to normal massage or shiatsu. It is helpful to explain to the client what the stroke involves and its effect; otherwise they may wonder why they are receiving such light and slow strokes. However, once the client understands the work, they usually find it extremely soothing and calming and it is a pleasant way to end the treatment.

Basic lymphatic principles

Strokes which support the lymphatic system are different from normal bodywork strokes. They are much slower and lighter. They flow in one direction only and they follow a specific sequence. Certified therapists have very specific strokes for all the different areas of the body, but basic principles of strokes can be learned and applied by other bodyworkers.

Remember to:

1. Keep the hand soft and relaxed.
2. Contact the skin.
3. Stretch the skin as far as it goes naturally but never slide over the skin during the movements. Maintain contact and gently stretch the skin to where it naturally goes then release.
4. Release the pressure between movements or strokes. There is a pressure phase and a relaxation phase to each stroke. Keep the pressure very light and alternating (on/off or milking actions).
5. Work slowly and rhythmically.
6. Avoid dragging or pulling back on the tissue as is often done in Swedish massage to complete the stroke. Move only in the direction of the lymph flow.
7. Always start with the neck. Start just superior to the clavicle at the terminal nodes. Use the index or middle finger to make a half moon shape; starting lateral and moving medially and down.
8. Massage/pump the regional lymph node next.
9. Always begin and finish every treatment with the neck (including the terminus).

Procedure for lymph work in pregnancy

This work is aimed at alleviating oedema in the legs, arms, face and neck during pregnancy.

First stimulate the terminus nodes (Fig. 9.37). Remember the left side does all the body apart from the right side of the head, neck, trunk, the right breast and

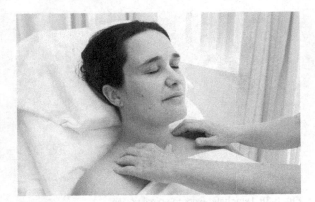

Fig. 9.37 Lymphatic work to terminus nodes.

arm, which are drained by the right side. These nodes lie just below the clavicle, but in many systems of training the strokes are focused on the area just above the clavicle. Work can therefore be done both below and above. The nodes can be felt by palpating along the inferior border of the clavicle from lateral to medial until a change in tissue is felt, which is the node. It is about midway along the clavicle. Stimulate the nodes with slow, light, gentle strokes. The most effective stroke is medial and pedial (half circle down and in). This can be repeated in sequences of five circling movements repeated three times. This encourages the therapist to work slowly and rhythmically. It can be repeated until there is some softening of the tissue.

Next work the neck. The neck has many lymph nodes. Light slow strokes can be applied down the side of the neck towards the lymph nodes.

Next stimulate the regional nodes of the limb (legs, inguinal nodes and spinal nodes, arms and breasts axillary). Some therapists have said that in pregnancy the lymph in the legs needs to be drained to the sacrum/spinal nodes, which lie each side of the spine, as well as the inguinal nodes (Fig. 9.38). The argument behind this is that excess fluid in the legs draining into the inguinal nodes may put too much fluid around the abdominal area. There is no research on this. It may be more of an issue with clients who have more extreme oedema and less of an issue for clients with mild oedema. It makes sense therefore to stimulate both the inguinal nodes and the spinal nodes as regional nodes for the legs. To stimulate the nodes direct strokes can be applied using finger pad pressure with light half-circling pressures.

For the groin and axilla (Fig. 9.39), the client may find this invasive and so it may feel more comfortable to be done through the sheet. An alternative is to use the leg and arm pumping techniques. With the pumping a series of pumping five times and then

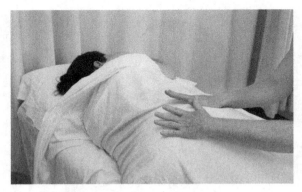

Fig. 9.38 Lymphatic work to spinal nodes.

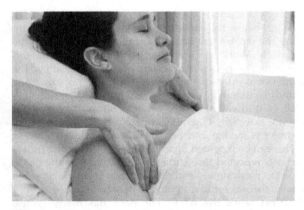

Fig. 9.39 Lymphatic work to axillary nodes.

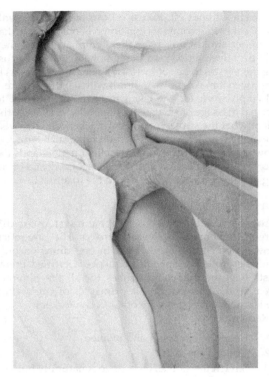

Fig. 9.40 Lymphatic: arm.

resting and repeating three times can be considered as a way of stimulating the node.

Next work on the affected limb. Work is done on the limb in sections – first proximal to the node and gradually moving out more distally, in gradually larger sections. Work is always done in one direction, namely towards the regional nodes, i.e. from distal to proximal. If the limb is elevated, this can support drainage. There are more lymph nodes on the medial aspect of the limb, but try to include work over the whole limb. Work with light strokes doing each section for a few minutes until the oedema has reduced before working more distally.

For the arm (Fig. 9.40)

After stimulating the terminal and axillary nodes work the upper arm in small sections, beginning close to the axilla and increasing the section as the tissue softens. Once the section being drained is from the elbow to the wrist, stimulate the supratrochleal (or cubital) nodes which are on the medial side of the

elbow with a few pumping strokes using the finger-tips; this can be a 'J' stroke using the flat surface of the fingers and making a J which is lateral and superior over the node. Alternatively the arm can be gently flexed in a pumping motion. Then continue the work in the lower arm in small sections, beginning close to the supratrochleal nodes and gradually increasing the sections as the tissue softens.

Once the section is from the wrist to the elbow, work the hand. Some pumping movements flexing the wrist or light pumps directly over the wrist help stimulate the nodes here (Fig. 9.41).

Work can then be done draining the hand in the same way as the arm – stroking towards the wrist (Fig. 9.42). The reflex zones for the lymphatic system lie between the fingers. Work can be done mobilising each joint and working towards the proximal joint. Modified thumb circles can also be used on the dorsum of the hand and fingers; these are half-circling movements with the thumb, with the stroke ending in the direction of the lymph flow.

To conclude, point TH5 (three thumb-widths from the wrist fold in the centre of the medial aspect of the arm) can be held. This point supports the lymphatic system. HC8 (in the centre of the palm) may also be held. Some slow gentle strokes working from the

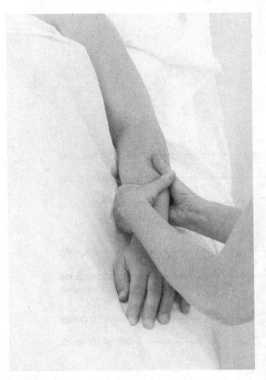

Fig. 9.41 Lymphatic: wrist.

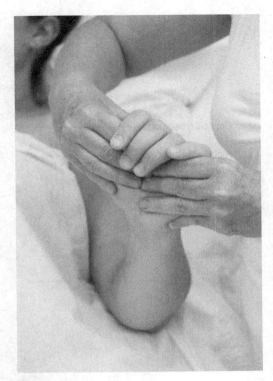

Fig. 9.42 Lymphatic: hand.

hand back to the wrist, from the wrist to the elbow, and from the elbow to the axilla can be included.

For the leg (Fig. 9.43)

After working the spinal and inguinal nodes, work in small sections starting close to the groin, progressing gradually out to the knee (popliteal nodes).

Stimulate the popliteal nodes with some gentle flexions of the knee or direct strokes pumping into the back of the knee. Then work in small sections starting close to the knee, increasing in length until the area from the ankle to the knee is being drained. At the foot, some gentle flexions or direct work around the ankle can be performed to stimulate the nodes here. The foot can then be drained in the same way as the hand. The foot can be finished with holding KD1 (just below the ball of the foot) to support fluid drainage. Work can then be done using strokes back along the sections ending at the spinal nodes.

Finish by stimulating the terminus nodes in the neck once more.

Specific pumping strokes

There are some slightly more complex strokes which involve a little more pumping.

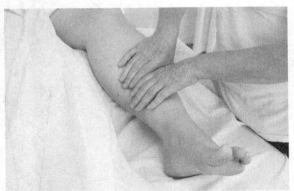

Fig. 9.43 Lymphatic: leg.

Butterfly

Open out the area between thumb and index finger and place the palmar surface of the hand on the tissue making full contact with the skin. Push upward and release. Pump lightly from the wrist upward, release, then lift wrist forward so as to hold skin and not allow lymph to flow back and then pump through again. Keep repeating this action.

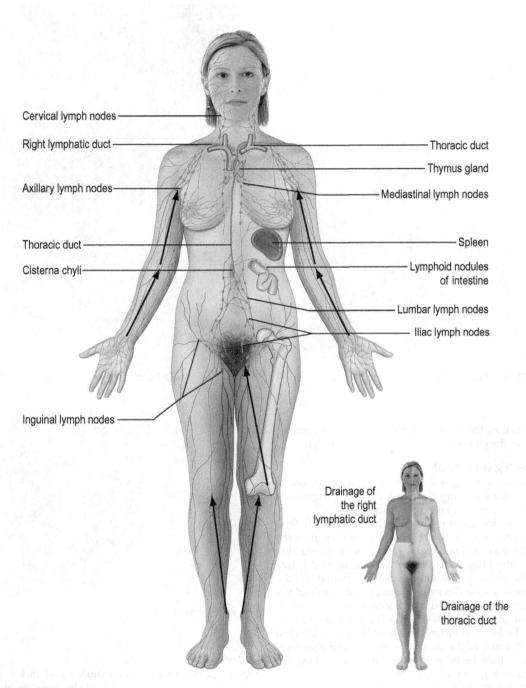

Cervical lymph nodes

Right lymphatic duct

Axillary lymph nodes

Thoracic duct

Cisterna chyli

Inguinal lymph nodes

Thoracic duct

Thymus gland

Mediastinal lymph nodes

Spleen

Lymphoid nodules
of intestine

Lumbar lymph nodes

Iliac lymph nodes

Drainage of
the right
lymphatic duct

Drainage of the
thoracic duct

Fig. 9.44 Lymphatic system.

Caterpillar

Slide the fingers along and then catch up with the heel of the hand.

Aftercare

Aftercare is important. It is important to drink water to help support the draining of the system. Warn the client that she may urinate more frequently than usual and with a greater volume. It is vital to avoid stimulants such as tea and coffee as the system will be more sensitive than normal for a few days. Self terminus lymph drainage can be taught.

Meridian work to support oedema

Meridians which support the lymph system and can be useful working with oedema are BL and Sp for the leg and TH and LU for the arms. Meridian work can be done even with lymphodynamic oedema, because it is working on the level of supporting the organ and energy, rather than physically moving lymph.

Legs – oedema, BL22 – promotes transformation and excretion of fluids in Lower Burner.

BL23 – benefits Kidneys and tonifies Kidney Yang.

ST36 – tonifies Qi and resolves oedema.

LV3, 14 and GB34 – move Liver Qi and eliminate stagnation.

References and further reading

Brady, L.H., Henry, K., Luth, J.F., et al., 2001. The effects of shiatsu on lower back pain. J. Holist. Nurs. 19 (1), 57–70.

Carlsson, C.P., Axemo, P., Bodin, A., 2000. Manual acupuncture reduces hyperemesis gravidarum: a placebo-controlled, randomised, single blind, crossover study. J. Pain Symptom Manage. 20 (4), 273–279.

Curties, D., 1999. Breast Massage. Curties-Overzet Publications, Canada.

Davis-Floyd, R., 1992. Birth as an American Rite of Passage. University of California Press, Berkeley.

De Aloysio, D., Penacchioni, P., 1992. Morning sickness control in early pregnancy by Neiguan point acupressure. Obstet. Gynecol. 80 (5), 852–854.

Diego, M.A., Field, T., Hernandez-Reif, M., et al., 2001. HIV adolescents show improved immune function following massage therapy. Int. J. Neurosci. 106, 35–45.

Dundee, J.W., Sourial, F.B.R., Ghaly, R.G., et al., 1988. P6 acupuncture reduces morning sickness. J. R. Soc. Med. 81 (8), 456–457.

Ernst, E., Matrai, A., Magyarosy, I., et al., 1987. Massage causes changes in blood fluidity. Physiotherapy 73 (1), 43–45.

Field, T., Grizzle, N., Scafidi, F., et al., 1996. Massage and relaxation therapies' effects on depressed adolescent mothers. Adolescence 31, 903–911.

Field, T., Hernandez-Reif, M., Hart, S., et al., 1999. Pregnant women benefit from massage therapy. J. Psychosom. Obstet. Gynecol. 20 (1), 31–38.

Field, T., Delage, J., Hernandez-Reif, M., 2003. Movement and massage therapy reduce fibromyalgia pain. J. Bodyw. Mov. Ther. 7, 49–52.

Goldsmith, J., 1984. Childbirth Wisdom. Congden and Weed, New York.

Hernandez-Reif, M., Field, T., Krasnegor, J., et al., 2000. High blood pressure and associated symptoms were reduced by massage therapy. J. Bodyw. Mov. Ther. 4 (1), 31–38.

Hernandez-Reif, M., Field, T., Krasnegor, J., et al., 2001. Low back pain is reduced and range of motion increased after massage therapy. Int. J. Neurosci. 106, 131–145.

Hovind, H., Nielsen, S.L., 1974. Effect of massage on blood flow in skeletal muscles. Scand. J. Rehabil. Med. 6, 74–77.

Hyde, E., 1989. Acupressure therapy for morning sickness: a controlled clinical trial. J. Nurse Midwifery 34 (4), 171–178.

Kitzinger, S., 2000. Rediscovering Birth. Simon and Schuster, New York.

Lafreniere, K.D., Mutus, B., Cameron, S., et al., 1999. Effects of therapeutic touch on biochemical and mood indicators in women. J. Altern. Complement. Med. 5 (4), 367–370.

Latka, M., Kline, J., Hatch, M., 1999. Exercise and spontaneous abortion of known karyotype. Epidemiology 6–7, 73–75.

Osborne-Sheets, C., 1998. Pre and Perinatal Massage Therapy. Body Therapy Associates, San Diego.

Priya, J.V., 1992. Birth Traditions and Modern Pregnancy Care. Element Books, Shaftsbury, Dorset.

Richards, K.C., 1998. The effect of a back massage and relaxation therapy on sleep. J. Crit. Care 7 (4), 288–299.

Royal College of Obstetricians and Gynaecologists (RCOG), 2006. Exercise in pregnancy. Available at: <www.rcog.what-we-do/campaign-and-opinions/statement/rcog-statement-exercise-during-pregnancy> (accessed 20.04.09).

Smith, C., Crowther, C., Beilby, J., 2002. Acupuncture to treat nausea and vomiting in early pregnancy: a randomized controlled trial. Birth 29 (1), 1–9.

Stillerman, E., 2008. Prenatal Massage: A Textbook of Pregnancy, Labor, and Postpartum Bodywork. Mosby, St Louis.

Thomas, C.T., Napolitano, P.G., 2000. Use of acupuncture for managing chronic pelvic pain in pregnancy: a case report. J. Reprod. Med. 45 (11), 944–946.

Verney, T., 2002. Preparenting. Simon and Schuster, New York.

Weinberg, R., Jackson, A., Kolodny, K., 1988. The relationship of massage and exercise to mood enhancement. Sport Psychol. 2, 202–211.

Yamazaki, Z., Idezuki, Y., Nemoto, T., et al., 1988. Clinical experiences using pneumatic massage therapy for edematous limbs over the last 10 years. Angiology 39 (2), 154–163.

CHAPTER 10

Practical bodywork in labour

Chapter contents

Refer to professional issues (Chapter 15)

For more information on:

Qualities of therapists attending births
Issues relating to working in home or hospital
How to charge for support in labour
Working alongside medical professionals in labour, especially related to working when interventions are utilised
Self-care for the therapist/doula during labour

Refer to labour theory (Chapters 2 and 13)

For more information on:

What happens during labour
Different types of medical interventions

Learning outcomes

- Demonstrate bodywork techniques which can be used to support a woman during different stages of labour
- Demonstrate bodywork techniques which the woman's partner can learn
- Describe other comfort measures such as breathing and birthing positions

Introduction

Bodywork during labour is quite unlike bodywork at any other time. The therapist does not know when or for how long they will need to be working with the client. It could be for a few hours or over the course of several days. It can be anytime within a month-long period (from 2 weeks before the due date and up to 2 weeks after) and during this time the therapist needs to be in relative proximity to the client. This means curtailing travel, late nights, loss of sleep and abstaining from partying or consuming alcoholic beverages. Being available 24 hours a day in this capacity involves making a substantial commitment to the woman/family having a baby.

In some respects professional boundaries become different at this intimate stage in a client's life. Work may need to be done while the client is experiencing nausea and vomiting, while she is on the toilet, or in situations where her realities of privacy and nudity are quite different from the clients seen in regular practice.

It is also essential that the therapist is able to communicate and work with the client's partner, who may or may not be the father of the baby. Partners may be unsure and frightened and just as much in need of support as the woman. Work may need to be done with both to provide the best care possible. If there is no partner, the therapist may be the only support person apart from the primary care providers. In all situations, body work needs to be appropriate to the environment and relevant to the tasks of all others attending the birth.

Once the baby is born, it may need to be held, especially if the woman needs medical attention such as suturing. Appropriately qualified therapists may provide bodywork for the baby.

Much of the therapist's role during labour may not be bodywork in the traditional sense. It may be that all that is done is to apply pressure to the sacrum or hold the woman's hands for minutes or hours. It may be that as much time is spent wiping the woman's face with a cool cloth, giving emotional reassurance, or helping her to get into supporting positions for labour as actually applying bodywork skills.

Knowing what to do, when – and when to do nothing – is essential.

The work may be provided in the client's home, or in the hospital – different environments in which to work and each with particular considerations.

It may be a time full of challenges, not only because it is not possible to plan in advance and is a process of continually responding to the unknown, but also because the length of labour may bring physical challenges to therapists as well as our clients. The therapist may become exhausted. Like the woman and partner in labour, the therapist must look after him- or herself, eating and resting where possible. This is both a personal responsibility and a responsibility to other clients.

Some therapists may decide that they do not want to take on the unpredictable and emotionally heightened opportunity of providing labour support. If the therapist has a young family or a complex schedule which can accommodate few alterations, it may simply not be practical to be out in the middle of the night or to drop everything at a moment's notice. It may be preferable to teach some useful bodywork techniques to the partner at an organised birth preparation session in the weeks leading up to the birth, or agree to be accessible for phone support, or to even drop by, if timing allows, to provide an hour or two of support without attending the birth in its entirety. Other therapists may enjoy birthing support work so much that they seize every opportunity to be present at this amazing moment in a woman's life and the life of the new baby. It truly teaches us a lot about the power, resilience and strength of the female body.

However, in deciding to work with women in labour, either helping them preparing before or by physically being at the birth, the therapist needs to be thoroughly familiar with the physiology of labour, including the different stages, and how to support the woman not only with bodywork, but also with positioning and breathing/visualisation. The therapist also needs to be aware of how to give appropriate emotional support. The power of the mind is as important as the power of the body during labour. Knowledge of types of medical intervention at different stages and their effects, as well as knowing the kind of bodywork which may or may not be appropriate if such interventions occur, is important.

In a sense, working with a woman in labour is one of the easiest times to do bodywork. A woman in labour is extremely sensitive to the kind of touch she needs and where she needs it. It is simply a matter of observing, watching the client's body language, and listening to her. However, it is important to be adaptable. One woman may want to be touched a lot, another not at all. The main difference between labour work and 'normal' bodywork is that often the woman simply wants to be held: held in a particular area, held on a particular point. The woman may have very different needs at different times during labour or she may want the same kind of support throughout. The only thing that can be said with certainty about labour is that it is unpredictable. No two labours are the same.

It is important to remember labour could be 1 hour long or more than 30 hours long. It could be painful or pain-free. Essentially labour support is about accompanying the woman in a journey into the unknown. While the therapist is present, he or she needs to be able to stay with the process of that journey as it unfolds.

This kind of approach was often a form of traditional labour support. The birth partner would often be a wise woman in the village, experienced in giving emotional and physical support. It is a pity that some aspects of this approach are missing from much current intrapartum care. Modern medical care is indispensable and potentially life saving when things go wrong but is not as well developed in supporting the natural processes of women's bodies. Rather than ensuring women's bodies function at their best during birth, it has achieved some of its benefits at the cost of causing women to have less trust in their own inner resources. Body processes sometimes do go awry. In this regard women today are luckier than their ancestors – they can turn to drugs and medical interventions if they are needed. However, currently drugs and interventions are often seen as the first way to approach birth, not the last.

What has to be remembered, which is often forgotten, is that birth is essentially a natural process and one that women's bodies are designed to be able to cope with, even in this technological age. In many cultures, birth was considered a spiritual process, a gateway between adulthood and womanhood, a key life transition. In modern cultures, where the emphasis tends to be on controlling many things, including our bodies, the simplicity, power and miraculousness of birth has been forgotten. One of the aspects of the therapist's role is to support this amazing process as much as possible.

Summary of benefits of work preparing for and during labour

For woman and partner
Offers tools to support the woman to:

- Tune in to her body and learn to pace herself and prepare for labour physically and emotionally.

- Be more aware of her baby.
- Trust in birth and increase her confidence that she can have a positive birth experience.
- Examine her attitudes, needs and hopes for her birthing experience.
- Provide strategies for working with pain.
- Include her partner by offering practical strategies for them to be involved during labour.

For baby

- May help the baby get in good position for labour (optimal fetal position).
- If the woman is more relaxed it will tend to create a more relaxing environment for the baby.
- Helps support prenatal bonding between the parents and their baby.

Other potential benefits

- Shorter labour, decreased need for caesarean deliveries, forceps, vacuum extraction, oxytocin augmentation and analgesia.
- Less difficult and less painful labour.
- Reduction in anxiety scores, positive feelings about the birth experience, increased rates of breastfeeding initiation.

Postpartum benefits

These include decreased symptoms of depression, improved self-esteem, exclusive breastfeeding, and sensitivity of the woman to her child's needs.

10.1 Overview of practical labour work themes

Supporting the physiological process of labour

As a bodyworker, a prime aim is to support the woman in whatever choice she makes in relation to her pregnancy and her birth. However, a key aspect of birth work is knowing how best to support the physiological process. This will include knowing which positions and movements best support this process, and what type of bodywork is likely to be most effective. The birthing positions utilised by the client will affect the type of work which is possible. For example, if the client is leaning forward, the therapist may need to be physically supporting her, which will limit the possibilities for hands-on work. If the woman is leaning forward in a pool, then the therapist may be unable to reach her back.

Working if medical intervention becomes necessary

Even if the client needs medical interventions it is often possible to continue to support her. Depending on when, why and how an intervention is chosen, the woman may be experiencing stress and/or pain and she will still need support. It is necessary to know how to change the focus of work. It is possible to enable a woman to maintain elements of her preferred birthing strategies in the face of medical decision making. For example, although the woman may be monitored throughout her birth, the therapist may be able to help her remain in an upright position. If a caesarean section becomes necessary, then the woman may want some support, regardless of whether the therapist is allowed into the actual delivery room. This may include giving emotional and/or physical support both immediately prior to and as soon as possible after the surgery.

Working with the breath

Breathing well is a fundamental part of labouring well. It ensures both woman and baby get an adequate supply of oxygen. The woman is more likely to stay calm and relaxed, thus increasing the hormones of oxytocin and endorphins which help her during labour. As the woman and baby are so connected this may have a positive effect on the baby too.

Childbirth classes in the 1970s tended to emphasise techniques of 'psychoprophylactic breathing', which are primarily dissociation techniques. These use breathing methods which try to get the woman to disconnect from pain in her body and focus on something outside. However, the current emphasis in childbirth education courses is to emphasise simple techniques which focus on connecting to the body. These tend to utilise a slow, deep relaxed pattern of breathing, often focusing on the out-breath. Prior to the birth, the therapist can help the woman explore what works best for her and if present during labour continue to support the woman to be able to focus on finding the most effective rhythm of breathing. It may be supportive to breathe with her. Using pressure and holding techniques alongside breath awareness can be additionally effective. If the woman prefers to focus on something outside her body – a technique, an image, a movement – the therapist needs to be able to support her to do so.

Working with contractions

Women usually find that they manage better if they focus on one contraction at a time – one contraction is not so overwhelming to successfully cope with. The therapist can support and encourage this.

In a labour which starts naturally (i.e. not induced), the contractions often start by being weaker in intensity, although some women experience intense contractions early on in labour. Some women are very aware of the uterus/abdomen tightening and it may or may not be painful to them. Some women feel pain from the contractions referred down into their back or their legs. Most women find it best to accept and work with the feelings of each contraction.

Contractions are often experienced as wave-like – building up in the body to reach a peak of intensity and then fading away gradually, so that the woman has time to get used to each contraction before it reaches its most intense moment. It is usually helpful to use comfort strategies as the contraction is beginning, so that the peak of it does not take the woman by surprise. Highly important is that for most women there is some space between the contractions which need to be used for rest, recovery, and to prepare for the next contraction. This will help to prevent exhaustion and conserve energy for both the woman and her support person.

An induced labour tends to be more intense, depending on how it is facilitated and how the medication is administered. With induction via oxytocin, the contractions are less like waves and have a more constant intensity, so that there is not the same kind of build up at the peak of a contraction, nor the rest in between. Some women can cope with these contractions without the need for medical pain relief, but they may require more focus to cope with them effectively.

As labour progresses, many women begin to find their own rhythm. This may suggest a dance-like activity with its creative, repetitive, appearance.

Some women find that focusing on something outside themselves such as an external object or a word or phrase may help block pain out (dissociation). However, many women find it is more helpful to use something related to what the contraction is doing (association). This could be a mental image such as a cresting wave or climbing and descending a mountain in the first stage, or a bulb pushing through the ground for the second stage. It is important to spend some time exploring with the client in advance what images she thinks are likely to work best for her if possible.

Some women find that certain bodywork techniques help the contraction to be less painful, or less frightening, and they allow them to relate to it in a positive way.

Many women can keep an intense focus for at least 24 hours but after this they tend to get more tired, especially if they have not been able to rest or eat much. However, women can focus for a lot longer. Some women keep going for 30 or 40 hours or more. If the woman is prepared well, has good support and keeps her focus it is amazing what inner strengths she may find to draw upon. Bodywork is a powerful tool for supporting this process.

Working with 'pain'

Many people argue that defining what happens during the birthing process as 'pain' immediately sets up certain expectations. Birth is certainly intense but its sensations may be unlike what is normally associated with 'pain'. Pain usually indicates that something is wrong with the body, whereas for the most part, birth is about the body doing what it is designed to do. Of course sometimes the body runs into difficulty; the baby may not descend, is positioned awkwardly, or the uterus becomes fatigued, and this can create sensations of pain.

Rather than feeling pain, some women feel intense sensations. Many childbirth methods emphasise seeing contractions as 'rushes', thanks to the excellent midwifery work of Ina May Gaskin and the midwives of The Farm in Tennessee (Gaskin 2002). Others call them 'surges' rather than 'pain' (hypnobirthing term). This certainly gives a more positive focus to birth. However, most women do experience pain or at least discomfort during labour and it is worth being prepared for that reality. In terms of bodywork for pain relief, if the woman is supported to be as relaxed as possible, she tends to feel less pain or is able to cope with it better.

Both traditionally and even today in Japan, where shiatsu originates, women were just expected to get on with labour and, not surprisingly, with that expectation, they often do. The aim of bodywork is not necessarily to take away all pain. Sometimes pain serves a purpose, for example in making the woman aware that she needs to change position to get more comfortable. The ultimate aim is to enable the woman to work with her body, whatever happens. Working with a woman during pregnancy helps prepare for this.

Working with an awareness of the baby and fetal position

Working with an awareness not only of the woman, but also of the baby is important. After all, it is an unknown journey for the baby as much as the woman. Often for the woman, focusing on her baby, rather than on pain, gives a more positive perspective.

The position that the baby is in at the start of labour will have an effect on the outcome of birth.

It cannot be known with any certainty how much the baby is emotionally aware of the process of labour, but certainly it is actively engaged with the process. Babies have been shown to release oxytocin in the womb and therefore may contribute to initiating the process of labour (Odent 2001, Hitchcok 1980). As the baby progresses down the birth canal it is getting into the optimal position for birth, and it is the pressure of the head on the perineum which releases the prostaglandins, which in turn stimulate the production of more maternal oxytocin to strengthen expulsive contractions.

It makes sense for both therapist and woman to be aware of what is happening for the baby and to try to support it, either through including it with touch or through talking to it.

Working with involvement of the partner

Introducing the partner to bodywork for labour during the last trimester is helpful, whether or not the bodyworker has been invited to be at the birth. If the bodyworker will not be present then the role is to identify with the couple what they want to learn. What can be taught will depend on what the partner wants to use as well as their prior knowledge. They could be taught shiatsu labour focus points and other aspects of labour support. The most important aspect is to teach them to work with feedback from the woman so that if it does not feel right, then they alter or discontinue the technique until they have re-checked with the therapist.

If the therapist is going to be present, often the woman's partner will also be present. It is vital to establish the role of the bodyworker/doula and the role of the partner as much as possible prior to labour. It may be that the partner wants to give emotional support while the therapist is there to give the hands-on support. However, the partner may be interested in learning bodywork skills in order to work alongside the therapist.

Working with awareness of the importance of the birth environment

The type of environment will affect the process of labour. Most therapists try their best to create a lovely space in which to give treatments. Similar aesthetic and supportive environments can be created during labour if possible. For those therapists working in hospital settings or places where there is little control of the surroundings, it is still worthwhile being aware of the setting and how best to encourage the creation of a supportive environment. It is worth talking to the woman before labour about how she can create the kind of space she wants, whether she is at home or in hospital.

I was once working with a family in the hospital setting. The lights were dim, my client was comfortably positioned in semi-reclining, and we were doing a repetitive, soothing massage. The nurse came vibrantly through the door and then instantly slowed her movements and tone of voice down to match the setting in the room. Later she told me she felt like a Tasmanian Devil – the hectic pace in the unit outside led to a level of frantic activity which was in direct contrast to the peace within our birthing room.

(Cindy)

Supporting a woman at home

This may be the easiest place to support the woman as she is in her own familiar environment. She has the benefit of knowing her own space, using her own possessions, and can do exactly what she wants. If the birth is going to be at home, then communication with the midwife and support people is needed to let them know the state of her labour when it begins.

If the woman is going to give birth in the hospital, she needs to know at what point her care provider wishes her to travel to the hospital.

Positions which support the physiological process of labour

If the woman is aiming for a natural birth, then the therapist will be working with the woman in positions which support the physiological process of labour.

These are:

- Upright, forward and leaning.
- Using gravity.
- Allowing the sacrum to move.

Common positions are:

- Standing: rocking, leaning against something.
- Squatting: full squat, supported squat or standing squat.
- Forward leaning: for example over a ball.
- Forward sitting.
- Lateral.

The basic positions are the same for the first and second stage of labour, and to some extent the third stage, to facilitate the delivery of the placenta. The main differences are that during the first stage of labour the emphasis is on relaxation and opening up the pelvis. In the second stage the emphasis is more on bearing down with a little more effort and focus.

These tend to be the same positions which women find comfortable at the end of their pregnancy, particularly the forward leaning positions (Fig. 10.1). The main difference in labour, however, is that the woman is likely to be moving around. The woman will need to practise these positions in the weeks leading up to labour and the therapist can support her to do this. The

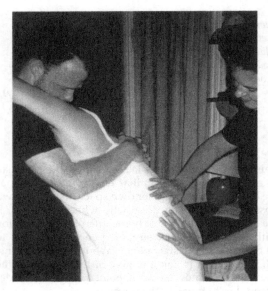

Fig. 10.1 Birth: direct hands-on technique.

role of the therapist or support person during labour is often to offer suggestions regarding positioning, to help support her in these positions, and to help her change positions when desired. Resting versions of each position need to be encouraged so that the woman can rest as much as possible during labour, particularly during the quiet space between contractions. If any position appears to be slowing down labour, or labour is not progressing, it is often wise to suggest a change of position.

If the woman needs to have some medical intervention then she may be placed in a position which is more convenient for the care provider. However, if the woman is uncomfortable, the therapist may be able to help the woman negotiate alterations for comfort. The therapist may also need to remind both the woman and caregiver to aware of PGI/SPD issues.

Supporting a woman to labour in water

The birth positions are essentially the same, except of course the woman cannot rest with her head lower than her hips. Water is especially good if the woman has pelvic girdle instability issues, provided she can get in and out of the pool in such a way that she does not aggravate the problem.

The therapist should not get into the pool with the woman for reasons of health and safety (blood and other body fluids and risk of infection). This means that most of the work is done with the neck and the shoulder and arms, and perhaps the back, if reachable. If the partner is in the pool with the woman s/he can be encouraged to do the work on the abdomen and sacrum.

The woman may use this for first stage or she may decide to stay in to give birth in the water. Midwives who have experience delivering babies in water should be sought for the client's primary care if the woman wants to consider this as an option.

Testimonial of birth support

S.H., birthing client/RMT, doula, Canada

Having spent 2 years at massage school and having learned the benefits of massage during labour, it felt natural that we would have a massage therapist friend attend the birth of our first child. I called her to come to our home when we realised that 'this was it' and after a brief adjustment to a new Energy in our midst, I relaxed into her repetitive strokes. It was the first birth for my friend and although a bit nervous she was very happy to be told (at times in no uncertain terms!) what felt good and what did not. As she had no previous birth support experience, it was necessary for me to offer direction vs her responding intuitively to my needs. It was the pressure on the sacrum that really worked for me, with the strokes matching rhythm with the contractions. It took a bit of experimentation to figure out what felt best but once there I would not let her hands leave my back; in fact I was amused to find after it all that my low back was raw from so much rubbing. And so, I had my team – the RMT gave some physical relief of rubbing and touch, my husband guided me through the breathing and provided me with a circle of focus and the midwife was a constant presence of calm reassurance. It was only during pushing that I asked the RMT to stop as I felt the need to be upright and wanted pure physical support at that point. She stayed in the background after the birth, helping with the 'clean up' and bringing me fresh strawberries. I don't think she said more than 10 words during the whole process and this for me was part of the beauty as she did not demand attention or care. I cannot imagine not having had her at the birth.

With our second birth, I again enlisted the services of another RMT friend but when we came to call her when it was 'time', we found she was ill and so could not come. We were very sad about this but we had no back up and so were left with no alternative. Honestly, I was not too worried as the midwife had a student with her and so I thought that with two of them present that there would be lots of support. However, it was so different from the first time around. The midwives were more interested in discussing with each other as it was a teaching situation but I felt left out of the loop. This time, I felt that my husband and I were on an island alone, trying to deal with the mounting waves. The midwives were out there somewhere, outside my focus talking about things I did not or could not relate to and yet which had the potential to be scary. I don't even remember if either of them touched me except to examine my dilation and being in the middle of labour I felt so unable to ask for more connection from them. That birth was not so smooth and I truly feel it is due to the fact that there was no 'bridging the gap' person there between me and my husband and what we were dealing with so intensely on the one hand, and the midwives who seemed more interested in the medical side of things than with creating an overall good vibe on the other.

With birth number 3 we knew what we wanted and what we did not want. We were prepared with the commitment of our regular RMT (with whom I had enjoyed massage throughout the pregnancy), a lovely midwife, a back-up midwife whom we had requested, and a host of labour aids. Subsequent to my first two labour experiences, I had attended two births as RMT/doula support and had experienced the positive effect of a RMT/doula presence from the other side. I was eager to try new positions, strokes, methods, etc. from the position of the receiver again and so when our RMT arrived it took very little time to start on her bag of tricks. She massaged me on the exercise ball, on the bed, in a waist-deep paddling pool that we had set up in my son's bedroom, with her hands, with a rolling pin. It was a wonderful situation as she had a lot of birth experience and I felt extremely confident in her abilities and attitude. Unlike my first birth experience when I felt I had to be in constant communication with the RMT to express my needs, Cindy seemed to respond intuitively to my non-verbal signals, and I was not afraid of hurting her feelings if I needed to communicate a sudden aversion to a particular method. The midwife was a calm presence as well and although initially resistant in our prenatal visits to us having another professional at the birth, when it came to the 'big event' she could see the benefits of having someone there who could give full undiverted attention to the needs of the labourer. As wonderful as midwives are, they have a medical job to do which occasionally demands taking a step back from supporting the labourer directly to check on dilation, the baby's heart rate, etc. She was used to doing some massage herself and so was surprised I think to see the power of the focused massage an RMT could give versus

her intermittent touch. We chose our team carefully and wonderfully everyone supported each other to the fullest.

I feel extremely fortunate to have had three peaceful home births but also to have had the chance to experience different situations with regards to support. With the combination of an experienced RMT/doula, a caring midwife and family support I feel with birth number 3 we came as close as possible to the perfect experience of birth.

Pelvic girdle instability (PGI) with symphysis pubis laxity (SPL)

If the woman has this problem, she should consider giving birth in water or using all fours positions to minimise stress on the joint. Birth may be easy because the bones of the pelvis move easily; however, pain may be an issue. Bodywork is advisable for an initial pain relief option as it is best to avoid anaesthetics such as epidurals, because then the woman will not be able to feel when she is putting pressure on the bones. Often women aggravate their condition through stressing the joint in labour. If an epidural becomes necessary then it is important for the birth support people to have established beforehand how wide apart the woman can place her legs without placing strain on the pubic bone and then monitor her positions carefully.

Forceps delivery will tend to aggravate the problem as the woman will have her feet in stirrups which may excessively stress the joint. If it becomes necessary, care needs to be taken both in placing the woman in lithotomy and also to minimise the amount of time she is in the position.

If care is taken to minimise stress on the joint in labour, then the problem usually begins to resolve quickly postnatally. If the joint is further stressed during labour then it may take a long time to heal postnatally, sometimes even years, especially if appropriate support and aftercare is lacking.

10.2 Birth preparation work

This includes work preparing for birth, supporting optimal fetal positioning, and working with 'induction' (initiation). Working with an awareness of the position of the baby can be an important focus of bodywork during the third trimester of pregnancy and becomes increasingly important as the trimester progresses. Work with the more specific 'labour focus' points can be initiated from 37 weeks onwards.

Encouraging optimal fetal positioning

If the baby is in an 'optimal' position at the start of labour it is likely to have a beneficial effect on the progress of labour. The most beneficial position is considered to be LOA (left occiput anterior).

Encourage the woman to be aware of the position of her baby during the third trimester, when the baby begins to settle more into a particular position. She needs to be aware that she cannot 'fix' the baby in any position as they will continue to move right up to and during labour. As the pregnancy progresses, and the baby gets bigger, they will have more fully filled the abdominal space and are therefore able to move less. However, babies continue to shift position, especially from posterior to anterior, even during labour. Transverse babies often shift to cephalic in late pregnancy. Breech babies find it the hardest to move later on, as they need more space and research indicates that 32–34 weeks is an optimal time to encourage a breech baby to move.

Maternal position and movement may help encourage the baby to move, especially forward leaning. Work to encourage anterior cephalic positioning with the woman in forward leaning positions. The type of work to include is work to mobilise the sacrum and release the sacral uterine ligaments as tightness here may impede movement and descent of the fetus. It can be valuable to check pelvic alignment (sacrum, coccyx, sacroiliac, hips, and pubic bones). Misalignments may affect the position of the baby. The shoulders and neck compensate or reflect imbalances in the pelvis and these areas may also need mobilising/realigning in order to support good fetal positioning. Be aware, however, that for a small number of women the shape and position of the uterus and the pelvis may influence the baby's position and it may not be possible for the baby to settle in an anterior position.

Working on an energy level will include work with the Bladder meridian. Bladder is about stimulating Water, transition and movement. Include BL 31–4 (sacral foramen points) to support releasing of the sacrum and pelvis. Include BL 67 (base of little toe) to help stimulate the baby to move. BL 67 is traditionally used with moxa for turning breech babies; however, as it stimulates fetal movement it may be used in all cases of malposition. In these other cases, holding pressures or rubbing to warm the point, or simply working intuitively all seem effective. Contrary to some beliefs, it will not turn a cephalic baby into breech.

The connection between the woman and her baby may also influence position. Encourage the woman to tune in to her baby and connect with him/her. This can be done through bodywork, visualisation, conversing with baby, writing, or artwork. If the baby is in a less optimal position then perhaps some stress is affecting it. Either the woman or baby may be afraid of the next steps in their journey. A Chinese view is that a breech baby is 'clutching at the woman's heart'.

Poor positioning may be partly due to modern sedentary lifestyle and certainly if the woman has a desk job, then it is important in the evening to spend time in other positions, if only resting forwards over some cushions. Even if it simply helps relieve low back ache, it will help the woman learn to relax in this kind of position which is helpful to use during labour itself.

Breech work

If the baby is breech at 32–34 weeks, encourage the woman to massage her own belly, talking to her baby and gently encouraging it to turn. This type of work can be included as part of abdominal bodywork – but it is a gentle movement. Do not attempt to rotate the baby (attempting an external version). ECV is a medical technique that needs to be done in a medical setting by primary care providers in order to be prepared should complications arise. Bear in mind that the closer to the due date the woman gets, the less room there is for the baby to turn from a breech position. If the baby is still breech at 34 weeks, a skilled practitioner can initiate moxa stimulation to BL 67. If the therapist is not trained in the use of moxa, then heat stimulation created by simply rubbing or pulling on the little toe can be effective.

One guideline for the use of moxa is the following:

Moxa BL 67 on both feet for 15 minutes, once a day for 10 days in all; initially for 5 days only, then waiting a few days and monitoring the position of the fetus, and then, if its position has not been corrected, repeating the treatment for another 5 days. It is important to pause and to monitor the position of the fetus rather than applying the treatment continuously, because the fetus may turn into the correct position and then, if the treatment is continued, may turn back into its previous position. Most research papers on moxibustion show that the 34th week of gestation is the optimal time to carry out the technique and gives a higher success rate.

(Budd 2006)

The optimum time to start acupuncture appears to be 33–34 weeks (Cardini & Weixin 1998, Neri et al 2004). Grabowska (2005) suggests that this time is when the uterus contains its maximum amniotic fluid, and before the breech starts to descend into the pelvis.

In contrast to the advice given above, other guidance suggests that up to 10 times a day may be fine. The frequency is best determined by the woman, usually with the proviso that it should only be done if she is 100% sure that the baby has not turned.

However, Betts feels that even that proviso is unnecessary as acupuncture only supports the body to do what is best for it (Betts 2006).

It is important not only to focus on more symptomatic treatment, such as the selection of only one point, but also to work with the overall energy patterns of the woman.

Many of the women with breech babies I see show signs of general heat or more commonly Heart heat, red papillae on the tongue tip. Moxa is still applicable but with cooling and calming treatment and I advise not doing the moxa within the 2 hours before bed.

(Lea Papworth)

The client needs to avoid deep squats in the third trimester if the baby is breech as they could encourage the baby to move deeper down in the pelvis, making it harder to turn.

Supporting the initiation of the birth process

It is better not to use the term 'induction' of labour for bodywork which is done in supporting the woman to go into labour. Changing the name of applying bodywork to energy points from 'induction points' to 'initiation points' helps to distinguish medical procedures from bodywork applications. Work is aimed at much more than stimulating hormonal release: it is about physical and emotional preparation, addressing issues that may block the woman's comfort with going into labour, such as fear of pain, and helping to support her to move into her birthing experience with excitement, readiness, and as much confidence as is possible.

Many factors can prevent the woman from going into labour: stress, anxiety/fear, simply not feeling ready, for example not having things organised/finished, not feeling emotionally ready, or being in difficult personal or interpersonal situations. She may simply be tired, especially when so many women currently work right up to their due date. The woman may also have enjoyed being pregnant, feels very connected to her baby inside her, and is reluctant for the pregnancy to end. A holistic approach enables the therapist to discuss and consider the woman's reality from varied angles.

While the 'initiation' points can be used, other strategies may also help. This may include working with the Extraordinary Vessels, general bodywork to help with relaxation and well-being and connecting with the baby. A full bodywork session is usually given addressing the many issues which may be going on for the woman, with the inclusion of 'initiation' points as appropriate. The focus is on supporting the woman to move from the state of pregnancy into giving birth.

Of course there are no guarantees that this work will result in turning the baby into a different position or initiate the onset of labour. However, clinically, many practitioners have witnessed success in seeing shifts in the woman's situation, and at the very least they believe these techniques help to prepare their clients both emotionally and physically for their birthing process (Ingram et al 2005, Smith & Crowther 2004).

Before proceeding with a labour focus approach, it is important to check with the primary caregiver that there is no medical reason why the woman has not gone into labour. For example, if the baby is still high in the pelvis and is not engaged it may be unsafe to utilise techniques which could stimulate contractions.

If the baby is not in the optimal position then the first focus might be to support the baby to position itself in alignment for good descent. If the baby is in a transverse or oblique position, the labour initiation approach is unwise because unless the baby changes position there is no chance of progressing to a vaginal delivery.

'Natural induction' does not carry the risk of overstimulating the uterus which could be an issue for women who have previously had a caesarean section (in contrast to induction via Syntocinon). This group of women would be carefully monitored by the primary care provider during their labour and indeed many hospitals do not perform medical induction for these clients because of the potential risk of uterine rupture. Therefore, unless there are additional factors which would make the client at higher risk for onset of labour, applying 'initiation' techniques should not be contraindicated for a client who is wishing to experience a VBAC (vaginal birth after caesarean).

Support for the initiation of the birth process for the woman

- Relaxation and touch encourage release of oxytocin and endorphins, which support the process.
- Energy wise, work to balance the CV and GV is important; Yin, Yang and Hormonal balance. Work with their associated points is particularly effective; KD 6 and BL 62 held simultaneously.
- Work with Girdle Vessel, to encourage it to open and using the opening and associated points GB 41 and TH 5.
- Labour focus points can be used when appropriate as they can have a strong effect on initiating the process.
- Supporting the woman/baby connection.
- Ensuring that the baby is in a good position for labour.
- Relaxed pelvis and sacrum.

Inhibitors to the birth process for the woman

It is the midbrain and the brainstem which set in motion the processes mediated by the hormones and prostaglandins. This is what is known as the 'old part' of the brain. Stress affects prostaglandin production; energy wise this relates to the Extraordinary Vessels.

Stress and adrenaline release constrict blood flow to the uterus which reduces the release of prostaglandins.

Labour focus/initiation points: SP6, LV3, BL60, GB21, LI4

Each point has a different effect. Some women will respond to some points, because that is the effect they need, and other women will respond to other points. This means that they do not all necessarily need to be used, as only some may work. If the point is the right point for the woman, she is likely to know. It may simply 'feel right' and induce relaxation. It may stimulate movement of the baby and even contractions.

There is much controversy around the use of these points prior to term, based on the fear that they could stimulate miscarriage or premature labour. Indeed many people include lots of other so-called 'forbidden points', although these five are the most effective labour stimulation points. It is unclear why there is so much fear around the use of certain points. Simply because a point is effective in labour does not mean it will create labour in a person whose body is not ready to go into labour; that is not how energy works. However, if a pregnancy has a predisposition toward premature labour, using these points might support that inclination, although some people have

anecdotally reported using these points to stop premature labour. The same is true of miscarriage in the first trimester. With a healthy gestation, there is no mechanism by which they could cause a miscarriage. Indeed, if they were that efficacious they would be widely used for supporting women in terminations. However, if the woman has an inclination for pregnancy loss, stimulating these points might add support to the process. Indeed they are useful to use in the first trimester if the fetus has died but is still inside the uterus in order to support natural miscarriage.

There are many anecdotal examples of therapists or women using the points because they are late with their period, and then afterwards realising that they were pregnant and carrying their babies to term. The following story illustrates how the points do not affect a healthy baby adversely.

We feel that the prohibition of these points is not especially founded in clinical reality, and it is up to each individual therapist to make their decisions regarding their use.

From 37/38 weeks the body and baby are preparing for labour and this is a time when these points are likely to be effective. They can be used as often as feels comfortable and the woman can be encouraged to practise them. A clear explanation should be given about why the points are being stimulated and the type of techniques which will be employed. If the woman does not feel comfortable with their use, do not use them. If the pregnancy is post term and medical induction is being proposed, then use these points as often and for as long as possible. In these circumstances, it is helpful to show the points to both the woman and her partner, so that they can practice them at home. The cumulative effect may be more powerful than just using them once. Try combining points. Sometimes this is more effective than using individual points but be guided by the woman. They may feel more powerful and therefore more effective. However, the combination may feel unhelpful or even strange, in which case do not proceed with them.

As 'induction' points they tend to be very effective. If the woman is ready to begin labour, they do not need to be stimulated much. However, the further away the woman is from labour, the more they tend to need to be worked and the less responsive they are likely to be.

Some women find some of the points helpful for pain relief during labour because they are allowing energy to flow. In labour they can be used as long and as often as the woman wants. This could be for short periods of time, or sometimes the whole of labour. Sometimes women want just one of the points held for hours. Sometimes they want different points stimulated at different stages. Each point has slightly different indications, but they all potentially help at any stage of labour,

---

Testimonial: Suzanne

One of my shiatsu colleagues, A, had been trying for some time to become pregnant. Her first pregnancy ended at 9 weeks, but she did not miscarry and had to go to hospital for a dilatation and curettage. In the ninth week of her second pregnancy she began to bleed quite heavily and assumed that she must be miscarrying. She instructed her husband, a large strong man, to work all the 'labour focus' points as strongly and as long as he could. They worked them a lot for a day or so but A carried on bleeding and so they decided to go to hospital. A heart beat was heard, but it took several weeks for the caregivers to establish what was happening. A had a bicornuate uterus and the septum was bleeding as the uterus grew. She bled for several weeks and was hospitalised during that time. The pregnancy continued and she now has a healthy young child.

both to help labour flow and to ease pain. The best way to use them is to try them out: no harm will be caused by using the 'wrong' point. If a point is not effective, it will not feel right to use. Stop using it and there will be no adverse effects. Often women find that at least one of the points does help their body to focus and get on with what it needs to do: 'labour focus' points.

Labour focus points: SP6, LV3, GB21 LI4 BL60

Labour focus points help to focus the woman and baby on getting ready for labour and they also support the process of labour itself. They do not put anything into the body and are simply working to balance energy. This means they can be used alongside drugs if necessary as there will be no interaction. They can be used to help with: initiation of labour, pain relief during labour, progressing a prolonged labour, strengthening ineffectual contractions, fetal positioning, delivering a retained placenta, delivering a placenta without the use of Syntometrine.

Remember – use them as often and as long as feels right for the woman. If they do not feel right – stop using them.

Locating and working the points

Women can practice using them on their partner, prior to 37 weeks, to learn the location of the points. As their effect is not limited to labour they may have an effect on men and on non-pregnant women. If they feel comfortable they can be practised, but if they feel sore or uncomfortable, do not use them.

Once the point has been located, it is often easiest to work with the thumb into the point. Make sure that the rest of the hand is comfortable. It can often be good to wrap the other fingers around the area being worked. The points on both sides can be worked simultaneously or one at a time. If working one point, place the free hand on another area of the woman's body where it feels comfortable. This hand can offer reassurance. It can often be helpful to have this other hand, the woman hand, over the woman's abdomen, in connection with the baby. This way the baby's response can be monitored. Do what feels best for the woman, but do work the point on each side, even if one side is stimulated for longer.

Try working them with the woman in the different labour positions, as emotionally this can help her feel more connected with labour.

How long should the points be worked?

It is not possible to say definitively as women respond differently. A minimum of 1 minute is suggested in order to produce an effect and to be able to assess whether it is an appropriate point to work. Some women do not feel any response initially and the point may need to be held for longer. If nothing is felt then either the point is incorrect, and so the location needs to be verified, or it may need to be held for longer. If nothing is felt after a couple of minutes, then it is probably an ineffective point.

After some time the woman will feel she has had enough. Before labour this might be after a few minutes. If she is nearly ready to go into labour and the point is really helping to focus her energy, then she may appreciate work for as long as 20 minutes. During labour, some women find they literally do want the points held for hours. However, other women may find after 5 or 10 minutes they do not want more work done on a point, but then a few minutes or hours later they want the point worked again. It is important to be guided by the woman's response.

Bladder 60 (Fig. 10.2)

This lies between the posterior border of the external malleolus and the medial aspect of tendocalcaneus, at the same level as the tip of malleolus (in the hollow midway between the knob of the ankle bone on the outside of the ankle and Achilles tendon).

This point is the Fire point on the Bladder meridian and has the useful effect of clearing heat and excess energy, especially from the head. Due to its relationship with the Heart, it can be used for physical or emotional pain. It can therefore be used to help calm an anxious woman in labour. It activates the whole length of the Bladder meridian and may ease tightness in the head, spine and legs. It has a strong downward effect and so is very useful for inducing and augmenting labour and for the expulsion of the placenta.

Spleen 6 and Liver 3

They can be incorporated into foot and ankle massage, which is beneficial both during pregnancy and labour.

Spleen 6 (Fig. 10.3)

Place the tip of the little finger on top of the medial aspect of the anklebone of the opposite leg, fingers pointing away from the medial aspect of the leg. SP6 lies beneath the second joint of the forefinger, under the shin (3 *cun* (thumbwidth) above the tip of the medial malleolus just posterior to the tibial border).

This is an important point for maternity applications as well as digestive, sexual, urinary problems and emotional balancing. Although it is on the Spleen meridian it is where Spleen meets Liver and Kidney and so affects all these energies – Earth, Wood and Water – which are important in labour. SP6 has

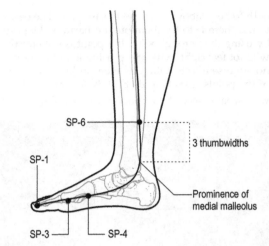

Fig. 10.3 Spleen 6.

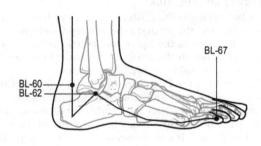

Fig. 10.2 Bladder 60.

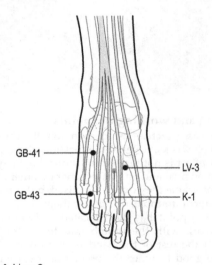

Fig. 10.4 Liver 3.

extremely wide applications and can be used for anything to do with deficiency of Qi, Blood, Yin, Yang or Kidney Essence, failure of Spleen Qi to hold the blood in the vessels, too much Qi, Blood or dampness. It is worth trying at any stage of labour, including initiation. It can help change fetal position and is useful for regulating uterine bleeding. In Japan SP6 is often used during the whole of the last trimester to prepare the uterus for birth and is often useful in cases where the uterus is tired.

Liver 3 (Fig. 10.4)

On top of the foot in the hollow between the first and second metatarsal bones. Place the finger on the space between the two bones and slide towards the ankle. It is in the depression before the junction of the bases of the first and second metatarsals.

This point is good for clearing Wood energy, both by bringing more energy into Liver or taking excess energy away. The emotion associated with Wood is anger and when any emotions are suppressed it is often Wood energy which gets stuck. It can help women release suppressed emotions and feel more in touch with what they are feeling in labour. Suppressed emotions are often what blocks the movement from first to second stage. It can therefore be a good point for transition. It can help draw energy down from where Wood energy tends to get stuck in the shoulders and so is helpful for headaches. It is often useful

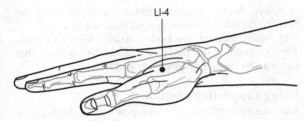

Fig. 10.5 Large Intestine 4.

if the woman finds the neck and shoulder points too intense. This point has an anti-spasmodic effect on the cervix, so it is useful in cases where the cervix is tense and not dilating with contractions.

Large intestine 4 (Fig. 10.5)

This lies between the thumb and forefinger on the back of the hand. To locate, either

(i) have the thumb and index finger closed and the point is at the highest spot of the muscle

(ii) stretch the thumb and the index finger.

The point is midway between the junction of the first and second metacarpal bones and the border of the web, slightly towards the second metacarpal bone.

It is known as the 'great eliminator' and is often used to relieve pain, including headaches. It is especially useful if the woman is feeling sick or has diarrhoea.

Gall Bladder 21 (Fig. 10.6)

In the hollow on top of the shoulder, straight up from the nipple when standing. It is in the highest point of the trapezius.

This can be incorporated in a shoulder massage which is relaxing for the woman in labour. It relaxes tension in the shoulder, neck and jaw. It can also help with poor lactation.

Point combinations

Combining points is about bringing two different energies together. It is a bit like finding the most Kyo and Jitsu points and balancing the energy from these. There have been found to be some useful point combinations in labour, although potentially any two points can be linked. Try any potential combination if it is helpful for the client.

The magic triangle Ikuyo Hosaka refers in her work to this combination of points (Yates 2003). It is SP 6, BL 60 and a point on the Gall Bladder. This is useful for initiating labour and augmenting contractions.

Joining above and below It is often useful if there are two birth support people to combine LV 3 with

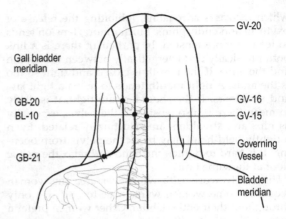

Fig. 10.6 Gall Bladder 21.

GB 21 – GB 21 sends Wood energy down and LV 3 draws Wood energy down. It is useful as a focus to stimulate second stage contractions.

LV 3 and LI 4 is another point combination.

10.3 Specific considerations for supporting different stages of labour

First stage

What is happening

Contractions serve to thin and dilate/open the cervix to 10 cm:

- Latent phase: 1–3 cm dilatation.
- Active phase: 3–10 cm dilatation.

Key words to support this stage

Opening up, going with the flow, relaxation, surrender.

Key elements

Water – movement from Yin to Yang aspect, i.e. Kidney Yin to Kidney Yang and Bladder.

Bodywork focus

Tension in any area may slow down the process of opening up. The main area which needs to open is the pelvis/uterus/cervix and it is often in the sacral or abdominal areas where women experience discomfort and appreciate bodywork. However, if there is tension in any part of the body: shoulders or hands, legs or feet, it is likely to: increase tiredness, divert blood and energy away from the pelvis, constrict movement and may be part of the tension cycle which increases adrenaline, inhibiting the release of oxytocin and endorphins. Furthermore, tension tends to lead to more tension. In particular, there is a link both physically and energetically between the mouth and the anus. If the mouth is closed and tight so too is the anus. A tight mouth tends to mean a tight jaw and shoulders. If the shoulders are tight, it is likely to mean there is also tension in the pelvis, especially as hips and shoulders are structurally related. Even a tightly held hand may block the pelvis from opening. It is hard to tighten the hand and relax the pelvic floor at the same time.

Ultimately work with whichever area the woman requests. Some women want focus to one area only throughout their entire labour. Other women prefer a focus with several different areas.

Some women respond more positively to pressure or holding work, while others prefer effleurage and stroking movements. Typically during a contraction, women respond more to holding or pressure work: often on the sacrum or abdomen. In between contractions they may still want static contact or they may want a more active stroke application. Often strokes down the back and down the legs may be comforting as women may perceive them as drawing pain and discomfort out of the body.

Labour focus points can be used with a focus of encouraging opening up of the cervix or with a focus of supporting the baby to move into an optimal position.

The focus of body work in the first stage tends to be:

• Releasing tension and keeping muscles as relaxed as possible, with any area of the back, sacrum, neck and shoulders, abdomen, arms or legs including hands and feet as possible areas of focus.
• Encouraging the relaxation of the pelvis and the opening up of the cervix.

Other ways to help support the process of first stage
Increase relaxation
Breathing is a key tool in supporting relaxation. By breathing deeply, the woman helps her body produce endorphins and oxytocin, which are the body's natural painkillers. The woman may need to be encouraged to find her own rhythm of breathing and visualisations and words may be appropriate tools to support this (see breathing in aftercare, section 12.2 p. 340).

Of course, being relaxed in labour is not what is normally thought of as 'relaxation'. In contrast to the quiet, slumbering, non-labouring client, a labouring woman is often moving around and may be making sounds or noises. Being relaxed in labour, means allowing the body to do what it needs to without resisting.

By being relaxed, the body actually feels less pain. The converse if the body is in pain and tenses, this can lead to fear and more pain and tension.

Using supportive positions
The woman will need to use positions which allow the pelvis and baby to move and facilitate the process of opening. These could be more upright and active positions but could also include side-lying or sitting.

Make sure that the woman is not blocking off blood flow to her limbs. She may need to move her legs or change how she is using her arms to support her. The therapist may need to give physical support to the woman or use effleurage techniques to promote circulation. Lying in the left lateral positions tends to encourage better blood flow to the fetus and maximise renal plasma flow.

Conserving energy
As this stage of labour is the longest, and since no one can anticipate its length, it is important that everyone, including the birthing woman, her partner and the therapist, conserve their energy as well as possible. The best way to do this is to provide attention and support while exerting the minimum amount of energy needed to care for the needs of the birthing woman. Also crucial is using the space between contractions to let go and rest. If the woman goes into labour in the middle of the night, this is even more important.

Using minimum expenditure usually means beginning with breathing and relaxation techniques so that the woman and baby are getting oxygen and restorative rest. This may be all the woman needs in early labour. She may even be able to carry on with attempts to sleep if it is in the middle of the night. As labour progresses then the woman will tend to need to move more. At some point the woman may feel the need of more support, which could be a clear physical or emotional presence from her support people, reassurance, or exploring positions and bodywork for increasing comfort.

Be aware of the baby
Helping the family focus on the energy of bonding with their baby can be helpful in bringing their attention to the importance of the woman's birthing work and lend a positive focus. Since babies are aware of touch and sound, this is likely to be reassuring for the baby as well as the woman.

The key is:

Keep focused and only use what is needed to support the process.
- Begin with the breathing and visualisations – create a safe, relaxed space.
- Support the woman to stay positive and focused on what her body is doing.
- Use positions and movement as required, but make sure everyone rests when they can.
- Use whatever type of bodywork the woman needs, when she needs it: this may be simple holding techniques or more involved bodywork.
- Encourage work which supports the woman to open up – breathing out and letting go. Lung energy work.
- Support the woman to 'go with the flow' – the Yin aspect of water to support the Yang.
- Work to relax muscles to release unnecessary tension which may prevent the uterus dilating effectively.
- If the woman is using water, try to keep the pool for when she really needs it as then it will be appreciated. If the woman gets in too early it may slow labour down. However, if the woman really wants to be in the bath or pool, it may be helpful.

Transition

What is happening

This indicates the end of first stage as the body is beginning to get ready for second stage. The cervix is completing its final stages of dilation (8–10 cm).

Key words to support this stage

Intensity.
Feelings of being overwhelmed OR a need for rest and quiet.

Key element

Transition from Water to Wood.

Bodywork focus

The woman and her support team may keep doing what they were doing in the first stage but in a more intense way – the woman may need more pressure, more reassurance, more reminders of her progress through her labour. On the other hand, some women may need more space and may not want any bodywork at this time. Touch may feel too intense.

More work may need to be done on the neck and shoulders, which are often areas where women hold tension. Often women pull away from the intensity of feeling in the perineum and this may involve tensing the upper body.

Women may get stuck at this stage in different ways. The therapist can observe how the client is getting stuck. Is it physical or emotional? Is it frustration, fear, pain or fatigue? These realities can express themselves in different energy presentations.

The focus of bodywork in transition is:

- Continuing to release tension in the body, but this may include more of a focus on the neck and shoulders.
- Supporting the woman to begin to focus down into the perineum, rather than resisting.
- Give space if needed.
- Support rest if needed.

Other ways to help the woman's body support this process

Supporting relaxation and emotional release

Staying relaxed and focused in whatever way helps support this stage of labour. The woman will still need to focus on the out breath and on relaxing but she needs to have more of a focus into the perineum.

Give reassurance and encouragement as the woman may become overwhelmed by the intensity and start to bear down before she is ready. If anything, encourage her to stay calm. If the urge to bear down is overwhelming, the woman can go with these sensations, but often she realises that her body is not quite ready for active second stage.

Using supportive positions

Support the woman to continue using positions where gravity helps but continuing to relax into these positions, even though there may be more intensity to them.

Continue to be aware of the baby

Second stage

What is happening

The contractions are called expulsive contractions as they are now working to push the baby down the birth canal and out into the world.

Key words to support this stage

Down and out, focus down, perineum opening up.

Key element

Wood.

Bodywork focus

As the woman often has a definite focus at this stage, she may not need the support of touch. Instead, she may require more physical support in sustaining birthing positions.

While some women may find they do not want as much bodywork in this stage of labour, others may find that it helps them to stay relaxed, focused and in contact with their support people. Some women want to continue receiving the same kind of bodywork they have received up till now or they may want different work.

Many women prefer more of a focus on the neck and shoulders. As the woman is 'learning' how to push effectively, and may be afraid of the strong bearing down sensations, she may resist them. This 'unproductive pushing' can be a bearing down using the upper body, tensing the neck and shoulders. The bodyworker can encourage the woman to keep her jaw loose and relaxed, to drop her shoulders and focus her attention down into the pelvis and perineum.

In between the urges to push, the bodyworker can encourage the woman to fully let go.

Labour focus points can be used with the focus of supporting the process of bearing down.

If second stage is long then there may be a need to do some stroking work in the limbs to improve circulation. However, monitor that the woman does not find this work too fussy and that it is not distracting her from the downward focus.

Bodywork focus in second stage:

- Release tension from jaw, neck, and shoulders.
- Encourage the woman to bear down into the perineum.
- Massage to legs and arms if tension builds with bearing down.

Other ways to help the woman's body support this process

Help the woman stay relaxed and keep breathing

Help her to stay relaxed, remind her of her baby, try to keep her calm and not panicked, and help her stay focused on her breathing.

Help the woman to listen to her body and to her baby

This stage can be portrayed as difficult with much straining and pushing. In fact attuning to the body and responding to its urges can result in the baby being born more easily. The therapist can encourage the woman to tune in to her baby, to listen to what her body wants to do, and to be patient with the process allowing her baby to be born as it is ready. The woman needs to focus on feeling the baby coming down onto the perineum and going with the feelings of pressure. Some women find that if they can visualise the perineum stretching open, this can help to allow this to happen. Perineal massage

done prior to labour can be a tool to support this process. Some women find it helpful to utilise something which helps them visualise the baby coming down, such as holding on to a rope and pulling down.

Help the woman to continue to use upright positions

The woman may need additional physical support in order to be able to continue to use the upright positions. It is important to continue to keep the pelvis free from compression as the coccyx needs to be able to move. If second stage is long then the mother may need to be encouraged to mobilise to promote circulation to the limbs.

The standing squat can be particularly useful at this stage and so the therapist may need to help the woman to get into this position.

The woman may need to be encouraged to shift the emphasis in the birthing positions from opening, and circling the hips to bearing down.

Summary of second stage work

- The woman needs to be able to stay focused and relaxed and allow her baby to be born; to trust that her body and her baby know what to do.
- Often physical support is needed to help the woman stay in more physically demanding upright birth positions.
- Less bodywork may be needed although some women may want bodywork to continue.
- There may be a shift from bodywork to the pelvis to bodywork for the shoulders.
- Labour focus points may be needed to help the descent of the baby.
- The woman needs to focus on what her body is doing so she does not force.
- The woman needs to continue to focus on her baby.
- The woman can focus on the Yang, Wood energy.
- The woman can focus on the bearing down sensations.

Third stage

What is happening
The delivery of the placenta.

Key words to support this stage
Staying focused.

Key element
Wood going into Fire.

Bodywork focus

At this time, attention is more focused on the woman and baby connecting with one another and giving the woman time to welcome her baby into the world. This is a time for the therapist to respectfully give space to the new family. Bonding rather than bodywork is the primary goal at this time. Encouraging the baby to nuzzle or latch is also valuable because it helps the placenta to release due to the increase in oxytocin. If the placenta is not delivered in a timely manner, relevant shiatsu points can be utilised in consultation with the primary caregiver. The most important points are GB 21, followed by LI 4 and SP 6.

Other ways to help the woman's body support this process

In order to have a natural delivery of the placenta, the woman needs to remain focused and relaxed. The therapist can help remind her client to breathe, to keep the baby close to her for the facilitation of the oxytocin release, as well as to relax and focus on the contractions which release the placenta.

If the woman has a full bladder this can interfere with the delivery of the placenta, so she may need to empty it. Usually the primary caregiver will remind the woman to do this, but the therapist can also encourage the woman to do so, especially as it is likely to be the last thing she feels like doing.

Fourth stage

What is happening

Getting to know the baby and bonding as a family – preparation for the rest of the family's life.

Key words to support this process

Getting to know the baby, connection, communication.

Key element

Fire.

Bodywork focus

Usually it is best to find an appropriate moment to leave the family so that they can have quiet, bonding time with their newborn. However, some women may wish to have their labour support person remain on hand, especially if they have special needs related to bonding and feeding their baby, or postpartum issues such as bleeding or stress in the birthing process. Now the woman can rest, hold and feed her baby. It is helpful for her to be able to do this in a comfortable position, not only for her, but to facilitate comfort for the baby, and also a good latch. Gently reminding the woman to relax her shoulders when holding her baby can be helpful.

> ### Summary of fourth stage work
>
> Standing back and allowing bonding to occur as much as possible

> ### Key points for supporting women in labour
>
> - Relaxation and focus is important in all stages.
> - Breathing is fundamental to this.
> - Use positions which support the process.
> - Encourage the mother to be aware of and in touch with her body and her baby.
> - Use massage and touch as appropriate: give space as needed.
> - Encourage the mother to welcome each contraction rather than resisting it.
> - Encourage the mother to get to know her contractions.
> - Encourage the mother to go with any pain rather than blocking it out.
> - Encourage the mother to ultimately do whatever feels right for her.

Other ways to help the woman's body support this stage of labour

Support the mother to be able to tune in to what feels right to her so that she can connect with the intense emotions she is feeling.

10.4 Bodywork techniques for different stages of labour

The usual precautions apply for all these techniques. It may be that the client does not want to be touched at all during labour. Often women prefer the more still type of techniques such as holding during contractions and more active ones between contractions. However, each client is different.

Stroking effleurage (Swedish massage), saka (shiatsu)

In early labour, or in a stop and start labour with a lengthy space between contractions, women may appreciate effleurage as a familiar comforting stroke. In active labour, some women like effleurage between contractions, as though it is helping to draw away any discomfort and encourage energy to flow. Effleurage can be good if the client has poor circulation or blocked energy, especially in the arms or legs, due to remaining in different positions for a while. There is often a stage in labour when women experience shaky legs and effleurage may be appreciated at this time. Sometimes, however, women find these types of techniques too fussy, especially during a contraction.

Kneading/petrissage (Swedish massage), kenbiki (shiatsu)

This may be done on specific areas, such as the shoulders and the gluteals if excessive tension builds up. It is usually quite effective. As with effleurage, it tends to be used more in early labour or between contractions. It may feel too fussy and 'busy' in more established labour and during a contraction.

Frictions

As above, for petrissage.

Tapotement

Light tapotement may be used to relieve tension in the legs but tapotement anywhere else would tend to feel too active and stimulating during labour.

Breathing

This is fundamental to all stages of labour. Breathing is a useful tool to support self-help visualisation techniques. Usually simple breathing, focusing on the out-breath and often using an open throat, is more appropriate than complex breathing techniques. Some women like to vocalise and others not.

Lymph drainage techniques

These would be less used during labour, except in a long labour if the legs started getting oedematous.

Static pressure and holds including soft tissue manipulation and Neuromuscular technique (NMT)

These are often the most appreciated techniques of all during labour – especially deep pressure and appropriate holding on the sacrum and shoulders. Static pressure on the labour focus points and other acupuncture points to balance energy in labour is often extremely effective. Women tend to like this type of work during the contractions themselves as well as between contractions. The pressure and holds tend to be more physically strong during the contractions and less strong in between.

Pressure on the abdomen at the appropriate depth can be comforting, both during and between contractions, although usually more between contractions to keep a focus on the baby and the breath.

Stretches/passive movements/ joint mobilisations

These are generally not used in active labour as the woman would be moving around and mobilising

herself in the way which feels most appropriate. However, if she is sat on a bed or chair for a long time then it may be helpful to mobilise her legs or arms, although probably with fairly gentle strokes. This would tend to be more in early labour and generally for the hands and feet rather than the whole arm or leg.

Women with SPI need especially to be careful of not destabilising their hips too much in labour. Often it may be advisable to try labouring in water, as this gives the joints additional support, provided the woman can get into the pool. Of course for the actual delivery she will need to abduct her legs, but it is better if she does not squat but uses the all fours position instead.

Fascial techniques and soft tissue release

Some of the more holding techniques may be helpful in labour, for example cranial-sacral hold. The more vigorous ones, including stretches, would be less suitable.

Use of oil in labour

The client may be undressed or partly clothed in labour. The use of oil depends on what she feels comfortable with. Often oil can be beneficial and even a non-aromatherapist may be working with oils if the client brings a blend pre-made by a trained aromatherapist. It can feel very comforting to have oil rubbed over the lower back or abdomen.

10.5 Approach and techniques for different areas of the body

Since each woman labours so differently most of the techniques can potentially be done at any stage of labour, during contractions or between contractions depending on the client's preference, state of health, type of labour and so on.

Main postural patterns

Women tend to be in many different types of positions in labour so there is not a typical pattern. However, we explore some of the main areas where tension may be stored in the section on different stages of labour.

Head, face, neck and shoulders

The neck and head are important to work because tension is often stored here. In labour, women often clench their jaws and tighten and elevate their shoulders. This can give rise not only to generalised tightness in the neck and shoulders, but also to specific symptoms such as headaches, nasal congestion and emotional tension. In shiatsu, the side of the neck and top of shoulder and around the shoulder blade (muscles SCM, scalenes, trapezius) relate to the Gall

Bladder meridian. This Wood energy tends to rise and get stuck in the shoulders expressing itself as Jitsu. In labour, if women are leaning forward or using all fours positions, then they may be holding tension in their shoulders as they support themselves.

If the shoulders are expressing patterns of tightness, then often this is reflected in the hips through tightness in the gluteus and piriformis muscles. The hips also relate to Gall Bladder energy. If the hips are too tight, or too loose, energy may not flow well in second stage and delivery may be more difficult.

There is a relationship between the neck and the sacrum, both structurally (due to being at each end of the spine and through the membranes) and energetically. The Bladder meridian runs down from the inner corner of the eye, through the length of the erector spinae from the neck to the sacrum. If the client is experiencing pain in the sacrum and working directly on the points there seems too intense or uncomfortable, then working in the neck is a good alternative.

The throat is related to the cervix and the perineum. This relationship is largely through the link with the digestive tract, beginning with the mouth and ending with the anus and urethra. There is also a link on a cellular developmental level with the primitive mouth and anus being the first orifices to form. This is in large part, Governing Vessel and Conception Vessel energy. The starting and ending points of these meridians are on the perineum and around the mouth. It also links with metal energy – Lung and Large Intestine – the taking in of nutrients in the form of food and letting go at the other end in the form of body wastes. Primary caregivers often refer to the relationship between the throat and the cervix: 'if the throat is open then the cervix is also open'.

Neck work can be useful at all stages of labour. It may help with pain relief and allowing energy to flow will also help the body to do whatever it needs to. It is especially important to support Wood energy in the second stage. If there is a big difference in tightness, Jitsu, between the two sides or if it is very Jitsu it may be an indication of the fetus being stuck. As with this kind of tightness in the sacrum, by balancing the Kyo and Jitsu it is often possible to support changes in the fetal position during the labour.

Of course, the amount of pressure used on the neck is going to be much less than the sacrum. Work can be done close to the vertebrae but it must be confirmed that there is no discomfort. Women tend to love or hate their neck being worked – it is a more sensitive area than the lower back, so good feedback is essential. Some women really do not like their necks being worked and this needs to be respected.

The neck is often worked if the client is in the pool, as, since the therapist cannot be in the pool, the main areas where the client can receive bodywork are the neck, shoulders, arms and hands.

Types of techniques

Often pressure type techniques are most appreciated, especially for the neck and shoulders.

Women tend not to like much work being done on the face. If they do want work here, it is often simply holding a cold flannel over the forehead.

Effleurage type techniques may be appreciated for the sides of the neck.

Working positions

The neck and shoulders can be accessed in most positions. If the client is leaning forward over something then the therapist will need to work more around the back of the neck and notice what kind of support the face and head need.

It can feel more comfortable if the client rests her head over something such as a pillow or a ball or the back of the bed or chair.

Cautions

Other than the usual, there are no specific cautions; however, if the client has pre-existing neck issues such as damage to the vertebrae or pre-existing injury such as whiplash, it may well be an area which is too sensitive to work.

Suggested techniques for the neck

The body position for most of these techniques is facing the base of the neck. The client will be in position, leaning over a ball, sitting on a chair, leaning on the side of the pool.

Begin by generally relaxing the neck through cupping the base of the occiput with the 'web' of one hand – i.e. the area between the thumb and index finger. Place the other hand over the client's forehead, being careful not to cover her eyes. Gently use the mother hand (the hand on the forehead) to ease the head back on to the working hand. This gives a generalised pressure on the base of the skull (Fig. 10.7).

Stroking

- Light hand over hand stroking can be done over the head and down the shoulders to move energy and relax.
- Slower stroking is more tonifying – to bring energy in.
- Faster strokes are more sedating – to take energy away.
- Usually there tends to be too much energy in the head so the stroke direction tends to be downwards over the top of the head and over the shoulders.

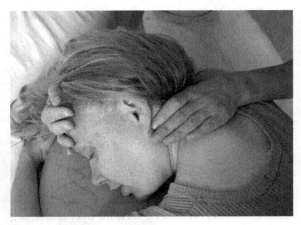

Fig. 10.7 Working neck holding points.

Palming

If the head is held, this can help bring energy here. Focus on the two hands. Find a Kyo point and a Jitsu point and hold the two. Meridians which can be worked include GB, BL or TH, GV.

Following meridian pathways

There are some specific meridians and points which are useful in the neck. Palming or stroking along the most relevant one can be done.

Point release techniques

These points release tension in the shoulder, neck and jaw. By relaxing the neck, the throat and the cervix may also relax.

BL 10

Location To locate this place the thumbs each side of the cervical vertebrae about 1½ thumb-widths from the centre. Slide up to the base of the skull where there is a hollow. It is on the side of the trapezius muscle about ½ inch above the hairline in the slight depression about an inch to each side of the spinal groove.

How to work it Hold the thumb in one side, with the fingers of this hand resting where they are comfortable on the head. Place the mother hand on the forehead. Use the mother hand to guide the head into the working thumb. Since the point lies under the occiput, then instead of a 90° angle, the pressure needs to be angled so as to hook under the occiput. Do this slowly, building up to maximum pressure. Repeat a few times and then repeat on the other side.

Why It is a point of the Sea of Qi and known as the Celestial Pillar. It clears the head, and is a useful point for occipital or vertical headaches. It can ease stiff necks and headaches. Because of its close

relationship to the brain, it clears the brain, stimulates memory and concentration. It has a special effect on the eyes, helping increase vision, and can clear nasal congestion. It can help with backache and wobbly legs which seem unable to support the body. It helps with Water energy flow and can therefore be very calming and relaxing.

Governing Vessel 15 and GV 16

Location GV 15 is in the dip between BL 10 and GV 15 is ½ thumb-width up.

How to work it Work in the same way as Bladder 10, although applying a little less pressure.

Why Both these points affect Governing Vessel energy and benefit the neck and spine. They can gather the energy of the body at times of change or when things are blocked.

GV 15

Clears the mind, stimulates speech and is indicated for heaviness of the head or loss of consciousness.

GV 16

It is said to nourish the brain and clear headaches.

GV 20

Location Right at the top of the head. To find it, place the heels of the hands on the anterior and posterior hairlines and extend the middle fingers towards each other. It is one thumb-width anterior to where the middle fingers meet. This is usually just in front of the crown of the head.

How to work it Place one thumb on top of the other on the point and cup the head with the rest of the hand and fingers. The thumbs are the 'working hand' and the rest of the hand the 'mother hand'. Gentle pressure can either be focused down the body, towards the feet, along the spine. Or a focus can be made on drawing the energy up – depending on what the client needs.

Why It is the meeting point of all the Yang channels which carry Yang to the head and therefore has the effect of clearing the mind and lifting the spirits. It also strengthens the ascending function of Spleen and is used for prolapse of internal organs such as stomach, uterus, bladder, anus or vagina and can also be used to revive an unconscious person. It has a powerful effect on either raising or lower blood pressure, depending on whether the intention in using it is to send energy down the body, or draw energy up the body.

This is quite a powerful point for exhaustion and can be very deeply relaxing.

Gall Bladder 20

Location This is an inch above the hairline in the depression between the sternocleidomastoid and the upper portion of the trapezius muscles. Locate Bladder 10 then slide up and slightly out until a protrusion of the skull is reached. The point lies just inferior and lateral.

How to work it Work in the same way as Bladder 10, except that the angle of pressure is at 45°, diagonally, while also hooking under the bone.

Why This releases tension in the head, especially relating to headaches in the side of the head. It helps release tightness in the Wood energy.

Five-point head hold technique (Fig. 10.8)

This was used traditionally by midwives in Japan and still used today.

The best position for the therapist if possible is to be facing the head so that the weight can go down the spine. Place the index fingers one on top of each other into GV 15, then place the middle fingers each side in BL 20, then the ring fingers in GB 20. Hook the fingers under the bone and bring the palms onto the skull so that they are cupping it. The palms act as the mother hand so a supporting connection needs to be made with them. Gently lean the Hara back so that the hands are drawn away and pressure is applied into the points with a gentle traction of the client's spine. This way all five points are stimulated at the same time. Notice which is most Kyo and Jitsu – hold the Kyo and use more dispersing techniques for the Jitsu. To disperse while holding the pressure can be a little quicker and sharper, as gentle vibration movements can be made with the thumbs/fingers.

If it is not possible to face the head, then simply hold as many of the points as possible, applying as much pressure as is comfortable.

Techniques for the shoulders

Shoulder leaning

A good way of working the shoulders is with the forearms. This way strong pressure can be applied. The therapist needs to be facing the shoulders with the weight able to lean down the spine. Place the forearms over the top of the shoulders and lean in the direction of the spine down towards the client's feet. As well as pressure, the shoulders can be used to roll and stroke the top of the shoulder. This is a good way of releasing Jitsu and relaxing the top of the shoulder which is often tight.

Gall Bladder 21 (Fig. 10.9)

This has already been described in the labour focus section (see p. 290).

Benefits It relaxes tension in the shoulder, neck and jaw. It is one of the points which should not be stimulated in pregnancy except after 37 weeks to prepare for birth, as it moves energy downward very strongly and can stimulate contractions. It can therefore be

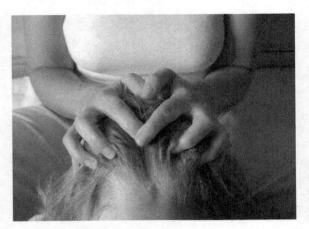
Fig. 10.8 Neck: five-point hold technique.

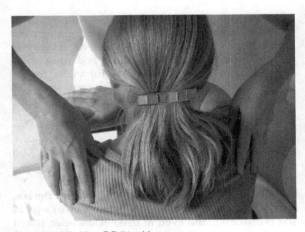
Fig. 10.9 Working GB 21 with pressure.

used to support the process of labour initiation or at any stage of labour to stimulate downward movement of the baby or contractions. It is an extremely effective point. Some women can enjoy this point for pain relief for hours in labour. It can also be used in the third stage for helping deliver retained placentas. It can help with poor lactation.

How to work This can be incorporated in a shoulder massage which can be relaxing for the woman in labour. The thumbs can be placed directly in the points and pressure can be applied through the therapist leaning down in the same way as for the general shoulder relaxing.

Scapula release – three-point hold – from Naoko (Yates 2003) (Fig. 10.10)

Standing behind the woman, the therapist places the hands on the top of the woman's shoulders.

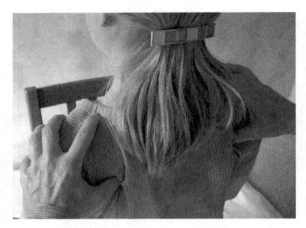

Fig. 10.10 Scapula release: labour three-point shoulder hold.

The middle finger is placed on the top, around GB 21; the other fingers grasp around the scapula and the thumb is placed on the scapula. As the client breathes out the fingers retract the scapula and pressure is applied by the thumb. It is a powerful release for the scapula and can be done in between contractions to release tension which may have built up.

Techniques for the face

The client will tend to prefer holding of the forehead, especially during a contraction. If she is hot, then cool flannels can be held on the forehead. However, she may like some gentle stroking over the face.

The main focus for the face is to check that the jaw is relaxed. Getting the client to open her mouth as she is breathing and even to make some open throat sounds ('aaaaah' sounds) will help to achieve this. Gentle frictions could also be done around the jaw if the woman feels comfortable with this.

The back torso

The spine is an area where tension can be stored in labour, especially in the sacrum, as the fetus pushes deeper down into the pelvis. It tends to be more painful if the woman is lying on her back and compressing the sacrum or if the baby is in the occipito posterior position, as pressure from the fetal spine may cause discomfort. During the first stage, the sacrum is often an area where women appreciate bodywork. Even during second stage, some women want these techniques continuing.

Energetically, the back is important to work in labour because the spine relates to Governing Vessel energy which is the main source of Yang energy and regulates Essence in the body. Further, the Bladder meridian in the back relates to all organs on the

body and thus may help balance the many different changes which occur. Water energy (Bladder) is especially important during the first stage when fear may block the process of labour.

Types of techniques

It is often holding and pressure techniques on the sacrum which the woman most appreciates. Effleurage style work can also be welcome over the whole back, often utilising downward strokes as though to draw the pain out from the body and bring it down to the earth, the Yin.

Working positions

The back is the more exposed area of the body in a physiological labour and is often worked fairly extensively. If the woman needs medical interventions, and especially if she has to lie down on the bed, then the back would not be able to be accessed so readily.

Cautions

In forward leaning positions be careful not to apply strong pressure to unsupported areas of the back, especially the lumbar area.

Technique suggestions

All these techniques can potentially be used at any stage of labour but they are especially helpful between first stage contractions to help the woman to fully use the space to relax and let go of the pain of the previous contraction and be ready for the next contraction. They can also help her to regain her energy, so can be useful if she is tired. They help her feel more in touch with herself and can help her to feel less anxious. This can also apply to the space between the contractions of second and third stages.

Occipitosacral rocking/balance

Benefits A connection is being made with the spinal column and the cerebrospinal fluid which is the energy of the Governing Vessel meridian. This runs right through the spinal column and some important points (GV 15 and GV 2) may be underneath the hands. The coccyx is an important area on the Governing Vessel. If energy is blocked here then there can be lower backache or blockages in the process of labour, especially in second stage when the coccyx needs to move. The sacrum also relates to Bladder energy and to the flow of Essence and the Governing Vessel. Both holds can be useful if the client is very exhausted, especially if she has a depletion of Yang energy. If the Yang energy of the woman is too active, she may be feeling agitated and frightened and the neocortex is being over-stimulated. The hold may quieten the energy, or it may be that some more dispersing type work such as faster palming or stroking needs to be included.

One hand is placed on the woman's occiput and the other on her sacrum. The therapist responds to any rhythm they may feel in an intuitive way.

Palming GV and BL

Benefits Both these meridians are important in labour. They represent the Water element which is drawn upon a lot in labour and can be used at any time the client is feeling tired or exhausted or fearful. They help promote a sense of flow. If the client is having problems urinating, then they may help. They are useful for backache in labour.

The GV can be gently palmed or stroked, keeping the mother hand over the coccyx, or moving it slightly higher, as feels appropriate. The pressure will tend to be quite light, especially in the middle of the back, because strong pressure in this position would be too strong, especially if this area of the spine was unsupported. The Bladder meridian, which has two branches each side of GV, one at one and a half thumb-widths distance and the other at three thumb-widths distance, can also be palmed or stroked.

Hand-over-hand stroking

Benefits This is a deeply relaxing stroke and can be used at any time in labour when the woman needs to be supported to relax and let go.

Stroking can be used over the neck, shoulders, back and down into the legs, ending with holding at the feet. A continuous hand-over-hand stroking movement can be used, starting at the neck and working down to the feet. The direction is important as with the downward focus, it tends to feel that tension is being drawn away from the neck and shoulders, down the spine and into the feet and the ground. Make sure that the wrists and shoulders are relaxed. Work can be done lightly over the neck, more firmly over the shoulders, more lightly down the spine, and quite firmly down the legs. It can be relaxing to finish by holding the feet.

The stroking can be focused on the GV/BL/KI meridians or on areas of musculoskeletal tension in the back or legs. It can be done as slowly or quickly, deeply or lightly, as feels appropriate to the client. It can provide a hypnotic rhythmical movement which can provide a focus for a client.

The sacrum

Massage of the lower back and sacrum can be beneficial – firm, slow effleurage can be pain-relieving. It is an extremely helpful area to apply pressure to, both in a general way and specifically working with the four pairs of points in the bony indentations of the sacrum. It directly relaxes this area, which can often feel painful in labour. It also relaxes the whole pelvis and can provide pain relief as well as allowing labour to progress. Between contractions, gentle stroking or lighter general pressure can help with relaxation.

General sacral pressures

In labour, the client often feels tightness, pressure or pain in the sacrum. She may feel the pain of the contractions directly in this area – a pain which often spreads down the legs. This relates to the Water energy in the body. With pressure this pain can be eased.

The sacrum is also related to the neck: tension in the neck can often be expressed in the sacrum. Sometimes the neck can be too painful to work on directly, so work on the sacrum is useful. The same also holds true the other way round, so work on the neck may be indicated if pressure on the sacrum is too strong.

As labour progresses, then direct pressure on the sacrum may feel too intense and may tend to block the movement of the sacrum. This is when work in the sacral indentations is used.

To give general pressure on the sacrum, place one hand on top of the other directly over the sacrum in a criss-cross pattern, the fingers of the lower hand facing up the spine and the fingers of the upper hand at 90° to the fingers of the lower hand. Lean the bodyweight into the sacrum, gradually building up to the maximum pressure which is comfortable for the client. The pressure can be quite intense. Make sure that the pressure applied is at an angle of 90° to the client's body.

This type of pressure can also be applied into each buttock. One hand can be placed into the centre of the gluteals and pressure can be applied between the two hands.

Sacral opening/gathering

This can be useful for backaches, especially those caused by the sacroiliac (SI) joint. Often the joint becomes overly compressed, or due to laxity of the tissue, can move out of alignment. Sometimes both movements help to realign the SI joint and ease discomfort. Sometimes one of the two movements feels more beneficial. This can be assessed through doing the movements. This work can also help to focus the energy, particularly of the Girdle Vessel, either to the back or the front. The sacral opening can be especially useful for women with SPI as it draws energy to the front and brings an awareness to the pubic bone. The sacral gathering tends to bring energy into the sacrum, while gently opening up the symphysis pubis. This can be helpful if the fetus is slightly stuck.

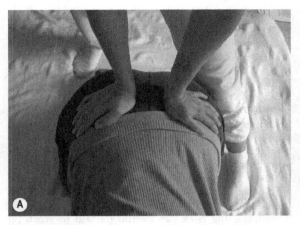 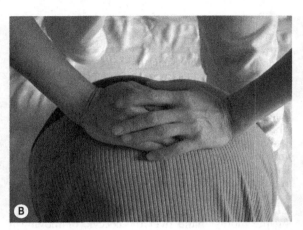

Fig. 10.11A (A) Sacral opening. (B) Sacral gathering.

Caution needs to be applied with this technique when is the client is suffering from SPI and it should only be used minimally in this case.

They can be used at any stage of labour, but usually more in first stage and often between rather than during contractions.

Sacral opening (Fig. 10.11A)

Pressure can be applied to each side of the sacrum. Place the hands so that the heel of each hand lies across the sacroiliac joint and lies in line with the lateral border of the sacrum and the fingers point out laterally. Apply pressure at a 90° angle to the client's body and then ease the elbows laterally so the pressure is also applied laterally. This has the effect of gently opening out the sacroiliac joint and closing in the symphysis pubis. There is not much physical movement on the joints but none the less this can help to bring more of a focus to the front.

Sacral gathering (Fig. 10.11B)

The opposite of this is to place the hands so that the fingers are pointing to the centre and the heel of the hands is as it was in the previous technique – along the edge of the sacrum and covering the SI joint. The hands may overlap. As the client breathes out, lean down at a 90° angle and then gently squeeze the heels of the hands medially.

Specific sacral groove work (Fig. 10.12)

Although the general sacral pressure can be very effective, sometimes it does not provide enough pain relief. Further, general pressure may start to feel uncomfortable as labour progresses as it may block movement of the sacrum. This is when it is helpful to apply pressure into the sacral grooves/foramen.

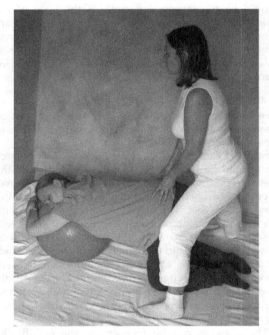

Fig. 10.12 Work into the sacral foramen in all fours.

These points are most commonly used during first stage contractions for pain relief and may help the contractions to be more effective. Usually they are used during contractions – many women find that this is all the work they need for the whole labour. They can be useful to teach the partner. Work can be as intense and for as long as the client requires. Often between contractions the client may appreciate stroking techniques or she may want pressure work continued in the points, although often with less intensity than during a contraction. They can also be used in second stage if the contractions seem ineffective to focus the woman's energy and in third stage for uterine bleeding.

Applying pressure into the sacral foramen can gently allow the sacrum to move in the way it needs to and thus be useful for helping the whole pelvis gently move and realign. These points also relate to the sacral nerves and thus may help with pain relief in labour. As labour progresses and the lower segment of the uterus and the perineum and lower vagina become more involved the sacral nerves supply this area. This means that usually in labour work tends to be in the points lower down as labour progresses.

Tightness in these points, especially more on one side than the other, can often indicate the fetus is stuck on the side where it is tighter. By releasing this tightness, the fetus may be encouraged to move.

The sacral points are on the Bladder meridian. They are important points for genital issues for women. They all tonify the Kidneys and benefit Essence and so tonify the whole body. As energy is released through to the uterus, women often feel a comforting warmth in the uterus. They are also used to strengthen the lower back, knees and for difficult urination.

- BL31 is in the most superior sacral groove.
- BL32 is in the second most superior sacral groove, counting downwards towards the coccyx. It is considered the most important as it tonifies the Kidneys and the Essence. It is used for infertility, prolapse of anus and uterus, and stimulates ascending Qi.
- BL33 has more of an effect on Bladder, and promotes, with BL20 formation of Blood in Blood deficiency.
- BL34 regulates Qi and Blood and can be used for uterine bleeding, especially useful for third stage bleeding, or indeed bleeding at any time.

The sacral grooves are four pairs of points on the sacrum – the four sacral foramen – usually about a thumb-width out from the midline, although it varies from woman to woman depending on the size of their bones. On some women they are easy to find, on others not so. They can either be located by feeling from the hip bone, following its curve down until the top points are reached or by locating the tail bone and feeling up for the first set of points. Begin at the top or the bottom and place the thumbs in a pair of points. Start gently massaging around the dip with small circling movements; this allows the thumbs to settle in the centre of the point. Then lean in with body weight to apply static pressure.

To increase the pressure in the points, they can be worked one at a time. In this case, place one thumb on top of the other. Lean in deeply. Make sure that the fingers support your hand by making contact with the body. The fingers act as the mother hand.

Knuckles can also be used in these points, either one at a time or in pairs. Work all pairs of points – some points are easier to feel, some feel more tender to touch, and some benefit from deep pressure.

The same technique can be used with the client in the side position. Turn and face the body and work the grooves on the side uppermost.

After working it is often beneficial to do some of the hand-over-hand stroking over the buttocks and down the legs to allow the energy released to flow and be integrated by the rest of the body. This can also be calming for the client. Work can be done on the feet as well.

Buttock point

It is a point for strengthening the Kidneys and supporting the lumbar spine. It can be helpful for exhaustion, backache and pain relief.

This point is an extra point and is not on any particular meridian. It is known as the lumbar eye and is level with the fourth lumbar vertebra, about three and a half thumb-widths from the midline. It is often seen quite clearly as a dimple in the buttock below the iliac crest.

Work can be done in a similar way to the sacral points. Place a thumb in each side and use the fingers to cup round the top of the iliac crest. The fingers act as the mother hand. Lean in at 90° with the thumbs. One point can be worked at a time with one thumb on top of the other. It is often effective during contractions of either first or second stage.

Chest/abdomen front of the body

Contrary to the perception in many countries, women often appreciate being held on the abdomen. In many traditional cultures, abdominal work is still a key part of labour support. It often involves quite physical techniques with the aim of shaking and moving the fetus and aiding birth.

Our experience of work with women in modern societies is that while they do appreciate work on the abdomen in labour, they tend to prefer lighter holding and connecting techniques, often linked in with breathing and connecting with the baby, rather than a more physically vigorous approach.

Work on the abdomen can provide a useful focus for breathing and visualisations in labour. The woman could visualise the pressure on the abdomen helping the uterus to contract and open up the cervix.

The woman may want to place her own hands over the abdomen, or she may find the touch of the therapist or her partner helpful. Often techniques which involve simply holding and responding to the movements of the abdomen with the breath are sufficient.

The client may appreciate gentle clockwise stroking or some gentle pressures. Effleurage techniques can include strokes from the back towards the abdomen and may be linked with work on the sacrum. This can be done with or without oil as the stroking would tend not to be overly vigorous.

Work on the Hara/abdomen can be used for helping the woman (and partner/therapist) make emotional connections with her baby – prenatal bonding – and through this may be potentially calming for the baby also.

As the Hara is the physical centre of the body and centre is the direction of the Earth energy, work with the abdomen tends to be centring and calming and linked with supporting Earth energy. In this regard it supports all other meridians and energies. Abdominal touch may help with pain relief.

Types of techniques

These could be holding or stroking techniques. The same principles for working the abdomen as outlined in pregnancy apply.

Working positions

The abdomen can be accessed in most positions. If the client is on all fours, on the floor or kneeling over the back of the bed, the therapist can stand or kneel behind or to the side and work the abdomen. It can be worked in the side or semi-reclining positions.

Cautions

Refer to the pregnancy section (p. 234) for cautions as the same cautions apply in labour. In labour, if a woman who has had a previous caesarean section experiences discomfort at any time this potentially could be the scar rupturing. This is rare (NICE 2004), but advise the primary care provider immediately.

Technique suggestions

Refer to the pregnancy section 9.8 p. 251 for some of the abdominal techniques. If the client has been used to abdominal work in pregnancy it can often be comforting in labour.

General abdominal pressures

Benefits

- It helps the client to connect with her breathing and to breathe deeper.

- It helps to bring the focus on to the baby as opposed to the pain.
- It may have a calming effect on the baby.

Obviously there may well be times in labour when the client does not want any contact with her abdomen, and for some women this could be throughout labour. However, some women do appreciate holding on the abdomen.

It can be done with the client in a variety of different positions. The most helpful position for labour is in all fours, but the client could be in left lateral or even standing. For the therapist/partner, the main thing is to be in a comfortable position where the practitioner's Hara is close to the client.

Refer to pregnancy chapter for description of technique.

Different places can be worked by moving the hand. Clockwise stroking movements on the abdomen can be interspersed with pressures. Stroking is energetically more dispersing, although it can be done with more of a focus of calming, in which case it is more tonifying.

Other holds

These are described in the pregnancy chapter; see p. 257 for details. These would usually be done in the all fours version.

Kidney, Uterus, Girdle Vessel

Benefits

As the Girdle Vessel is about linking from front to back, it can help balance the two. It can be useful if the client has strong backache where you feel she is holding on and the energy is stuck in the uterus, so that the uterus is not dilating. This is often the case if the baby is stuck, in either first or second stage, in an awkward position. By moving the energy from front to back, the baby may be freed to move. It is also often the case with uncoordinated contractions in either first or second stage or at any time when you feel energy is stuck in some way in the pelvis.

It can also be very calming for woman and baby as it is working to balance deep energies in the body.

For the technique refer to pregnancy chapter, p. 259. Work with a focus of 'opening up' the Girdle Vessel – working from CV 2–8 to GV 4. This can be done by holding the points, or some stroking movements can be included, stroking from the abdomen to the sacrum. For a stronger 'opening' place the fingers on the front of the anterior superior iliac spine (GB 27 and 28) and rest the thumb wherever it is comfortable on the gluteals. Next pivot the fingers back onto the

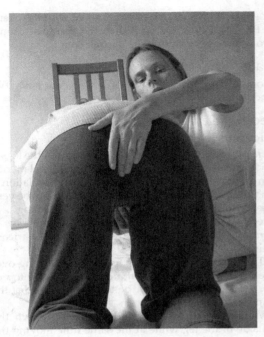

Fig. 10.13 Client on all fours with CV 2, GV 2 connection.

thumb, applying as much pressure as feels comfortable and appropriate.

This is rather like the shoulder opening (p. 301) and helps the hips to open and relax.

Pelvic floor support: connecting CV and GV through their lower pathways (Fig. 10.13)

Benefits

This can be an area where women feel disconnected in labour. Although the primary care provider may touch the perineum during labour often women find that direct touch on this area in labour feels invasive. This is often the case for women who may have experienced sexual abuse for whom it may feel very traumatic. This technique offers a safe, gentle way of getting energy to flow along here and can be especially useful in second stage for helping the mum to focus her energy onto the perineum.

This can be done while the woman is on all fours.

Working specific points in the Hara

Benefits

These points can be held when doing abdominal work in labour. All these points are on the lower part of the Conception Vessel and relate closely to Original Qi, Essence, the Uterus, Spleen, Liver and Kidney energy.

They are all good for exhaustion and depletion of these energies. They can all regulate uterine bleeding.

CV 3, CV 4 and CV 5

CV 3 is four cun below the navel on the midline.
CV 4 is three cun below the navel on the midline.
CV 5 is two cun below the navel on the midline.

- CV 5 – this tends to be more important for regulating heat as it is the Bo point of the Three Burners/Triple Heater.
- CV 4 – some traditions consider this to be one of the most important points in the body. It can be used for retention of urine, especially if it is due to fetal pressure. It has especial importance on the uterus and can be useful for easing the pain of contractions, as well as encouraging them to be more effective.
- CV 3 – relates to the Bladder and is the Bo point of the Bladder. It can be used for retention of urine, swelling of the cervix, retention of the placenta, pain in the abdomen.

Baomen (door of uterus) and zihu (door of baby) These coincide with ST 28 – 2 *cun* lateral to CV 4 Baomen on left and Zihu on right; retained placenta, difficult childbirth.

Jueyun (terminating pregnancy) 3/10 *cun* below CV 5. Meant to make a woman infertile. Forbidden absolutely in pregnancy, but may be used to induce childbirth. It is often stimulated with moxa cones but warm hands or towels, or some oil/lotion can also be used to generate heat.

Chest and breasts

The front of the body is generally less exposed in a more physiological labour. It is not usually an area where women would want to receive work. If the client was lying on her side and was feeling panicky then it might be appropriate to do some work with the CV or PV or ST in their upper pathways. It tends to be more exposed and therefore accessible in a more medicalised labour when the woman may be lying on her side or semi-reclining. In this case, she might appreciate CV, PV or ST work.

Cautions

It is thought that stimulation of the nipple may strengthen contractions, due to its release of oxytocin, but this caution applies to stimulation from the partner rather than the therapist who would not be touching the nipple.

Suggestions of techniques

We are not outlining any techniques as it is not an area which is often worked in labour and there are no specific techniques in addition to any outlined in pregnancy or birth.

Legs and feet

The legs may have to work hard in labour, especially if the woman is using upright birthing positions. If she is upright and moving around, engaging her muscles, it is less appropriate to work with petrissage style strokes. Effleurage work may, however, feel supportive and relieve tension and support circulation of both energy and blood and lymph, particularly if the client stays in one position for a while. Often, especially during transition, the legs may become wobbly or tremble. The legs can be a good area to work if the woman wants touch, but not as intensely as work on the abdomen or back. Work to the legs can provide a sense of support while also giving some space. Work to the feet is often appreciated for the same reason.

It is often the case that there is too much energy or tension in the neck and shoulders and to balance this, work is needed in the legs, to draw this energy down.

If the woman is in more static positions, or lying down, then she may appreciate some work to the legs for both relaxation and circulation. Depending on where in the labour she is at and how intense and close together the contractions are, she may or may not appreciate petrissage work.

If the toes are clenched this tightens the muscles and meridians in the legs which tends to have an effect of tightening and blocking energy flow to the pelvis. In Japan in the last few weeks of pregnancy, women are often encouraged to massage their toes to free up this energy and it may be helpful to continue this opening during labour as well. Shiatsu points on the feet are extremely important as distal points are considered some of the most powerful. Many of the labour focus points (SP6, LV3 and BL60) are around the feet and they are related to the Earth and Wood energy which is about downward movement and grounding. Work to the feet through the reflex zones in the feet which correspond to the uterus or the pituitary may support the process of labour. Many women find that having the feet held is extremely calming and relaxing for them and helps them to focus. It is work that the partner can easily do.

Types of techniques

Holding or stroking to the depth to which the woman wants. If the woman is suffering from oedema then the work would be lighter. Petrissage and more physical work may be appropriate at some stages.

Working positions

The client could be walking around or standing and so the therapist needs to find various comfortable positions in which to work and move with the client. If the client is in the pool then the therapist cannot work the legs, although the partner could.

Cautions

Normal cautions apply re varicose veins and DVT and oedema.

Technique suggestions

Vigorous leg stroking (Fig. 10.14)

Benefits This stimulates all the meridians in the legs and focuses on their direction in the traditional meridian system. It also helps to support blood circulation and release muscular tension in the legs. It can be very useful during labour itself if the woman is feeling tired and particularly if her legs are feeling wobbly.
Caution Do not work directly over areas of varicose veins.

The client can be standing or kneeling, leaning over the back of a chair. Start with one hand at the top of the leg and one hand at the bottom. Make sure that the hands and wrists are relaxed.

Vigorously stroke the hand at the top down the outside of the leg while at the same time moving the hand at the bottom up the inside of the leg.

Keep the movement flowing while lightly moving the hand which is now at the bottom and the hand which is now at the top, back to where they started.

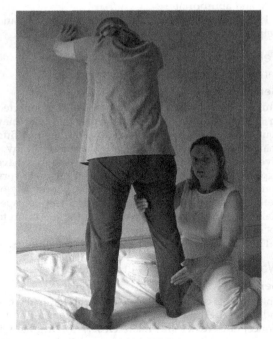

Fig. 10.14 Vigorous leg stroking in labour.

This technique can be done quite vigorously, provided there are no areas of varicose veins. It is an invigorating technique; however, it can also be done lightly if appropriate. It tends not to be done for very long.

Holding techniques for the legs

Benefits Stroking techniques could feel too vigorous and dispersing. Palming and holding provide a more calming approach.

Holding the legs can often feel calming and grounding for the woman. Energy often fails to flow well in different meridian channels and these can be focused on to support their flow. The Bladder meridian which relates to fear and palming the meridian in the legs can help with grounding and calming. Gall Bladder can help with moving physical energy. Spleen may help if the client is tired.

The technique Place one hand on the woman's sacrum and use the other hand to palm down the woman's legs, focusing on whichever meridian/aspect of the legs feels appropriate. Stay on each place for as long as feels appropriate. At the level of the knee, move the hand from the sacrum and place it at the level of the knee. Continue to work down the lower leg.

Specific shiatsu points in the legs

Bladder 67 On the lateral side of the base of the little toe nail. This is the point which is used to turn breech babies – it has the effect of promoting downward movement of the head of the fetus, especially when followed by Bladder 60.

Gall bladder 34 This lies close to Stomach 36. It is below the outside of the knee in the depression about one thumb width below and to the front of the head of the fibula. It is a little bit above and to the outside of Stomach 36. This is known as the 'Gathering point of the sinews' so it has the effect of dilating a scarred or tight cervix.

Stomach 36 This lies in the groove beside the tibia, one finger width below the knob at the top of the tibia (the anterior crest of the tibia). One way of locating it is to start at GB 34 first and it is one thumb-width below that point and one finger-breadth out from the crest of the tibia. Another way is to rest the thumb against the tibia from below the knee and slide the thumb along the lateral border of the tibia. Where it stops – just below the crest of the tibia – is the point.

This point has a strong effect of tonifying Qi and nourishing Blood and Yin energy. It can be used in almost any case of exhaustion or stuck energy. It balances earth energy and is very grounding and settling. It is not an exaggeration to say that this is one of the most important points in the body and can be useful for almost anything. Indeed Qin Cheng-zu of the Song dynasty wrote nearly 1000 years ago that by using it 'all diseases can be treated'.

Along with Bladder 60, this point helps relax the vaginal area which is good for pain relief and an aid to dilatation. Care must be taken to check that they are not shortening the length of the contractions and other points should be chosen if this is happening. It is known as the leg three miles point and links with Large Intestine 10 (arm three miles).

Feet

Benefits

In reflexology the foot represents the whole body. In labour this can be used if the mother feels too sensitive to touch in other areas. All areas, including the baby, can be accessed by working on the foot.

As there are many points which start or end on the feet, it is helpful to allow the toes to open up.

Toe opening

Placing your fingers between the toes and then wiggling the toes around. This helps to open up the pelvis.

Heel opening

This helps to open up the pelvis. Cup the heel in the palm of the hand and then use the fingers to ease it open.

Kidney 1

It is just below the centre of the ball of the foot, in a depression formed when the foot is plantarflexed.

This point is known as the bubbling spring and is the only point on the sole of the foot so it is the lowest point on the body. As the lowest point it links in to Earth energy and is said to help the body absorb the Yin energy of the earth. In this respect it is a very calming point. As the first point of the Kidney channel it has an effect on the whole Kidney meridian and is especially useful for drawing Kidney energy down. It can also be good in cases of exhaustion. It is also the Wood point on the Kidney channel and therefore is helpful for balancing Water and Wood energies – the main two energies involved in labour.

It is often a very good point to hold between contractions, at any stage.

Hands and arms

The arms may become tense or tired during labour if the woman is using them to support her in various birthing positions and gentle work to the arms may help to ease tension. Like the legs, if she wants the reassurance of touch but without the intensity of work around the pelvis she may appreciate stroking of the arms down into the hands or holding of the hands. The arms, like the legs and feet, represent the extension of energy outwards and acupuncture points around the hands tend to have a deep internal effect. Energy wise, the legs relate more to Earth energy of grounding, while the arms relate more to the Fire element and its energy of communication and connecting with others. They also relate to taking in of energy which relates to Lungs. The ability to breathe deeply is extremely important in labour. Holding the woman's hands may be relaxing and provide a communication link.

In a more medicalised labour they can help provide reassurance and calming.

Working position

The arms and hands can be worked in most positions, including in the pool and with medical interventions.

Cautions

No specific cautions other than the usual for labour.

Technique suggestions

Arm stroking

Simply stroking down the arms from over the shoulders and finishing by holding the hands.

Specific points

Heart protector 8 This is in the centre of the palm of the hand. It is said to be the mirror of Kidney 1 on the feet. Linked with the energy of the Heart and Fire, it has the effect of calming the emotions. It can be effective if the woman is feeling panicky and uneasy. It can be useful if the woman is not feeling comfortable in her environment or is feeling disconnected from her baby. It can be good to hold during contractions, and indeed at any time of labour to help calm the woman.

Stroking down the arms

As with stroking down the legs, this can have the effect of feeling as though tension is being drawn out of the body.

Reflective questions

- Think about which of these techniques you are mostly likely to use in labour.
- Consider how the work in labour differs from usual bodywork and any further training or skills you will need to access.

References and further reading

Betts, D., 2006. The essential guide to acupuncture in pregnancy and childbirth. J. Chin. Med. UK.

Budd, S., 2006. Obstetrics 2. Pregnancy and Labour: The Evidence for Effectiveness of Acupuncture. British Acupuncture Council, London.

Cardini, F., Weixin, H., 1998. Moxibustion for correction of breech presentation: a randomized controlled trial. JAMA 280 (18), 1580–1584.

Chang, M.Y., Wang, S.Y., Chen, C.H., 2002. Effects of massage on pain and anxiety during labour: a randomised controlled trial in Taiwan. J. Adv. Nurs. 38 (1), 68–73.

Gaskin, I.M., 2002. Spiritual Midwifery, fourth ed. Book Publishing Company, Summertown, TN.

Grabowska, C., 2005. The development of a study on 'turning the breech using moxibustion'. MIDIRS Midwifery Dig. 15 (2 Suppl. 1), S32–S34.

Hitchcok, D.A., Sutphen, J.H., Scholly, T.A., 1980. Demonstration of fetal penile erection in utero. Perinatalol. Neonatol. 4, 59–60.

Ingram, J., Domagal, C., Yates, S., 2005. The effects of shiatsu on post term pregnancy. Comp. Ther. Med. 13, 11–15.

Keenan, P., 2000. Benefits of massage therapy and use of a doula during labor and childbirth. Altern. Ther. Health Med. 6 (1), 66–74.

Kennell, J., Klaus, M., McGrath, S., et al., 1991. Continuous emotional support during labor in a US hospital: a randomized controlled trial. J. Am. Med. Assoc. 265 (17), 2197–2201.

Khoda, M., Karami, A., Safarzadeh, F.N., 2002. Effect of massage therapy on severity of pain and outcome of labour in primapara. Iran. J. Nurs. Midwifery Res. 12 (1), 6–9.

Langer, A., Campero, L., Garcia, C., et al., 1998. Effects of psychosocial support during labour and childbirth on breastfeeding, medical interventions, and women's wellbeing in a Mexican public hospital: a randomised clinical trial. Br. J. Obstet. Gynaecol. 105 (10), 1056–1063.

Maciocia, G., 1998. Obstetrics and Gynaecology in Chinese Medicine. Churchill Livingstone, Philadelphia.

McNabb, M.T., Kimber, L., Haines, A., et al., 2006. Does regular massage from late pregnancy to birth decrease maternal pain perception during labour and birth? A feasibility study to investigate a programme of massage, controlled breathing and visualization, from 36 weeks of pregnancy until birth. Complement. Ther. Clin. Pract. 12 (3), 222–231.

National Institute for Health and Clinical Excellence (NICE), 2004. Clinical guideline: caesarean section, <http://www.nice.org.uk/Guidance/CG13>.

Neri, I., Airola, G., Contu, G., et al., 2004. Acupuncture plus moxibustion to resolve breech presentation: a randomized controlled study. J. Matern. Fetal Neonatal Med. 15 (4), 247–252.

Odent, M., 2001. The Scientification of Love, revised ed. Free Association Books, London.

Scott, K.D., Klaus, P.H., Klaus, M.H., 1999. The obstetrical and postpartum benefits of continuous support during childbirth. J. Womens Health Gend. Based Med. 8 (10), 1257–1264.

Smith, C.A., Crowther, C.A., 2004. Acupuncture for induction of labour (Cochrane review). The Cochrane library, Vol 2. Oxford Update Software.

Yates, S., 2003. Shiatsu for Midwives. Books for Midwives, Oxford.

CHAPTER 11

Practical bodywork in the postpartum

Chapter contents

Refer to Chapter 14

For more information on:
Higher-risk clients

Refer to Chapter 15

For more information on:
Case history taking and qualities of therapists

Refer to postpartum theory (Chapters 3 and 7), Effects of medical interventions during labour (ch 13)

The theory of underlying some of the conditions including references

Learning outcomes

- Describe the benefits of bodywork in the postpartum period
- Outline different approaches and considerations for:
  - the early postnatal period (first 6 weeks postpartum)
  - the later postnatal period (week 6 to 6 months)
  - longer-term postnatal patterns (6 months plus)
- Describe special issues relating to the postnatal period: work to support different types of birth experience, work if the newborn is in a special care unit, pelvic girdle issues, postpartum depression and breastfeeding
- Evaluate different techniques and their suitability through the postpartum time
- Approach each area of the body, understanding the changes and considerations on how to work

Introduction

The focus in conventional postnatal care is primarily on the health of the newborn and less so on the mother, especially if she has no obvious health issues. Postnatal care for the mother has often been described as the 'Cinderella' of the maternity services (Clift-Matthews 2007, Fraser & Cullen 2006), yet it is at this time the foundations of the future health of both mother and baby are laid. A traditional Japanese view was that if the baby was ill the mother should first be treated, because it is the mother who gives support to the baby. Naturally this would not apply in cases where the newborn was experiencing severe illness. Modern cultures are now beginning to value the importance of good support in the postpartum period and the phrase 'Mothering the mother' helps describe this emphasis (Kennell et al 1993). Bodywork provides a wonderful way of 'mothering'.

Both physically and emotionally the postpartum is a time of great change. In many traditional cultures the new mother would get support and there was the 'lying in' or 'confinement' period of usually a month. Examples of this can still be seen, particularly among Asian families in the West. While family support can sometimes be overbearing, particularly if there are tensions, aspects of this idea of resting for a few weeks are useful to consider. Indeed, at the Birth Centre in south London, new mothers are advised by their midwives to stay at home for a month to rest and get to know their baby.

One client of mine decided not to have any visitors for a week or so, even close family, to support this process and called it her 'baby moon'. I thought this was a nice way of creating intimate family bonding space.

(Suzanne Yates)

This is a welcome antidote to a current cultural trend of the 'yummy mummy' where celebrities parade their slim bodies in front of cameras days after giving birth. Many women feel under pressure to recover as quickly as possible and bounce back to 'normal', whatever 'normal' means. New mothers need to be encouraged to recognise that it takes time to recover, even from an 'easy' birth. It is unrealistic to expect the body to bounce back within days. The body is recovering not only from labour, but from the whole 9 months of being pregnant. At the same time, new demands are placed on it with all the physical and emotional adaptations of being a mother. It is common in the first few days, with the euphoria of birth, for the mother to do too much. Bodywork provides an excellent tool in this first week to help her rest and encourage her to stay in tune with her body. The bodyworker needs to liaise with the primary care provider as the risk of infection and complication is high and referral may be needed, but appropriate bodywork can offer support for the recovery process.

The mother's living situation will be a major factor in this recovery. Factors such as whether she has a good support network; whether she has a supportive or unsupportive partner, or is on her own; the number of other children she has; her financial and housing situation, will all affect her experience of the postpartum.

In the weeks following birth, without the emphasis on the 1 month recovery time, many women tend to get caught up in the demands of adapting to a new baby and changing relationships in their family, so that they often neglect their own needs.

As well as the living situation, the mother's experience of the early postnatal period (first 6 weeks) will depend greatly on the type of pregnancy and birth that she has experienced. For the bodyworker, knowing a woman's pregnancy and birth history is important and having worked with a client throughout their pregnancy and even during their labour may help to facilitate optimal support being offered. The early postnatal period is a sensitive time and many mothers may benefit from this continuity of care, or certainly a therapist who knows the issues of this time.

Work in this early period, as indeed the whole postnatal period, will also be affected by the needs of the baby. If the baby is premature or spending some time in hospital this will impact significantly on the mother and the rest of the family. However, throughout the first year, and indeed beyond, how the baby feeds, sleeps and settles will hugely affect the emotional and physical state of both the mother and family. The therapist needs to be sensitive to these issues and include the baby, or not, as appropriate during the sessions. Infant work may help address some of the issues for the newborn and if the therapist is trained in infant massage, this can be a useful additional skill to be able to offer.

In some European countries the mother has 2–3 years' maternity leave. However, in many other countries, particularly in the UK and USA, there is increased pressure for women to go back to work within 6 months or even earlier. In some cases women are working again at 6 weeks. This places additional strains on having to recover quickly while also getting the most out of the few precious weeks or months the mother has with her baby.

After 6 weeks the initial 'recovery' period is over, but the body still needs to recover from the many changes of pregnancy, birth and being a new mother. Many mothers experience health issues in this period, especially musculoskeletal or digestive issues, and even if they feel well physically, they are usually tired and need support and time out and need to be encouraged to continue looking after themselves. Bodywork can play a key part in this process, especially in establishing long-term patterns of good self-care – it is not simply a luxury. For many women having children signals a period of focusing on the needs of others and may lead to self-neglect. They may not begin to focus on their own needs until many years later when their children leave home.

As time goes by the mother may become pregnant again and then the therapist would be working with a woman who has both postnatal and pregnancy needs simultaneously. Some mothers may even conceive during the first 6 weeks. This places additional demands on the body which ideally needs at least 1–2 years to recover from a pregnancy/birth.

After having a baby, a mother's life and her body are changed forever. Bodyworkers can support these changes and help lay the foundations for long-term emotional and physical health for both mother and baby. Indeed one of the best ways of supporting the long-term health of society would be to give mothers and babies regular bodywork during the first year, especially weekly for the first 6 weeks. It can make a huge difference in helping mothers come to terms with their changing bodies and emotions, which in turn affects their relationships with their whole family.

11.1 Benefits of postnatal work

For mother and partner

- Helps promote postnatal recovery, facilitating the restoration of pre-pregnancy physiology, for example by supporting abdominal and pelvic floor toning, relieving back and shoulder aches, improving circulation and lymphatic flow, supporting energy flows.
- May help prevent and provide support in cases of postnatal depression.
- Touch may help in the birthing recovery process by helping relieve stress and trauma, especially if the birth experience differed from the woman's expectations. It may also help promote physical recovery and support healing from the effects of any strains or medical interventions experienced during birth.
- Helps promote a positive relationship with her partner and baby: the partner can be involved in providing bodywork for mother and baby. The partner could also receive bodywork to support them in their adjustment to parenthood.
- Provides support for the emotional demands of early mothering.
- Provides a relaxed environment.
- Helps promote sleep, giving space for rest, easing fatigue.
- Offers support for breastfeeding.

For baby

- Can offer a space for the mother to be with the baby without other demands.
- Offers support for bonding and feeding.
- Can include direct work for the baby, to support baby's physical and emotional development.

Long-term implications

- Supports the family unit in making the transitions.
- Helps lays foundations to support the long-term emotional and physical health of mother, father and baby.

11.2 Overview of practical postnatal bodywork themes

The impact of birth

Postnatal bodywork includes being aware of the effects of birth including the effects of different types of instrumental delivery, working with awareness of scar tissue and the effects of different drugs and interventions.

Whatever kind of birth the mother has experienced she needs time to 'recover' – even from an uncomplicated vaginal birth. Emotionally and physically, birth is a major life event for women. However, if there has been medical intervention, especially if the mother had not anticipated it, there may be additional physical and emotional effects to process.

It is important to gather appropriate information about the mother's personal emotional and physical response to her birth as each woman has different expectations and responses to her birth. Do not assume that a fast vaginal birth was 'easy' or that the mother is disappointed because she had to have an elective caesarean. Consider each mother's needs on an individual basis.

Many women have some form of medical intervention during the birthing process. The therapist needs to understand the physical and emotional implications of different interventions, both in the short and long term, and the most appropriate form of work along with any relevant aftercare issues.

Space for the emotional processing of birth and being a mother

As it is a key time of change for the mother, the therapist needs to create an environment for the woman to describe or discuss her experiences within the context of the bodywork session. Bodywork sessions can provide a valuable space to debrief after the birth, especially if the therapist had been supporting the mother in the antenatal period. It can also provide an opportunity for the mother to air issues about how she is feeling about herself and her baby, how breastfeeding is going, sleeping issues, partner relationships and so on.

Working with awareness of the baby

This includes bonding with and feeding the baby and postural demands on the mother.

The mother and baby are very much a unit and it can be good to encourage the mother to bring the baby to the bodywork sessions, if she wants to. Work can be done while the mother is breastfeeding or while the baby is sleeping. In this way the baby is less likely to be fussy and distract from the work. Work on the floor may provide a slightly roomier space for the baby to lie down next to the mother. If the therapist is appropriately trained, bodywork can also be included for the baby. Once the baby starts becoming more physically active, especially crawling, they usually become too 'disruptive' to remain present.

Having the baby present may help the therapist observe how the mother holds and carries the baby and the postural effects of this. However, it is also important to recognise that, for some mothers, the bodywork session is providing time and space away from the baby, where her own needs can be focused on.

Bodywork can support the establishment of breastfeeding, help prevent mastitis and support changes in the ribs and breasts.

11.3 Specific considerations for supporting different postnatal periods

Energetically, the woman starts from a state of relative 'weakness' and 'depletion' immediately after birth and gradually her emotional and physical strength start to build. There is considerable variation in terms of length of time of recovery. Recovery tends to be longer after instrumental and surgical deliveries, longer labours and for multiparous women. Recovery tends to be quicker for fit and healthy women who have had natural deliveries.

The first 6 weeks

In many traditions the first 4–6 weeks was the period of 'lying in'. In contrast, in modern cultures many women tend to be up and about too quickly and resuming their normal life patterns. Often, in the excitement of wanting to 'show off' a new baby, families invite too many visitors round. This can be tiring for both mother and baby and place additional strains on the family.

The early postnatal period is a sensitive time where the mother is recovering from the experience of pregnancy and the effects of birth and is getting to know her baby. She needs good nutrition and adequate rest to support this process. Inadequate nutrition may result in slower recovery, difficulties breastfeeding and conditions such as anaemia.

The uterus is contracting and only goes back into the true pelvis by around day 10, resuming its prepregnant size around week 6. The lochial discharge has usually become colourless by 3–4 weeks, indicating that healing is nearing completion. However, if there is still red lochia present at 6–8 weeks this may indicate problems, so it is important to refer the mother back to her primary caregiver. If there is odour this is especially important as it indicates the possibility of infection. How long the mother will be monitored by the primary caregiver differs from country to country.

Until recently the mother would spend most of the first week in hospital after birth, but currently there is an emphasis on early discharge in many countries, primarily as a cost-saving measure. With an uncomplicated vaginal birth, discharge can be as early as within 6–24 hours. After an instrumental delivery or a caesarean, discharge typically ranges from 3–5 days, if there are no complications. Some women prefer to return home as soon as possible as they find their own space more restful, while others find the support and observation of the hospital setting to be more reassuring both physically and emotionally. Both possibilities have advantages and disadvantages. In the hospital the mother may not be able to sleep that well and is potentially exposed to infection. However, she can be monitored closely and given appropriate treatment and support. At home the mother may get back too quickly into her normal routine and may miss out on appropriate breastfeeding and exercise/self-care support. Bodyworkers may find it useful to have some basic training in these fields so they can at least give some support and know when and where to refer. It is important to work in collaboration with the primary care provider.

The end of this period coincides with the 6 week medical check which is offered in most countries. From the western point of view the mother is considered to be 'back to normal'. The gross physical (hormonal, cardiovascular, reproductive) changes have occurred by this time. By 2–3 weeks the perineum is usually healed, even after an episiotomy. However, in reality it is only the beginning of the body's recovery. Some of the organ changes take longer (for example the intestines) and the musculoskeletal changes will impact on the mother for the rest of her life. There will always be a tendency to weakness in the abdominal and pelvic floor. Some women feel quite well by the end of 6 weeks, some may still be recovering from the effects of surgery, and some may be feeling exhausted or overwhelmed. Some women may still be experiencing ligamentous or musculoskeletal problems such as pelvic girdle instability or diastasis recti. Others may be dealing with more serious health issues such as scar tissue healing, infection or fever. Bodywork will need to reflect the individual reality of each mother but work in this period is important as it sets the foundation for the rest of the postnatal period and therefore for the rest of life.

The baby might not be sleeping much during the night or the mother might not be able to sleep as she might be preoccupied by her baby. The mother may start to suffer effects of sleepless nights. If she gets overly tired then this may trigger depression. This is a time when it is ideal for the bodyworker to be able to visit the mother where she is, whether it is home or hospital, so that she can rest as much as possible and not have to worry about getting her baby ready to go out or be looked after.

Feeding patterns are being established. Many women experience the discomfort of 'after pains' in the first couple of weeks, especially after more than one pregnancy or if they have had medication for third stage labour. The mother may develop sore nipples, especially if the baby is not attaching properly. Milk comes in around days 3–5 and engorgement may be a problem with the breasts becoming full, hard, hot and painful. Engorgement can be relieved by removing some of the excess milk by hand or expressing with a pump, or through massage. It is important to develop good patterns as otherwise issues may become more severe. Sore or sensitive nipples or blocked milk ducts could lead to infection and mastitis. If the bodyworker cannot give sufficient support then refer to experienced care providers to create success and confidence in establishing breastfeeding.

If the mother is not breastfeeding, then she and the baby are still getting used to feeding patterns and she may experience breast tenderness as the milk supply dries up. For all women there are hormonal changes and the mother is getting used to feeding her new baby. This means she may feel quite emotional as well as concerned about whether her baby is putting on enough weight.

It is an important family bonding time. If the mother already has a child, s/he will be getting used to the new baby and this may raise some issues and possibly cause some stress for the mother. If the mother is in a relationship there are big adaptations for the partner to make and feelings of jealousy may arise as the mother focuses attention intently on her newborn. Resuming sex may become an issue. Often the partner will be at home for the first couple of weeks, depending on the paternity leave of the country.

Emotionally this can be an intense period. Hormones are adjusting at a rapid rate. There is often, especially after an 'easy' birth, an initial elation, the surge of oxytocin bonding, followed by a 'down' around days 3–5 as the hormones settle back to their pre-pregnancy levels. These days are known as the 'baby blues'. It is normal for the woman to feel emotional and important for the therapist to reassure and validate these feelings. However, for some women, these huge emotional changes may trigger longer-term feelings of depression and it is important for the therapist to be alert to that possibility.

Bodywork

Due to the focus on the baby, mothers usually need to be encouraged by the therapist to book appointments.

It can be a good idea to book a postnatal appointment at the last antenatal appointment. The therapist may want to offer a home visit at the clinic price for clients who have come regularly through their pregnancies, to encourage them to continue looking after themselves once they have their baby. The first 6 weeks is a good time to give mothers regular, ideally at least weekly, bodywork sessions. In some cultural traditions women would have massage daily for the first week (Japan, India, Asia; Davis-Floyd 1992, Priya 1992) and some women would benefit from that. However, the reality is that most women tend to only manage one or two sessions a week. During weeks 2–6 it is still of great benefit to have a session once a week.

Whatever kind of birth she has had, the woman's body has had to open up and deliver a baby, whether vaginally or abdominally. In some respects the approach is similar to that of the first trimester, with a focus on gathering in energies and structures with the goal of supporting the uterus to contract and the pelvis to become strong.

In the early part of this period especially, be careful not to over-stimulate the body. Although the mother's pre-pregnancy and pregnancy fitness will influence the type of work done, work tends to be gentle and often involves the use of energy and holding techniques to help the body recover. It is unlikely that the mother will want any vigorous physical work. The levels of relaxin remain high for the first 6–8 weeks and even longer. This means that caution still needs to be taken in terms of softness of the tissue and laxity of joints and ligaments, especially in the pelvic and lumbar areas.

If the mother has had a vaginal birth, she may have given birth squatting, which will have placed demands on the pelvis to expand and the joints to move, especially the sacroiliac (SIJ) and symphysis pubis and the hips. If the mother had a forceps or ventouse delivery, or delivered lying on her back, she may have displaced or even fractured the pubic bone, or had damage to the coccyx. There may be sensitivity around the epidural site in the lumbar region. Issues of pelvic girdle instability may therefore be aggravated.

It is vital to include work which can help strengthen the abdominal muscles, pelvic floor muscles and muscles of the lower back to support pelvic strengthening. The abdominal muscles need to be encouraged both to contract and the rectus abdominis muscles to draw back together. If the mother feels comfortable, the recti can be checked for separation and appropriate work given. If there is no scar tissue, abdominal work can be done to help encourage involution of the uterus. In many cultures this is done quite vigorously and it often results in an initial increase in bleeding. This style of deeper work needs to be done by the primary caregiver rather than the bodyworker. The bodyworker can, however, work with more of an energy focus and through encouraging the mother to massage her own abdomen.

In the early days the abdomen often has a buzzy quality to it as it is contracting. Gradually, an underlying pattern of emptiness in the abdomen begins to emerge. Once the uterus is in the pelvis and lochial discharge has stopped, with a vaginal birth some gentle physical abdominal work can be begun. If the mother has had a caesarean section more physical abdominal work can only be done once the incision has healed. After a caesarean, the abdomen will be more weakened and recovering so extra care needs to be taken even with energy techniques. Any work on the abdomen needs to avoid putting strain on the incision.

The pelvic floor needs to be encouraged to regain its strength, even if the mother has had a caesarean section. While no direct work would be done, energy work can support this process. The Girdle Vessel and Conception Vessel are particularly beneficial for this.

The upper body often has tightness in the musculature, due to feeding or the birth, so some passive movements of the shoulders can be indicated. Fairly physical work can be done here, even in this early period. Work involving the breasts may be needed to support breastfeeding. Massage of the breasts, either performed by the therapist with the mother's consent or self-taught massage, can help. Lymphatic work in the arms and for the breasts may be very useful in helping with blocked milk ducts as well as relieving tension/fullness in the breasts and shoulders.

The legs may be tired and tight and it is important to do some gentle work to support circulation and minimise the risk of thrombosis, from the earliest opportunity. The use of stretching and mobilisations is likely to be minimal or absent, especially after surgery, but as the mother regains her fitness and strength it can be included and more physically deep work can begin.

Energy work to the Penetrating Vessel to support the Blood and recovery is likely to be beneficial. Heart work to support the Shen, Blood and the emotions may also be indicated.

The back often has issues related to either pregnancy or birth.

Positioning

The mother often likes to lie prone, although she may need pillowing under her chest. It may be comforting while the uterus is contracting and the pressure can bring energy and attention here. Supine is safe to resume again. Side is an excellent position if the mother comes with her baby, particularly on the floor, so the mother can lie with the baby next to her and feed and comfort as needed. Forward leaning tends to be avoided as the mother is not likely to be comfortable in this position after the birth and will not receive the benefits she did in pregnancy.

Bodywork cautions

- Care with work to the abdomen, especially for the less experienced practitioner and after a caesarean section.
- Monitor for signs of infection and fever and excessive bleeding for possible haemorrhage. Refer.
- Be aware of issues relating to scar tissue: abdomen (caesarean), pelvic floor (episiotomy).
- Be aware of potential thrombosis signs.
- Be aware that for the first 48 hours there is still the possibility of eclampsia developing.
- Be aware of continued laxity of the joints, especially in the pelvis.

Self-care
Breathing

It is important for the mother to continue to value the importance of relaxation and breath work. She can do her breathing exercises while feeding the baby and incorporate breathing techniques while exercising the abdominal and pelvic floor muscles as well as for overall tension release.

In the early period, gentle 'huffing' breathing can be helpful to clear the lungs for women who have had a caesarean section.

Exercise

During the first week or so Early ambulation is important to reduce the incidence of thromboembolic disorders. For women who have had an epidural or a caesarean, ambulation may take longer, but gentle leg mobilisations can be done, possibly in bed and with supervision.

Abdominal muscles: during the first few days these need to shorten vertically as well as horizontally. They need to be checked for recti muscle separation and the mother can begin to do the corrective exercises within a couple of days if she has not had a caesarean section.

Pelvic floor: gentle exercise can be begun with these in the first few days. The aim is to encourage gentle tightening and awareness of the musculature. These are best done initially in the supine position to avoid the forces of gravity. It often takes the mother a few days to feel the muscles. After an episiotomy it is still valuable to gently contract the muscles.

As the mother increases her awareness, she can gradually build up to stronger exercises. As the pelvic floor begins to recover the mother can gradually start to tighten the muscles more readily, hold them for longer and begin to use upright positions.

Gentle pelvic tilts can be suggested with breathing awareness to begin to work the abdomen and pelvic floor. These are initially begun while lying down supine or in side or sitting on a chair or on a ball rather than standing, in order to minimise the effects of gravity. They tend not to be performed on all fours, while the mother is bleeding due to its effects of tilting the uterus forward and opening up the pelvis.

Gentle mobilisations of the shoulders are beneficial to help release tension in the breast area.

After week one, depending on recovery and pre pregnancy levels of fitness

- The mother can begin to do stronger versions of exercises.
- Pelvic tilts could be done using gravity, for example standing as opposed to lying down.
- Squatting is probably still too strong for most mothers.

Postural awareness and including the baby in the exercises As the mother recovers, it can be helpful to introduce more awareness of how she is holding her baby and how this affects her posture. Encourage exercise where the mother holds the baby on the opposite hip to the usual one as well as with her holding the baby in the centre of her body.

Cautions

- Forward leaning exercises, such as the cat or all fours, tend to be less advised, certainly while the mother is bleeding.
- Inverted positions tend to be less advised because they encourage lochial discharge to flow inwards rather than be discharged.

Massage

- Self-massage of the breasts may help prevent blockage of milk in ducts and reduce risk of mastitis developing.
- Gentle massage of the abdomen as appropriate.

General

Good nutrition and adequate rest are paramount.

Week 6 to 6 months

Recovery continues and patterns are set for the rest of the woman's life. During this time, depending on the country in which she lives, the mother may go

---

Summary box: the first 6 weeks postnatally

- Work in collaboration with primary care provider.
- Be aware of the risk of infections, especially uterine infection. Monitor lochial discharge through questioning the mother. If it is still red by 2–3 weeks refer to primary care provider.
- The mother may want a 'familiar' therapist to work with her.
- Encourage rest. Offer home or hospital visits rather than clinic.
- Be aware of emotional changes due to hormonal changes and lifestyle changes. Heart/Shen work may be helpful.
- Include the newborn if appropriate and support bonding.
- The bodywork focus is to support recovery. There is more emphasis on gentler type techniques. Holding and energy work are particularly effective.
- Support the mother in her feeding choices.
- Breast work is important to include to help prevent mastitis and encourage relaxation. Lymph work can also be included.
- The mother may need support with feeding: for example, advice re physical positions and relaxation, emotional support, support re nutrition and fluid intake.
- Bodywork generally can begin to get stronger and more physical techniques can be used as the mother recovers.
- Be aware of encouraging good postural awareness in order to prevent poor long-term posture and associated issues.
- Be aware of changes in blood flow and the risk of uterine haemorrhage and thrombosis. Gentle work to the legs is important to reduce risk of thrombosis formation.
- Work to the arms and shoulders is helpful to promote relaxation in feeding and to help prevent carpal tunnel syndrome from developing.
- Be aware of the possibility of anaemia and the importance of adequate nutrition. ST and PV work helpful.
- Use positions as per the mother's choice, although forward leaning is less favoured.
- Work with Extraordinary Vessels to support changes in blood and hormonal flows. Especially CV and PV blood and breastfeeding.
- Work to support the shift of energy from the Lower to the Upper Burner.

---

back to work. In the UK/USA it is often at 6 months. In many European countries it may not be during the first few years of the child's life. Some women go back to work within weeks of having a baby.

If the mother is going back to work within the first 6 months, she will be thinking about this impending change in her life with her baby. From the physical point of view, depending on the kind of work and the kind of support the woman has in her life, this may be challenging. Women who go back to work early often say they do not have time for bodywork, although they may be even more in need of it than those who stay at home.

In terms of emotional and physical recovery it is still early days, even though many women expect to be 'back to normal' by now. This can increase feelings of frustration with the healing process and lead to lack of appropriate self-care and support. Being back at work during this period may place additional strain on the mother, especially if the baby is not sleeping well and she is tired. Chronic tiredness may contribute to feelings of depression. On the other hand, some women bounce back and feel quite healthy and strong by 6 months.

With each week postnatally the baby is growing and their weight gain places more strain on the mother's body. Posture becomes a key factor. Women are often so busy thinking about picking up the baby or moving around they do not think about how they are carrying their baby and the effects on their own body. They often use their backs to bend down, or hold their baby on one hip so that hip/shoulder issues may develop. It is important to address these postural factors and suggest appropriate exercises as well as addressing the issues through bodywork, otherwise the mother will continue to create the problems. Usually with one child, the body copes but it is likely to be more of an issue with each child the mother has.

The mother may begin to wean her baby, perhaps towards the end of this 6 month period. This heralds another period of changes in feeding and sleeping patterns as adjustments are made. If the mother is not breastfeeding her baby she will resume menstruation by around 15 weeks.

The partner will be back at work by now. Usually family support diminishes and the mother may be left more on her own. Life begins to settle into a new pattern. The baby is likely to be more settled, although not always.

During this time the scar tissue of the caesarean is likely to heal, although for some women there may be continued sensitivity or numbness.

The mother may want to continue to bring baby with her, but as time goes on she may find she wants to have the session as a space in which to relax on her own. Respect each woman's needs. Although the mother might not come as frequently for bodywork, regular sessions every 2–3 weeks continue to be beneficial.

Bodywork

As the body is further on in the recovery process and getting stronger, then deeper and more physical work is often appropriate, especially in the abdominal and lower back areas. As deeper work is begun, the therapist needs to elicit good feedback from the client, particularly if they have had a caesarean or epidural. Feedback is helpful also to engage the client in the process of learning to reconnect with areas of their body and build up strength in them.

Muscles such as the psoas and quadratus lumborum, which cannot receive much direct bodywork during pregnancy but which have played, and continue to play, an important role in stabilising the pelvic and lumbar regions, can now be focused on more directly.

The mother often suffers from constipation postnatally and deeper colon work and ileocaecal work, which was not suitable in pregnancy, can begin. Work varies individually and the therapist needs to gauge appropriate pressure. It can take several months for the intestines to return to pre-pregnancy positioning.

Hip, shoulder and postural issues continue to be a focus due to the increasing demands of carrying a growing baby.

Bodywork cautions

- The major cautions re infection and thrombosis are over, but still be alert to that possibility.
- The cautions now are mostly to do with varicose veins, healing of scar tissue, sensitivity in the abdomen and digestive issues.
- If the woman has a caesarean section scar then deeper abdominal techniques should not be attempted until the scar is well healed and caution must be taken with the pressure.
- Monitor for continuing signs of pelvic girdle instability.

Aftercare

Exercise

- The mother can begin to do gentle cat and forward leaning exercises, depending on her recovery.
- Exercises can gradually begin to get stronger, with focus on strengthening the abdomen and lower back and releasing tension from the hips and shoulders.
- In case of pelvic girdle instability and extreme diastasis recti (abdominal separation), monitoring still needs to continue regarding the effects of

increasing exercise regimes, especially around the premenstrual time.

- Abdominal and pelvic floor exercises can be stronger, and regularity for the rest of the woman's life needs to be emphasised.
- It is beneficial to include the baby with the exercises to support bonding and add weight to the exercise challenge, as well as providing the time to do the exercises as the mother does not have to wait for the baby to sleep.

Six months and beyond – themes for the rest of life

The same themes continue, but as the baby becomes more alert it may be harder for the mother to rest during the day, although she may begin to be able to get more sleep at night. The mother may be feeling more tired, especially if she is back to work or has other children to look after. By the end of the first year, the baby will be mobile and may have started to walk. This can create more physical demands. During the infant years the mother will be lifting and carrying a lot and potentially straining her body if she does not pay attention to good postural habits. Long-term patterns of body imbalance can arise without good self-care.

It is important to recognise that the body will never be as it was. The ribs and intestines have altered their positions. The mother may find weaker areas become more obvious premenstrually, especially

pelvic instability or aggravation of caesarean or episiotomy scar tissue. The abdominal muscles and pelvic floor will always have a tendency to be slightly weaker without appropriate care. It is important to continue to work with these areas, both with bodywork and with appropriate exercise and postural suggestions, otherwise there may be issues in later life particularly after menopause. Later issues may include uterine prolapse, bowel problems and stress incontinence. It is much better to set up good habits at this point, rather than wait for women to return in the peri/postmenopausal period with these issues.

If the mother is considering having other children then she needs to think about preparing her body for another pregnancy. The better state of health a woman is in when she conceives the less strain the pregnancy will be for her. Recent research suggests that it is better for the mother to wait at least 2 years before conceiving again.

The relationship with the partner may be difficult if the mother does not feel like resuming sex because she is tired or because she is still processing the birth. Sometimes, rather than bringing partners together, having children may place strains on relationships.

The mother will probably want to leave the infant with someone else while she has her bodywork sessions as they probably provide a rare space for her to connect with herself.

Bodywork

- The main themes are likely to be tension in the hips and shoulders and weakness in the abdomen, pelvic floor and lower back.
- By 6 months the body has often recovered well but the therapist still needs to pay some attention to patterns of tiredness and weakness.
- The treatments gradually become more similar to work with women who are not in their childbearing phase.

Cautions

- The body should be healed physically from the birth although continue to be aware of any issues and areas of weakness.
- Emotional trauma relating to the birth can take longer to process and can still be there years after the birth if unresolved.

Aftercare

Gradually the mother will be resuming normal exercise routines but ligamentous laxity especially in the pelvis still need to be monitored, especially premenstrually.

Summary box: 6 months and beyond – patterns for life

- Long-term patterns of exhaustion may set in.
- Good or poor health patterns can be established.
- Regular patterns of exercise to be encouraged to maintain good posture.
- Stress incontinence may be an issue and pelvic floor exercise is important to continue for the rest of life.
- Good nutrition continues to be important.
- Be aware that having children changes the body forever: ribs changed, long-term patterns of weak abdominals and pelvic floor are often the reality.
- If there has been surgery the body may compensate with protective patterns and it is always advisable to be aware of the effects.
- Caesarean scar tissue may affect menstruation. Scar tissue may remain an issue.
- There is a continued tendency for varicose veins and haemorrhoids.
- The type of birth experienced will have emotional and physical implications for the rest of the mother's life. It is important to evaluate with each client the potential impact of her birthing experience (positive or negative, processed or unprocessed) and the continuing implications (musculoskeletal, reproductive or emotional).
- Caring for a young child places certain physical and emotional demands on the body. Be aware of common poor posture habits which mothers may develop.

Potential postnatal emergency situations

After diagnosis bodywork may be an adjunctive therapy to support the healing process.

Immediate referral to primary caregiver without bodywork

- Fever: may indicate uterine infection, bladder or kidney infection, breast infection (mastitis), or other illness.
- Burning with urination, or blood in the urine: could indicate bladder infection.
- Inability to urinate: swelling or trauma of urethral sphincter.
- Swollen, red painful area on leg (especially calf) which is hot to touch: thrombophlebitis – development of blood clot in blood vessel. However, remember that DVTs are not always symptomatic.
- Sore reddened painful area on the breast in addition to fever and flu-like symptoms: breast infection, mastitis.
- Passage of large red clots, pieces of tissue or return of bright red vaginal bleeding after flow (lochia) has decreased and changed to brownish, pink or yellow: retained fragment of placenta, uterine infection, overexertion.
- Foul odour to vaginal discharge, vaginal soreness or itching: uterine infection, vaginal infection.
- Increase in pain in episiotomy site, may be accompanied by bleeding or foul-smelling discharge: infection of episiotomy, reopening of incision or tear, stitches give way.
- Slight opening of caesarean incision, may be accompanied by foul discharge and blood.

11.4 Special issues of the early postnatal period

Early risk

The early postnatal period (first 6 weeks) is potentially a time of risk for the mother and this is why she is usually under medical supervision, at least for the first 10 days and, if there are complications, for the first month. The uterus is contracting and the placental site healing, so there is a risk of infection or haemorrhage. There are changes in the breasts, especially if the mother is breastfeeding, and there is a risk of breast infection and mastitis. The substantial changes in the circulatory system also mean this period is at highest risk for thromboembolitic disorders. If undiagnosed some of these can result in severe illness and even death. It is important if the therapist is aware of any concerns and can recognise warning signs so that they can refer the mother immediately back to her primary care provider.

Normal precautions and considerations always apply.

Supporting the mother with PGI (pelvic girdle instability) complications

The PGD could have been caused by the birth itself – most frequently after a forceps or ventouse delivery when the mother has been in stirrups. In these cases the injury caused to the symphysis pubis is likely to be more extreme as it is caused by trauma, rather than that which has come on gradually during pregnancy due to the softening of the tissues. It is important to recognise this and advise the mother appropriately. The pain may persist for months and it is important that the mother knows the correct exercises to support the pelvic girdle and help it to recover.

Care for mothers with pre-term babies or babies with medical health issues; work with the baby in special care unit

With these clients the baby may be in the hospital and the mother may want the therapist to go and visit her there, especially if they offer infant bodywork. The mother is encouraged to have as much contact as possible with her baby as promoting bonding and non-invasive touch between mother and baby is essential. Bonding may be difficult in the hospital setting, especially if the mother is not staying in the hospital which she usually is not after the first few days, unless she also has medical needs.

If working in the hospital on the postpartum unit the therapist needs to be aware of the protocols of the hospital environment (see Ch. 15).

Be aware that a mother's main feeling is likely to be one of anxiety, or at least concern, over her baby's health. Be sensitive to her emotional state, which may include feelings of failure, disappointment, distress and guilt. It can be helpful to give the mother space to express her fears and work them through in a constructive way.

If appropriately trained, and depending on the health status of the baby, the therapist can teach appropriate massage techniques and energy based on or off the body holding techniques, in consultation with medical practitioners. The mother may be very tense herself, so in teaching infant work the therapist can encourage her to relax and even do some work, for example on the shoulders, while the mother is working with her baby. The therapist can encourage the mother to breathe and look after herself, as often her attention is taken up with worry about the baby's health and her own recovery process becomes ignored.

Arrangements are usually made for the mother to feed her baby herself but feeding a newborn in the hospital setting may not be that easy. Emotionally it can be difficult for the mother as she may feel tired and frustrated as well as anxious about her baby and may find that she is not producing enough milk. She may need additional breastfeeding support.

The mother may prefer the therapist to visit her at home as she may find it more relaxing to receive bodywork in this setting.

Postpartum depression

It is quite common in the first week for the mother to experience extreme emotions which are known as the 'baby blues'. The therapist needs to support this reality and allow the mother to release and process her emotions while reassuring her that this is often a 'normal' part of the postpartum process and she is not experiencing a nervous breakdown.

However, if the 'baby blues' is becoming more chronic this may indicate that the mother is beginning to suffer from depression. The therapist should be aware of the kind of support the mother has and accept that the bodyworker's role is not to offer emotional and practical support beyond the bodywork session, although it can be helpful to facilitate the mother to identify what she needs. It is important to have a good resource network so that the mother can be referred to her primary care provider or to another health professional who has expertise in counselling or psychotherapy.

Be alert for the signs of a range of postpartum psychological issues ranging from uncontrollable crying, inability to sleep or eat, extreme anxiety or agitation. These may include signs of obsessive compulsive disorder and extreme depression or even puerperal psychosis. Puerperal psychosis is the most extreme postpartum mental health issue and the mother will need to receive medical attention as it may lead to her harming either herself or her baby. She may be admitted to a specialist mother and baby unit of a hospital. In this case it can be supportive to continue to work in the hospital setting.

Type of work

The eastern view of postpartum psychological issues is an imbalance in the Heart can be balanced by work with the Stomach, Penetrating Vessel, Heart, Uterus.

From a western point of view relaxation work and work to address tense areas in the body would be of benefit.

Supporting breastfeeding

Most bodyworkers will not be fully trained breastfeeding counsellors. However, any existing issues may be compounded if the mother and baby are not relaxed. Bodyworkers can be crucial in providing a relaxing environment which may reduce stress. Sometimes the issue may be to do with positioning and if the mother decides to feed the baby during the treatment, the therapist may need to help the mother and baby get into comfortable positions. It is useful to understand some of the basic mechanics of breastfeeding such as how the baby latches on so that if the baby is feeding poorly during the treatment simple ideas can be suggested without contradicting other breastfeeding advice. If breastfeeding is not going well then the mother may ask the therapist for 'advice'. Simple things can be checked, such as basic diet and rest, without overstepping the therapist's scope of practice. If mother is not producing enough milk or having other difficulties, it is often related to lack of rest, insufficient fluid intake and issues related to adequate nutrition.

Breastfeeding technique (Fig. 11.1)

Current breastfeeding attitudes tend to support the view of feeding the baby on demand, with no limit to the frequency and duration of feeds. This can be encouraged by supporting the mother to be able to tune in to her body and be relaxed so that she can better tune in to her baby.

Many problems with breastfeeding are caused by poor positioning and the bodyworker can promote relaxation during this process. The baby is held close to the mother with their head and shoulders at her breast. As the baby opens its mouth and begins to root then it is moved to the breast with the mouth wide open and lower lip well below the nipple so it grasps as much breast tissue as possible. The nipple and as much of the areola as possible should be in the baby's mouth. The nipple needs to be well back in the baby's mouth to avoid damage to it. If the baby is not feeding well then this can cause sore or cracked nipples which can be incredibly painful and may stop a woman from breastfeeding. They may also allow infection to enter and so the therapist needs to be able to recognise signs of local infection, general infection and mastitis and refer if necessary. If any pain is felt by the mother while breastfeeding, she should stop and check the position of the baby and attachment at breast to prevent any damage. The fat content of the hind milk is higher than that of the foremilk and so the baby needs to be encouraged to empty the breast.

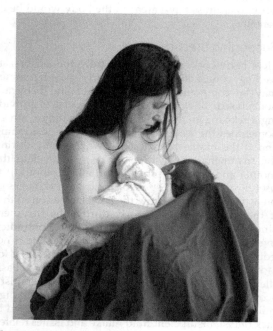

Fig. 11.1 Woman breastfeeding.

If the baby is not thriving then check that the mother does not:

- Have a blocked duct.
- Experience breast compression from tight clothes.
- Hold the breast too tightly while feeding.
- Have the baby in a poor position.
- Restrict feeding.

However, also encourage referral to the primary care provider in such a manner that the mother does not become overly anxious and that adequate support is given.

Practical work to support breastfeeding

This includes:

- Work with the lymph system, to stimulate terminal nodes, axillary nodes, and work with the breast (either directly or teaching the mother to work herself). This helps the body process minor infections so that they are less likely to develop into more serious conditions.
- Encouraging the mother to be aware of and relaxed about her breasts – achieved by simple breast massage techniques (self-help or performed by practitioner).
- Encouraging postural awareness. If the mother is tense in any area of her body, but especially in the shoulders and mid-thoracics, then this may interfere with breastfeeding. The baby may pick up on the mother's tension which in turn may affect the success of feeding.
- Encouraging the mother to massage her baby which will support bonding and the baby to be more relaxed.
- Encouraging the mother to ensure that she is eating properly and drinking enough fluids.

Other issues

The therapist needs to be aware that there is a possibility of leakage of breast milk. Breast milk is a body fluid and could contain the HIV virus. Universal precautions of infectious control need to be followed with respect to the handling and disposal and cleaning of equipment and linens.

The mother may want to keep her bra on when prone so that breast pads can absorb leaking breast milk or she could undo her bra at the back to make back work possible. Alternatively towels can be used for absorption.

Supporting the non-breastfeeding mother

For the mother who does not want to breastfeed, the production of milk is suppressed naturally by not feeding. If the baby does not feed, the release of prolactin ceases and the breasts stop producing milk. They become engorged on the third or fourth day with blood which causes pressure on the milk-producing cells (acini) and milk engorgement may follow. If the mother is sore, then some milk can be expressed to relieve the discomfort. This will not increase lactation because prolactin levels remain low, but it will help reduce mastitis and subsequent breast abscesses. The therapist can encourage the mother to massage her breasts to reduce this discomfort.

It is important to support the mother in whatever choice she makes. The therapist needs to recognise that, while breastfeeding is the healthiest way to feed a baby, not all mothers are able to choose this as an option. They may have tried and found it too difficult. They may not be in a situation where they feel supported to breastfeed. They may have issues around breastfeeding. While encouraging mothers to breastfeed where possible and supporting them in that choice, mothers also need to be supported who are not able to, or choose not to, breastfeed.

Supporting the mother who wants to breastfeed but is unable to

It is important to recognise issues such as pain and discomfort; for example a sore nipple which does not heal. The mother is likely to be quite stressed by the whole process, as she is likely to be aware of the benefits of breastfeeding and feel guilty that she is not able to offer this to her baby. However, she may be in considerable pain when she is feeding and this may in itself be disturbing the bonding process.

It is up to each mother to determine how long she wants to try to continue to breastfeed and up to the therapist to support the mother in the choices she makes. It is important to monitor for signs of infection

and refer as it is often repeated infections and mastitis which eventually force the mother to stop.

11.5 Overview of practical techniques and their suitability at different stages postnatally

General precautions apply for all these techniques and specific cautions for areas of the body are listed under that area of the body.

Specific postnatal cautions:

- Increased incidence of varicose veins.
- Thrombosis.
- Infection.
- Pressure on scar; caesarean section.

Effleurage (Swedish massage), saka (shiatsu)

These types of techniques are generally suitable at all stages postnatally. They can be used to facilitate circulation, whether of lymph, blood or energy. Lighter effleurage for the legs is particularly beneficial during the early postnatal period to encourage circulation and prevent thrombosis. Effleurage for the arms and breasts is beneficial to encourage lymph and circulatory flow, to prevent carpal tunnel and mastitis from developing and to support breastfeeding.

Cautions

Care always needs to be taken with any work to the abdomen after a caesarean section.

Kneading/petrissage (Swedish massage), kenbiki (shiatsu)

These types of techniques remain important for addressing areas of tightness which are common postnatally. They are particularly beneficial for tightness around the shoulders, tight gluteus muscles, piriformis and iliotibial band.

Special issues

Supporting women whose baby is in hospital, women with postpartum depression, breastfeeding women

- Be aware of issues relating to working in the hospital.
- Be aware of issues relating to breastfeeding.
- Be sensitive to and support mothers who are trying to breastfeed but in a lot of pain. Support them in their choice if they decide to stop.
- Be aware that while some transient degree of 'depression' is common, sometimes it may develop into longer patterns and women may need support.

Summary of maternal changes with most implications for bodyworkers

- Continued softness of tissue for breastfeeding mothers.
- Quicker recovery for non-breastfeeding mothers.
- Changes around menstruation.
- Continued potential weakness of pelvic area including abdominal and pelvic floor muscles.

In the early postnatal period the mother may be more sensitive to deeper work around the pelvic area, although she will probably appreciate deeper work on the upper body. As the time after birth increases there is more physical strain on the body, especially the lower back, shoulders and legs. These techniques are important modalities for addressing tension in these areas.

Cautions

- Deeper work on the abdomen should not be undertaken while the mother is bleeding.
- Care will always need to be taken with the abdomen after a caesarean section and with the lower back after an epidural, to monitor depth of these stronger strokes, even potentially years later.

Friction

As per kneading.

Tapotement

Light tapotement to stimulate the terminal lymph nodes, thymus and chest may be useful in the first few days postnatally, especially for caesarean section clients. This work will support the immune system which may be prone to infections for the whole of the first year.

Moderate tapotement can be useful to address tension in the shoulders from immediately after birth. It can be used with caution in the hip area.

Stronger tapotement can be used progressively more in other areas as the woman recovers and levels of relaxin diminish. Usually this is during the first 6 weeks, but could still be high for the first 6–9 months. The softness of the tissue remains an issue for longer than 6 weeks if the mother is breastfeeding.

Cautions

- Do not perform tapotement in the abdominal area while the mother is bleeding and always be careful regarding a caesarean incision.
- Bear in mind that even by the end of the first year the mother may still be experiencing underlying patterns of tiredness and so relaxation rather than more intense work may be more appropriate.

Breathing

This is an important tool which is to be encouraged throughout the postnatal period. It is usually more effective and easier for the mother to integrate if she is building on techniques she has been using in pregnancy. It is excellent for stress reduction and can be used with postnatal visualisations. It can be used to encourage connection with the baby and to support breastfeeding, especially if the mother has sore nipples. It can be used as part of early abdominal and pelvic floor work.

Lymph drainage techniques

These can be particularly beneficial in the early postnatal period, as there may be some oedema in both arms and legs. They can help with sinus congestion. They also offer useful techniques to support changes in the breasts postnatally for both lactating and non-lactating mothers. Work on the breasts will support breastfeeding and help prevent breast congestion/breast engorgement and therefore may help reduce the incidence of mastitis.

Abdominal work can support circulation and aid abdominal recovery.

Cautions

- Do not do lymphatic work if there is any indication of infection as it could potentially spread and worsen the infection. If there is infective mastitis then no lymphatic work should be done.
- Be aware of the increased risk of thrombosis for the first 6 weeks and of the risk of PET during the first 48 hours. In both cases no lymph work should be done.
- For post section recovery, after consulting the client's physician/midwife to establish when to safely work with the client, work can be done to help remove cellular debris and increase circulation.

Static pressure and holds including soft tissue manipulation and neuromuscular technique (NMT)

Generally these techniques are suitable even in the early period. The holding of acupuncture points for balancing energy can be extremely beneficial. Light pressure, even off the body holding, can be done to support scar healing.

These techniques can be especially useful to address tension in the sacral and gluteal area even during the early postnatal phase.

Cautions

- Be careful in the early period not to apply pressure directly over a caesarean scar and use pressure only as desired by the mother over the abdomen.
- While the mother is still bleeding do not do deep work over the abdomen.
- Do not use pressure on varicose veins.

Stretches/passive movements/ joint mobilisations

These techniques can be beneficial from immediately after birth for the arms and upper body. They would tend not to be done for the pelvic area as it is likely to be unstable after all the movements it has undergone during labour and needs time to recover rather than be stretched out. As the body recovers then they can be beneficial for all areas of the body and resisted type stretches can be included once more.

Cautions

- During the first few days, avoid mobilising the pelvis. Movements can gradually be introduced depending on the level of recovery.
- During the first year, especially the first 8 weeks, if the mother is breastfeeding be aware of the potential instability of the joints created by the softening of tissue due to the continued high levels of relaxin. Continue to be cautious of movements of the joints, especially those of the pelvis (sacroiliac and symphysis pubis) which may have continued laxity. These techniques need to be performed slowly, with care not to overextend the movement, or use resistance techniques.
- Be aware that premenstruation, hormonal changes may re-trigger the instability of the joints for a few days each month.

Fascial techniques and soft tissue release

During the early postnatal period the fascia is affected by the huge levels of changes which are occurring. Fascial techniques offer excellent modalities in supporting the process of recovery.

11.6 Approach and techniques for different areas of the body

Main postural patterns in postnatal period

This is outlined in the assessment section (p. 190).

Head, face, neck and shoulders

While the mother is establishing breastfeeding and bonding with her baby, she may experience muscular tightness in the shoulders and neck due to feeding in awkward positions at night and lack of sleep. She may also have built up tension in the shoulders from the different positions she was in during labour. The increased weight of the breasts in the early days may add additional tension to the shoulders and the pectorals.

Women may suffer from headaches due both to tension and to hormonal changes. They may also experience carpal tunnel syndrome due to tightness in the shoulders. The sinuses may be congested.

The mother may continue to experience jaw clenching and temporomandibular joint (TMJ) issues.

Types of techniques

This area can be worked from the earliest time with most types of techniques. It may have been an area where the mother received work during labour. Work here can be calming, reassuring and provide nurturing touch and support when the rest of the body may still be quite sensitive to touch.

GB 21 is an excellent point for freeing up tension in the breast, shoulder and neck and stimulating the flow of milk.

Working positions

The mother will usually be able to lie comfortably supine and this is an excellent option for upper body work. The side can also be continued. It provides excellent access to the shoulders and can be useful if the mother has the baby with her.

Cautions

None apart from the usual general cautions.

Technique suggestions

All of the techniques outlined in pregnancy are suitable.

The back torso

It takes time for the back to recover from the demands placed on it during pregnancy. Energetically and structurally, work can be done to support this process.

The main patterns for the spine in the postnatal period are a continuing tendency to lordosis and tension in the lower back due to weakened abdominal muscles and carrying the baby. The upper back can be tight due to compensation for heavier breasts. There is a tendency for hyperkyphosis due to the increased weight and size of the breasts for breastfeeding mothers.

In addition to this, mothers often develop unbalanced carrying and lifting postures with their babies, carrying them solely on one side. This can cause problems of left/right imbalances especially with the hip and quadratus lumborum, iliopsoas. These issues tend to be more exaggerated in women with more than one child.

It is important to encourage good postural awareness in this first year to set up good patterns for the back later on, especially when lifting older children. These can include rhythmic movements into the mother's posture of ease, while either not holding the infant or with the infant in a sling in the midline. This will aid the proprioceptive postural positioning into an optimum posture for that state of her health. The repetition of full body movements reduces the reliance on a small number of muscles.

Positions

Often mothers enjoy work on the back being done in the prone position although it is not suitable for all mothers. Some mothers find that prone is uncomfortable for their breasts or it may put pressure on the scar if they have had a caesarean. Furthermore if the mother is bringing the baby with them, then the side position may continue to be a preferred position to work the back.

Cautions

Watch for any potential damage to the vertebrae due to the extra load of carrying a baby. This may be a problem for mothers with pre-existing back problems and for multiparae.

Assess sensitivity of the epidural site if relevant and use appropriate techniques.

Suggestions of techniques

All of the pregnancy techniques are suitable. In the early period it is usually preferable to minimise or avoid work such as stretches or spinal rocking. An energy approach, or utilising gentle effleurage may be preferable for most mothers during the first week.

The techniques shown here are stronger techniques for the later postnatal period. These can be performed after a minimum of 4 weeks, depending on the health and recovery of the mother. These are shown as they are techniques which are too strong to use during pregnancy, but which can have benefit in the postnatal period.

Quadratus lumborum (QL) release – cross fibre

Benefits

There is often one-sided contraction due to balancing the baby on one hip. This is likely to be exaggerated with each subsequent pregnancy unless the mother has become aware of her poor posture.

It has to be worked with care in pregnancy because many techniques place too much strain on the uterus and its ligaments due to its proximity and its function in stabilising the pelvis. This cross fibre release is not used in pregnancy because of its potential pull on the uterus and its ligaments. For this reason it would not be used in the early postnatal period while the uterus is involuting.

When is it suitable?

It can be used from a few weeks postnatally if the mother is recovering well from a vaginal birth. It is used later after a caesarean section and depending on the mother's recovery.

The technique

The client can be prone or in side (Fig. 11.2). First use some effleurage and friction over the muscle to warm it.

With side, start with one hand on top of the other and with the fingers resting on the superior side of the body and draw the hand towards the spine, holding firmly. As the edge of the muscle is reached, gently lift and lengthen it. The work will need to be fairly deep in order to engage the QL. Let the muscle slide through the fingers very slowly. This can be repeated up to three times if necessary. Repeat on the other side.

One side is likely to be more contracted than the other.

Cautions

Watch that there is no pulling on the caesarean section scar.

Chest/abdomen/front of body/breasts

This area is undergoing many changes in the early postnatal period and is important to include in the treatment. The abdomen has been weakened, energetically and physically, through the work it had to do during the pregnancy and in labour. Stronger abdominal tone will help to prevent longer-term issues such as those connected with digestion and prolapse of the abdominal organs. It is important to

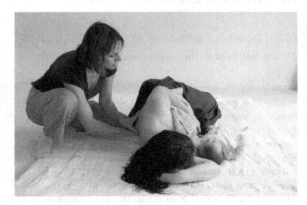

Fig. 11.2 Quadratus lumborum release, side.

help to strengthen it in order to give support to the lower back and pelvic floor which have also been weakened. Women often assume that the muscles will simply become stronger again, but the reality is that work usually needs to be done to help them regain their tone. Advising on appropriate self-care exercises is an important part of this process. The rectus abdominis muscles need to be the first to go back together before work is done to strengthen the transverse and obliques.

For women who have PGI issues, abdominal work is especially important as the abdominal muscles give support to the pelvis. The pelvic joints will continue to be less stable for at least the first 6 weeks, and longer if the mother is breastfeeding. Immediately after birth, it would not be so suitable to do movements which involve mobilisations of the pelvis due to this relative weakness. Furthermore, during birth the pelvis has often been destabilised and so needs to be strengthened through appropriate work such as strengthening muscles and energy rather than stretches and movements. However, as the mother recovers it is an important area to work with stretches and mobilisations, especially as postural imbalances are often set up through one-sided carrying of the baby.

The psoas is likely to be contracted in order to compensate for this weakness in the pelvis. In the early days care needs to be taken not to over-release the psoas, but as the pelvis becomes more stable then deeper work can be done with the psoas.

For mothers post caesarean section there may be body image issues associated with the abdominal scar, including numbness or pain and an awareness that the abdomen is weaker.

If the mother is breastfeeding, then she is likely to be experiencing fullness and tension in the breasts. She may have issues about her body and the changed size and shape of her breasts; some women love the changes, others find them difficult to come to terms with. There are often issues of blocked milk ducts or lymphatic issues. If the mother is not feeding, or unable to feed, she may also be experiencing issues with engorgement or soreness. Appropriate work may support her in this process of the changing of the breasts.

Informed consent with clear client communication will determine if breast work is an appropriate treatment. It depends on the mother, and on the therapist's relationship to the mother, whether it would be appropriate to provide work directly on the breasts or whether it is better to show the mother work to do herself. Another option can be to work through the sheet so that there is no direct physical contact over the breast. As well as a personal issue, it is also a cultural issue. In some countries working directly with the breast is not considered controversial, indeed in Japan work with white sesame oil antenatally as well as postnatally was considered part of preparation for being a mother. The male therapist may find that the woman is less happy to receive breast massage from him than from a female therapist.

Types of techniques

In the first week or so, energy work can be done over the uterus to help with involution and for helping with the healing of the perineum.

Abdominal muscle-gathering techniques can be incorporated to help strengthen the abdominal wall as well as work to emphasise support from obliques and transverse. It is important to include exercise which the mother can do herself.

Breast techniques may be beneficial at all stages.

Positions for work

Either side or supine may be used.

Cautions

- Monitor caesarean section incision and do not work directly over it while it is healing. Do not do any techniques which would put pressure on it.
- If there is mastitis with infection then do not work at all, and do not do lymphatic work or work on the breasts if there is a suspicion of infection.
- Caution needs to be paid to mothers who are suffering from SPI as this can continue for months, even years, if the mother does not receive appropriate care and support.

Principles for postnatal work on the abdomen

- During the time when the mother is still bleeding (discharging lochia) it is important to be more cautious and to do less vigorous physical techniques as the bleeding indicates that the placental site and uterus are still healing. Bodywork should not increase blood loss and, if it does, techniques used should be re-evaluated. During this period collaboration with the primary care giver is fundamental in order to monitor any health issues which may arise.
- It is important to make sure the rectus abdominis muscles have gone back together before doing stronger techniques on the abdomen.
- Work needs to be done in a clockwise direction to support the digestive flow.
- Remember that the abdominal wall will be weaker after childbearing and so it is always important to include work here and remind the mother of exercises.

- Take into account any scar tissue.
- Be aware of mother's sensitivity, especially if she has a caesarean section (overhang, lax, saggy abdominal muscles), with regard to her abdomen. Many women feel quite embarrassed by the state of their abdominal muscles, stretch marks, scars and so on.

Cautions

- Discontinue physical techniques if bleeding is increased.
- If there has been a caesarean section then no pressure should be applied on the scar until the wound has healed. Energy work can be used to promote healing. Cup the hand so that there is no direct contact over scar and focus on allowing energy to flow to the scar.
- If infection is suspected, refer to the primary caregiver.
- Minimise use of forward leaning techniques while the uterus is still contracting (i.e. for first few weeks). This includes exercises.

Abdominal techniques

Depending on the level of recovery, many of the antenatal techniques are suitable.

Girdle Vessel

Benefits

- Work here holding the points brings energy together and can be done very gently or more physically.
- Refer to pregnancy Girdle Vessel work in pregnancy practical (p. 259).
- Postnatally this would be done more in the supine and side position and in the early period rather than the forward leaning positions.

Conception Vessel and Penetrating Vessel work (Figs 11.3, 11.4)

This work, described in the pregnancy section (chapter 9), is vital postnatally.

Pelvic floor support

This work is relevant postnatally to aid recovery and is especially important after an episiotomy.

Connecting the lower pathways of CV, GV, PV

This is done without directly contacting the pelvic floor. It can be done in semi-reclining, side-lying or forward leaning.

Following on from the previous work with the PV (p. 261) place the thumb in the centre point just on the superior border of the pubic bone (CV 2), with the

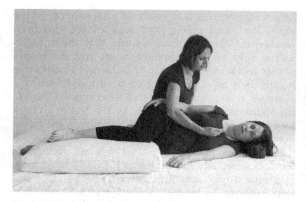

Fig. 11.3 Palming CV side, through sheet.

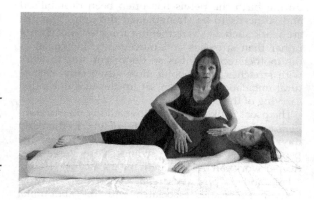

Fig. 11.4 Working CV facing the body.

other hand cupping the sacrum with the middle finger over the coccyx.

Try to imagine a connection between these two points which passes directly through the perineum (Fig. 11.5). As these points are held, warmth may be felt spreading between the two hands. The client usually finds this relaxing.

Uterus involution

Benefits

This is a modified energy version of a physical technique often used by midwives in the past and still used in many cultures today. The physical version is outside the scope of practice of bodyworkers but the physical movements can be mimicked in a gentle energetic way with the aim of helping the uterus contract. It should not be done if there has been a caesarean section.

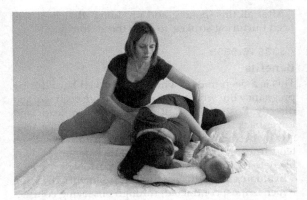

Fig. 11.5 Holding pelvic floor in side, visualising the connection between CV 2 and GV 1.5.

The technique

Mimic the following movements without pressure. When working the points use more of an intention than actual pressure. Touch/pressure must be monitored carefully with feedback from the mother.

Make a clockwise circular movement over the abdomen.

Roll the knuckles down from the fundus of the uterus to the pubic bone.

Use energy focus 'pressure' on points from CV 8 to CV 2 – i.e. from navel to pubic bone.

Gentle abdominal strokes for early abdominal work

Benefits

- This is the area that is usually Kyo postnatally. The Chinese would focus extensively on the points between CV 8 and CV 2 to bring more energy here.
- Work here may help the uterus contract.
- Gathering strokes toward the midline help the rectus abdominis muscles draw back together and also 'gather' energy to the midline.

Cautions

- Do not work directly over any caesarean section scar or do anything to pull on the scar, even light effleurage.
- Beware of over-stimulating the uterus and thus potentially stimulating blood loss. 'Less' is definitely better than 'more' to begin with.

Circling technique

Use either large sweeping strokes covering the whole abdomen, or smaller ones around the navel.

Gathering stroke

The first part of the movement, which is a lateral movement, is very gentle as it is important not to lengthen the abdominals. The hands start together at the base of the sternum. They separate and pass right under the back, the fingertips almost meeting at the spine. The next part can be strong. With a lifting movement the hands pass back round to the front of the body, moving over the ASISs and down the iliac crest to the pubic bone. Repetition of this is usually soothing.

Lymphatic work for abdomen

For post caesarean section recovery, gentle lymphatic strokes can be applied to the abdomen to help remove cellular debris and increase circulation. The work would be from peripheral to central to peripheral – focusing on modified thumb kneading and 'J' strokes. This would need to be done after consultation with the client's physician/midwife to establish when work could be safely done with the client.

Deeper abdominal techniques

Before undertaking any of the following techniques, the abdominal muscles and organs need to have received warming nurturing massage and the client should be happy and accepting of the touch. Many women may be carrying emotional issues in the abdomen, especially if they have had a traumatic birth. These are all techniques which should be performed only after at least 6 weeks, when the uterus is back to its pre-pregnancy size, there is no bleeding and there is healing of the abdominal wall. If there is any issue with caesarean section scar, then the techniques should not be performed. *None of these techniques is suitable in pregnancy.*

Liver/spleen balance

Benefits

This is a stroke which helps to balance the energy of the organs of the spleen and liver, which had to work hard during pregnancy and which continue to work hard due to changes in the blood flow.

Cautions

Do not perform this technique if there is any inflammation of either organ, soreness in the abdomen, bleeding, or any of the usual precautions of working on the abdomen.

The technique

Stand on the right of the client. Place the hands over the area of the spleen, and with swift light strokes 'pull' the energy of the spleen over to the liver. When a feeling of heat building is sensed, hold the hands over the liver, and rest them there for a short time.

Swap to the left side, and repeat this process, 'pulling' the energy from the liver to the spleen. Hold the hands over the spleen to finish.

Colon rocking
Benefits
Postnatally, women often experience digestive problems such as gas and constipation. While it is important to be aware of any dietary factors affecting the mother, direct bodywork is likely to be beneficial in supporting good peristaltic functioning.

The technique
Laying the hand flat across the ascending or descending colon with the fingers pointing to the side of the client's body. Let the hand sink down into the abdomen with the out-breath and then gently curl the fingers so that the edge of the colon is taken in a light grasp. Accentuate this with a gentle rocking action. Release gently and move along the edge of the colon. To work the other side, the therapist will have to move to that side.

Work can only be done effectively on the ascending and descending colon in this manner.

Ileocaecal valve release
Benefits
The ileocaecal valve is found in the lower right quadrant of the abdomen. It forms the junction between the ileum of the small intestine, and the caecum of the large bowel. It regulates and controls movement of liquid waste from the small to the large bowel and is prone to blockage, often in the postnatal period due to the changes and the laxity in the tissue.

It is a useful area to work if there are problems with excess mucus secretion throughout the body. It is in close proximity to the psoas, and so it is worth assessing if the psoas is also contracted and thus blocking the valve, in which case a release here to balance would be indicated.

The technique
Trace the gut from the central line across to the right where the large intestine lies. If this is repeated two or three times an area is usually felt which feels 'different'. This may well coincide with a tender spot for the client. It is usually about 3 inches to the right of the midline in the lower right quadrant.

Once this spot has been located, it is the same technique as for a gallbladder release. Apply pressure with the client's out-breath, hold for a few in-breaths, and on an in-breath suddenly release. If it releases, there may be some gurgling and movement in the area. Repeat 1 or 2 times. However, this may need to be repeated over several treatments.

After all this 'poking and prodding' the client will need nurturing strokes, to calm the abdomen.

Psoas release
Benefits
This is a deep muscle which has worked hard during pregnancy but which is too deep to have been worked directly. Postnatally, as it is the main hip flexor and lower back stabiliser it often goes out of balance, usually by becoming hypertonic. Often, as most mothers tend to carry their children on one side, one side is likely to be comparatively more hypertonic.

Evaluate, through postural assessment, the side which is most contracted, through observing contraction in the hips, legs, and shoulders. The client may be bending forwards complaining of back pain, leaning over to one side.

The technique
Client supine.

On the contracted side, palpate the psoas muscle in the abdomen. Bend the knee on the affected side and rotate the hip gently while compressing the muscle. Once there is good contact with the muscle, ask the client to raise the leg in the air, and slowly lower the leg to the couch, while maintaining a gentle but firm pressure on the muscle.

Palpate the muscle again to check for any release.

This may need to be repeated once or twice at weekly intervals for clients with chronic muscle contraction.

SPI correction technique
Benefits
This is a gentle technique to support the symphysis pubis to realign itself so is helpful in cases of PGD. It involves the mother and engages her in the work.

SPI check
The mother lies supine. She extends her opposite arm and leg and the therapist gently pushes down against their resistance. Repeat for both sides. If the limbs move easily this tends to indicate weakness in the pubic bone.

Re-check after doing this and there is often a marked change.

The technique (Fig. 11.6)
In the supine position the mother bends her legs so that her knees and feet are together on the table/floor. The therapist sits at the mother's feet and wraps their arms around the mother's knees, crossing the hands so that the fingers rest on the mother's adductors.

The therapist instructs the mother to push her pubic bone together without using the adductors.

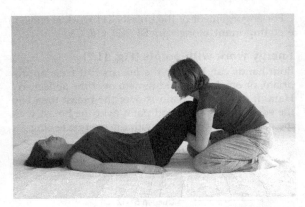

Fig. 11.6 Symphysis pubis laxity (SPL) support technique.

The therapist's hands on the adductors are initially there to ensure that the mother does not use the belly of the muscle – she has to use the pelvic attachments of the adductors only and the pelvic floor muscles. It is experienced as a subtle movement by the client.

It takes some explanation here and involvement of the client. Once the client understands the instructions, the therapist can give a little resistance with their fingers along the adductors.

Chest and breasts: practical techniques
Useful acupuncture points
ST 36 and SP 6 tonify Qi and Blood.

LV 8 nourishes Liver Blood.

GB 41 removes obstructions from the Breast Connecting Channels.

ST 12 influences the breast.

SI 1 is an empirical point for insufficient lactation.

BL 20 and 23 tonify Qi and Blood.

CV 17 tonifies Qi in the chest.

SP 4 and HC 6 regulate PV.

GB 34 and LV 3 move Qi.

LV 4 affects Liver.

GB 21 moves Liver Qi.

TH 3 moves Qi and removes obstructions from upper burner.

BL 51 moves Qi of Triple Burner in the breast region.

Important points directly on the breast
LV 14 – sixth intercostal space: LV channel has strong influence on breast area.

GB 24 – seventh intercostal space: harmonises middle burner, benefits GB and spreads Liver Qi.

ST 18 is a local point for the breast.

HC 1 – benefits the breast and often used for insufficient lactation.

KD 25 – second intercostal space; unbinds the chest and lowers rebellious ST and SP Qi.

SP 20 – also second intercostal space, 6 *cun* lateral to midline: regulates and descends Qi and unbinds chest.

Benefits
Working on the breasts, will help with postural concerns, and the mother to feel more at ease with the physical changes which occur to the breast tissue as well as their new role in feeding and bonding with her newborn. It may also be of benefit in helping to prevent mastitis.

Work with the Chong Mai (PV)
The Chong Mai has connecting channels which pass through the breast, as well as the main channel which passes over the breast tissue. When work is being done with the PV, although there are no specific points to follow, try to feel for where the connecting channels pass. It helps to keep the mother hand somewhere on the PV and with the working hand do some holding and connecting work on the pathways.

Local work on the breast
First make a connection with the breast. A potentially less threatening way, certainly initially, to do this is to connect with one hand on the Hara/abdomen and the other directly over the breast. This dual connection helps to establish the links between the breast and the abdomen. It can be done through the sheet if the mother is unsure and it can also be combined with some breathing work to help establish a sense of ease. Initially one hand could be placed over the sternum rather than the breast.

Rest the hand on the breast for a few breaths, feeling how much pressure to give. The breast tissue is sensitive and the pressure should never be strong; breasts respond better to light work. Do not work directly on the areola. Do not work if there is infection.

Work with direct strokes on the breast
Direct strokes over the breast can also be included. The strokes should not be too firm. If there are issues with milk being blocked in the ducts, then some light effleurage strokes can be done over the breast towards the nipple, to help promote the flow of milk and ease blockages. This is like a gentle 'milking' action towards the duct.

To support the flow of lymph then some light slow strokes can be done working towards the axilla. This is part of the lymph work (see pregnancy chapter). This means that before the lymph strokes are done then work first needs to have been done to stimulate the terminal lymph nodes (under the clavicle on each side), the neck and the axilla to stimulate the main drainage nodes for the breast. The lymph draining can include some gentle 'J' strokes or modified palmar kneading from the areola to the chest wall for blocked ducts.

For engorgement of the breasts TH work is considered important, along with ST, KD, GB, CV.

Energy work with points (Fig. 11.7)

Both hands can be over the breasts if it feels appropriate, or one hand could remain over the abdomen/Hara. If the mother hand is over the breast then cup the edge of the breast and palm over the breast with the other hand to connect with the energy, feeling for

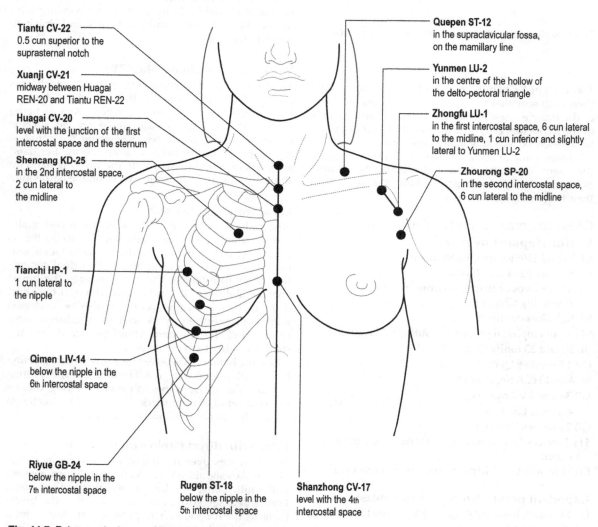

Tiantu CV-22
0.5 cun superior to the suprasternal notch

Xuanji CV-21
midway between Huagai REN-20 and Tiantu REN-22

Huagai CV-20
level with the junction of the first intercostal space and the sternum

Shencang KD-25
in the 2nd intercostal space, 2 cun lateral to the midline

Tianchi HP-1
1 cun lateral to the nipple

Qimen LIV-14
below the nipple in the 6th intercostal space

Riyue GB-24
below the nipple in the 7th intercostal space

Quepen ST-12
in the supraclavicular fossa, on the mamillary line

Yunmen LU-2
in the centre of the hollow of the delto-pectoral triangle

Zhongfu LU-1
in the first intercostal space, 6 cun lateral to the midline, 1 cun inferior and slightly lateral to Yunmen LU-2

Zhourong SP-20
in the second intercostal space, 6 cun lateral to the midline

Rugen ST-18
below the nipple in the 5th intercostal space

Shanzhong CV-17
level with the 4th intercostal space

Fig. 11.7 Points on the breast: ST, LV, SP, HT, HC meridians and points.

Kyo and Jitsu and also assessing the energy of the meridians passing through the breast:

- ST – passed in a vertical line directly through the breast.
- LV – the traditional branch goes to LV 14. In Zen shiatsu extended meridians, it continues up, to the outside of SP to third rib where it has two branches, the first going to the arm and the second going to the clavicle.
- SP – the traditional branch goes to SP 21. The Zen branch continues lateral to ST on the chest to the third intercostal space where one branch goes to the arm and the other up to neck.
- Zen HT – goes from the edge of the sternum following in the third intercostal space to the axilla.
- Heart Protector flows from the fifth intercostal space until it reaches the pectoralis when it flows into the arm.
- Lung is on the upper border of the breast tissue.

Any points which particularly draw attention can be worked on with a focus of balancing Kyo and Jitsu. Be aware also of areas/points below and above the breast and make appropriate meridian or muscle connections.

Work with the diaphragm and the lungs

Lung release technique

Benefits
Often there is congestion in this area due to feeding.

Technique
One hand cups under the diaphragm, the other hand goes under the clavicle with the middle finger resting over L1. As the client breathes in, the hand under the diaphragm gives a little resistance to expand the ribs; as the client breathes out, the finger puts a little pressure into L1.

Stronger diaphragm release
This can gradually be included, depending on the recovery of the mother. It is often done in the supine position.

First use some holding or stroking to warm and prepare the area. Encourage the client to breathe deeply. The thumbs are placed under the diaphragm on both sides, lateral to the xiphoid process. The rest of the hand cups where comfortable around the ribs. As the client breathes out they hook under. Repeat this a few times. Once the area has released slide the thumbs laterally and repeat the release.

Legs/feet

In the early postnatal period, the mother's legs are recovering from the effects of pregnancy and birth. If the mother used strong birth positions such as squatting

or standing the legs can be tired and tight or strained. If the mother had an epidural then they may even be slightly numb. Due to the cardiovascular and haematological changes, it is important to mobilise the legs to reduce the risk of potential thrombosis, especially after an instrumental delivery. The veins of the legs take about 6–8 weeks to return to tone due to blood and hormonal changes. The muscles will tend to be softer during the first few weeks while hormone levels rebalance – longer if the mother is breastfeeding – and due to the changes in the blood may be more sensitive than usual. It is important to elicit good feedback from the mother with stronger techniques.

As the baby gains weight then the mother's body will be working harder. It is important to encourage leg-strengthening work to support these demands. Stronger legs will give support to the lower back. If the lower back is weak then this often affects the hamstrings.

Types of techniques

It is important to do early mobilisations but without excessively abducting the legs in order to improve muscle tone, release tension and improve circulatory and lymphatic flow. The mother needs to be educated to use her legs rather than her back when lifting and carrying her baby. Stronger work with more mobilisations and postural awareness can begin as the pelvis begins to regain its strength. Ultimately all leg muscles can be worked.

Spleen energy work is beneficial to support building up of muscle tone, as well as supporting the mother/baby bond.

Breathing which exaggerates the pelvic floor relaxation on inhalation helps the venous return and lymph flow via the inguinal canals and internal iliac vessels (personal correspondence with Averille Morgan, 2005).

Positions

The mother can be in whatever position she finds comfortable for the leg work.

Cautions

Immediately after birth, it would be less suitable to do strong leg and hip mobilisations because of the relative weakness of the pelvic girdle. As the mother recovers from birth, this type of work can begin to be included once more.

Be aware of leg issues which may indicate thrombosis. The risk is highest in the first few days and greater after operative delivery and for women who do not mobilise. Be aware that thrombosis may be asymptomatic.

The same cautions therefore apply as in pregnancy:

- Woman needs to be referred to primary care provider immediately if suspected DVT (see pregnancy bodywork, Ch. 9).
- Homan's sign is often taught to bodyworkers, but is an unreliable test.
- If DVT is suspected, refer immediately so it can be checked with ultrasound.
- If DVT is diagnosed and the mother is taking blood-thinning drugs, the therapist can work once the mother has been given the medical diagnosis that the thrombosis has cleared. When working, it is important to be aware that one of the effects of blood-thinning drugs is to increase sensitivity to bruising which means that lighter work to the legs is indicated for these clients.
- Varicose veins may have developed during the pregnancy. They tend to improve with the postnatal blood alterations, but often remain. The therapist needs to be alert to this common reality and know how to work with it (refer pregnancy practical p. 264–267).

PGI support with leg work: quadriceps and hamstring strengthening

After having done symphysis pubis strengthening work, leg work is beneficial to support the pelvic girdle. Often the quadriceps muscles and adductors are weaker and the hamstrings and iliotibial band more contracted when there is a weak symphysis pubis. Work to all these muscles, both direct work and mobilisations and stretches, is potentially indicated. Flexing the knee of one or both (floor only) legs and drawing the knee into the chest (quads), internally rotating the hip to stretch the IT band with either one or both legs flexed, or resting the legs on the floor/table and stretching out the hamstrings, and the extended hamstring stretch can all be included. These stretches can help realign the supporting musculature.

Hands and arms

Typically, during the whole postnatal period, the arms are an area where the mother is likely to experience tension. During labour she may have been supporting herself or resting in awkward positions. In the early postnatal period she may be sleeping or lying awkwardly due to feeding or holding her baby. As time goes on most women find they are doing a lot more lifting and carrying than prior to having children. There may be a tendency for tendon issues in the wrist and forearm, including carpal tunnel and tenosynovitis, to develop through repetitive movements or wrist deviation caused by holding

and carrying the baby or the car seat, or through undertaking the many demanding household tasks. Continued tightness in the shoulders may contribute to conditions such as de Quervain's and thoracic outlet syndrome.

Techniques

Arm stretches and mobilisations are especially helpful in the postnatal period. Deeper physical work, due to the physical demands placed on the arms, is often required. Axilla decongestion via breathing and hand and arm pumping and lymphatic strokes will help draw the lymph towards the terminus nodes.

Cautions

- Be aware of carpal tunnel and thoracic outlet syndromes.
- Place the arm in comfortable positions which neutralise strain on the mother.

11.7 Working with scars

Many people have some kind of scar, whether it is minor injury, such as a broken wrist or ankle, or more severe, for example abdominal or back surgery. Scar tissue tends to block the flow of energy and the movement of fascia and muscle. It is important to address these blockages. The effects of a scar can be lifelong, especially the effects of a caesarean section scar.

During the maternity period the two most common scars which will be encountered are the horizontal scar in the lower abdomen due to a caesarean section and the vertical incision in the perineum due to an episiotomy. With clients who birthed their children 15 years or more ago then cases of the vertical incision caesarean section scar may be encountered.

Direct work can be done with the caesarean section scar once it has healed. Massage and shiatsu therapists would not work directly with an episiotomy scar, although indirect energy work can be included. Additionally self-care suggestions for clients can be given, or the client can be referred to an osteopath qualified in this type of work.

Work is different for scars which are still in the process of active healing than for scars which have healed. Although there are certain basic principles, it is important to remember that each mother is different in terms of how quickly she heals. This depends to some extent on the degree of trauma she has suffered and the skill of the person carrying out the suturing. If the scar becomes infected or is poorly sutured, it is going to take longer for it to heal.

Working with scars while they are still in the process of healing

As a general guideline, it will take approximately 6–8 weeks for an incision to heal. The main principle during this time of acute healing is to work with an energetic focus rather than doing physical work directly over the scar.

Work here includes:

- Holding the palm a short distance off the body over the scar or cupping the palm over the scar so no physical contact is made, while visualising the scar healing and approximately energetically the knitting together of tissue
- Working the areas or points superior, inferior or distal to the scar with the focus of allowing energy to flow.

Work to reduce oedema can also be done. This includes stimulation of the terminal nodes, light work in the inguinal nodes and work at the edges of the scar tissue. No work should be done which challenges the integrity of scar tissue in any way.

Working with older scars

After a scar has healed there are two common responses by women to how they relate to their scar: either they experience a feeling of numbness or a feeling of increased sensitivity.

There may be adhesions which can result in compensatory patterns of muscular and fascial tension and which can cause blockages in energy. Work which can be done to address these patterns includes:

- Working physically over the scar with techniques which gently break down adhesions in the tissue.
- Working energetically with points directly on the scar.
- Working superior and inferior to the scar, either with points to allow energy to flow, or working with the fascia and tissue around the scar.
- Lymphatic work.

Often the patterns may link in with pre-existing scar tissue patterns. Holding other scars at the same time as working on the caesarean section or episiotomy scar may release both energy and fascia.

The numbness can be associated with a scenario of empty energy and the sensitivity with a scenario of full energy. This means that energy work may be either tonifying or sedating.

Aftercare work can include suggestions of scar creams, such as vitamin E.

Fascial work, which includes energy work, can be beneficial.

With all work, follow with passive stretching of the scar and the surrounding tissue. This promotes the alignment of collagen fibres which are laid down as part of the healing process and also the development of more supple scar tissue which will allow for movement.

Working with scar tissue on the abdomen: caesarean section scar (Fig. 11.8)

The caesarean section incision involves complex suturing. There are many layers. The most superficial is the incision in the abdominal wall which cuts through the skin and muscle layers. The deeper incision then goes into the uterine wall itself. It is not just the most superficial scar which must be included in the work. Concerns have been raised recently (by Ina May Gaskin among others) of short-cuts being taken in the USA in suturing, as a result of the larger numbers of caesarean sections being carried out, which reduce the future integrity of the scar.

Effects of the caesarean section

The net effect of the caesarean section is to reduce the strength of the abdominal wall, which in turn affects the integrity of the body. A weak abdominal wall may link in with weakened lower back and pelvic girdle weakness. This may express as lower back or hip pain or restriction in movement.

Pain in the pelvic girdle is often referred to the hip flexors (psoas). The psoas has attachments to T12–L5 and pain and restriction can often be experienced here due to the psoas restriction as well as to its other attachments at the lesser trochanter of the femur and groin.

The deeper scar layers may affect deeper functioning of abdominal organs. It is not uncommon for

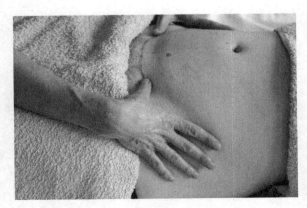

Fig. 11.8 Working with connecting with a recently healed caesarean section scar (6 weeks).

women to experience issues with digestion. Mothers also often experience increased period pains, fibroids and excessive menstrual bleeding due to the scarring of the uterus.

All the Yin meridians SP, LV, KD and CV and PV will have been affected energetically by the incision.

A caesarean section is often performed with epidural anaesthesia. This affects the GV as well as the spine itself.

Work to integrate the effect of a caesarean section

The mother will need to be assessed to see the effects on her individually, and appropriate work begun.

Working with perineal scar tissue

This is an area where most bodyworkers would not work directly. However, it is important to encourage the mother to do so. Pelvic floor exercises are important.

Work that can be done is to support the CV and GV meridians as previously described.

References and further reading

Clift-Matthews, V., 2007. Let Cinderella go to the ball. Br. J. Midwifery 15 (7), 396.

Davis-Floyd, R., 1992. Birth as an American Rite of Passage. University of California Press, Berkeley.

Fraser, L., Cullen, D., 2006. Postnatal management and breastfeeding. Curr. Obstet. Gynaecol. 16 (2), 65–71.

Kennell, J.H., Klaus, P.H., Klaus, M.H., 1993. Mothering the Mother: How a Doula Can Help You Have a Shorter, Easier, and Healthier Birth. Perseus Publishing, New York.

Priya, J.V., 1992. Birth Traditions and Modern Pregnancy Care. Element Books, Shaftsbury, Dorset.

CHAPTER **12**

Chapter contents

Learning outcomes

- Describe some relevant breathing and relaxation exercises
- Describe simple appropriate exercises
- Identify bodywork skills which the mother and her partner may use

Introduction

Aftercare/self-care is an important part of bodywork in the maternity period as there are so many changes, both physical and emotional, which can be supported. It is important for each therapist to establish what they are competent to teach and to know when to refer to another therapist or class.

Diet and nutrition form an important aspect of aftercare, but as the focus of this book is bodywork then there is no space to cover these here. We have chosen to focus primarily on tools which are in essence an extension of the bodywork which is done in the session, namely breathing, exercise (stretches) and simple bodywork techniques which can be easily taught to the mother and her partner. Often, though, in the safe space which is created, mothers may take the opportunity to explore their emotions and feelings. It is important to give them that space, while at the same time being aware that counselling is not part of the bodywork session. However, the client can be encouraged to talk, to identify additional sources of support

they may need, to consider keeping a journal, or to write down their feelings about what is going on.

Of course, some clients may not be interested in these suggestions and the therapist has to be sensitive as to how to address these issues. Often presenting self-care in the form of a relaxation position (e.g. 'relax over a ball') rather than an exercise ('let's do some all fours exercises') can be a useful way around this. Introducing simple exercises gradually and checking the client has understood them is also important.

The primary focus is to encourage women to listen to their body and their baby and to support the work of the bodywork session. If, at any point, the client is uncomfortable doing exercises then, depending on their level of expertise, the therapist needs to suggest alternatives or stop working with that exercise. However, do bear in mind that women's energy levels vary daily at this time. On different days they may be comfortable with different things.

It may be helpful to encourage partners to be involved in aftercare work and so suggestions are given on how to include them.

12.1 Benefits of aftercare

Pregnancy

Pregnancy, possibly more than any other time in one's life, is a time when changes are happening in the body on an almost daily basis. In order to support these changes, and to prevent them becoming 'problems' as much as possible, it is vital to guide clients to look after themselves properly during pregnancy. Especially in the third trimester, good self-care may help alleviate many of the minor discomforts as well as help prepare for birth.

Birth

Birth is an important milestone in the maternity journey. Due to sedentary habits and cultural fear around childbirth, most women need to be encouraged to prepare both emotionally and physically.

Postnatal

Recovering after birth and becoming fit is vital in order to support the family and the mother for the rest of her life.

12.2 Breathing and visualisation

Breathing is probably the most fundamental, and in a way the simplest, self-care exercise. It underlies all the others. It is important to include breathing with massage and exercise.

Benefits

General

- Gives a quiet focused time.
- Aids relaxation – for stress reduction and calming.
- Can be used as a tool with visualisations.
- Provides good oxygen supply to the baby and mother.
- It is a way of spending quality time with the partner.
- Is a helpful focus when exercising.

Birth

- Prepares the mother and partner for labour.
- It can provide a focus for the mother.
- It can allow the throat to open which will support the opening of the cervix.

Postnatal

- In the early days the mother often does not feel like exercising much; breathing can be done which helps focus on drawing in the abdominal exercises and pelvic floor.
- Breathing can help relax tight areas of the body, for example shoulders.
- Breathing can aid relaxation and bonding with baby and incorporating the huge changes.

What kind of breathing is most helpful?

The approach we prefer to teach is simple, the emphasis being on deep abdominal and diaphragmatic breathing. In yoga there is more of an emphasis on abdominal breathing and in pilates on diaphragmatic breathing. Both are important. Breathing can be taught while teaching exercises or can be done while the mother is lying down to receive bodywork. It can be a good way to start or finish the bodywork session. Another time to work with the breathing is during a partner session. The mother and partner can be encouraged to become more aware of their own and each other's breathing.

Encourage the mother to focus on her out-breath and to find her own deep breathing pattern with which she is comfortable. Emphasise a long, slow out-breath, pausing until she needs to breathe in again, and then a long slow in-breath. Ideally, as the mother breathes in, her abdominal muscles should contract. However, often people breathe the 'wrong way'.

It is of benefit to continue this during labour and to continue into the postnatal period so that the mother is not having to learn new techniques but building on a fundamental skill.

Labour

Association techniques and simple techniques which help the mother connect with her own breathing are more helpful rather than the dissociation techniques which were more popular in the past.

It is important for the partner to practice as well as the mother and can be a useful tool to help the mother and the partner connect with each other.

Basic deep breathing for mothers and partners

Once the couple are in a comfortable position, with eyes closed or open, encourage them to first observe their breathing without altering it any way. Encourage them to notice the length of the in- and out-breaths and any pauses or holding between the breaths, how deep they are breathing, and if they breathe through the mouth or the nose.

Then encourage them to deepen each out-breath and find their own rhythm of breathing. It can be helpful to place the hands on the lower abdomen, below the navel, while doing this and feel the muscles gently drawing the hands in on the out-breath and pushing the hands gently away on the in-breath.

Visualisation

Various images can be added to the basic deep breathing. It is important to be sensitive to each client's needs. Some mothers like the images to be quite firmly based in reality, such as images of the particular stage of development their baby is at in the womb. Other mothers may want to connect with how their baby might be feeling, with different types of energy or sensation, colour or light. Some suggestions are given below.

Pregnancy

Connecting with the baby

From the deep state of relaxation and focus on the out-breath, they can visualise their baby in their womb at its different developmental stages.

First trimester Some women may not want to connect with their baby, due to the high rate of miscarriage.

Others love to tune into what is happening. These visualisations can also be useful when working with fertility clients.

They can visualise the egg travelling down the fallopian tube into the womb and finding a place to implant on the wall of the uterus and then starting to form into the baby's body, the amniotic sac and the placenta.

Talk the woman through the main changes, such as the development of the primitive spine, digestive system, mouth, anus. Visualise the heart beating and all the other organs developing, limb buds growing into legs and arms. Imagine the baby moving, even though the movements cannot be felt, the baby swallowing amniotic fluid and at around week 8 becoming aware of touch.

Second trimester The woman is more aware of the movements of the baby. They might feel them as a tiny flutter, like a butterfly, or like a paint brush brushing gently against the inside of the womb.

They can be encouraged to be aware of the space around their baby, the baby hiccupping, contractions, the water surrounding the baby, the baby swallowing amniotic fluid, the baby growing and becoming more aware of the space around them.

They can be aware of how their baby gradually becomes aware of sounds outside the womb. Talking and singing can become more relevant now.

They can be aware of how the placenta is nourishing the baby.

Third trimester/pre-labour This can focus on visualising the baby being in a good position for labour or readying the baby for birth.

The client can be encouraged to be aware of the position of their baby. Do they know where their baby's spine is? Can they sense his/her arms and legs?

If their baby is in a good position, head down and back around the front, they can visualise their baby's head gradually going deeper down into the pelvis, as s/he engages in preparation for birth. They can become aware how their baby's time in their womb is gradually coming to an end and allow themselves to feel comfortable with the thought of letting their baby be born and moving out into the world.

If their baby is not in such a good position, head away from their pelvis or back against their back, they can visualise how their baby might be able to get into a better position. They can be encouraged to talk to the baby about why they feel comfortable in the position they are in and how, if they move, it will be easier for their journey out of their mother's body.

Preparing for birth

The client can be encouraged to explore fears, hopes and expectations in a safe, relaxing space.

Breathing and relaxing while moving

This is an important skill to have during labour. It is also a useful to skill at any time but especially during the postnatal period when the mother may not have much time for herself. While she is holding the baby she can focus on her deep out-breath and relaxing her body.

It can be helpful for the mother and partner to try practicing this in different positions – for example all fours, sitting, standing, lying next to each other. In each position they can notice the pattern of breathing, how comfortable they are and how their baby is.

Encourage the mother to practice breathing deeply while breastfeeding.

Breathing for labour: first stage breathing

During first stage, the woman may find that all she needs to do is simply to focus on the movement of the breath, to breathe out slowly and deeply and allow the in-breath to come into her body. As the contractions get stronger and more intense, she can continue to focus on the breath, especially the out-breath. Simply by doing this, she may find a rhythm which supports first stage. If that is all she needs to do, then she does not have to feel that she has to do anything else.

Some women find that they like to use the out-breath as a focus. It can be used to:

- Help relax any tense parts of the body.
- Open up the hands or feet.
- Make open throat sounds or simply open and relax the jaw and throat.

Exploring images for first stage

Some women like to have words or images to focus on.

The wave

The wave is often an image which mothers tune in to instinctively in labour because it links into the energy of Water. The wave allows mothers to contact the Yang, dynamic, moving aspects of Water. The mother can visualise the rise and fall of a wave flowing through her body and opening up the cervix. The wave can be used as a focus for each contraction, building slowly, reaching a peak and then fading away.

The cervix opening up, like a flower

Some women find it helpful to visualise the cervix opening and thinning as the contraction gets intense. They may say the words, 'opening up, thinning out' as they breathe out during the contraction.

Some women find they like to visualise the cervix like a flower opening up, the petals of the flower unfurling as the power of the contraction builds.

Surrender

Some women like to say words with each contraction, such as 'surrender' as they allow their body to relax and open up.

Transition breathing

The most important thing during transition is for the woman to keep listening to her breathing and not give up. If transition is very intense, she will probably need to focus with more intensity on her breathing. It is usually best not to change what she has been doing up to that point, if it has been working for her. However, if it is not working, then she may want to try something different.

On the other hand, transition may simply be a time when the woman needs to rest and focus on her breathing in a calm way.

Second stage breathing

It is still important to focus on the out-breath, but it has a little more power about it. As the woman breathes out there is a sense of strength behind the breath, which is helping her to focus her attention down to the pelvis, cervix and perineum and help ease or push her baby out into the world. She still needs to stay relaxed as she breathes out. Often women feel that they are pushing/bearing down, but they are tensing their jaw, neck and shoulders and holding the breath in their throat. As the woman breathes, she still needs to use the open throat sounds (aaah), allowing the jaw to open and relax. As she does this, she can focus the attention of the breath down to the perineum and feel that she is using the breath to push her baby out.

Exploring images for second stage

The kind of images which may help in this stage are:

- Imagining the baby coming down the birth canal and moving out into the world.
- Visualising the perineum opening and stretching.

Some women find it helpful to physically hold on to a rope which is hanging from the ceiling. As they hold on with their hands, they imagine feeling the strength and power of the rope moving down into their body.

Postnatal

It is helpful to talk the mother through remembering to continue to use breathing she may have practised during pregnancy and birth. It can be beneficial to remind her of the breathing she did with awareness of her baby and encourage her to continue to do this. She can focus on relaxed breathing while she is feeding her baby, or resting. She can be aware of her newborn's breath.

Deep breathing

After any kind of birth, deep abdominal breathing will help venous return as well as loosen any secretions in the chest. The mother can begin this as soon as possible after birth. She can simply sit and hold her hands over her abdomen, breathing deeply.

Huffing breathing

A huffing cough is beneficial to release any mucous which may have built up during the birth or in the early postnatal period. Huffing is an outward breath forcefully using the diaphragm to expel air from the lungs, pulling in rather than pushing out the abdominal wall. Since the diaphragm is moving up in the chest, and the abdominal muscles are shortening but not tensing, pressure is decreased in the abdominal cavity. These means that if there is an incision it is not under any strain. The huffing needs to be done quickly so that some force is generated to dislodge mucus. It is rather like saying 'ha' but briskly and with force from the abdominal muscles. The mouth is opened wide and the jaw relaxed. Any expectorate which is generated needs to be spat into a tissue or paper cup. For women with an incision, as a comfort measure, they can support the incision area with their hands or with a pillow. However, be reassured, the stitches will not pop out.

Huffing is an ideal way of clearing the chest at any time of life. It can be especially useful in pregnancy, as coughing strains the abdominal wall and pelvic floor whereas huffing helps strengthen them (Noble 1982: 155).

Breathing to draw the abdominal muscles together

Breathing can be done to support the rehabilitation of the abdominal muscles. Initially the breathing is to focus on shortening them vertically and then to draw them together horizontally. Breathing is also vital for working with pelvic floor exercises.

Making sounds with the breath

This can be useful at different times:

- In pregnancy some women like to sing to their baby.
- Some women like to make lots of sounds with the breath during their labour, others are quieter and tend to go inside themselves.
- Postnatally the mother can continue some of the songs she has sung during her pregnancy. These often help to calm the baby.

- Open throat sounds are especially useful for relaxing the jaw and can be used during labour. The woman can be encouraged to open her mouth and relax her jaw while making an 'aah' sound. This may help some women breathe more deeply. They may also feel a connection between the jaw and the cervix/perineum. By letting go of the jaw, the perineum relaxes.

Ba ba, pa pa, maaa

There is a Sanskrit mantra which many women find helpful. It uses the sounds

Baaa baaa
Paaa paaa
Maaaaa.

It is interesting that these are the basic sounds that Hindus said that babies make in the womb. In most cultures they form the root of the words for:

Ba ba: Baby
Pa pa: Father
Ma ma: Mother.

The client can be encouraged to repeat these sounds in whatever way she wants. They can be said or sung. The woman can experiment with different tones, longer or shorter, higher or lower, feeling the vibration of the sound in her body and her baby's response.

12.3 Exercise

Benefits of exercise

- To promote body awareness.
- To promote relaxation and well-being during pregnancy and the postpartum.
- To alleviate aches and pains, such as backache and shoulder tension.
- To prepare the mother, baby and partner for the physical demands of birth.
- To help with postnatal recovery. Whatever kind of birth the mother may have, whether natural or caesarean section, if she has prepared antenatally, she will recover better.

Exercises

There has long been controversy over the amount of exercise that pregnant women can do. ACOG guidelines (ACOG 2002), which are generally considered relatively conservative and safe, suggest moderate exercise in pregnancy is of benefit and may even help prevent miscarriage.

Several postpartum concerns are addressed. They note that there are no known complications of return to training. Although rapid resumption has not demonstrated adverse effects, a gradual return to activity is advised. Moderate weight reduction while nursing does not compromise neonatal weight gain and exercise has been associated with decreased incidence of postpartum depression – but only if the exercise is not stress provoking (ACOG 2002).

Pregnancy

As soon as the woman knows she is pregnant, encourage her to begin with some level of exercise. Of course the amount depends on how tired or not she is, and on her level of fitness before she was pregnant. The key in all exercise is to encourage the client to listen to her body. She will find some days she can do more and others less. An important area to focus on is building strength in the pelvis.

It is best to suggest moderate levels of aerobic activity, rather than high intensity. Step classes are not a good idea, especially as they also include ballistic movement.

In terms of walking, swimming or cycling, encourage the woman to pay attention to her body and check that none of these aggravate any conditions she may have. If she suffers from symphysis pubis problems, then she may have to wear a support belt to help with walking. She will probably have to give up swimming and will not be able to ride a bike.

There are myths around breaststroke: many women are advised as a blanket guideline not to do it while they are pregnant. It is true that it may aggravate problems in the neck and lower back, and it is certainly not advisable if the client has SPI. However, if the woman feels that this is the best stroke for her and she does not suffer from any adverse effects afterwards, then she can be encouraged to carry on for as long as she feels comfortable. It is usually advisable to aim to do a mix of strokes if possible, rather than many lengths of one stroke, especially breaststroke.

It can be useful to suggest that the client attend specific pregnancy exercise classes, such as yoga or aqua-natal. It is wise, if suggesting classes, to visit and see which ones seem good. As with any profession, some people are better teachers than others. The type of questions which can give an idea of the teacher's expertise are:

- What sort of exercise modifications do they offer if the client has symphysis pubis instability?
- What kind of abdominal and pelvic floor work do they do?

- How do they include the baby, especially in terms of supporting good fetal positioning?
- What exercises do they include on preparing for birth?

It can be helpful to suggest that the partner is involved with exercise: that way they can help motivate the woman.

For specific trimester considerations refer to the pregnancy trimester summaries (p. 228–235).

Postnatally

It depends on the type of birth that the woman has and her recovery. Encourage the client to begin with gentle exercises as soon as possible after birth and gradually build up to stronger ones. Many women find it hard to make time, and need to be encouraged to see exercise as an activity that can be done while doing other things, for example while sitting with their baby or brushing their teeth.

The main focus of early postnatal work is to promote perineal healing, prevent thrombosis, support abdominal healing and breastfeeding as appropriate (relax neck and shoulders). Pelvic ligaments are still lax and abdominal muscles and pelvic floor recovering, so it is important not to do any strenuous exercises for the first few weeks and certainly to avoid lifting. Encourage the client to get her housework done by someone else.

As the baby gets a little older they may want to go to a postnatal mother and baby class. It is helpful to have information about local classes available for clients.

Teaching exercises

The therapist must only teach exercises they are qualified to show. With all the exercises ensure that the client does not experience discomfort and modify the exercises appropriately.

Many types of exercise can be shown to the client. Here we outline a few exercises which are of particular relevance in the maternity period:

- Postural awareness.
- Abdominal and pelvic floor.
- Exercising with a partner.
- Integrating exercise into daily activity.

Postural awareness exercises

Good posture is fundamental to good health in pregnancy and supporting health postnatally. It may help alleviate many of the so-called 'minor ailments' of pregnancy, aid postnatal recovery and support long-term health patterns. The type of conditions which may be helped range from back ache, including sciatica and shoulder tension, indigestion and heartburn, rib flare and carpal tunnel syndrome, and puffy legs and arms. Postural awareness may be introduced at any time the client is comfortable.

Pelvic tilting

Pelvic tilting is the key to good posture. Encourage the woman to focus on tucking her pelvis under, as though she is drawing the bottom of her back, the sacrum and tail bone down to the ground.

This is the starting point for all the other exercises, because without a good basic posture none of the other exercises are going to be as effective.

Standing

Encourage the client to be aware of their breathing. They can then check their pelvic tilt. Get the woman to breathe out and gently tilt the pelvis so that the lower back flattens out. Encourage the client to feel the work that is happening in the abdominal muscles as they shorten slightly to allow the back to flatten. Make sure that they are not tightening their buttocks. They can also focus on drawing up the pelvic floor as well.

Encourage them to notice that as they move the pelvis, the spine begins to lengthen and this helps to relax out the shoulders. They may also find shifts in the weight and relaxation of the legs and feet.

In pregnancy they can imagine that the pelvis is like a basin in which they need to keep their baby nicely supported. Postnatally they can continue tilting with or without their baby. If they are holding their baby encourage them to try different positions while tilting the pelvis: holding on the front of the abdomen, holding on one hip and then on the other. It is helpful to encourage women to notice if they have a habit of holding their baby only on hip, which they often do. This is a cause of postnatal structural issues. It usually feels slightly odd for the mother to hold the baby on the opposite hip, but it is important to encourage them to do so.

The client can be encouraged to do pelvic tilting exercise every day and incorporate it into daily activities. It can be done while waiting for a bus, or the kettle to boil, sitting on a chair or a ball. Postnatally the mother can be encouraged to be aware of her posture while feeding.

All fours (Fig. 12.1)

Awareness of the tilt of the pelvis can also be included in the all fours positions. This is useful from the second trimester and after a few weeks postnatally. It can be a great one to do with baby underneath after a couple of weeks (see Fig. 12.1). All fours awareness can be simply resting over a ball or cushions, every day for at least 10 minutes, if possible, during pregnancy. If the wrists feel uncomfortable or the client

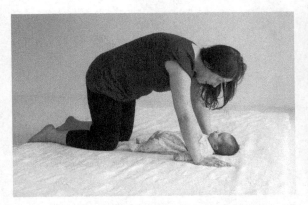

Fig. 12.1 All fours with baby underneath; cat stretch.

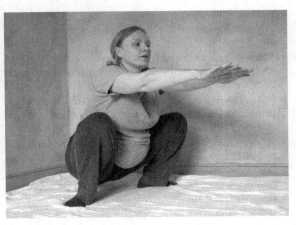

Fig. 12.2 Squatting.

has carpal tunnel syndrome then she will need to do it this way.

The woman can also be encouraged to do the yoga cat exercise, or rocking forward and backwards. There are many other exercises which can be done in this position, including crawling.

Squatting (Fig. 12.2)

This is another exercise/position which is potentially beneficial for posture. In many traditional cultures women would squat for many daily activities. In modern culture, in some circles, squatting is considered controversial. It is true that for many women it may presents a challenge and there are some situations when it should not be done, such as:

• Varicose veins
• Breech baby
• Low-lying placenta
• SPL
• Vaginal bleeding
• Knee and ankle problems.

However, for a client with none of the above issues who is comfortable in the squat it offers key postural benefits of strengthening the pelvis and legs. Encourage the client to find a version of the squat with which she is comfortable. She may need the support of books under her heels or need to hold on to a door handle. Once in the squat she can be encouraged to move. She can rock or be encouraged to stand and then go down into the squat and vice versa. As it is good for strengthening the legs, it can be beneficial to suggest a modified version for the client with SPL. This can be done by standing with legs together against a wall, supported by a ball. The client can then lean against the ball and try going down and up again as far as she is comfortable and stable.

Abdominal exercises

These are important in order to give support to the pelvis. Simply doing pelvic tilting and being on all fours help to strengthen the abdominal muscles. Breathing out deeply in any position while focusing on drawing up the pelvic floor and drawing in the abdominal muscles is also helpful. Traditional abdominal work may not be suitable during pregnancy as the woman may be unable to lie on her back. However, during the first trimester, it is worth encouraging clients to continue with supine abdominal work if they have been doing it prior to pregnancy. There are some myths about overly exercising the abdominal muscles; however, appropriate exercise is vital to support them. The issue is more that often abdominal exercises are done incorrectly. It is important for the therapist to be aware of some of the basic principles of abdominal work, even if they do not specialise in exercise. It is important to check the separation of the rectus abdominis muscles as this will determine which exercises the client can do. If the muscles are more than two fingers apart then she should not do any curl ups. The check for recti muscle separation is in assessment (p. 197).

Basic principles of abdominal work

• Exercise needs to be done with engaging the muscles on the out-breath so that the abdominal muscles draw in.
• It is important to engage the pelvic floor at the same time by lifting up from the perineum as the abdominals contract.
• It is important not to hold, block or force the breath.

- Relax while exercising the muscles; it is important not to strain and not to do more than is comfortable.
- The movements need to be done smoothly, slowly and working with the body. Movements should not be forced or jerky.
- In supine work, have the legs bent. This allows the lumbar spine to lengthen and aids the focus on drawing up the pelvic floor muscles.
- Allow the back to lengthen. The vertebrae should not be compressed. The shoulders and hips should not be brought together.
- Exercises working with the abdominal muscles involve small subtle movements. Bigger movements tend to engage the hip flexors.

Level 1 – easy: abdominal breathing

In any position work with abdominal breathing and drawing in the muscles. Focus especially on CV 4 and points in the lower Hara.

Level 2 onwards – fairly easy: lying supine or side, pelvic tilting

In supine, feet must be placed in front of the buttocks so that the knees are bent. This allows the lower back to relax. It is important then to focus on gently making contact with the lower back and the floor, without straining. Allow the ribs to feel relaxed and soft. Engage the pelvic floor muscles as well by drawing them up. Tilting the pelvis can also be done in the side and it is important to work in both sides. This is the first stage of engaging the abdominal, especially the lower, muscles.

Level 3: exercise for separated rectus abdominis muscles (Fig. 12.3)

Part 1

This needs to be done supine. Breathing out, gently and slowly curl the head, but not the shoulders, away from the ground. At the same time, have the hands crossed around the navel area and draw the hands together, while allowing the breath to draw in the abdominal muscles. It can be helpful to picture the recti muscles being drawn together. Try to feel the lateral border of the recti muscles with the fingers and draw to the midline from here. With the in-breath, release the hands and curl back down. This can be repeated as many times as is comfortable. It probably will not be more than 15 repetitions but may be as few as 5–10. Encourage the client to keep the neck as relaxed as possible.

Part 2

Lying supine, keeping the lower back in contact with the ground, breathing out, slowly slide one foot

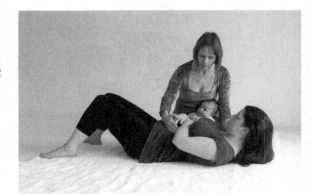

Fig. 12.3 Corrective exercise.

along the ground so the leg comes towards the fully extended position. Only extend as much as possible, keeping the lower back pushed into the ground. If the lower back starts to lift away, do not lower the leg any more. On the in-breath draw the leg back to its starting position. Repeat with the other leg. Repeat as many times without straining, up to 15 times each side.

Level 4 – harder levels for non-separated recti muscles

Part 1: the upper abdomen

Lying supine, breathing out, slowly and gently curl up and forwards as far as is comfortable, just using the abdominal muscles. On the in-breath, curl back down again. To engage the transverse muscles repeat curling to the left and down and then to the right and down. Repeat as many times as is comfortable, up to 15 of each.

Progressions:

- The easiest version of this is with the arms crossed across the chest.
- The less easy version is with the arms extended reaching forwards.
- The hardest version is with the hands behind the head (but be careful not to have them pulling on the neck).

These can be done postnatally with the baby sat on the mother's abdomen (Fig. 12.4).

Part 2: the lower abdomen

Begin by bringing the knees into the chest, so that the knee is at 90° to the hip and the knee is at 90° to the ankle. Slowly lower one knee down, breathing out, keeping the 90° between knee and ankle and keeping the lower back pushed into the ground. Stop just before the foot touches the ground. Breathe in

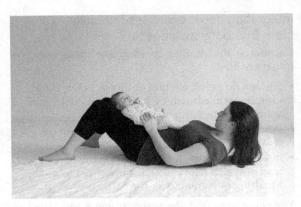

Fig. 12.4 Abdominal curl up with baby.

and rest. On the next out-breath slowly bring the leg back to the starting position, keeping the lower back pushed in to the ground.

Repeat as many times as comfortable, up to 15 times.

Journal of abdominal exercises

Encourage women to keep a journal of the different exercises they do. How do they feel doing them? At what point do muscles separate? How quickly does the abdomen recover postnatally? It is important to encourage an awareness of the importance of the abdomen for the rest of the woman's life.

Pelvic floor exercises

Most women are aware that they need to do some pelvic floor exercises – however, many women do not actually do them.

Squatting is key to pelvic floor strength. The pelvic floor assumes support and has to work in this position. If squatting is not practised then the skeletal muscles do not develop, causing the smooth muscles to thin out in an effort to support the pelvic floor. As not many women squat much in modern life, the pelvic floor is often weak.

In day-to-day activities and exercises women often do not pay attention to the pelvic floor and the muscles do not get worked. However, they can be exercised at any time, for example while doing other exercises. Different positions place different work loads on the muscles: lying down is the easiest and squatting is the hardest. Encourage the client to do pelvic floor exercises in different positions. They can do them while they are waiting for the kettle to boil, at red traffic lights, each time they open the fridge door, or at any time.

It is easy to substitute other muscles like the buttocks and thighs. To prevent this, encourage the client to exercise in positions where the legs are abducted.

The exercise most people know for the pelvic floor is to contract the outer layers. In fact, it is important to work up into the deeper layers of the pelvic diaphragm. However, if the client is not used to doing the exercises, or immediately after birth, she can begin with the outer layer and, over a week or two, gradually build up to the deeper layers.

Sometimes women have been told that they should try doing this exercise when they are actually urinating. This is not a good idea, as it may tend to push the urine back inside the bladder and potentially cause kidney and bladder problems. Some women like to do this to check that they are exercising the muscles and in this case, it is important not to do it on a full bladder (i.e. not first thing in the morning) and wait until the bladder is almost emptied, so that there is less pressure to force urine back up. It probably will not cause problems if just done once or twice but it is important not to use that as the exercise.

A better way to check is to get the client to practice at home by putting their fingers inside the vagina. This could even be combined with doing perineal massage. The woman's partner could also help check, even while having sex.

With all the pelvic floor exercises, it is helpful to tighten the muscles on the out-breath. This helps surrounding muscles to relax and for the focus to be on the layer of pelvic floor muscles which are being worked. It is helpful to work with the contraction of the abdomen as the two muscle groups work together.

When exercising the pelvic floor the muscles should only be contracted for a short while (10 seconds is long enough) and not repeated more than two or three times in one go. Allow 10 minutes before exercising them again. The pelvic floor consists of fast-twitch muscles which tire easily. Holding for longer only causes the muscles to tire and go into spasm, rather than increasing endurance.

To do all three levels in one go is sufficient. If only level one is being done, then this can be repeated a few more times. If just doing levels 1 and 2 then repeat each a few times.

Pelvic floor exercises can be done within the first 24 hours after birth, but gently. They help move Blood and can help prevent infection as well as strengthening the muscles.

Level 1: the outer layer – the perineum

This focuses on the outer layer of the pelvic floor, the perineum, which forms a figure of eight around the vagina, urethra and anus.

It is done on a slow out-breath; the muscles around the vagina are tightened, and then released slowly two or three times. The muscles are relaxed on the in-breath. This is repeated once or twice. It can be repeated with a focus of tightening and releasing around the anus; especially good for piles. This works the slow-twitch fibres.

It can be repeated with tightening and releasing as fast as possible on the out-breath.

Level 2: the middle layer

Once the client is used to working the outer layer, they can try drawing up a little bit higher. This can be done in any position, but a good way to start is to sit with legs apart or extended.

Starting either around the vagina or the anus, tighten the muscles gradually on the out-breath. If working with focusing on the anus, extend the awareness behind to exercise the coccygeal muscle.

Imagine that the muscles are being tightened in levels, e.g. going up one floor in a lift at a time. For example, on the out-breath, tighten around the vagina and, continuing to breathe out, gradually tighten as though going up from the first floor, continuing to breathe out, a little higher to the second floor, continuing to breathe out, a little higher to the third floor and if possible, going higher to the fourth floor. Try to hold the muscles drawn up as much as possible. If they fade a little, try to draw them up a little more; keep holding as much as possible until the need to breathe in. Then on the in-breath, gradually release back down to the third floor, gradually back down to the second, gradually back down to the first floor and the ground floor.

This is usually done only once as it is quite a strong exercise.

Level 3: the deepest layer – reaching up to around the public bone

This continues from the previous exercise, level 2.

From the highest point of the lift, while breathing out, draw the muscles up as high possible towards the pubic bone. On the in-breath gradually release to the starting point.

Again it may be helpful for the woman to record her pelvic floor exercises and note changes in the pelvic floor during pregnancy and post delivery.

Partner exercises

Exercising together can be useful, relaxing and fun. Encourage the mother to practise exercises with her partner and do some partner exercises such as the standing squat, full squat, all fours leaning together. This is a useful way to practice birth positions together.

Integrating pelvic exercises into daily life – true body awareness

Encourage the mother to integrate these exercises into daily life:

- She can do pelvic circling or tilts or pelvic floor exercises while brushing her teeth, or cooking or waiting for the kettle to boil.
- When she bends to pick things up, she can go down into the squat.
- Instead of always sitting to chat on the phone, read or watch television, encourage her to do this squatting or leaning over the ball.

The client may find she wants to get a little stool to use for squatting.

Postnatally she can include the baby in the exercises. An example is the following:

Back/leg sitting BL/KD stretch

Benefits
- An excellent exercise for women with SPL as it is strengthening the energy of the midline of the body and places no pressure on the symphysis pubis.
- It is good for strengthening the back.
- It stretches out the legs and can be good for cramp and oedema.
- It supports the Kidney and Bladder meridian energy.

Cautions

If the client cannot touch her toes easily in pregnancy, she will need to use a dynaband or belt around her feet in order to experience the stretch in the back without rounding it.

Exercise

Sit on the ischial tuberosities and have the spine extended. Extend the legs so that they are straight and together. Slightly dorsiflex the toes to lengthen the back of the leg. Some ankle circling can be included. If the client has oedema, she could rest her knees over some cushions to slightly elevate the legs.

This is also an excellent exercise to do with a newborn (Fig. 12.5).

Exercising for women with symphysis pubis issues

While it is important not to do exercise which aggravates the condition – essentially avoiding abduction, balancing and strong involvement of gravity – women still need to exercise. Work on all fours, such as the cat, is excellent.

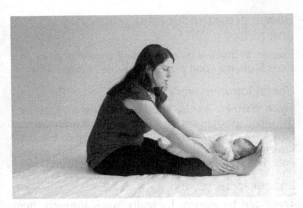

Fig. 12.5 BL/KD with baby.

12.4 Touch, including shiatsu and massage techniques

Introduction

There are many simple massage techniques which the partner can learn to use with the mother. The benefit of showing these are that massage is a way for the partner to become involved and sometimes the mother may need daily massages, for specific issues such as oedema, backache or breast issues.

These techniques can be built on from the basic deep breathing. The partner can be taught to listen to the mother's breathing and then begin to work with simple pressures on the abdomen, connecting with the baby during pregnancy or labour. This can then be extended to touching the back and introducing sacral pressures and the sacral points, from the second trimester. The partner's position in all of the suggested massage techniques is important, and so this can be incorporated into partner exercise. Emphasise to the partner the importance of good body posture and relaxation. A typical mistake is for the partner to tense the shoulders rather than lean their body weight in a relaxed manner.

Techniques for the first trimester

Often in the first trimester, the woman may feel quite sensitive and vulnerable. She may or may not want to be touched. Techniques can be done without the use of oil, so that if the woman does not want to get undressed, she can remain clothed.

The partner might also be anxious about doing bodywork, especially if there has been a history of miscarriage. However, if both woman and partner are open then some simple holds may be introduced.

Kidney/Uterus – baby breath

The woman and partner can sit close together and breathe together. The partner can place their hands over the woman's abdomen and feel her breathing and the movement of the abdomen.

Face/sinus/neck/shoulders

Women in the first trimester often suffer from headaches, sinus congestion and shoulder tension. It is helpful to teach a simple sequence addressing these concerns. The woman could be lying supine or sitting and the partner can learn simply cupping the skull. The partner could use oil or no oil. Encourage the partner to find a comfortable position and then show them some simple facial work.

The partner could also be shown:

- Conception Vessel and Heart Protector for nausea; palm or side palm pressures.
- Working ST 36 for nausea: holding with the thumb.

Techniques for the second and third trimesters

This can be a more exciting time to work with the woman, as the partner can start to feel the baby. The client may be a lot happier with being touched and she may or may not want to be massaged with oil.

Teach the partner to do some of the work in the side position.

As the woman advances more into the third trimester, then work can be done with more of a focus on preparing for birth and incorporating the forward leaning and all fours positions.

Massaging the woman's abdomen and baby in the womb

Once the woman can feel the baby move, she usually instinctively rubs her own abdomen. It is lovely for the partner to become involved with this from early on. This technique can be done with or without oil, depending on the woman's preference.

Abdominal pressures

When the partner feels relaxed s/he can begin to follow the woman's breathing and gradually build up to abdominal pressures. Often the partner is slightly anxious and needs to be encouraged to make a sufficiently deep contact.

This work can be taught with the woman in different positions such as sitting or forward leaning. This can also be useful for teaching for labour work.

Simple lymph sequence

Since work for oedema ideally needs to be done every day, it can be helpful to show the partner how to do this. Ensure that the partner does not do this if there is any possibility that the mother may have pre-eclampsia.

Simple work is often effective. Begin by showing the partner how to use light pressures on both terminal nodes under the clavicles for a minute or so and then how to do some light slow stroking along the back and side of the neck. S/he can then be shown some simple lymphatic stroking along the limb, with an emphasis on direction, pressure and slowness.

Backache routine

It can be helpful to teach the partner a simple routine for working the back in the side position. This can be useful not only in pregnancy and birth but the partner can be encouraged to continue caring for the mother in the postnatal period, especially if she is having difficulties feeding her baby. She could lie with the baby and the partner could massage her back.

Teach some simple effleurage strokes each side of the spine and how to do some kneading in tighter areas. Pressures each side of the spine can also be shown.

Over the years I have run a variety of birth preparation sessions for partners ranging from one day workshops, to evening classes and individual sessions. What I teach depends on the amount of time I have to teach it, and the starting point of skill for the partner. If the partner has never done any kind of massage at all before, then it will probably take a couple of hours simply to teach the sacral work well. If they have done some work before and are comfortable in their body, then they can be taught more.

It is important to practice massage techniques in different birthing positions. Practising birth positions can be used as a warm up before beginning the massage techniques. These can also be incorporated with the breathing techniques and I often start the massage with some of the abdominal breathing and the simple abdominal holds. I use this as an opportunity to get the woman and partner connected both with each other and with their baby.

I then usually teach the sacral work in the all fours position, linking it in with some of the abdominal holds.

What I teach of the rest of the work depends then on how the woman and partner get on with all of that. I try to teach some of the labour focus points if I can, showing them on the partner if the mother is before 37 weeks.

An ideal time for teaching is some time in the third trimester, not far enough away from the birth to forget but not so close that there is no time to practice.

Suzanne

Sacral pressure for later pregnancy and birth

Prepare to practise by establishing a good position. All fours is often a good position in which to teach this.

Sacral foramen work

Teach partners to use thumb pressure directly into the sacral grooves and to feel how much pressure and how long to stay. They can also be taught to use their knuckles. Unless they have prior bodywork experience, it is usually best not to teach elbow leaning.

Labour focus points

These can be shown. I usually work through them all and then show the ones which have had the most response.

Perineal massage

This is something that is not for everyone, but if the woman can do it, preparing the perineum for labour will help prepare it for the huge amount of stretching it has to do. It may also help the woman feel more connected and hopefully less afraid of what is going to happen, especially if it is her first labour or if she tore badly in a previous labour. It is a good idea to involve the partner with the massage, as part of their preparation. If either partner does not feel comfortable about it then it may be helpful to explore why. With a first labour, many women find the stretching of the perineum at the birth of the baby the most 'painful' time of labour. It can be experienced as a strong burning sensation.

(With thanks to Alice Lyon, midwife, for first writing out some class notes for me in 1991 and to Penny Simkin, to whose work she referred.)

Explain and locate the perineum

Firstly explain to the client where the perineum is and how it is going to stretch as the baby's head crowns. Then explain simply what she needs to do, using diagrams if necessary. It can be useful to create a handout for this so she can take it away and think about it before practising it in the privacy of her home.

The exercise

It can be done from about 32–34 weeks. The partner can be encouraged to do it.

Encourage the woman not to be embarrassed, and think positively about what you are hoping to achieve. Deep breathing can help with relaxation.

She will need to lubricate her fingers well with oil. Any vegetable oil will be suitable (i.e. not petroleum based), but oils rich in vitamin E such as evening primrose and wheatgerm are particularly good, although they are usually diluted with a vegetable oil such as jojoba, sunflower in a ratio of 25% to 75% of the vegetable oil. She will then need to rub enough oil into the outside of the perineum to allow her fingers to move smoothly: this is feeding the skin and helping to make it more supple.

Once the client is confident with this stage she can move on.

Next, she will need to use her fingers to stretch out the skin of the perineum in different directions – from the medial to lateral, from anterior to posterior, moving it around.

Then she needs to oil her index finger or thumb thoroughly; she may need to experiment to see which suits her best. She then places the finger or thumb inside the vagina up to the second knuckle and gently massages in a rhythmic U or sling-shaped movement from 3 o'clock to 9 o'clock. This will gently stretch the vaginal tissues and muscles.

Once she is confident and comfortable, she can increase the pressure and introduce a stretch downwards. This may sting slightly; this stinging sensation occurs when the baby's head is born.

The perineum is like any other muscle in the body, and with use and practise it gets more supple and stretchy.

The client can do some pelvic floor exercises while doing her perineal massage.

Caution

The woman should not do perineal massage if she has vaginal herpes, thrush or any other vaginal infections. Massage could worsen and spread the infection.

Techniques for the postnatal period

Often at this time, the focus switches to the baby and away from the mother. Parents go to infant massage classes to learn work to do with the baby. However, the mother needs work as much in this period as in any of the others and massage can be a good way of continuing to support the bond between the parents. Indeed the mother could even begin to do some work on her partner.

Abdominal work

After a vaginal birth

The mother could do this herself, or the partner could be encouraged to do this. As soon as possible after birth the mother or partner can do some gentle stroking over the abdomen, with some gentle 'energetic' hacking. Mother or partner may cradle the lower abdomen with their hands. As time goes on, deeper work can be shown and even included as part of the abdominal exercises.

Post caesarean

Often gently breathing into the lower abdomen is sufficient to begin with, but the mother or partner could gently cup over the incision without directly making contact. Encourage the mother and partner, as the incision heals, to gradually make more contact.

Breast care for breastfeeding mums

Self-massage of breast, partner massage of breast

Many issues with breastfeeding are due to milk getting blocked in milk ducts. This may be prevented by teaching the mother or partner to gently massage the breast tissue, in the direction of the milk ducts, stroking towards the nipple. If lumps do develop then teach them to gently massage sore lumps within the mother's comfort zone. If there is inflammation beginning to develop then a simple lymphatic sequence can be taught. This begins with gentle stimulation of the lymphatic ducts in the neck and clavicle, followed by stimulation of the axillary node and then lighter strokes from nipple to lymph ducts (axillary or terminal).

Infant massage and massage of other siblings

It is important to consider how to include older children so that they do not feel left out. It is helpful to get the mother to continue with massaging of the older child or to include the older child in massaging the new baby. The older child could even be given the role of massaging the mother.

Reflective questions

- Consider the training you have for offering aftercare suggestions.
- How can you include this as a component of your maternity work?
- Is there further training which you could undertake which can enhance your work?

References

ACOG 2002, ACOG Committee on Obstetric Practice. Exercise During Pregnancy and the Postpartum Period. Committee Opinion No. 267, January 2002. Int. J. Gynecol. Obstet. 77 (1), 79–81.

Noble, E., 1982. Essential Exercises for the Childbearing Year, second ed. John Murray, London.

CHAPTER 13

The medical approach to labour

Chapter contents

Learning outcomes

- Describe the components of the medical model of labour
- Describe the benefits and side-effects of medical interventions in labour
- Describe the type of bodywork which can support the client in labour, if relevant, and in the postnatal recovery period

Introduction

Most births include some form of medical intervention. Medicine saves lives and has other health benefits. However, there is a general agreement that healthy women and fetuses do not usually need much intervention and that birth has become overly medicalised in the past 50 years.

An example is the rising caesarean rate. This varies considerably from country to country, indicating that social and cultural factors play just as much of a role as medical factors in determining the use of medicine. In parts of some countries such as Brazil the rate is as high as 85–100% with rates of 47.7% not being uncommon (Ratner 1996).

Nationally in the UK the rate is 23% (in 2003–4; RCOG 2004), in Canada 25% (Anderson & Lomas 1984, but still approximately this rate), while in the Scandinavian countries the rate is 10% (Wagner 2000). In 1985, the WHO suggested that 10–15% should be the highest rate. In the work of Ina May Gaskin, an American lay midwife who specialises in supporting natural births, fewer than 2% of women needed a caesarean. No one knows what the optimal rate should be, although Mukherjee (2006) still feels that the rate should be kept between 10 and 15%.

There is increasing concern about rising rates in medical circles as well as among advocates of natural birth, as unnecessary caesareans carry health risks to both woman and fetus.

The reasons for the spiralling rate are multifactorial and include:

1. Patient choice (about 8%).
2. Increased incidence of twins, due to assisted reproductive technologies.
3. Reluctance to undergo trial of labour if there is scar from a previous caesarean because of potential risk of uterine rupture.
4. Medico-legal pressure on practitioners.
5. Increasing safety of procedure.
6. Increasing age of women having children.
7. Increasing obesity rates.
8. Use of caesarean for breech deliveries.

Even in what are recorded as 'normal' births there is a high degree of intervention. In a recent study in the Trent region of the UK in over 60% of the 956 deliveries recorded as 'normal' or 'spontaneous' (i.e. excluding instrumental or caesarean section deliveries) interventions had occurred. These included amniotomy, induction, augmentation of labour, episiotomy and epidural anaesthesia. In about a third, induction or augmentation of labour had taken place, while in 89% amniotomies were performed before the cervix was fully dilated (Downe et al 2001). There is current debate about how to 'adopt the truly scientific approach of seeking the evidence base of all methods old and new' (Henderson & Macdonald 2004: 1096).

Some practitioners argue that we are beginning to forget what 'normal' birth is and that anything which interferes with the natural process of birth can be considered an intervention. This includes vaginal examinations, telling the woman to push (or not to push if the obstetrician is not available), and monitoring the fetus (especially electronic fetal monitoring), because they rely on external sources for assessing and progressing labour and because they may interfere with the interaction between the woman and her baby.

While bodyworkers are not the professionals making the decisions about the use of medicine in labour, in this current climate they need to understand the implications of the different types of procedure in order that they can support their clients during labour and in the postnatal recovery period.

Bodywork during labour if there is medical intervention

The bodyworker must recognise that they are always secondary to the primary caregiver and should not interfere with their role. However, they may be able to continue to give emotional and physical support to their client in appropriate ways.

This may include:

Reducing stress for mother

This can include continuing to work with massage, holding techniques, breathing and visualisations.

Continuing to support the physiological process of labour as much as is possible

This may include:

- Supporting the mother to be in birth positions which support the process of labour.
- Using bodywork for a pain relief option to reduce the use of pharmacological pain relief which may lead to further interventions.

Including the baby

Doctors and midwives tend to communicate with the woman about what is going on. However, they often forget about the baby. The baby is aware and appreciates some form of communication. This could be through touch or sound. It is important to encourage the woman or her partner to talk to the baby and continue to touch the abdomen. If the woman and partner are too stressed then it may be appropriate for the bodyworker to touch the abdomen and communicate with the baby.

Bodywork to support postnatal recovery after intervention

Each intervention carries different effects which the bodyworker needs to take into account when working with women in the postnatal period. Some of

the emotional effects of an intervention, particularly if it was a stressful time, or the mother felt disempowered during the process, may last for years, if unprocessed.

In understanding the implications of each intervention, the bodyworker must be careful not to make the client feel 'guilty' about not having achieved a natural birth. While interventions have effects on the body, without relevant interventions it must be remembered that sometimes mothers and babies might die or be severely injured.

13.1 The medical model of labour

Progress is determined by:

- Dilatation of the cervix.
- Descent of fetal head, measured in fifths palpable per abdomen above or below the ischial spines.

  Assessments are made to check:

- The condition of the woman: pulse rate, temperature, blood pressure, urine output, urinary protein and ketones and psychological state.
- The condition of the fetus: auscultation of heart rate, meconium in amniotic fluids, cardiotocography and measurement of fetal scalp blood pH.

The partogram

Labour is usually charted on a 'partograph' where cervical dilatation is plotted against time.

The 'normal' parameters are often defined as such: 6 hours for latent phase and 6 hours for active phase, making a total of about 12 hours for the acceptable normal duration of the first stage of labour in a primipara; multiparas do not take this long.

When labour does not fit into these parameters a diagnosis of 'prolonged labour' is made.

Prolonged labour: 'failure to progress'

A main cause given for failure to progress is cephalopelvic disproportion (CPD), when the fetal head seems too big for the birth canal. This is hard to be sure of as CPD is often relative and may be due to fetal position more than size.

Other causes include:

Fetal causes

- Fetal malposition (which can often be corrected).
- Fetal malformation (e.g. hydrocephaly). These days this is very rare and is often known prior to the

onset of labour due to the prevalence of ultrasound as a routine part of antenatal care in developed countries.

- Macrosomia or a large fetus. This is often due to congenital or developmental abnormalities.

Maternal causes

- Contracted pelvis, e.g. deformed through rickets.
- Pelvic tumour.
- Stenosis or scarring of the cervix which means that the cervix may not dilate effectively.
- Septae or stenosis of the vagina.
- Uterine dysfunction; this could be due to many causes.

Medical treatment

Allow labour to continue with the goal of a vaginal delivery,
OR
Intervene with instrumental delivery.

Bodywork

This can be appropriate if labour is being allowed to continue.

The woman and baby are both likely to be exhausted. Work to relax the client wherever she is experiencing tension. Work to revitalise the client: this may include energy work with the leg meridians, supporting the Kidneys and the Extraordinary Vessels, especially the Conception Vessel.

13.2 Monitoring in labour

Assessing fetal condition

Different checks are regularly made on the fetus to monitor how they are coping with labour. If it is deemed that the fetus is not coping, then interventions may be made either to speed up labour or deliver the fetus instrumentally.

Status of amniotic fluid

This provides some indication of fetal well-being. If there is thick meconium (fetal faecal excretion) at the onset of labour there is a five- to sevenfold increase in risk of perinatal death (MacDonald et al 1985) as well as morbidity resulting from the risk of meconium aspiration. The recent passage of meconium will be indicated by dark greenish-black-coloured amniotic fluid. Old or stale meconium is a paler greenish-brown. If there is fresh meconium the fetal heart is checked more frequently.

Pinard/manual monitoring

This is a hollow instrument (Pinard fetal stethoscope) placed on the woman's abdomen. It involves no ultrasound and is done intermittently. It is a traditional midwifery tool and often used in home births. Its accuracy depends on the skill of the individual caregiver. It is the least invasive form of fetal monitoring.

Electronic fetal monitoring

This can be hand held and intermittent or continuous.

An electronic fetal heart monitor or cardiotocograph (CTG), ultrasound, is placed over the woman's abdomen near the fetus's heart. It measures the fetal heart rate and gives a readout. It need not necessarily interfere with maternal position as the woman may still be able to utilise forward leaning or upright positions, although if she moves much the printout will be inaccurate. Some care providers prefer the woman to be semi-recumbent or side-lying. It cannot be used if the woman is in water.

Hand-held monitors, also called fetal Dopplers or sonicaids, which are not attached to a graphic record can be used. These can be used in the pool and the woman can remain more mobile than with the CTG.

The fetal heart rate is usually measured every 15–30 min in early labour and every 5 min in active labour. The normal rate is between 120 and 160 beats per minute.

Fetal scalp monitoring

This is done if more accurate monitoring is needed, which may be the case if there are risk factors present such as the use of oxytocin.

It involves inserting a spinal wire electrode through the cervix and attaching it to the fetal scalp. The heart rate is measured by calculating the intervals between R waves in the fetal electrocardiographic cycles. This method of monitoring is only possible when the waters have broken and if it is needed then the membranes need to be ruptured (ARM).

Fetal blood sampling (FBS)

When the fetal heart rate pattern is suspicious then FBS should be carried out (NICE 2001). The woman is placed in the left lateral position while a sample of blood is taken from the fetus's skull. This is sent for analysis and gives a more accurate indication of fetal distress than monitoring heart rate as it assesses oxygen levels in the brain.

Benefits

Monitoring in labour may enable the early detection of potential risks to fetal health.

Drawbacks

- Continuous monitoring may interfere with the woman's ability to move and remain comfortable, thus increasing the need for pharmacological pain relief.
- There is variation in the clinical interpretation of the data and altered heart rate does not necessarily mean fetal compromise.
- Increased monitoring is associated with an increase in the rate of caesarean section, especially if it is used without fetal blood sampling.
- Its increased use has not been linked with a decrease in maternal or fetal mortality or morbidity. Many clinicians believe that fetuses are just as safe if someone listens to the fetal heart just after a contraction has finished and in the interval between contractions with a Pinard stethoscope or hand-held Doppler machine.
- No one fully understands the effects of ultrasound monitoring on the fetus although some small studies have postulated possible adverse effects (American Institute of Ultrasound in Medicine 2000).
- Current NICE guidelines in the UK do not recommend continuous fetal monitoring in normal labour although many hospitals worldwide still employ it.

Bodywork implications

- The client may need more support to get into comfortable positions.
- The client may need emotional support as she may get worried about her baby.

13.3 Induction

Augmentation of labour often uses similar procedures to induction but they are made during a labour which has already begun, in order to strengthen uterine contractions.

Maternal indications for induction

1. Post-term pregnancy. In the Cochrane systematic review, trials demonstrated an effect of reducing perinatal mortality only for induction conducted after 42 weeks of gestation (Crowley 1999). There are, however, variations in different clinical opinions, with some clinicians inducing before 42 weeks.
2. Hypertension, primary or pregnancy-related, which may adversely affect the continuation of the pregnancy.
3. Renal and heart disease where there is concern about the pregnancy continuing.
4. Pre-labour at term spontaneous rupture of the membranes (PROM), due to increased risk of infection. There are variations: some hospitals induce after 24 hours whereas others allow up to 96 hours (RCOG 2001) if there are no other causes for concern such as raised temperature. Research (Savitz et al 1997) shows that 86% of women go into labour within 24 hours and 91% within 47 hours spontaneously.
5. Placental abruption or other placental issues.

Fetal indications

1. Fetal compromise.
2. Fetal death.
3. Rhesus iso-immunisation.

Contraindications

The following indicate that a caesarean section is needed rather than induction:

1. Placenta praevia – vaginal birth is too dangerous.
2. CPD (cephalopelvic disproportion).
3. Oblique or transverse lie of the fetus as normal labour is not able to proceed.
4. Severe fetal compromise necessitating immediate delivery.
5. VBAC (vaginal birth after caesarean section). Induction may cause excessive uterine contractions which could be too strong for the scar.

Methods

An assessment is made of how ripe the cervix is using the Bishop score. This is a way of grading softness and effacement.

Sweeping the membranes

The membranes are stripped from the lower uterine segment at term. The maternity care provider places a finger inside the cervix and makes a circular sweeping action to separate the membranes from the cervix. The theory behind this is that the localised prostaglandin production is increased (Mitchell et al 1977). It is not associated with an increase in infection but women may feel discomfort both during and after the procedure. It is routinely offered in the UK from 40 weeks of gestation.

Prostaglandin gel (PGE2)

The next method is to use prostaglandin (PGE2) gel/tablets to ripen the cervix. Gel is applied to the cervix in the form of a pessary. This is one of the most commonly used methods of induction worldwide. It is more likely than placebo to start labour and tends to reduce the need for induction with oxytocin (Enkin et al 2000).

Benefits

- It may be a fairly gentle way of getting labour started and then labour can proceed naturally.
- It may reduce the need for oxytocin.
- It is considered the most efficacious induction agent (Henderson & Macdonald 2004: 872).

Drawbacks and risks

- Side-effects include diarrhoea and nausea. Vomiting is less common. This affects LU/LI energy.
- Sometimes the uterus responds by producing excessive contractions. Contractions may be painful and emotionally difficult for the mother to process.
- The fetus may go into distress.
- There is a sudden onset of Yang energy affecting Yang Heel, Small Intestine, Heart, GV and CV.
- Sometimes there is maternal pyrexia due to the effect on the thermoregulating centre in the brain.

Rupturing the membranes (breaking the waters/amniotic sac) – amniotomy

This involves rupturing the membranes to accelerate or initiate labour. An amnio hook is introduced into the cervix and the amniotic sac is ruptured. This requires a firm commitment to delivery (Enkin et al 2000) as it increases the risk of intrauterine infection, early decelerations of the fetal heart rate, umbilical cord prolapse and bleeding from the cervix.

It is more usually done during labour to speed it up, often after prostaglandin gel when there are signs that labour is beginning, rather than to start labour off.

Benefits

This method does not introduce hormones into the body and if the woman is nearly ready to go into labour, may help speed up progress.

Drawbacks

- It may stimulate excessive contractions.
- The fetus is no longer protected by the amniotic sac and may show an increase in fetal heart rate decelerations.
- It may be unsuccessful in establishing labour, in which case the woman is on a time frame to deliver, which may in turn lead to more intervention.

Oxytocic drugs

This is the most common induction agent used worldwide. Intravenous infusion is the licensed and most common method of administration.

Synthetic oxytocin (syntocinon or pitocin)

This is a synthetic preparation of oxytocin administered through an electronic infusion pump. It is also used to augment labour and a version (Syntometrine) is given in the third stage of labour for the preventative treatment of postpartum haemorrhage.

Benefits

Usually labour will begin.

Drawbacks

1. Uterine hyperstimulation.
2. As the woman needs to be monitored continuously, her ability to move freely will be interfered with which may also affect her ability to cope with the pain.
3. It may produce strong contractions which are not able to effectively dilate the cervix, meaning that a LSCS becomes necessary (Bidgood & Steer 1987).
4. Water retention and hyponatraemia (low levels of sodium in blood) due to the antidiuretic effect of oxytocin. Symptoms are weakness and lethargy, muscle cramps and postural hypotension.
5. It may increase the risk of postpartum haemorrhage (Stones et al 1993).
6. It may affect the complex hormonal changes for the mother, affecting the energy of the Extraordinary Vessels, especially GV.
7. Some observational studies have shown a reduced rate of breastfeeding following induced labour even among women who intended to breastfeed and when controlled for low breastfeeding rates (Out et al 1988).
8. Neonatal hyperbilirubinaemia (jaundice).

Bodywork implications

Bodywork can often be continued. Many people assume that medical induction of labour happens quickly but it often involves a lot of waiting around and medical staff are reluctant to give any pain relief because they do not know how long it will take to get labour established.

Bodywork will not only help the woman be more relaxed while waiting, thus helping her to be more likely to go into labour, but this waiting time can also be used to work on the labour focus points as much as possible to try to get labour going naturally. Once the woman has started on whatever regimen she is having, it is still possible to continue to work the labour focus points.

Postnatally work with the effects of the drugs

Bodywork can also help with pain relief. Postnatally work with the effects of the drugs.

13.4 Pain relief

This is a key part of the medical approach to labour which assumes that women need help. Some practitioners believe that the hormones released naturally by women offer more effective pain relief without the potential side-effects of medical pain relief (Buckley 2005).

In the UK the obstetrician James Young Simpson was the first person to use chloroform for the relief of pain in labour in 1847. Dr John Snow administered it to Queen Victoria during the birth of her two youngest children and it became a popular analgesia. It was also introduced in the USA at around the same time.

Entonox (gas and air, nitrous oxide)

This is nitrous oxide inhaled through a mask. It provides partial relief of pain through its sedative effect. It is used fairly extensively in the UK but not so much worldwide, as in some countries such as Canada its use has been associated with an increase in abortion in caregivers.

Benefits

- It may take the edge off contractions by encouraging the woman to be less focused which can help her 'let go', relax and go with the contractions.
- It can be stopped easily if not suited to the woman.
- It has no long term side-effects for the mother.

Drawbacks

- It may make the woman feel sick, light-headed and disconnected: LU and LI energy.
- In second stage it may make it harder for the woman to focus on bearing down. There is excessive Yin energy.

Implications for bodywork

- Bodywork can usually be continued.
- Support can be given for relieving sickness; LI 4 and HC 6 particularly effective.
- The woman may need help with being focused, especially in second stage.

- Breathing can be supported to focus although it will probably need to be adapted, as the woman is having to focus more on the in-breath.

Analgesics: morphine, pethidine (Demerol, meperidine), Meptid; opiate painkillers

The most commonly used pain-relieving drugs are synthetic opioid drugs: pethidine, Demerol, meperidine, Meptid or Nubain. Introduced in 1939, these are powerful analgesic, sedative and antispasmodic drugs. They are less effective than morphine but have less of a depressant effect on the respiratory centre of the newborn. Their effects are rapid and last for approximately 3–4 hours. They may be given intramuscularly or as an intravenous injection or infusion.

Benefits

- Can numb the woman so she can rest, without slowing labour down: this can be useful in a long labour.
- The loss of control may be helpful to some women to let go.

Drawbacks
Woman

- May include nausea, reduction in blood pressure and sweating.
- The woman may feel unable to be active and less able to communicate.
- They may interfere with the woman's own opioid hormone production (Thomas et al 1982) which may slow labour (Thomson & Hillier 1994) and interfere with bonding (Stafisso-Sandoz et al 1998).
- Energy-wise, they affect the Blood.
- Postnatal feelings of nausea and sickness may interfere with breastfeeding.

Side-effects for the fetus

The drugs cross the placenta and may depress the fetal respiratory centre. Changes in fetal heart rate pattern and a loss of baseline variability may be noted within 40 minutes of maternal administration. To avoid the greatest depressant effect on the fetus the drugs should not be given to the woman within 2–3 hours prior to delivery.

Peak effects of the drug on the fetus are observed on the seventh day postnatally – newborns are found to be less alert, quicker to cry when disturbed, and less able to settle themselves. The opioid receptor antagonist naloxone (Narcan) may be administered to the woman prior to delivery or to the fetus at birth to minimise these effects.

These effects may interfere with bonding and breastfeeding.

Some research indicates that the adult is 4.7 times more likely to become addicted to opiate drugs (Jacobson et al 1990).

Bodywork implications

- As the woman may not be so 'with it' she may need extra support in birth positions. It is probably advisable not to use more challenging positions such as the standing squat.
- As these drugs are not anaesthetics the woman may still need the support of bodywork – indeed, some areas of the body may be tense and benefit from it.
- Work to address feelings of nausea and sickness may be required.
- Postnatally, work with the Extraordinary Vessels can support hormonal changes, bonding and breastfeeding, especially Penetrating Vessel.

TENS

Transcutaneous electrical nerve stimulation (TENS) sends nerve impulses to the skin via electrode pads linked to a battery-powered unit. The electrode pads are placed on the tenth thoracic to the first lumbar and from the second to fourth sacral vertebrae. It is thought to assist in the prevention of the perception of pain sensations, based on the gate control theory, by blocking nerve pathways and preventing pain signals travelling to the brain. It is best used from early labour. It is said to stimulate the production of naturally occurring endorphins (Simkin 1989).

Benefits

- It does not affect the chemical balance within the woman's body in the same way as drugs.
- It has limited side-effects.
- It may be enough to control pain.
- It can be useful during a move from home to hospital as the woman operates it herself and a bodyworker is often unable to reach back points at this time.

Drawbacks

- It may be ineffective in distracting from the pain.
- It may interfere with the use of shiatsu and pressure techniques to the lower back.
- It cannot be used in water.
- It may interfere with the reading of the internal fetal scalp electrode.

Bodywork implications

- As it is similar to shiatsu, be cautious of work to the lower back as it may be too much stimulation. However, many women find that work still feels appropriate.

- Bodywork anywhere else, if appropriate, is likely to be of benefit. Often neck work is indicated to balance out the lower back.
- The woman can still be encouraged to mobilise and use breathing techniques.

Anaesthetics

These are more powerful than analgesics and block pain.

Epidural anaesthesia

Local anaesthetic is introduced into the epidural space, the outermost layer of the meninges, in the spine. The anaesthetics are usually cocaine derivatives (e.g. bupivacaine, ropivicaine and lidocaine) which numb the motor as well as the sensory nerves making lower limb movement impossible. Lower-dose opiates reduce the motor block effect so that the woman can move – the 'walking epidural'. An epidural may be given as a single dose, or, more commonly, as a continuous technique in which a catheter is inserted into the epidural space so that further doses of anaesthetic may be given. One dose is effective for 4–6 hours.

The woman's blood pressure and the fetal heart beat are monitored frequently and a primary care provider is constantly present. With a full epidural the woman will be on her side or sitting so as to maximise blood flow to the fetus via the placenta.

An epidural is usually given if a caesarean section is indicated unless there is insufficient time, in which case general anaesthetic will be given. It is often used with vaginal operative procedures such as rotation and forceps delivery of a head in the occipito posterior position. It may be used in cases of prolonged labour caused by incoordinate uterine contractions or for severe cases of hypertension.

It is introduced by the lumbar or caudal route:

Lumbar route

The needle is inserted between L1 and L2, sometimes L2 and L3 or L3 and L4 and rarely L4 and L5. It is similar to a lumbar puncture except that the meninges must not be punctured. Sensory fibres from the uterus and upper third of the vagina enter the spinal cord at the level of the tenth, eleventh and twelfth thoracic segments. A lumbar epidural block usually anaesthetises T10–T12 and is most effective for pain during first stage.

Caudal route

This is less used. Local anaesthetic is injected via the sacral hiatus into the caudal canal. It is quicker acting but more painful and requires a higher dose of anaesthetic. The risk of toxicity and placental transfer of the local anaesthetic is therefore increased. As it blocks the sacral nerves perineal sensation is lost and the woman loses the reflex urge to bear down in second stage of labour. This makes the need for forceps delivery more likely. Pain sensations from the lower two-thirds of the vagina and perineum are transmitted to S2, S3 and S4 nerve roots, so the caudal route is most suitable for perineal pain in the second stage of labour.

Pudendal block

This is used in second stage with forceps or vacuum or for the repair of an episiotomy or perineal tear. The pudendal nerve is derived from the second to fourth sacral nerve roots which unite above the level of the ischial spine. Anaesthetic here blocks sensations to the skin around the anus, the perineal muscles and skin and the labia majora.

Benefits of epidurals

- The woman will not feel pain when it is working, but can still feel touch and the fetus being born.
- Mobile epidurals do not block the nerves supplying the bladder, abdominal and leg muscles, so the woman can still move around and have a vaginal birth.
- It can take the edge off the pain while the woman remains conscious.
- The woman can rest.
- It reduces high blood pressure.
- The woman has to have a caregiver with her constantly because of possible side-effects and this has the positive advantage of additional support.

Drawbacks and risks

- A full epidural will inhibit abdominal and leg movements and sensation from waist down.
- The drugs have effects on all the hormones of labour, inhibiting beta-endorphin production (Bacigalupo et al 1990, Räisänen et al 1984).
- Hypotension.
- Retention of urine.
- It is not always effective: sometimes it is completely ineffective or partially ineffective (it leaves a window of pain).
- It may decrease the strength of contractions due to the numbing effect on the stretch receptors of the lower vagina, increasing the need for forceps and synthetic oxytocin (Lieberman & O'Donoghue 2002, Thorp et al 1993).
- The musculature of the pelvic floor loses some of its resistance. This may increase the incidence of failure to rotate when a vertex in the occipito-posterior position meets the pelvic floor. This

increases the likelihood of low forceps delivery.
- Labour may be longer with an increased risk of instrumental delivery, perineal tear (Leighton & Halpern 2002) and risk of caesarean section (Lieberman & O'Donoghue 2002).
- If the needle enters the dural space it will cause a drop in CSF (cerebrospinal fluid) pressure, causing headaches which can last for days.
- Back pain at the site of injection may persist for years (Lieberman & O'Donoghue 2002).
- Occasional serious effects include nerve damage, in extremely rare cases leading to paralysis.
- It affects some of the most important points in the body along the Governing Vessel in the lumbar area:
  - L1–2 – GV5 Suspended Pivot – affects lumbar spine and lower burner.
  - L2–3 – Ming Men GV4 – gate of life – Jinggong – Place of Essence and BL23.
  - L3–L4 – between GV4 and GV3.
- It affects the Jing and Kidney energy on a deep level, and is considered to have a cooling effect. It may be that the energetic effects last for 7 years.
- It anaesthetises T10–T12, affecting Spleen and Stomach energy.
- It introduces Yin; Yin Heel.

Fetal effects

- May compromise fetal blood and oxygen supply (Mueller et al 1997, Roberts et al 1995).
- It may cause fetal distress due to lowered heart rate.
- Deficits have been found in newborn abilities consistent with toxicity from the drugs (Lieberman & O'Donoghue 2002).
- May affect breastfeeding due to diminished sucking reflexes and capacity (Riordan et al 2000, Walker 1997).

Bodywork implications

The type of bodywork required depends on the type of epidural the woman has had and how effective it has been. Bodywork would tend to be more focused on techniques which relieve tension in the neck and shoulders rather than the back. Work can be done to address the side-effects such as trembly legs, cold or sickness (e.g. LI4 and/or HC6). For the cold feelings, Heart Protector points are effective; holding the cold areas or simply holding the woman wherever she wants to be held can help with the focus of warming her up.

Although the woman will be on the bed, she can still choose the side position rather than lying on her back or lean forward over the back of the bed with some physical support. It is wise to continue to support the natural process of labour as much as possible because the epidural can be allowed to wear off so that the woman can deliver her baby herself, without having to use forceps or ventouse.

She may also find that she feels anxious, especially if pain relief is not complete, so any work which can help her stay calm and focused can be used.

Postnatally, there are many potential longer-term effects of epidurals, which the therapist may help to address, particularly the energy flows.

General anaesthesia (GA)

This is avoided where possible as a number of fatalities occur each year from complications. These are usually caused by inhalation of vomit when solid particles obstruct the bronchioles. This is why women have often been denied food in labour. However, a gastric tube can be inserted to prevent inhalation from occurring. Cricoid pressure is applied to compress the oesophagus and prevent regurgitation into the stomach until the tube is effective.

Woman

- The slowing down of respiration affects the Lungs. Energetically most GA drugs are considered cold in nature.
- There may be too much Yin; Yin Heel.
- All the Extraordinary Vessels will be affected.
- Warming the mother after a GA is important. It is generally done with moxa on CV 8 and GV 4 and Bladder 23 'but it can be done very simply by placing warm towels over the navel (using a small towel to avoid warming the caesarean section scar), lower back and feet a few times a day' (Jacky).

Baby

There is not so much direct effect on the baby from the GA itself but its use means that the baby has been delivered by caesarean section.

Implications for bodywork

As GA is given in an emergency medical situation, there is little that the bodyworker can do at the time. However, work can be done to support the recovery from the effects of a GA.

13.5 Assisted delivery

Episiotomy

This is a cut in the perineum between the anus and the vagina, to enlarge the vaginal opening in order to assist in second stage. Local anaesthetic is given and suturing is required. In some countries it is done routinely but many care providers believe that it is better for the perineum to stretch and tear minimally rather than be cut and that a tear with its jagged tissue repairs more easily than a cut.

Benefits

It may be necessary if birth needs to be speeded up because of fetal distress, or the tissues are too tight, the head is particularly large or an extra pulling force such as forceps or ventouse is needed.

Drawbacks
Mother

- It does not prevent deep tears into the vagina or anal muscles.
- It does not necessarily prevent birth injury.
- It can increase maternal blood loss and increase the incidence of anaemia; affects Blood and PV.
- It may lead to an increase in pain after birth, especially during intercourse.
- It heals more slowly than a tear and is harder to repair. Tears of the anal sphincter are more common and may lead to flatulence or anal incontinence.
- Infection may occur.
- The mother may feel a sense of invasion of boundaries (HT, LU), pain, and later fear of urinating because of pain (KD/BL energy).
- It cuts across CV/GV interrupting the circular flow of energy and the microcosmic orbit and Spleen energy.
- It involves use of anaesthetic.
- It creates scar tissue.

Fetus

The fetus no longer has symmetrical pressure from the perineum on its cranium and this often causes problems with the cranium and neck. This affects the GV (especially GV 20-Baihui) the Gall Bladder and Bladder plus the shock of the sudden change of pressure – Heart and LU and the Yin (Jacky).

Bodywork implications

There is not so much that can be done to support this while it is happening other than to encourage the woman to relax. The therapist may be able to hold the woman's hands.

It is important to ensure that the legs are placed evenly in the lithotomy position, especially if there is a history of SPD, to ensure that the pelvis is not put out of alignment.

After birth, the mother may need to be encouraged to do pelvic floor exercise and perinal massage and bodywork can be done to support the healing.

Forceps and ventouse

These are used during second stage to assist delivery. Forceps tends to be used less frequently due to the increased use of the ventouse (vacuum extractor) or suction cap. The ventouse is thought to cause less trauma to the fetus's head. However, as it is more gentle it is more likely to fail than forceps and some people argue that the effect on the neonate is similar. The obstetrician pulls while the woman pushes. It can only be used when the fetus's head has fully entered and engaged in the pelvis. Now that caesareans are safer, high forceps deliveries are less frequently utilised as the further away from the perineum the fetus is, the greater the chance of injury. In these cases caesareans are now the preferred choice.

The woman will usually need pain relief (epidural or pudendal block). She will need to lie on her back with her legs in stirrups (lithotomy position). It is important that both legs are placed in the stirrups together to avoid strain to the sacroiliac joint and pubic bone. It is a less advisable position for women with SPD and its use should be minimised. A catheter is inserted to empty the bladder and protect it from damage during delivery. Forceps usually also involves episiotomy, although not always.

Benefits

Used instead of caesarean section to deliver the fetus quickly if the fetus has got stuck or is in distress or if the woman is tired and unable to push effectively.

Drawbacks

Mother

- Internal bruising from the introduction of forceps between the fetus's head and the birth canal, combined sometimes with a strong pulling force.
- SPD and lower back problems are likely to be exaggerated or initiated. There is a sudden shift of the GV energy. This may lead to feelings of distress and loss of control, KD (fear), LU (boundaries), SI (trauma), HT or Pericardium.

Fetus

- It may affect the fetus's head and spine: GV.
- Less compression – affects the Yin and Earth element.

Bodywork implications

- It is still helpful for the woman to focus on bodywork which supports the second stage of labour to ensure the greatest chance of success. This includes the downward focus work, especially points such as GB21.
- Postnatally the mother will be recovering from bruising and pain.

Caesarean (planned/elective and emergency)

The fetus is delivered through an incision in the abdominal wall and uterus. Its history is uncertain but there are references to it in rabbinical writings of about 140 BC, and it was practised on dead women before that. Numa Pompilius (760–715 BC) forbade the burying of a woman who died during labour until the fetus had been cut out. This law later became the Lex Caesarean and so the term was born. However, it remained a dangerous operation until the 20th century when in 1906 Frank devised the transverse abdominal and lower segment incisions which are used today.

The operation can be either elective (planned in advance) or emergency (decision made during labour). An elective LSCS is much safer for the mother than an emergency LSCS.

There are two main types:

Classical upper segment caesarean section (USCS)

This involves a longitudinal incision in the upper uterine segment and is rarely performed because of the higher risk of scar rupture in a subsequent pregnancy (incidence 2.2%; Henderson & Macdonald 2004: 977). It may be used in the case of a major degree of placenta praevia, cervical carcinoma, lower segment uterine myomas, or for delivery of pre-term infants prior to the 28th week when the lower segment has not fully formed (Crichton et al 1991).

Lower segment caesarean section (LSCS)

This is most commonly used and is performed, once the bladder is emptied, through a suprapubic transverse incision to open the peritoneal cavity. The peritoneum is divided and the bladder pushed gently down off the lower segment. A transverse incision about 2 cm long is made in the midline of the lower uterine segment and deepened until the membranes bulge. The amniotic sac is kept intact if possible. Two index fingers are slipped in to the incision and finger traction is used to extend it to about 10 cm. The membranes are ruptured and the head is delivered by slipping a hand below it and applying fundal pressure. Sometimes a vacuum or forceps may be used. Next, the shoulders are eased out and the fetus held head down at the same level as the placenta while the mouth and pharynx are cleared of fluid. The cord is clamped and divided. If there are no complications for woman or fetus, then the fetus can lie on the woman's chest. The placenta separates soon afterwards and may be delivered though the incision or left in place. The uterine incision is sutured with two layers of catgut or Dexon. The abdominal wound is closed in the ordinary way.

Benefits

- The only way a transverse or oblique fetus can be delivered.
- It is necessary in cases of placenta praevia, or severe pre-eclampsia/eclampsia, high blood pressure or certain medical conditions where the stress of labour could be too much for the woman or fetus.
- It is needed where emergency delivery of the fetus is necessary, e.g. prolapse of umbilical cord, or if the fetus is stuck but not low enough for forceps or ventouse.
- It is also used to avoid the maternal transmission of certain infections such as when the woman has active herpes genitalis or HIV.
- The mother is relieved that her baby is delivered safely.
- The mother can plan when her birth is going to be.

Drawbacks

For the woman

Studies show that over 90% of women prefer a vaginal birth to a caesarean section.

Short-term implications

- The mother has to recover from major abdominal surgery with its associated health risks such as pain, infection, anaesthetic complications, excessive postnatal bleeding, thrombosis, haemorrhage (Liu et al 2007).
- Milk production and breastfeeding may be affected, especially with an elective section.

Long-term implications

- It is possible that the scarring to the uterus (uterine adhesions) may affect fertility (LaSala & Berkeley 1987) and the menstrual cycle and increase the risk of placenta abruptio and praevia (Gilliam et al 2002, Wagner 2000).
- There is double the risk of peripartum hysterectomy (Knight et al 2008).
- Hillan (2000) noted that 9–15% of women suffer serious maternal morbidity while another 65% do not feel fully recovered 3 months after caesarean section.
- Energetically it cuts across LV, CV, PV, KD, SP, ST meridians.
- There is some weakening of the abdominal muscles, the presence of scar tissue and adhesions in the uterus affecting HT/UT, Girdle Vessel,

the Extraordinary Vessels, potentially causing stagnation, especially in the lower burner (TH).
- Emergency caesareans impede the natural energy flow of birth from Yin to Yang and elective caesareans eliminate it. This affects the labour hormones, regulated by the Extraordinary Vessels and the movement of Water to Wood energy.
- With an emergency there may be the feelings of fear and shock; HT, SI, LU energy.

For the newborn

- With an elective LSCS, newborns are more likely to have breathing difficulties as they do not release the same hormones as during a vaginal birth and the amniotic fluid is not forced out of the lungs as it is during natural birth. Transient tachypnoea is four times greater in fetuses delivered by caesarean section than in those delivered vaginally (Strang 1991).
- Babies do not have any bacteria when they are born. They must receive these beneficial bacteria from their woman on their way through the birth canal and, after birth, from breast milk and their environment. If an infant's bacteria is off balance, colic and thrush can develop, both of which are more common in caesarean section fetuses (Grönlund et al 1999).

Bodywork implications

Planned

Encourage the woman to be relaxed and maintain her connection with the baby. She may want to think about how to make the caesarean as enjoyable as possible for her, her partner and the baby. Even in this highly medicalised environment there are often choices which can be made, such as bringing in special objects or playing a particular kind of music, deciding who is the first to hold the baby.

The woman is still going to give birth and it is important to prepare for it and for the recovery. It is beneficial to continue doing exercises and visualisations.

Emergency

There is not so much that can be done other than to help the woman be relaxed. It is important to include an awareness of the baby. The therapist may be present and offer a sense of calm as much as is possible. They can also help remind the woman to have immediate skin-to-skin contact with the baby if possible. They may need to reassure and support the father.

Postanatally

Support is crucial. Work needs to be done for the abdomen and uterus, both physically and to encourage the flow of energy. Gentle exercise is important to prevent stagnation of Qi, but care must be taken not to over-exercise and thus deplete the energy. There are more likely to be patterns of exhaustion and Blood deficiency.

Work can be done to support breastfeeding, bonding and hormonal changes. Encourage ambulation and work on the legs to reduce the risk of thrombosis.

Do not assume that a LSCS is traumatic; it may be for some women, but on the other hand vaginal birth can also be traumatic for women and babies. Many women are relieved to have got through birth, and grateful for the medical support which may have saved their own and their baby's life. Support the mother with where she is at and do not emphasise the negative aspects.

13.6 Management of third stage

Cutting and clamping the cord

Modern management of third stage usually involves clamping the cord immediately after the birth of the fetus in order to reduce the risk of haemorrhage to the mother. It has its place if there are high risks of haemorrhage or complications but its routine use is being questioned.

Without clamping, there is a reservoir of blood in the umbilical cord and placenta which is gradually transferred to the fetus during third stage which happens while the cord pulsates. This cord blood contains stem cells which are important in the future development of the immune system.

In one study, premature fetuses experienced delayed cord clamping of 60 seconds and showed a reduced need for transfusion, less severe breathing problems, better oxygen levels and indications of improved long-term outcomes compared to those whose cords were clamped immediately. This shows that this could be a way of helping fetuses in their initial adaptation to life outside the womb and possibly has implications for their long-term health (Lagercrantz & Slotkin 1986).

Early clamping is required if the mother wants to bank the cord blood.

Use of syntocinon for managed third stage

Versions of Syntocinon, including Syntometrine, are combined with controlled traction on the umbilical cord to hasten the process of separation and delivery of the placenta and reduce blood loss. It was traditionally given with the delivery of the shoulder but can be delayed until the baby has been born to minimise transfusion of the drug. Until recently this method was very common in the UK (Garcia et al 1987, Turnbull 1976) but physiological third stage is increasingly practised (Levy 1990). The practice of 'active management' is recommended by the WHO in developing countries where postpartum haemorrhage is the biggest cause of maternal death, due to ill health and lack of appropriate medical facilities.

Bodywork implications

At this stage of labour the bodyworker will be in a secondary role to the primary care giver if intervention is required. Postnatally there will be the effects of the use of oxytocic drugs, but not to the same extent as induction or augmentation.

Reflective questions

- Explore your feelings about how you feel working in the hospital setting alongside a high degree of medical intervention and involvement from the medical professions.
- Do you feel you would be able to communicate effectively?
- Do you feel you would be able to hold your space and therefore hold a good space for the woman and baby, and partner?
- Think about the implications of the different interventions for your postnatal work with clients.

References and further reading

American Institute of Ultrasound in Medicine, 2000 Section 4 – bioeffects in tissues with gas bodies. J. Ultrasound Med. 19 (2), 97–108.

Anderson, G.M., Lomas, J., 1984. Determinants of the increasing cesarean birth rate. Ontario data 1979–1982. N. Engl. J. Med. 311 (14), 887–892.

Bacigalupo, G., Riese, S., Rosendahl, H., et al., 1990. Quantitative relationships between pain intensities during labor and beta-endorphin and cortisol concentrations in plasma. Decline of the hormone concentrations in the early postpartum period. J. Perinat. Med. 18 (4), 289–296.

Bidgood, K.A., Steer, P.J., 1987. A randomized control study of oxytocin augmentation of labour 2, uterine activity. Br. J. Obstet. Gynaecol. 94 (6), 518–522.

Buckley, S.J., 2005. Gentle Birth, Gentle Mothering. One Moon Press, Brisbane.

Crichton, S.M., Pierce, J.M., Stanton, S.L., 1991. Complications of caesarean section. In: Studd, J.W. (Ed.), Progress in Obstetrics and Gynaecology, vol. 9. Churchill Livingstone, Edinburgh.

Crowley, P., 1999. Interventions for Preventing or Improving the Outcome of Delivery at or Beyond Term. Cochrane Review. Cochrane Library, Issue 1. Update Software, Oxford.

Department of Health, 2005. Statistics Bulletin 10: NHS Maternity Statistics England 2003–4. Government Statistical Service for DOH, London.

Downe, S., McCormick, C., Beech, B.L., 2001. Labour interventions associated with normal birth. Br. J. Midwifery 9 (10), 602–606.

Enkin, M., Keirse, M.J.N.C., Neilson, J., et al., 2000. A Guide to Effective Care in Pregnancy and Childbirth, third ed. Oxford University Press, Oxford.

Garcia, J., Garforth, S., Ayers, S., 1987. The policy and practice of midwifery study: introduction and methods. Midwifery 3 (1), 2–9.

Gilliam, M., Rosenberg, D., Davis, F., 2002. The likelihood of placenta previa with greater number of cesarean deliveries and higher parity. Obstet. Gynecol. 99 (6), 976–980.

Grönlund, M.M., Lehtonen, O.P., Eerola, E., et al., 1999. Fecal microflora in healthy infants born by different methods of delivery; permanent changes in intestinal flora after cesarean delivery. J. Pediatr. Gastroenterol. Nutr. 28 (1), 19–25.

Henderson, C., Macdonald, S. (Eds.), 2004. Mayes' Midwifery: A Textbook for Midwives, thirteen ed. Baillière Tindall, Edinburgh.

Hillan, E., 2000. The aftermath of caesarean delivery. MIDIRS Midwifery Dig. 10 (1), 70–72.

Jacobson, B., Nyberg, K., Grönbladh, L., Eklund, G., et al., 1990. Opiate addiction in adult offspring through possible imprinting after obstetric treatment. Br. Med. J. 301 (6760), 1067–1070.

Knight, M., Kurinczuk, J.J., Spark, P., et al., 2008. Cesarean delivery and peripartum hysterectomy. Obstet. Gynecol. 111 (1), 97–105.

Lagercrantz, H., Slotkin, T., 1986. The stress of being born. Sci. Am. 254, 100–107.

LaSala, A.P., Berkeley, A.S., 1987. Primary cesarean section and subsequent fertility. Am. J. Obstet. Gynecol. 157 (2), 379–383.

Leighton, B.L., Halpern, S.H., 2002. The effects of epidural analgesia on labor, maternal and neonatal outcomes: a systematic review. Am. J. Obstet. Gynecol. 186 (5 Suppl. Nature), S69–S77.

Levy, V., 1990. The midwife's management of the third stage of labour. In: Alexander, J., Levy, V., Roch, S. (Eds.) Midwifery Practice – Intrapartum Care, a Research Based Approach. MacMillan Press, Basingstoke.

Lieberman, E., O'Donoghue, C., 2002. Unintended effects of epidural analgesia during labor: a systematic review. Am. J. Obstet. Gynecol. 186 (5 Suppl. Nature), S31–S68.

Liu, S., Liston, R.M., Joseph, K.S., et al., 2007. For the Maternal Health Study Group of the Canadian Perinatal Surveillance System, Maternal mortality and severe morbidity associated with low-risk planned caesarean delivery versus planned vaginal delivery at term. Can. Med. Assoc. J. 176 (4), 455–460.

MacDonald, D., Grant, A., Sheridan-Pereira, M., et al., 1985. The Dublin randomised controlled trial of intrapartum fetal heart rate monitoring. Am. J. Obstet. Gynecol. 152, 524–539.

Mitchell, M.D., Flint, A.P.F., Bibby, J., et al., 1997. Rapid increases in plasma prostaglandin concentrations after vaginal examination and amniotomy. Br. Med. J. 2 (6096), 1183–1185.

Mueller, M.D., Brühwiler, H., Schüpfer, G.K., et al., 1997. Higher rate of fetal acidemia after regional anesthesia for elective cesarean delivery. Obstet. Gynecol. 90 (1), 131–134.

Mukherjee, S.N., 2006. Rising caesarean section rate. J. Obstet. Gynaecol. India 56 (4), 298–300.

National Institute for Clinical Excellence (NICE), 2001. The Use of Electronic Fetal Monitoring; the Use and Interpretation of Cardiotocography in Intra Partum Fetal Surveillance Guidelines. NICE, London.

National Institute for Health and Clinical Excellence (NICE), 2007. NICE Clinical Guideline 55. Intrapartum Care: Care of Healthy Women and their Babies During Childbirth. NICE, London.

Out, J.J., Vierhout, M.E., Wallenburg, H.C., 1988. Breast-feeding following spontaneous and induced labour. Eur. J. Obstet. Gynecol. Reprod. Biol. 29 (4), 275–279.

Räisänen, I., Paatero, H., Salminen, K., et al., 1984. Pain and plasma beta-endorphin level during labor. Obstet. Gynecol. 64 (6), 783–786.

Ratner, D., 1996. Sobre a hipotese de establizacao das taxas de cesarean do Estado de Sao Paulo, Brasil. Revista de Saúde Pública 30, 19–33.

Riordan, J., Gross, A., Angeron, J., et al., 2000. The effect of labor pain relief medication on neonatal suckling and breastfeeding duration. J. Hum. Lact. 16 (1), 7–12.

Roberts, S.W., Leveno, K.J., Sidawi, J.E., et al., 1995. Fetal acidemia associated with regional anesthesia for elective cesarean delivery. Obstet. Gynecol. 85 (1), 79–83.

Royal College of Obstetricians and Gynaecologists (RCOG), 2001. Induction of Labour. Evidence Based Clinical Guideline No. 9. RCOG Press, London.

Royal College of Obstetricians and Gynaecologists (RCOG), 2004. Clinical Effectiveness Support Unit. The National Sentinel Caesarean Section Audit Report. RCOG Press, London.

Savitz, D.A., Ananth, C.V., Luther, E.R., et al., 1997. Influence of gestational age on the time from spontaneous rupture of the chorioamniotic membranes to the onset of labor. Am. J. Perinatol. 14 (3), 129–133.

Simkin, P., 1989. Non pharmacological methods of pain relief during labour. In: Chalmers, I., Enkin, M., Keirse, M.J.N.C. (Eds.) Effective Care in Pregnancy and Child Birth, vol. 2. Oxford University Press, Oxford.

Stafisso-Sandoz, G., Polley, D., Holt, E., et al., 1998. Opiate disruption of maternal behavior: morphine reduces, and naloxone restores, c-fos activity in the medial preoptic area of lactating rats. Brain Res. Bull. 45 (3), 307–313.

Stones, R.W., Paterson, C.M., Saunders, N.J., 1993. Risk factors for major obstetric haemorrhage. Eur. J. Obstet. Gynecol. Reprod. Biol. 48 (1), 15–18.

Strang, L.B., 1991. Fetal lung fluid: secretion and reabsorption. Physiol. Rev. 71, 991–1016.

Thomas, T.A., Fletcher, J.E., Hill, R.G., 1982. Influence of medication, pain and progress in labour on plasma beta-endorphin-like immunoreactivity. Br. J. Anaesth. 54 (4), 401–408.

Thomson, A.M., Hillier, V.F., 1994. A re-evaluation of the effect of pethidine on the length of labour. J. Adv. Nurs. 19 (3), 448–456.

Thorp, J.A., Hu, D.H., Albin, R.M., et al., 1993. The effects of intrapartum epidural analgesia on nulliparous labor: a randomised, controlled, prospective trial. Am. J. Obstet. Gynecol. 169 (4), 851–858.

Turnbull, A.C., 1976. Obstetrics – traditional uses of ergot compounds. Postgrad. Med. J. 52 (Suppl. 1), 15–16.

Wagner, M., 2000. Choosing caesarean section. Lancet 356 (9242), 1677–1680.

Walker, M., 1997. Do labor medications affect breastfeeding? J. Hum. Lact. 13 (2), 131–137.

World Health Organization, 1985. Appropriate technology for birth. Lancet 2 (8452), 436–437.

CHAPTER 14

Working with higher-risk maternity clients

Chapter contents

Learning outcomes

- Outline global maternity healthcare realities for pregnant women and children
- Define 'higher-risk pregnancy'
- Describe common conditions encountered by the bodyworker including incidence, aetiology, physiology, pathophysiology, medical management, psychosocial implications
- Describe implications for bodywork

Introduction

From the 20th century onwards many countries throughout the developed world have witnessed a major decline in maternal and infant death rates. For women and babies in these countries, pregnancy and birth, are now relatively 'safe' events. Few women and babies die (e.g. 64 deaths per 1 054 828 in Canada). However, therapists working in these countries should not lose sight of the fact that

More than half a million women die from the complications of pregnancy and childbirth each year and 15 million women suffer injuries, infections and disabilities in pregnancy or childbirth. 10.6 million children under 5 die each year, 40% of them in the first month after birth. 98% of these occur in developing countries.

(WHO 2005)

The World Health Organization (WHO) chose World Health Day 7 April 2005 to focus on mothers and children. Their slogan was: 'Make every mother and child count'. Other global initiatives such as 'The Millennium Development Goals', ratified by more than 189 nations, have set targets to reduce maternal deaths by 75% and child deaths by two-thirds by 2015 (WHO 2005). The goal of such initiatives is not only to reduce mortality, but also to ensure access to appropriate health care services during pregnancy and childbirth (WHO 2004).

The decline of mortality rates in developed countries is due to improved sanitation, nutrition, standards of living, and level of education along with advances in medicine, improved access to health care, and better surveillance and monitoring of disease (Center for Disease Control and Prevention 1999, Detels et al 2002). Because of the low incidence of death, an additional indicator, 'severe maternal illness/morbidity', has been established which 'places a woman at serious risk of death but is not fatal' (Public Health Agency of Canada 2006).

The reasons that women die vary from country to country. Canada has one of the lowest maternal mortality rates and one of the best early childhood survival rates in the world. The European fetal death rate ranges from 3.7 to 7.3 per 10 000 births (Zeitlin et al 2003). In Canada, the leading causes of direct maternal death are pulmonary embolism and pre-eclampsia/pregnancy-induced hypertension, amniotic fluid embolism, and intracranial haemorrhage. The leading cause of indirect maternal death is cardiovascular disease (Gilbert & Harmon 1993, Health Canada 2004).

In 1997 the leading causes of direct maternal death globally were haemorrhage, infection and unsafe abortion. The leading causes of indirect maternal death were anaemia, malaria and cardiovascular disease (WHO 2005).

For information on mortality and morbidity rates in specific countries, check websites for the World Health Organization and for governing bodies related to maternity healthcare within the therapist's location (e.g. SOGC, ACOG, RCOG, CDC).

The realities for therapists working in developing countries are different. In these countries, women are often younger, have many more children and may live in difficult conditions. They may not have access to basic facilities such as water, let alone healthcare or bodywork.

For therapists working in developed countries, the focus is not working with high mortality and morbidity rates since the majority of their clients will be healthy women. However, there will be a number of clients who have some kind of risk. It is important to identify those types of clients, understand the kinds of conditions they present with and how much or how little bodywork can support them.

14.1 Definition of 'higher-risk' pregnancy

A healthy pregnancy with no predictable risk is defined as:

- No pregnancy complications now or in the past.
- No significant maternal medical disease.
- No prior maternity morbidity or mortality.
- Adequate fetal growth.

(Ontario Medical Association 2005)

A pregnancy becomes 'at risk' when 'Closer observation of the pregnancy may be necessary.' These patients may be managed by continuing collaborative care and birth in an obstetrical unit with intermediate level of nursing facilities or they may be returned to the care of the referring provider with a suggested plan of management for the remainder of the pregnancy.

A pregnancy becomes high risk when 'the fetus and/or mother are obviously in danger'. These patients should be transferred to a regional maternity centre (level III) for intensive care and birth. Clearly, there are patients who deserve to be placed in this risk category (with problems such as excessive antepartum bleeding, cord prolapse, or advanced uncontrolled premature labour) who cannot be transferred safely or in time to benefit the fetus or mother.

(Ontario Medical Association 2005)

Risk factors can be divided into three main categories: (i) general health status and predisposing risk factors including systemic issues, (ii) obstetrical issues and (iii) socioeconomic-behavioural factors including psychological and emotional issues.

General health status and predisposing risk factors

- Current health issues, e.g. cardiac disease, hypertension, thyroid issues, anaemia, chronic lung disease, diabetes, seizure disorders.
- Past medical history: illnesses, surgeries.
- Reproductive issues, e.g. pap smear anomaly, sexually transmitted infections.
- Older or younger pregnant woman.
- Pre-pregnancy obesity.
- History of genetic disease or congenital anomalies: family history or self.
- History of infections, e.g. cytomegalovirus, rubella, toxoplasmosis.
- Current symptoms, e.g. nausea, vomiting, headache, musculoskeletal discomfort or pain, varicosities.
- Significant family history, e.g. DVT, phlebitis, pre-eclampsia.

Obstetrical issues

- Previous obstetrical history: gravida/para/ previous pregnancy losses.
- Previous history of pregnancy loss or termination including therapeutic abortion, spontaneous abortion (miscarriage), intrauterine death (IUD), or stillbirth.
- Fetal anomalies.
- History of pre-term labour (<36 weeks).
- History of placental issues, e.g. placenta praevia, abruptiae.
- History of high-risk pregnancy, e.g. gestational diabetes, gestational hypertension, pre-eclampsia, antepartum haemorrhage, cervical incompetence, premature rupture of membranes, poly- or oligohydramnios.
- History of fetal/infant weight issues, e.g. SGA (small for gestational age), LGA (large for gestational age), IUGR (intrauterine growth restriction).
- Multiple birth.
- History of issues related to previous or current births, e.g. fetal malposition, breech presentation, labour dystocia, length of labour, medical interventions (induction, epidural, forceps, vacuum, operative delivery), outcome of labour.

Socioeconomic and behavioural factors

- Demographic factors.
- Socioeconomic status.
- Lack of prenatal care.
- Maternal substance abuse, e.g. smoking, alcohol, drug usage both prescription and non-prescription.
- History of sexually transmitted infection.
- Psychological issues.

- Exposure to teratogens such as heavy metals, solvents, pollutants, radiation.
- Cultural practices, e.g. immunisation, nutrition.
- Occupation risks, e.g. exposure to adverse substances, heavy lifting.
- Nutritional status and supplementation, e.g. eating disorders, food restrictions.
- Exercise patterns and limitations if any.
- Sleep patterns.
- Teenage pregnancy.
- Stress issues.
- History of abuse or violence.

Some of the pregnancy outcomes related to these factors are low gestational weight gain, pre-term birth, small for gestational age births, intrauterine growth restriction, pregnancy-induced hypertension, gestational diabetes, higher risk of maternal death, as well as a range of adverse infant health outcomes including congenital anomalies (Public Health Agency of Canada 2006).

There are wide-ranging implications for pregnancy and birth outcomes related to the severity of the risk issue and how it is managed or treated. In some cases, for example with a multiple pregnancy, or with age as the 'risk factor', thorough monitoring is the outcome as opposed to a specific treatment and there may be no actual complication. It is important to remember that: 'Only 10 to 30 percent of women who are labelled high risk actually end up having the outcome for which they are at increased risk' (Pearson 1997).

One of the most important components for a healthy pregnancy outcome is adequate prenatal care. Many tests and observations are available to help assess risk factors, prevent complications from developing and assist with diagnosis and treatment.

Goals for bodyworkers when treating higher-risk population groups

Working with the higher-risk population requires additional skills, training and experience compared to working with the low-risk population. The therapist needs to know the specific adaptations and precautions including those on home or hospital bedrest.

Prior to undertaking bodywork, there needs to be a solid understanding of the circumstances which result in a woman being considered 'higher risk'. This includes: the woman's general and maternity health history, knowledge of the type of primary care she is receiving, liaising with primary caregivers if relevant, the specifics of the health issue and an evaluation of the type of bodywork which would be safest and most beneficial. Complete contraindications to bodywork

are rare, except in the obvious case of medical emergency or an unstable health situation. Once the situation has stabilised, bodywork can be a useful adjunct to the recovery process.

Some bodywork texts suggest that higher-risk clients should not receive any therapy, or advocate modifications that are not based on clinically researched documentation. These recommendations are often based on fear or concern for litigation rather than clear evidence-based practice. There are no existing collected data to suggest that bodywork is harmful in higher-risk situations, particularly if it is done according to sound training and careful clinical application. On the other hand, there have been numerous clinical programmes within antenatal hospital settings, some for over a decade, with wide-ranging positive effects for patients, hospital staff, and the professional and student massage therapists who have participated in the sessions.

Massage therapy within the maternity hospital setting

Cindy McNeely

Massage therapy colleges in Ontario, Canada, have been pioneers in creating maternity hospital programmes. The first programme of its kind in Canada began in 1991 at Guelph General Hospital. Under the supervision of Kathy McDonald RMT, students from a Toronto massage therapy college provided treatments for antenatal patients as well as for women who were in the labour and delivery and postpartum setting. Students also provided direct hands-on care for hospitalised babies within the nursery setting.

In 1995 another maternity massage therapy programme was piloted within an urban level III, high-risk maternity hospital setting. This hospital delivers 4000 babies each year, with one quarter of the deliveries related to high-risk pregnancies. Cindy McNeely RMT designed and implemented this programme which served pregnant clients in the hospital due to their high-risk pregnancy. In addition, students worked within the labour and delivery and postpartum units. Infant massage instruction was provided for parents, both out-patients and within the level II nursery setting.

To date, the programme has trained students from four massage therapy colleges as well as providing postgraduate experience for Registered Massage Therapists (RMTs) seeking skill development in working with higher-risk pregnant clients. Student training in Ontario encompasses 2200 hours of training: this is the highest level of training worldwide.

Approximately 400 treatments are administered to patients in the maternity units each year which has resulted in over 5000 treatments given in the 13 years the programme has been running. Some patients receive a single session of treatment, while others may receive several massage therapy treatments per week and/or a series of treatments over the prolonged time they are in the hospital for observation and treatment of complications of their pregnancies. Women have been treated who have been in the hospital for up to 5 months of their pregnancies.

Although formalised statistics have not been gathered from these patients, whenever possible an evaluation form is given to the recipient of the treatment in order to receive voluntary feedback about the effectiveness of the programme.

Information requested relates to the effects of the massage treatments with respect to muscle discomfort and tension, effect on mobility and stiffness of joints, swelling, pain, feelings of stress and anxiety and sleep patterns. Of thousands of evaluations gathered, an overwhelming majority of positive feedback has been received about the efficacy of the treatments received in all units.

General points

In addition to knowing the specifics of each individual condition and client, there are some general points to consider.

Work in close collaboration with the primary care provider

Always ensure that the client is receiving appropriate medical care for their condition. Consult with the care provider if unsure of approach.

Stress reduction – a primary component of care

Regardless of the condition or issue, documentation of preventative and treatment practices within nursing care highlight the importance of stress reduction. Gilbert and Harmon (1986, 1993, 2002) repeatedly list anxiety, stress, fatigue, and over-activity in their list of contributing factors to some of the issues resulting in a higher-risk pregnancy. They suggest rest, stress reduction, relaxation techniques, problem solving

and 'back rubs' as appropriate care strategies for the patient experiencing higher-risk pregnancy: 'plan daily rest periods to increase blood flow to the uterus which decreases the risk of prostaglandin release' (Gilbert & Harmon 1993: 281, 430).

Daily activity level

The bodyworker can be aided in assessing treatment approach by considering the daily activity level prescribed by the primary care providers and any modifications or limitations. If extra caution is desired, the level of intensity of bodywork should be slightly less in nature than the activities of daily living prescribed by the primary care provider.

Encourage listening to the body

The therapist can play a role in encouraging, nurturing, and supporting the client in listening to her body.

The client on bedrest

If the client is on bedrest, then bodywork should aim to provide comfort, increase relaxation and reduce stress, and help maintain tissue well-being. As these clients may be at higher risk of developing DVT they are usually prescribed dorsiflexion/plantarflexion exercises by the antenatal physiotherapist and advised to mobilise. Bodywork can support these protocols with gentle mobilisations and effleurage. Energy work can include LV to support blood flow.

Absolute contraindications to bodywork

When working with this client group, the therapist needs to be more alert to the times when not to use bodywork (refer to tables in assessment chapter).

Working in hospital

The therapist may need to visit the client in hospital, with agreement from the primary caregiver.

Specific needs groups

In addition to understanding specifics of medical conditions, therapists may need to educate themselves on the specific needs of specific client groups such as: teenagers, refugees, women with a history of abuse, women carrying twins, women who have conceived through assisted reproductive technologies.

Testimonial

C.B. (client of Suzanne Yates)

I had kidney disease before becoming pregnant and knew some of the risks. However, when I saw the consultant I was informed I had stage 4 renal failure and a

60–90% chance of a successful pregnancy (i.e. live birth) and a 10% chance of needing dialysis during the pregnancy. The outlook seemed bleak. It was hard to find a complementary practitioner who would support me but eventually I found Suzanne and had shiatsu regularly during the rest of the pregnancy, during my birth and in the immediate postpartum.

Possibly the most important benefit was that it gave me a space where I could come back to myself and be doing something that other pregnant women were doing. I think it had an impact on my blood pressure; I remember feeling the ground under my feet after my shiatsu and I felt a lot less stressed. It gave me time to be aware of my baby daughter; it was very reassuring to feel her kick. Suzanne showed me points to work on myself between sessions, which really helped calm me down. She encouraged me to continue with my meditation practice.

My whole pregnancy was quite stressful and I was continually being monitored. Suzanne helped me get things in perspective and be calm about all the tests. If I had gone along with all the worries I would have been a basket case. Suzanne gave me space to express my fears, without denying the situation and giving false reassurance. I also appreciated that she was not afraid of working with me.

The main risks were that I would miscarry, have a premature baby or develop PET and need an emergency caesarean section.

When I was in hospital towards the end with suspected PET, the hospital staff were more than happy for Suzanne to come in and provided us with a space where I could have my shiatsu. This helped me continue to stay calm and connected.

At 36 weeks, after some weeks in hospital, a decision was taken to induce me. It felt like it was a bit of a long shot, but there was not much choice as my creatinine levels were creeping up. Suzanne worked the labour focus points with me for about a week before. I was given prostaglandin gel but after 24 hours nothing much had happened and my waters were broken. By this time my partner and I were both exhausted and feeling very negative. Suzanne came and gave me about an hour of shiatsu and I was able to reconnect once more with the calm meditative space and be more aware of my body. When Suzanne worked the labour focus points I could feel that I was beginning to contract. My partner also managed to have a rest.

No one believed I was having contractions and so I was put on a drip which made the contractions even stronger. I managed to get them to check my blood pressure before giving me drugs to lower it and to everyone's astonishment it had gone down after the shiatsu. As the contractions got more intense I felt scared but Suzanne helped me

to focus and kept reminding me of my body. I managed to avoid having an epidural and things progressed quickly and I wanted to bear down. The midwife wanted to catheterise me as my bladder was full and give me drugs for third stage, but I did not want any more intervention. Suzanne explained the reasons so I did not resist. My daughter was born soon after with no other interventions.

I am sure I would have ended up with an emergency caesarean if Suzanne had not been there. I felt supported by her calm presence. She helped me stay with myself but also encouraged me to work with the medical team who were supporting me. It felt good that there was no conflict between those who were caring for me.

Suzanne

My main focus in pregnancy was to:

- Support Kidney function with energy work.
- Help C. stay connected with her feelings.
- Support the positive aspects of the pregnancy, especially her connection to her baby.
- Give C. support while she was going through tests.
- Create a supportive space in the hospital environment.

In labour:

I worked to keep her in tune with what she needed to do and support the positive aspects of birth and her connection with her body.

I see my main focus of work in labour to support someone to be in the moment with their body and not worry about what might happen. That is a luxury of being a bodyworker rather than a primary care provider. They have to try to predict what may happen and also deal with complications. I have immense respect for that. It was an amazing process to support C. through many months of stress and uncertainty to reach 36 weeks of gestation and deliver her baby vaginally. Sadly now her kidney function has degenerated more and she is on the list for a kidney transplant. She has found the first year of being a mum with a serious medical condition quite draining but has appreciated the support of her medical carers and bodywork therapy.

14.2 Medical conditions existing prior to pregnancy

- Pre-existing hypertension, gestational hypertension and pre-eclampsia.
- Pre-existing heart or kidney disease.
- Diabetes.

- Thyroid problems.
- Endometriosis.
- Immune system disease: e.g. fibromyalgia, lupus.
- Reproductive tract anomalies.
- Sexually transmitted diseases.
- Genetic factors.
- Other diseases.

The conditions listed above may or may not cause additional complications.

Heart or kidney conditions

These two systems are significantly challenged by the increased demands of pregnancy and, depending on the type and severity of the condition, there is an increased risk of complications. Bodywork may be completely contraindicated, or reduced with respect to the length of time of the treatment, the intensity or vigour of the work, and the position of the client.

Heart conditions

The primary care provider may prohibit the inclusion of any bodywork if there is any risk of overload to an already compromised cardiovascular system as in cases of unstable hypertension or thrombosis or imminent risk. Technique approach is soothing in nature. Energy approaches aim toward supporting the Conception Vessel, Heart, Heart Protector and Penetrating Vessel.

Kidney conditions

The woman is at increased risk of developing hypertension, including eclampsia and associated issues. Energy work, if appropriate, would focus on the Kidney and Extraordinary Vessels.

Effects on labour

Both the heart and kidney have extra demands placed on them during labour and a compromised heart or kidney may be especially challenged. Renal issues are associated with a risk of pre-term labour.

The type of delivery is determined by the primary care provider but vaginal delivery is generally considered preferable as it causes less haemodynamic fluctuation than a caesarean section (Gilbert & Harmon 1993). It is also advised that the second stage of labour be kept as short as possible to avoid excessive stress.

Implications for bodywork postnatally of heart conditions

Due to the strain of labour and early postnatal circulatory changes, heart failure may occur in the first few days postnatally. These clients are usually kept in the hospital after delivery for observation or treatment. They may be on orders for increased rest. Modified activity is usually advocated in order to prevent increased risk of onset of circulatory issues such as the formation of thromboembolic disorders.

There is no contraindication to breastfeeding; however, consultation would be made with the primary care provider in the event that the client is taking particular medications.

Bodywork, especially if it includes gentle leg work and mobilisation of the legs, may help to reduce the risk of thromboembolic disorders.

Postnatal kidney implications

The kidneys may be strained after the delivery, resulting in altered blood pressure (either higher or lower). Medications may be prescribed to normalise blood pressure. Energy work to GV, CV and KD may help support the normalisation of blood pressure and kidney function. Studies related to massage therapy and its effect on blood pressure are still preliminary.

Diabetes

The pregnant diabetic woman

Women who have diabetes and are considering becoming pregnant are advised to consult their primary care provider or specialist before becoming pregnant. Blood glucose levels should be stabilised before pregnancy as unstable levels during embryologic development may increase the risk of congenital anomalies.

Pregnant diabetic women experience an increase in insulin requirements by the end of pregnancy and may need up to four times their usual dose of insulin. Women with type II diabetes may require insulin during their pregnancy. Insulin requirements return to normal after delivery. During pregnancy, insulin levels become less stable and this may exacerbate some of the existing complications. There is an increased risk of pre-eclampsia, polyhydramnios, pre-term labour, fetal macrosomia (large baby) and fetal malformations, especially cardiac anomalies (Landon 1999). However, regular monitoring has proved successful in achieving good control.

Implications for bodywork

Refer to GDM (p. 381).

Thyroid issues

These may be exacerbated or improved by the changes in the endocrine system. Depending on the symptom presentation, therapists may need to adapt their bodywork or work. Energy work would include Extraordinary Vessel work.

Endometriosis

This is likely to be a cause of infertility, ectopic pregnancy and miscarriage, due to the presence of endometrial tissue outside the uterine cavity. Energy work can be done to support the Extraordinary Vessels and Spleen, Liver and Kidney.

Autoimmune disease

This may be related to the immune mechanism involved – if the disorder involves alterations in T_h1 responses which decrease in pregnancy or T_h2 responses which increase (Formby 1995).

Rheumatoid arthritis

Around 77% of women with rheumatoid arthritis (which is associated with increased T_h1 mediators which are decreased in pregnancy) experience improvement, generally beginning in the first trimester; 90% relapse between 6 weeks and 6 months after delivery (Formby 1995, Buyon 1998).

Systemic lupus erythematosus (SLE/lupus)

Lupus may be related to an increased incidence of miscarriage. It is often exacerbated, especially in women with renal involvement or active SLE at the time of conception. SLE involves the production of auto-antibodies of the IgC class and increases in T_h2 mediators which are increased in pregnancy. Women with SLE who have anticardiolipin antibodies or lupus anticoagulant antibodies have an increased risk of thrombosis, fetal loss and thrombocytopenia (Tseng & Buyon 1997).

Fibromyalgia

Fibromyalgia is a chronic condition which can affect the autoimmune and musculoskeletal system. It may improve or worsen during pregnancy. Massage therapy can be an effective treatment for easing symptoms of pain and chronic fatigue. Depth of pressure can vary significantly and relates to the client's previous experience with massage therapy. Feedback from the client is crucial to ensure improvement rather than exacerbation of musculoskeletal symptoms.

Overexertion can exacerbate symptoms, so good communication is important. Prenatal preparation taking into consideration the pregnant woman's stamina will help ensure an appropriate labouring process.

In the postnatal period, the mother may experience a worsening of her symptoms, and with increased demands postnatally, she may feel additionally tired.

Energy work will include Extraordinary Vessel and Spleen work.

Reproductive tract abnormalities

Approximately 3% of women have a developmental anomaly of the genital tract (Llewellyn-Jones 1990). Examples of such conditions are: double uterus (with or without a double cervix and vagina), bicornuate uterus or septate uterus and/or abnormalities of genital tract, cervix, vagina, malformation of the kidney and ureters (Rabinerson et al 1992, Tindall 1987).

A uterine malformation increases the risk of fetal malpresentation, spontaneous abortion and pre-term labour by four times (Llewellyn-Jones 1990). Some malformations may cause complications in labour.

Cervical incompetence is also common. The use of ultrasound scanning will usually reveal a uterine abnormality. However, if the cervix and vagina are structurally normal, the woman is usually fertile.

Women may also have displacements of the uterus, such as retroverted uterus or prolapsed uterus, which may cause complications. These may be indicated by severe abdominal pain.

Implications for bodywork

- Clients who have a history of miscarriage or pre-term labour may have structural abnormalities of the uterus.
- A less optimal position of a fetus may be due to a malformation of the uterus. Bodywork by a therapist with a goal to encourage optimal fetal positioning would not only be ineffective in changing fetal position but could cause increased risk of harm.
- Fetal positioning at term may affect the progress of labour and determine mode of delivery.
- The therapist needs to be cautious with abdominal work as there is an increased risk of other complications.
- Energy work may include supporting the Extraordinary Vessel energy, especially CV, GV and PV.

Fibroids and cysts

About 5 per 2000 Caucasian women have fibroids (Lewis & Chamberlain 1990), although the number varies among population groups and the incidence is higher in older women. Most fibroids cause little problem apart from pain and tenderness but sometimes they may prevent the descent of the fetus into the pelvis or obstruct labour. With the changes to the endocrine system during pregnancy, fibroids may either increase or decrease in size.

Cysts are less common (1 in 1000). They may obstruct labour if left untreated.

Cysts and fibroids are considered a result of Liver Qi stagnation which could be addressed from the second trimester once the pregnancy has become established.

Cervical incompetence

Cervical incompetence is loss of sphincter control resulting in dilatation or opening of the cervix. Rechberger describes an incompetent cervix as containing more smooth muscle than a normal cervix (Gilbert & Harmon 1993). 'It is usually caused by one of three factors a congenital defect, cervical trauma, or hormonal factors.' (Parisi 1988). It may cause miscarriage, usually in the second trimester, and is the cause of 15–20% of pregnancy losses as well as premature labour. There may be no warning signs of early dilatation in the second trimester and the diagnosis and treatment is given for subsequent pregnancies.

Treatment is to surgically insert a stitch or suture around the cervix – 'cervical cerclage'. Timing varies according to clinical practice with some clinicians believing that early insertion may prevent the miscarriage of an abnormal pregnancy. Risks include increased infection, rupture of the membranes, or onset of premature labour at the time of insertion. Research on the benefits is inconclusive and its use varies; it is not commonly performed in the UK, but is quite common in Canada, France and other European countries. The stitch may be removed in the last few weeks of pregnancy so that spontaneous labour can occur, or may be left in and a caesarean section performed.

Bodywork implications

Pregnancy
- Be alert to any signs of premature labour and refer immediately.
- Techniques utilising deep abdominal strokes, especially downward strokes, should be avoided.
- The woman may be placed on bedrest to diminish activity levels and prevent the weight of the gravid uterus from increasing downward pressure on the cervix. This may occur temporarily in the event of the insertion of a cerclage, or longer term depending on the client's history.
- Exercises such as squats which increase intra-abdominal pressure or downward pressure which could affect the cervix are contraindicated.
  This may include modifications to pelvic floor exercises.
- Visualisations to focus on drawing up and holding in may be appropriate.
- Cervical incompetence is a sign of weak Spleen energy and energy work would have a focus of drawing energy up and strengthening the cervix.

Postnatally Depending on mode of delivery, bodywork to help strengthen the abdominal muscles and pelvic floor may be appropriate. The emphasis of energy work would be work with Spleen and the Extraordinary Vessels, especially Girdle Vessel.

Sexually transmitted infections

Women who are considering becoming pregnant, or who are pregnant, may have a range of optional or mandatory tests which indicate the presence of sexually transmitted infections. Choosing to have such tests done, and/or awaiting results, may create stress for women.

Positive test results may have an impact not only on the woman but on her baby as well. Treatment options and delivery choices may both be affected by the presence of sexually transmitted infections.

Bodywork should not be done in the presence of an active infection and/or fever.

The presence of HIV raises issues regarding treatment possibilities, the type of delivery most suitable for the woman and her baby, and whether breastfeeding is an appropriate form of feeding for the baby.

The therapist needs to be aware of the emotional impact on the client, as well as the possibility that they may have challenging decisions to make. Universal Standards of Infection Control must be applied, especially in the presence of bodily fluids during delivery or during breastfeeding.

Female genital circumcision

Circumcision is still relatively common among some groups of African women (especially women from Nigeria, Ethiopia, Sudan and Egypt). Because of the large immigrant populations in most western countries and the fact that some bodyworkers may be working on the African continent, it is wise to be aware of the implications of this procedure, both emotionally and physically.

There are three main types of circumcision:

1. Simple excision of the clitoral hood and suturing of the labia majora.
2. Removal of the clitoris (clitoridectomy).
3. Infibulation or pharonic circumcision.

The third type is the most extensive and similar to a vulvectomy. The clitoris, labia minora and most of the labia majora are removed and the labial remnants are closed together, leaving a small orifice near the fourchette which allows the escape of urine and menstrual blood.

Although these practices are illegal in many western countries, including the UK and Canada/USA, they are often carried out by a traditional birth attendant illegally or young girls may be sent back to their country of origin for the circumcision. Types 1 and 2 present fewer complications, particularly for the maternity period; however, type 3 may cause major issues. The procedure itself carries a high risk of mortality from haemorrhage and sepsis. Lifelong morbidity from urinary infection, pelvic inflammatory disease, endometriosis and renal damage is common. Cervical smears cannot be obtained and psychological trauma and marital disharmony are common (Jordan 1994).

In pregnancy urinary tract infection is more likely. During labour, progress cannot be assessed by vaginal examination and second stage labour may be prolonged because of the rigidity of the scar tissue.

This may result in fetal hypoxia and brain damage (Thompson 1989). An episiotomy may be needed. If the perineum is not meticulously repaired then faecal incontinence may result, there is likely to be severe damage to the pelvic floor and uterine prolapse is not uncommon. The caregiver must not repair the labia to restore the infibulated state, which is illegal, although they may face pressure from relatives to do so.

14.3 Issues arising during pregnancy

- Hyperemesis gravidarum.
- Hypertensive disorders of pregnancy:
  - Gestational hypertension.
  - Pre-eclampsia.
  - Haemolysis, elevated liver enzymes and low platelet count (HELLP).
- Issues with the placenta;
  - Placenta praevia.
  - Abruptio placentae.
- Coagulation disorders in pregnancy:
  - Disseminated intravascular coagulation (DIC).
- Venous thromboembolism (VTE)/thromboembolic disorders (TED).
- Diabetes.
- Gestational diabetes mellitus (GDM).
- Poly-/oligohydramnios.
- Rho (D) isoimmunisation and ABO incompatibility.
- Infections during pregnancy.
- Renal and bladder conditions.
- Cholelithiasis (gallstones).
- Chromosomal and developmental abnormalities of the fetus.

Hyperemesis gravidarum

This is severe nausea and vomiting, which may be accompanied by ptyalism (excessive salivation) and is pathological. Its exact cause is unclear although it is thought to be related to the endocrine and hormonal changes of pregnancy. The client can become dehydrated and, more seriously, suffer electrolyte disturbances, ketosis and weight loss. Hospitalisation may be necessary if the woman is unable to retain fluids and nutrition and needs to receive them intravenously; otherwise, her condition could deteriorate resulting in liver and renal damage.

It is more likely to occur during the first trimester, although for some women it remains an issue throughout the pregnancy.

Implications for bodywork

- Energy-based techniques could be utilised, especially those that affect PV, SP, ST and LV, or reflex zones.
- A small study of 10 hospitalised women considered the effect of tactile massage for severe nausea and vomiting during pregnancy. After treatments were administered, an open interview was done with subjects commenting that the massage 'helped women obtain a relieving moment of rest access to the whole body when nausea rules life, promoted relaxation, and gave the subject an opportunity to regain access to her body' (Agren & Berg 2006).

Hypertensive disorders of pregnancy

The hypotensive client

Some women have reduced blood pressure, in the region of 110 over 60, throughout their pregnancy. There are no specific bodywork precautions for women with lower blood pressure except to ensure that they get off the table slowly in order to prevent light-headedness or dizziness from occurring. However, extremely low blood pressure may be linked with issues of placental abruption.

Energetic work to the Governing Vessel can be done with focus to GV 20 and an aim to draw energy upwards.

The hypertensive client

Terminology describing hypertensive orders varies within the medical community. The guidelines of the *Journal of Gynaecologists of Canada* are used in this text (Magee et al 2008).

Hypertension can be classified as chronic or existing prior to pregnancy, or may develop within pregnancy or the postpartum.

Gestational hypertension

Gestational hypertension is a diastolic blood pressure (dBP) equal to or greater than 90 mmHg based on at least two measurements, taken using the same arm. Above this level perinatal morbidity is increased in non-proteinuric hypertension.

While dBP is considered a better predictor of adverse pregnancy outcomes than systolic blood pressure (sBP), women with a systolic BP greater than or equal to 140 mmHg 'should be followed closely for development of diastolic hypertension'.

The onset of gestational hypertension usually occurs at or after 20 weeks.

Pregnancy-induced hypertension (PIH) is frequently referred to in the literature. However, the SOGC guidelines advise against using this term because 'its meaning in clinical practice is unclear' (Magee et al 2008).

Women with gestational hypertension of onset before 34 weeks are more likely to develop pre-eclampsia, with rates of about 35%, and the associated risks of serious maternal (2%) and perinatal complications (16%) are high.

Pre-eclampsia

Pre-eclampsia is a multi-system disorder that complicates 3–5% of all pregnancies. It usually arises after 32 weeks but may occur as early as 20–24 weeks (Dietl 2000, Higgins & de Swiet 2001).

The SOGC guidelines define pre-eclampsia as 'a hypertensive disorder most commonly defined by new-onset proteinuria, and potentially, other end-organ dysfunction'.

Oedema used to be included as one sign of pre-eclampsia but now is considered a feature of normal pregnancy, although it is a different type of oedema when linked with pre-eclampsia. Weight gain is also not included in the definition of pre-eclampsia.

Pre-eclampsia may develop into eclampsia. However, with adequate monitoring and treatment it rarely reaches this level of severity. Once an initial assessment has been made, through elevated blood pressure and proteinuria, further tests are undertaken to assess renal function, thrombocytopenia and liver enzymes.

Eclampsia is assessed with extreme oedema occurring throughout the body including the face, eyelids and neck and onset of headaches, visual disturbances, followed by seizures. The onset of convulsions (although in 38% cases there were no signs of pre-eclampsia) in the UK occurs about once in every 2000 births and represents severe risks to mother and fetus. Of these, 1 in 50 women died and 1 in 14 babies also died (Douglas & Redman 1994).

Eclampsia is characterised by decreased perfusion to all organ systems secondary to vasospasm (narrowing of the blood vessels). There is arteriolar vasoconstriction and disseminated intravascular coagulation (DIC). The effects are seen in the kidney, liver and placental bed. Other features of PET may include central nervous system irritability and at times coagulation or liver function abnormalities.

Past medical history
- Previous pre-eclampsia.
- Pre-existing medical conditions such as hypertension, diabetes, or renal disease.
- Family history of pre-eclampsia (mother, sister, grandmother).
- Obesity (30% body mass index (BMI)).

- History of autoimmune disorders such as lupus, rheumatoid arthritis or multiple sclerosis.

Current pregnancy
- Multiple pregnancy.
- First pregnancy.
- Inter-pregnancy interval greater than or equal to 10 years.
- Booking sBP greater than or equal to 130 mmHg.
- Booking dBP greater than or equal to 80 mmHg.
- Polycystic ovarian syndrome.
- Polyhydramnios.

Additional factors
- Over 40 or under 18 years of age.
- Smoker.
- Cocaine and methamphetamine use.
- Reproductive technologies.
- Excessive weight gain in pregnancy.
- Infection during pregnancy, e.g. UTI.

'Women are classified as low or increased risk based on the existence of one or more markers which vary in their weight of importance' (SOGC).

Causes
Because pre-eclampsia refers to a set of symptoms rather than any causative factor, there are various theories about the causes for pre-eclampsia:

1. *Uterine underperfusion, i.e. inadequate blood flow to the placenta*: possibly due to an inadequate remodelling of maternal uterine spiral arteries (development of blood vessels to placenta). This is related to how the placenta is formed in early pregnancy.

2. *Hormonal changes*: includes disruptions of prostacyclin/thromboxane which maintain the diameter of the blood vessels, the renin-angiotensin system, and factors influencing retention of salt and water such as antidiuretic/vasopressin hormones from the pituitary gland and aldosterone from the adrenal gland (Chamberlain 1991).

3. *Immunological factors* have been studied and there is evidence that genetic dissimilarity of the father and mother plays an important role. It is more common in first pregnancies; even if the first pregnancy resulted in abortion there is a reduced risk in subsequent pregnancies.

4. Pre-existing maternal conditions; described above in risk factors.

5. It may be more common in humid rather than dry conditions (Makhseed et al 1999) because of changes in fluid levels.
6. Insufficient magnesium oxide and B6. Magnesium stabilises vascular smooth muscles and helps regulate vascular tone.
7. Calcium deficiency.
8. Nutritional problems and poor diet.
9. Endothelial activation and dysfunction; damage to the lining of blood vessels.
10. Dietary aspects; there is a connection between long-chain omega 3 fatty acids (present in oily fish and certain oils), low dietary calcium and the development of pre-eclampsia (Odent 1994).

Treatment

Activity levels may be restricted at home, the woman may be monitored by clinic or hospital day units, or she may be placed in hospital on modified bedrest. Total activity restriction is not advised. SOGC states that there is 'insufficient evidence' to state the efficacy of bedrest, workload restriction, stress reduction or reduction in exercise levels although these lifestyle suggestions are often given to the pregnant patient who is experiencing elevated blood pressure.

Women with severe pre-eclampsia or severe hypertension will be hospitalised.

Treatment for women with severe hypertension (BP > 160 mmHg systolic or > or equal to 110 mmHg diastolic) will entail decreasing blood pressure using anti-hypertensive drugs. The fetal heart rate is monitored until the blood pressure is stabilised.

Blood pressure medications will also be utilised for non-severe hypertension with or without co-morbid conditions (SOGC S4). Magnesium sulphate may be utilised in cases of eclampsia or in some cases of non-severe pre-eclampsia and is administered intravenously.

For women who have been diagnosed with pre-eclampsia prior to 34 weeks antenatal corticosteroid therapy may be given in order to accelerate the lung maturity of the fetus in case of possible pre-term delivery.

Method of delivery

The aim is to continue pregnancy as long as the blood pressure is stable, but delivery may be initiated if deemed necessary. Vaginal delivery may occur with or without induction depending on the medical state of the woman, but a caesarean section may be considered.

Walker (2000) suggests that prior to 32 weeks caesarean section is appropriate and after 34 weeks vaginal delivery should be aimed for. Epidural anaesthesia or other anaesthesia methods are suggested

methods of pain relief provided no contraindications exist for their usage.

Blood pressure will also be closely monitored in the days and weeks following delivery for the woman who has experienced blood pressure issues.

Haemolysis, elevated liver enzymes and low platelet count (HELLP)

HELLP syndrome occurs in 4–12% of women who have pre-eclampsia and its incidence is reported as 0.2–0.6% of all pregnancies. HELLP usually begins during the third trimester but may occur in the second trimester or in the postpartum. HELLP is a life-threatening condition that can affect the lungs, heart, liver and kidneys, as well as causing possible intrauterine growth restriction, placental issues and premature birth.

The outcome for mothers with HELLP syndrome is generally good with treatment and maternal mortality is about 1%.

HELLP is a variant of pre-eclampsia characterised by abnormal liver function and *thrombocytopenia* (i.e. reduced platelet (thrombocyte) count). The term HELLP comes from this syndrome's characteristic clinical findings:

H – haemolysis (the breakdown of red blood cells).

EL – elevated liver enzymes.

LP – low platelet count.

The symptoms of HELLP syndrome are liver (upper right quadrant abdominal pain) and right shoulder pain. There also may be a gradual but marked onset of headaches (30%), blurred vision, malaise (90%), nausea/vomiting (30%), and tingling in the extremities. HELLP syndrome is dangerous because it can occur before the mother exhibits the classic symptoms of pre-eclampsia and be mistaken for the flu or gallbladder issues.

If untreated, rupture of the liver capsule and a resultant haematoma may occur.

Disseminated intravascular coagulation (DIC) is seen in about 20% of all women with HELLP (Sibai et al 1993) syndrome and in 84% HELLP is complicated by acute renal failure (Sibai & Ramadan 1993). Arterial hypertension is a diagnostic requirement but may be mild, therefore if HELLP is suspected, blood tests, liver enzyme, renal function, electrolyte and coagulation tests are performed.

The exact cause of HELLP is unknown, but general activation of the coagulation cascade is considered the main underlying problem.

Treatment

The only effective treatment is delivery of the baby. Several medications have been investigated for the treatment of HELLP syndrome, but evidence is conflicting as to whether magnesium sulphate decreases the risk of seizures and progress to eclampsia. DIC is treated with fresh frozen plasma to replenish the coagulation proteins, and anaemia may require blood transfusion. In mild cases, corticosteroids and antihypertensives may be sufficient. Intravenous fluids are generally required.

Implications for bodyworkers

- Every maternity client should be asked what their most recent blood pressure is at every visit and the response recorded.
- If the therapist has been trained and is skilled in accurate blood pressure assessment, they should maintain consistency of client positioning and arm measured, utilisation of an accurately calibrated BP device, and consistency of the phase assessed as per recommendations for standardised blood pressure technique (SOGC S9).
- If the therapist has any reason to suspect their client has developed symptoms that may indicate onset or exacerbation of hypertension, they should refer the client to their primary care provider immediately. If bodywork is deemed appropriate then:
  - Specific symptoms of headache, blurred vision, dizziness, right upper quadrant or abdominal pain, sudden weight gain, or sudden increase in oedema should be reported to the primary care provider immediately.
  - Contraindications include any treatment application that increases stress, overstimulates the client, creates pain, overburdens a circulatory system that is already compromised due to elevated blood pressure. This includes techniques such as lymphatic drainage and repetitive flushing strokes such as effleurage.
  - Any treatment that could exacerbate other existing adverse symptoms affecting either the mother or the fetus should be avoided.
  - The environment of the treatment should be as calming and relaxing as possible – dimmed lights, quiet with no interruptions and minimal discussion.
  - In energy work, high dBP indicates a failure of Kidney energy, often linked with Liver energy rising (headaches, dizziness and heat), abdominal tightness (Girdle Vessel) and Spleen energy failing to descend. This affects the Heart Meridian. It is useful to work these meridians even in extreme cases, provided the woman is in the hospital for medical care.
  - Energy work to balance the GV and CV may be helpful including their opening and associated

points. GV 20 may be worked with a focus on sending energy downward.
- Kidney, Conception Vessel and Governing Vessel: work palming downwards from GV 20 to Uterus. Palming up the legs along SP and KD. Girdle Vessel, Heart-Uterus, Kidney-Uterus, Penetrating Vessel. Some gantle work to release the neck and shoulders.
- Preliminary studies are being performed to determine the effects of bodywork for clients with high blood pressure but randomised controlled studies have yet to be completed.

Issues with the placenta

About 4% of all pregnant women experience some type of vaginal bleeding during the third trimester of pregnancy, with the major cause being placental abruption and placenta praevia (Gilbert & Harmon 1993: 321).

Placenta praevia

This occurs when the placenta implants in the lower part of the uterus (LUS), rather than the upper uterine segment (UUS). It is assessed through ultrasound. As the pregnancy progresses, the growth of the placental site tends to move away from the internal os of the cervix. The incidence of placenta praevia at term is around 0.5–1%, although for women with grand multiparity (more than four pregnancies) the incidence may be as high as 2% (Henderson & Macdonald 2004: 769).

With placenta praevia, particularly towards term, 'the lower segment of the uterus becomes elongated and the cervix begins to dilate and efface which can cause tearing or a separation of the placenta and result in bleeding' (Gilbert & Harmon 1993: 330).

Cases where the placenta overlies the internal os carry the greatest risk of haemorrhage (Sanderson & Milton 1991). Placenta praevia is classified according to the degree that the placenta covers the cervix and is described as marginal, partial or complete.

With a low-lying placenta, depending on its proximity to the cervix the woman may be able to labour naturally and a trial of vaginal labour may be allowed if the placenta is > 2.5 cm away from the cervix.

Complete placenta praevia (with the placenta fully covering the cervix) is a clear indicator for caesarean section in order to prevent maternal haemorrhage and fetal hypoxia.

Table 14.1 lists some causes of placenta praevia, and the reasons why it may occur.

Placental abruption or abruptio placentae

This is the separation of a normally implanted placenta at any stage of pregnancy or labour. It will result in bleeding that may be concealed, apparent,

Table 14.1 Causes of placenta praevia

Cause	Reason
Multiparity	The increased size of the uterine cavity may predispose to placenta praevia
Multiple pregnancy	A larger placental site is more likely to encroach upon the internal os
Age	Older mothers are at more risk, possibly due to the increase in other factors such as multiparity, scarring, etc.
Scarred uterus	This limits places for the blastocyst to embed. It can be due to: – previous caesarean section – previous uterine surgery or fibroids
Smoking	Pregnant women who smoke more than 20 cigarettes a day are twice as likely to develop placenta praevia

or a combination of both. The severity of the bleeding is defined as mild, moderate or severe. Concealed bleeding, due to bleeding occurring internally within the placenta, presents more complications as there is no visible blood loss, but pain and shock may be severe as intrauterine tension rises. It may become life threatening before a diagnosis is made. Signs of severe abdominal pain and a hard uterus could be present along with maternal hypotension and fetal distress.

Causes

The cause is unknown but there are risk factors associated with placental abruption. Maternal hypertension is the most consistent finding.

Risk factors

- Essential hypertension.
- Pre-eclampsia.
- Premature rupture of the membranes, especially if there was excessive fluid (polyhydramnios) as this may cause a sudden change of pressure in the uterus.
- Previous history of placental abruption.
- Trauma, for example following external cephalic version, road traffic accident, a fall or a blow.
- Smoking.
- Illegal drug use, e.g. cocaine, crack cocaine, marijuana.
- Folic acid deficiency (although this has not been confirmed).
- Placental abnormality.

Implications for bodywork

- Bleeding, abdominal pain and high or extremely low blood pressure are all potential indicators of placental issues and require immediate medical referral with no bodywork.
- If there is complete placenta praevia (type IV) a caesarean section will be needed.
- Once the immediate emergency situation has resolved then it may be possible to work. *Extreme caution* is required for abdominal work and any work should be on the level of light energy techniques with no physical work.
- Most early diagnoses of placenta praevia, with no history of bleeding, resolve by term and present no complications. For these clients moderate caution should be applied with regard to bodywork but in many cases the pregnancy and labour will proceed normally.
- Care needs to be taken with treating the legs, particularly with respect to using mobilisations and stretches which may be contraindicated due to their effect on the pelvis.
- Deep physical work to the lower back or sacrum should be avoided, with techniques being more energy based as the sacral nerve plexus innervates the uterus.
- It is best to focus bodywork on relaxation rather than on postural realignment.
- Energy techniques to support the CV and PV, GDV and Spleen may be appropriate but it is better to do work in areas other than the abdomen.

Placenta praevia
- No exercise should be done which puts downward pressure on the abdomen or pelvic floor or which increases intra-abdominal pressure (such as squats or strong standing exercises).
- Energy work may be done with a focus of encouraging the placenta to move away from the internal os. Spleen is particularly indicated.

Cervical bleeding/undiagnosed bleeding Sometimes no cause can be established for the bleeding even after extensive medical assessment. Establish what guidelines have been given regarding activity level, and modify work accordingly. Exercise suggestions and work to the abdomen are especially likely to need to be modified.

Coagulation disorders

This covers a range of disorders ranging from mild to more severe; 'venous thromboembolism remains a major cause of morbidity and mortality in pregnancy and the postpartum period' (Kent et al 2000). The risk of thromboembolic disorders (TED) is five times greater than in non-pregnancy (from 0.6 to 3 in 1000 pregnant woman) (De Swiet 1985).

This issue is particularly relevant given that the overall maternal mortality rate has significantly diminished in the developed world. There were 35 deaths caused by TED in the UK in 1997–9 (Lewis 2001). Of these 13 were in pregnancy (eight in the first trimester), seven following a caesarean and 10 following vaginal delivery (Gates 2000).

Friend & Kakkar (1970) estimate that deep vein thrombosis (DVT) is less common than thrombosis in superficial veins. About two-thirds of thromboembolitic disorders occur antenatally and one third postpartum. The onset of thrombophlebitis is three times more likely to occur in the postpartum period than antenatally because of postnatal changes in blood flow accompanied by reduced mobility and is higher following instrumental delivery, which may cause injury to blood vessels (Arafeh 1997, Bennhagen & Holmberg 1989).

Risk factors for all thromboembolic disorders

The risk of TED increases with:

- Each subsequent pregnancy.
- Increasing age.
- Lack of mobilisation.
- Obesity.
- Use of oral contraceptives prior to becoming pregnant.
- Sedentary work.
- History of a TED either prior to or during pregnancy: chance of recurrence is 5–30%.
- Pregnancy-induced hypertension (PIH).
- Vascular expansion anaemia.
- Artificial heart valves.
- Bed rest, dehydration or family history during the first trimester of pregnancy.

Risk factors postnatally include:

- Operative delivery; the risk is 3–16 times higher among women with caesarean than vaginal births.
- Dehydration following delivery.

Ambulation following delivery reduces the risk.

Thrombophlebitis

This is a thrombus in a superficial vein. The most common site of thrombus formation is in the saphenous vein supplying the calf of the leg on the left side.

Symptoms

Include a tender reddened area over the vein that has a thrombus with possibly a small increase in pulse and temperature. Motility and elevation of the legs at rest can reduce the risk of thrombus formation.

Treatment

Compression stockings may be helpful and can be prescribed by the primary care provider. Thrombophlebitis is unlikely to progress to pulmonary embolism as it is in a more superficial vein but bodyworkers still need to refer as drug treatment may be required.

Deep vein thrombosis

This is a thrombus in a deep vein. DVT is less common but carries the risk of the clot dislodging which can cause pulmonary embolism. It has been observed clinically that there is an increased risk of DVT in the left leg especially after caesarean section because blood flow velocity is reduced to a greater extent following surgical intervention.

Diagnosis

A positive diagnosis has implications for subsequent contraception and future pregnancies. The oestrogen-containing contraceptive pill is contraindicated and prophylactic anticoagulation will be required in any subsequent pregnancy.

Clinical signs

DVT may not display any symptoms or the woman may experience pain or tenderness in the calf, swelling over the affected area, which may be reddened (erythema), and occasionally pyrexia (fever). There may be marked differences in calf size or in extreme cases circulation to the leg below the thrombosis may be affected so that the leg appears cold, white and possibly oedematous.

Pain may be elicited with dorsal flexion of the foot (Homan's sign (Knuppel); see p. 197) but it is not a reliable test to determine a positive or negative indication of a DVT. Referral is necessary for diagnostic testing using a Doppler ultrasound, impedance plethysmography, ascending phlebography or isotope venography.

Treatment

Women assessed to be at increased risk for thrombus formation are treated with prophylactic anticoagulants such as heparin. Warfarin is contraindicated during pregnancy. Treatment is usually stopped prior to labour and resumed in the early postpartum until the acute signs are resolved (Howie 1995).

Pulmonary embolism (PE)

Pulmonary embolism occurs when a thrombus dislodges and travels to the lungs. This is an obstetric emergency that may follow DVT without warning. Pulmonary embolism is a condition that contributes towards maternal mortality associated with pregnancy. If a thrombosis breaks away and enters the venous system it is then carried to the right side of the heart and the pulmonary circulation. As the pulmonary arteries reduce in size the thrombus may occlude an arterial vessel within the lungs causing major damage. Symptoms are sudden collapse, acute severe chest pain, dyspnoea, cyanosis, haemoptysis and shock. A woman with PE will require intensive treatment and care. It occurs in 1–2 in 2000 pregnancies and is a major cause of maternal mortality (Hathaway & Bonnar 1987).

Disseminated intravascular coagulation (DIC)

DIC is an unregulated activation of the extrinsic or intrinsic pathways of coagulation which leads to persistent thrombin generation and fibrin production in circulating blood. This causes intravascular thrombosis formation, tissue hypoxia, activation of the fibrinolytic pathways, depletion of coagulation factors, inability to maintain haemostasis and overt bleeding. It is an extremely serious condition requiring immediate referral as it can lead to maternal and fetal death. It is usually associated with other complications such as: placental abruption, pre-eclampsia, intrauterine fetal death, amniotic fluid embolism and septic abortion (Arafeh 1997, De Boer et al 1989, Scholl et al 1992). Drug treatment will be required or in extreme cases, massive blood transfusions of stored blood.

Implications for bodyworkers

- Awareness of the client's potential risk factors is essential and should be determined during case history gathering and assessment.
- If the client presents with suspected blood clotting concerns she should be referred to her primary care provider immediately, with no bodywork.
- Once medical treatment has begun, dialogue with the primary care provider should occur to determine the appropriate time to recommence bodywork. Blood-thinning drugs may increase the risk of bruising and tissue damage so gentle work would be more appropriate.

Gestational diabetes mellitus (GDM)

GDM is defined as a carbohydrate intolerance 'characterised by the inability to produce or use sufficient endogenous insulin to metabolise glucose properly' (Gilbert & Harmon 1993: 178). It is due to the inability of the maternal pancreas to increase insulin secretion enough to counter the pregnancy-induced insulin resistance. This is probably due to limitations of the pancreatic beta cells. It occurs in 2–3% of pregnancies in the US (Borg & Sherwin 2000).

Women who suffer from GDM have an increased risk for later development of diabetes, primarily type 2. The risk is greater with weight gain after pregnancy or GDM in a subsequent pregnancy. Regular exercise and dietary modifications may help prevent future complications from diabetes.

Education in diet, glucose monitoring, and treatment with insulin if necessary, along with close monitoring of the fetus will be the primary care received by the diabetic woman.

An emphasis is placed on foods high in nutritional value consisting of complex carbohydrates and proteins rather than those high in sugar or fat or of limited nutritional value.

High levels of blood glucose increase risk of miscarriage, pre-eclampsia, pre-term labour, polyhydramnios and infection. For the fetus there is an increased risk of fetal distress or macrosomia due to potential placental insufficiency. A large baby with more fat may make delivery more difficult and be a cause of heart problems. There may be issues related to low fetal blood glucose at birth.

Depending on how well the diabetic condition is controlled and whether the woman has any additional complications, she may be able to deliver at term, may be induced, or delivered by caesarean section.

Symptoms of GDM

- Increased thirst.
- Increased urination.
- Sweet-smelling breath.

Labour

The aim is to keep blood sugar levels stable during labour. Blood glucose levels will be checked hourly and the rate of insulin infusion will be adjusted accordingly (Gillmer & Hurley 1999). Continuous fetal monitoring is likely, either with EFM or with a fetal scalp electrode, because of the increased risk of fetal distress or hypoxia. If the blood sugar level of the woman is stable intermittent fetal monitoring may be deemed sufficient.

Postpartum

Maternal insulin requirements can fall sharply after delivery and so the mother needs to be monitored for hypoglycaemia. The mother is encouraged to monitor her glucose levels carefully if breastfeeding. She may need additional carbohydrates of about 50 g per day (De Swiet 1995) with long-acting insulin at night to prevent nocturnal hypoglycaemia. 'Insulin does not cross into breast milk, however elevated blood glucose levels will be present in the breast milk if the mother's blood glucose level is high' (Gilbert & Harmon 1993: 206).

Care must be taken to monitor the postpartum woman for infection due to the effect of diabetes on the circulation. Any sign of vaginal, urinary, or incisional infection should be reported immediately to the primary care provider. Hygiene is also important.

Implications for bodyworkers

- When blood sugar levels have stabilised or the client has been advised by their primary care provider to maintain a moderate to normal level of exercise, bodywork can be an adjunctive tool to encourage self-care and minimise stress in pregnancy, labour and the postpartum.
- 'Exercise can affect glucose control and insulin sensitivity' (Gilbert & Harmon 1993: 197). Massage may also have this effect and the client needs to be informed that there may be fluctuations in their blood sugar levels in the 24 hours following bodywork and to monitor this.
- For the client with fluctuating blood sugar levels only gentle, localised, non-stimulating techniques are utilised. Techniques challenging to the circulatory system are avoided.
- For the client being treated with subcutaneous injections of insulin, massage to injection sites may be contraindicated because of sensitivity or discomfort in these areas.
- Therapists should have snack supplies on hand in the event that a diabetic client feels a change in their blood sugar level. Peanut butter, crackers, apples or orange juice may be helpful.
- Work to the Spleen, Stomach and Penetrating Vessel may help regulate blood sugar levels. ST 36 may be a useful point.

Issues related to amniotic fluid

Polyhydramnios is excess amniotic fluid (more than 2000 ml). It occurs more frequently in women with GDM; 10% of all diabetic women (Gilbert & Harmon 1993: 187). Polyhydramnios causes an increase in osmotic pressure and may be associated with premature rupture of the membranes and an increased incidence of fetal anomalies.

Oligohydramnios describes too little or decreased amniotic fluid (less than 500 ml). It is associated with post-term pregnancies (Leveno et al 1984, Silver 1987). This can cause issues for the fetus due to the diminishment of the cushioning effect for the baby and may be related to impaired fetal renal function.

Biophysical profiles (BPP) monitor the level of amniotic fluid volume in the uterus, and amniocentesis is also done to assess fetal well-being.

Implications for bodywork

- In cases where abnormal levels of amniotic fluid exist, abdominal massage may be contraindicated as the application of pressure may be inappropriate given issues related to fetal or maternal well-being.
- For the therapist experienced in energy work, Water Energy and Essence may help regulate fluid. Meridian work may be done on Bladder, Kidney, Heart Protector and Triple Heater:

BL 23 benefits Kidney
BL 25 benefits Bladder
BL 22 benefits Triple Heater
CV 4 benefits Essence.

Rho (D) isoimmunisation and ABO incompatibility

Rho(D) isoimmunisation occurs when a Rho (D) negative mother carrying a Rho (D) positive fetus produces antibody against the D antigen on the fetal RBC. This can trigger isoimmune haemolytic disease in the fetus (haemolytic disease of the newborn (HDN) or erythroblastosis fetalis). The effects of this may be minimal or may include severe anaemia, congestive heart failure and death. As the maternal antibody remains in the infant's circulation, this haemolytic process continues after birth. In many countries, the mother is given a blood product known as (D) immune globulin (RhIG) to stop her producing the antibody.

Isoimmunisation is rare in first pregnancies as the small amounts of fetal blood that cross the placenta and enter the maternal circulation are usually too small to trigger the production of antibodies by the woman's immune system, although approximately 1–2% of Rho (D) negative women develop anti-D antibodies during their first pregnancy (Crowther & Middleton 1999).

With delivery and placental separation, larger quantities of fetal blood may enter the maternal circulation and stimulate formation of anti-D antibody and memory cells resulting in lifelong immunisation. During subsequent pregnancies even small amounts of blood may be enough to trigger memory cells to produce antibodies against the D antigen on the fetal RBC. With each subsequent pregnancy the maternal immune system often responds more rapidly and intensely. However, overall the incidence of Rho (D) isoimmunisation is relatively low, ranging from 10–14% if the (D) immune globulin (RhIG) is not given after delivery to less than 2% if RhIG is given (Blackburn 1985). Fetal Rh status can be determined by polymer chain reaction analysis of amniotic fluid or chorionic villous samples, both of which are invasive procedures.

RhIG may be given prophylactically at 28–30 weeks to prevent immunisation during pregnancy or after any potential immunisation events such as abortion, ectopic pregnancy, amniocentesis or significant antenatal bleeding. A dose of RhiG given at 28 weeks gives protection until term. It acts by destroying fetal RBCs in the mother's system before the foreign D antigen can be recognised by her immune system. After birth it is generally given within 72 hours.

Routine use of anti D in all RhO (D) negative women is controversial as many women need to be treated who may not have developed immunisation, in order to prevent some cases developing. The Cochrane review (Crowther & Middleton 1999) indicates that more research needs to be done on the benefits and possible risks.

Implications for bodywork

Rhesus negative women face additional choices in their pregnancy on whether to have anti-D, especially in a first pregnancy. While the therapist cannot advise them in their choice of treatment, they need to be alert to supporting them during this potentially stressful time.

Maternal infection and disease

Pregnant women have increased susceptibility to influenza, varicella, rubella, herpes, listeriosis, hepatitis and human papillomavirus. Pregnancy-induced suppression of helper T-cell numbers may be permanent so pregnancy can cause a progression of HIV-related disease. Both acute and chronic maternal infections are associated with pre-term labour and there is increasing evidence of the role of vaginal and cervical organisms and chorioamnionitis in the initiation of pre-term labour and premature rupture of the membranes (Lockwood & Kuczynski 1999). If the mother is actively experiencing symptoms such as fever, then she is likely to be receiving antibiotic treatment.

Any acute maternal illness, particularly with a high temperature, may cause a miscarriage. This may be due to the general metabolic effect of a high fever or the result of transplacental passage of viruses. Influenza, rubella, appendicitis, pyelonephritis, pneumonia, toxoplasmosis, cytomegalovirus, listeriosis, syphilis and brucellosis may all cause abortion. Other medical disorders which may cause abortion include diabetes, thyroid disease, renal disease and hypertensive disorders.

Hepatitis

The baby will be given immunoglobulin and hepatitis B vaccination within 12 hours of birth.

Herpes

The mother will most likely be advised to have a caesarean section if there are active herpes lesions as it can be transmitted to the baby.

Group B streptococcus (GBS)

Women may need intravenous antibiotic therapy in labour or following rupture of the membranes to reduce the incidence of transmission. The standard practice in Canada is to routinely screen women at 35 weeks and to treat all those with PROM (premature rupture of membranes) or when in active labour (www.gbss.org.uk).

Chorea gravidarum

This condition is related to streptococcal infections and is most common in women with a history of rheumatic fever or heart disease. It consists of rapid, brief non-rhythmical, involuntary, jerky movements of the limbs and non-patterned facial grimacing. The incidence is 1 in 139 000 women. It may be associated with pre-eclampsia (Palanivelu 2007).

Implications for bodywork

Bodywork is generally contraindicated in the event of acute infection or fever. However, during labour, the therapist must consider whether localised bodywork could be done without increasing risk of harm while acting as a calming or supportive measure. No modalities should be used that could affect the circulatory system.

Energy work to nurture the connection between the mother and her baby may be appropriate along with techniques to help support a progressing labour. Energy work may also be done to support the immune system with attention to GV/CV and lung meridians.

Renal and bladder conditions

Urinary tract infections

Urinary tract infections (UTIs) are relatively common in pregnancy and if left untreated can progress to more serious issues affecting the bladder or kidneys and may be implicated in onset of pre-term labour. Bacteriuria in the urinary tract may be asymptomatic or symptomatic and urinary cultures are necessary to determine the presence of bacteria indicating infection. Medical treatment is usually with antibiotics. Cystitis is also relatively common due to engorgement of vessels in the pelvis.

Implications for bodywork

- Be aware of the symptoms: increased urgency, frequency, burning or pain with urination, low back or suprapubic pain.

- Signs of fever, chills, nausea, vomiting, malaise or flank pain may indicate the presence of kidney infection (pyelonephritis).
- If there are mild symptoms, then it may be possible for bodywork to proceed but the client should report to the primary care provider immediately afterwards.
- If the symptoms are more severe then immediate referral will be required.
- In milder cases, and to support in post medical treatment recovery, energy work may be done to help strengthen the BL and KD meridians and to support the immune system.
- The client should be advised about the importance of maintaining adequate hydration.

Renal disease

Renal disease may develop as a result of increased complications of the pregnancy such as with lupus, hypertensive disorders of the pregnancy, or with diabetes. Investigations related to renal function will be done and appropriate treatment will be given. Undiagnosed renal issues could lead to maternal mortality and IUGR or intrauterine fetal death and need to be recognised as soon as possible.

Digestive tract

Cholelithiasis (gallstones)

With an incidence of around 5–6%, this is the second most common non-obstetric surgical problem in pregnancy (acute appendicitis is the most common; Tsimoyiannis et al 1994). It is often the cause of pancreatitis. Elevated progesterone and oestrogen may be aggravating factors, along with increased bile stasis. Symptoms are nausea and vomiting and acute abdominal pain.

Biliary colic may be experienced. This is a crampy right upper abdominal pain that comes and goes repeatedly, due to gallstone in the gallbladder or anywhere along the pathway of the ducts that connect the gallbladder to the liver and small intestine.

Implications for bodywork
- Know the signs of biliary colic and refer immediately if suspected.
- Once the acute stage is completed bodywork may proceed.

Obstetric cholestasis (OC)

This is sometimes called 'cholestasis of pregnancy', or 'intrahepatic cholestasis of pregnancy' ('ICP'). It affects about 1 in 200 pregnant women each year in the UK, but may be slightly more common in women of Asian origin (Williamson et al 2004).

OC affects the liver, which in some women seems to be oversensitive to pregnancy hormones. The flow of bile into the intestines is reduced and bile salts build up in the blood. The excess bile salts are excreted through the sweat glands, causing itchiness (pruritis).

It usually occurs after 28 weeks of pregnancy and the first symptoms are extreme itching in the palms of the hands and soles of the feet (as they contain many sweat glands). It is often worse at night; so can result in fatigue and insomnia. It can become generalised. Some women are made so desperate by the itching that they scratch themselves until their skin is bleeding. Less commonly, women can develop jaundice. The itching completely disappears within a couple of weeks of giving birth. Other symptoms include dark urine, light stools and loss of appetite.

In most cases it is benign but it is associated with an increased risk of 15% of having a still birth and premature delivery. Nobody is quite sure why. It is hypothesised that the cause of death may be due to the increased bile salts affecting the fetal liver or as a result of sudden oxygen deprivation, perhaps due to placental problems.

Mothers with OC may be at risk of bleeding after the birth as they may have low levels of vitamin K. In some hospitals the mother is given vitamin K daily by mouth until delivery to protect her.

Diagnosis

Blood tests include a bile acid test and a liver function test. If these tests are negative but the mother is still itching, they are repeated. This is important as it is known that mothers may itch for some time before testing positive for OC.

Treatment

Two drugs are currently used to manage OC. Ursodeoxycholic acid is favoured in the specialist centres for OC as it appears to eliminate or reduce the itching and can result in the liver function and bile acid results returning to normal. Steroids (in particular dexamethasone) are sometimes used in cases of premature labour to mature the fetal lungs prior to inducing labour.

The principal aim of treatment for the fetus is to eliminate the risk of stillbirth by delivering them as soon as the lungs are mature enough to survive outside the womb. This usually means delivery of the baby between 35 and 38 weeks. If women with OC have their labour induced at this time their babies are very likely to survive, while if pregnancy is allowed to continue to 40 weeks the risk of stillbirth increases.

Implications for bodywork
- It is fairly common for pregnant women to experience some itching due to the changes in the

skin, especially around the abdomen. The therapist should be aware, however, if the client complains of very intense itching, especially around the hands and feet, as this may indicate obstetric cholestasis. Bodywork can proceed but refer the mother for accurate diagnosis.

- Bodywork may help ease symptoms but depending on the level of lesions, Swedish massage may not be the most appropriate method. The therapist should not work over any open lesions and use of gloves should be considered. Lubricants such as oil may aggravate the condition. Oat baths seem to help improve it.
- Energy work may be a more appropriate option; work to Liver and the Extraordinary Vessels Meridian is especially indicated.
- If the client is going to be induced bodywork can be used with the aim of supporting this process.

14.4 Chromosomal and developmental abnormalities of the fetus

Ectopic pregnancy

The Andalusian Arabic physician Abulcasis (936–1013) was the first to describe ectopic pregnancy. It occurs when the fertilised egg implants outside the uterine cavity. In 95% of cases this occurs in the fallopian tubes and is known as a tubal pregnancy. Occasionally the egg may implant in the ovaries, abdominal cavity or cervical canal, but this is very rare. The incidence of tubal pregnancy is 1 per 150 and varies geographically. In the West Indies 1 pregnancy in 28 is ectopic, while abdominal pregnancy is more common in African countries and cervical pregnancy is more common in Japan (Lewis & Chamberlain 1990, Stabile & Grudzinskas 1990).

Ectopic pregnancy is the major cause of maternal death before 20 weeks gestation in the industrialised world.

Tubal pregnancy

Its incidence is increasing – a two- to threefold increase has been reported in the past 25 years (Kadar 1999). This is thought to be largely due to the increasing incidence of sexually transmitted disease, the widespread use of the progestogen-only oral contraceptive pill and the intrauterine contraceptive device and the trend towards delaying pregnancy until later. Tubal pregnancy occurs when there is a delay in the transport of the zygote along the fallopian tube. This may be due to a congenital malformation of the fallopian tubes or more commonly scarring due to uterine

infection. The ovum implants and starts to grow in the tube. The conceptus is frequently abnormal and there is a higher incidence of 'blighted ovum' (Stabile & Grudzinskas 1990).

Risk factors

- Older mother.
- Mother of lower gravidity or parity.
- Tubal surgery.
- Hormonal stimulation of ovulation.
- Salpingitis (inflammation of the fallopian tubes), especially caused by chlamydial infections.
- Intrauterine contraceptive device.
- In vitro fertilisation.
- Tubal endometriosis.
- History of pelvic inflammatory disease.
- Appendectomy.
- Pelvic or abdominal surgery.
- Progesterone-only pill (appears to have a detrimental effect on tubal ciliation and peristalsis).

Diagnosis

This can be difficult as it may appear to be similar to pelvic inflammatory disease or threatened abortion. Delay in treatment may contribute to maternal mortality and morbidity. Diagnosis is made by measuring serum progesterone levels which tend to be low. Together with low or falling hCG levels this is strongly suggestive of ectopic gestation. Ultrasound may reveal fluid in the pelvis and the absence of an intrauterine pregnancy (Tin Chiu et al 1999).

As the conceptus develops the tube distends. Initially the woman will experience the usual signs of pregnancy such as nausea and breast tenderness although amenorrhoea is not always present. The uterus will soften and enlarge under the influence of pregnancy hormones. As the tube distends, the woman will experience abdominal pain and some vaginal bleeding. She may also experience pain and bleeding during/following intercourse. If the site of implantation is near the narrower proximal end of the tube, rupture is likely to occur between week 5 and week 7 of pregnancy. If it is located in the wider ampullary section the gestation may continue until week 10. Occasionally the gestational sac is expelled from the fimbriated end of the tube as a tubal abortion.

As the ovum separates from its attachment to the ampullary part of the tube, layers of blood may be deposited around the dead ovum to form a mass of blood clot similar to a uterine carneous mole – this is called a tubal mole. It may remain in the uterine tube or be expelled from the fimbriate end of the tube as a tubal abortion.

When the tube ruptures there will be severe intra-peritoneal haemorrhage and the woman will experience intense abdominal pain. There may also be referred pain as shoulder tip pain on lying down as blood tracks up to the diaphragm. The woman will appear pale, shocked and nauseous and may collapse. This is an acute surgical emergency and requires immediate treatment.

Treatment

If the tube ruptures then it will need to be removed. If the condition is detected in the early stages and before tubal rupture conservative management may be attempted with local injection of prostaglandins.

Implications for bodywork

- Know potential symptoms of tubal issues so that immediate referral can be made.
- Goals would be to support recovery after emergency treatment.

Hydatidiform mole (Fig. 14.1)

A hydatidiform mole is the result of the overgrowth of placental tissue, probably because fertilisation is not normal (for example, when two sperm fertilise one egg). Usually the embryo fails to develop but occasionally a hydatidiform mole may be found alongside a fetus. The incidence in the UK is about 1 per 1000 pregnancies and is more common in:

- Women under 20 and over 40.
- Multiparous women.
- Smokers.
- Women with a previous history of hydatidiform mole.
- Women in Asia, South-East Asia and Mexico (Lewis & Chamberlain 1990, Parazzini et al 1991, Symonds 1992).

Its appearance is rather like grapes or white currants. The villi become distended with fluid and may measure 1 cm in diameter. The outer layer is trophoblastic tissue and may become malignant if it is not completely removed. A complete mole shows degeneration of all villi. Partial moles occur when some vesicles develop within an otherwise normal placenta. In this case the fetus is normally present.

Signs

The first sign is excessive nausea and vomiting. The woman may complain of intermittent bleeding from the vagina around week 12. When the mole begins to abort there may be profuse haemorrhage. The uterus is large for the period of gestation and may

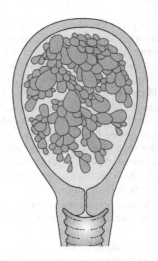

Fig. 14.1 Hydatidiform mole.

feel soft and doughy. There is no evidence of a fetal heart. There may be sign of mild thryotoxicosis due to the thyroid stimulating hormone (TSH)-like activity of human chorionic gonadatropin (hCG) which is secreted in large amounts by the molar vesicles. The diagnosis is confirmed with an ultrasound scan. Urinary or serum hCG level are higher than those of a multiple pregnancy. Occasionally the mole may be detected through maternal serum screening (triple test) for Down syndrome (Cuckle et al 1992).

Treatment

Once diagnosis is made curettage must be performed. The woman is then observed for about 1 year as about 3% of women will develop malignant trophoblastic disease (choriocarcinoma). If any molar tissue remains it will continue to grow and may invade the myometrium causing perforation of the uterine wall which may cause major haemorrhage. The woman must avoid further pregnancy until hCG levels have returned to normal.

Implications for bodywork

Refer women immediately if there is a suspicion of a molar pregnancy:

- Work to support recovery afterwards.

The fetus at risk

There are various issues which affect the well-being and development of the fetus such as placental issues, developmental or congenital abnormalities. About 3% of newborns have a 'major physical anomaly', meaning a physical anomaly that has cosmetic or functional significance (Kumar et al 2004).

The cause of 40–60% of congenital physical anomalies (birth defects) in humans is unknown. These are referred to as *sporadic birth defects*, a term that implies an unknown cause, random occurrence regardless of maternal living conditions, and a low recurrence risk for future children. For 20–25% of anomalies there seems to be a 'multifactorial' cause, meaning a complex interaction of multiple minor genetic abnormalities with environmental risk factors. Another 10–13% of anomalies have a purely environmental cause (e.g. infections, illness, or drug abuse in the mother). Only 12–25% of anomalies have a purely genetic cause. Of these, the majority are chromosomal abnormalities.

Environmental causes of congenital anomalies are referred to as teratogenic. Teratogens can include dietary deficiencies, toxins or maternal infections. The greatest risk of a malformation due to environmental exposure to a teratogen is between the third and eighth week of gestation. Before this time, any damage to the embryo is likely to result in fatality, and the baby will not survive. After 8 weeks, the fetus and its organs are more developed and less sensitive to teratogenic incidents.

Implications for bodywork

In all cases, work to support the connection between the mother and baby may be beneficial. It is important to be aware that the client faces additional potentially stressful choices about whether to keep a baby which may have developmental or congenital abnormalities. The therapist should also be aware of signs of fetal distress (e.g. the baby not moving). Energy work can be focused on supporting the Jing and the Blood. If the fetus dies, then work to support the mother in her grieving as well as recovery process.

14.5 Complications of labour and delivery

Cautions and complications arising in labour

Situations the therapist can support working alongside the primary care giver
Conditions
- Pre-labour rupture of the membranes
- Prolonged labour
- Fetal compromise (distress); mild
- Maternal exhaustion
- Fetal malposition/presentation
- Retained placenta (without haemorrhage)
- Planned caesarean section

Emergency when obstetrics take over
- Fetal compromise (distress); concerning
- Obstructed labour, depending on cause
- Shoulder dystocia
- Uterine rupture
- Lacerations
- Cord prolapse
- Haemorrhage
- Extreme fetal compromise
- Emergency caesarean section

Pre-labour rupture of membranes

If this occurs the client needs to be immediately referred to her primary care provider as it can increase the chance of infection entering the uterus.

Pre-term rupture

If the pregnancy is not term (i.e. before 37 weeks), usually the treatment is to try to stop labour as the risk of infection is outweighed by the risk of premature birth. The woman may be given drugs to stop her going into labour and will be monitored closely in hospital.

Bodywork can aim to support the woman to relax as much as she can, to support the baby and the woman's connection with the baby, to stop labour. This can include visualisations focusing on keeping the baby in the womb or the amniotic sac being re-sealed. Work has an emphasis on 'holding in'/'gathering' style approaches and techniques. This means avoiding strong vigorous physical strokes and working with more of an energy focus. Work with the Spleen meridian will help with the holding up and in. Work can also be done with the Extraordinary Vessels, especially the Girdle Vessel, to hold energies in.

Term rupture

If the woman is past 37 weeks, then labour needs to begin soon because there is an increased risk of infection. Most women go into labour within 3–5 days. There are varying policies on induction ranging from induction within 24 hours to waiting up to 96 hours, provided there are no signs of infection.

Bodywork during this time will be the labour focus work, provided there are no other complications.

Pre-term labour

This is when labour occurs before 37 weeks. It ranges from 6–10% of all deliveries in developed countries.
Pre-term labour may result from:

- Uncomplicated spontaneous pre-term labour of unknown cause – 40%.
- Premature rupture of the membranes – approximately 20%. This is often related to infection.

Elective pre-term labour: this is when labour is induced or a caesarean section is performed because the risk of continuing the pregnancy is greater, either for mother or baby, than the risk associated with early delivery. This can occur in conditions such as severe pre-eclampsia, maternal renal disease, or severe intra-uterine growth restriction.

Emergency delivery: approximately 25% of pre-term births and may occur due to placental abruption, rhesus isoimmunisation, eclampsia, maternal infection or prolapsed cord (Henderson & Macdonald 2004: 853).

Risk factors

Pre-term labour is associated with:

- Teenage or older pregnant women.
- Medical conditions.
- Infections.
- Bleeding.
- Uterine abnormality.
- Poor nutrition.
- DES-exposed daughters (diethylstillbestrol: a drug given to pregnant women in the 1950s and 1960s).

Survival of babies born prematurely

By week 25, and in some cases as early as 23 weeks, the fetus may survive. With the development of neonatal intensive care facilities, the survival of low birth-weight infants above 1500 g has become more common. High mortality rates are now found predominantly in babies under 1500 g and particularly in those under 1000 g. Research has shown that for babies under 28 weeks gestation mortality rates depend on gestational age, while neuro-developmental outcome relates more closely to birth weight. Mortality rates for babies under 29 weeks gestation are about 50% (Johnson et al 1993). Of the survivors 23% were found to have severe disabilities. The most common disability in very low birth-weight babies is cerebral palsy (CP) (Pharoah et al 1990). Although the number of very low birth-weight babies surviving is increasing, the percentage with major disabilities appears to have changed little (McGrath et al 2000). This raises many ethical issues.

If the woman is at risk for pre-term labour and there is a good chance the baby is going to be born between 24 and 32 weeks the doctor may prescribe steroidal medication to accelerate surfactant production in the fetal lungs and reduce the risk of respiratory distress syndrome (hyaline membrane disease) at birth. This drug is effective after 24 hours and for up to 7 days. Research has been done to determine its efficacy and the specific dosage and frequency that is most effective for the aim of promoting fetal lung maturity, and a number of randomised controlled trials have indicated its value (Crowley 2000).

Implications for bodywork

- The role of the therapist will depend on whether the labour is being induced, allowed to proceed without intervention, or will occur via caesarean section.
- Medical support for the newborn will occur and the therapist's role may be continued support for the mother while the partner focuses on staying in close proximity to the newborn. The baby may be transferred to a neonatal care setting rather than remaining with the mother. This could increase stress for the entire family and the presence of the therapist may help ease the situation.

Fetal malposition and malpresentation

- Occipito-posterior positions.
- Breech presentation.
- Transverse or oblique lie.

These may result in the following complications.

Deep transverse arrest of the head

This is when the fetal head has descended to the level of the ischial spines and the sagittal suture lies in the transverse diameter of the pelvis. The fetal head must be rotated so that the occiput comes to the front and then traction is applied with either forceps or vacuum.

Face presentation

This occurs in approximately 1 in 300 labours (Lewis & Chamberlain 1990: 186). It is most commonly caused by the baby's head being extended without any abnormality. It also occurs in conditions where the baby's head is malformed such as anencephaly. Many OA face presentations are delivered without difficulty but others may require a caesarean delivery.

Brow presentation

If the fetal head is of normal size and lies across the brim of a pelvis it cannot engage and obstructed labour occurs. However, a brow presentation is rare as membranes often rupture early in labour due to increased pressure, and there is then some risk of cord prolapse.

Implications for bodywork

It is best to try to work before labour, to help the fetus be in the best possible position. However, sometimes it is not, or it changes position to a less favourable one during labour. Work can also be done during labour to help the fetus get into a better position.

Obstructed labour

There is usually a reason for this and appropriate care needs to be determined as early as possible. Reasons include:

Maternal

- Deformity of pelvis.
- Uterine fibromyomata.
- Ovarian tumours.
- Tumours of rectum, bladder or pelvic bones.
- Abnormalities of uterus or vagina.
- Stenosis of the cervix of vagina.
- Obstruction of one horn of a double uterus.
- Contraction ring of uterus.

Fetal

- Fetal macrosomia. Issues tend to arise when the fetus is excessively large due to a medical condition (such as congenital abnormality or diabetes) or if the mother has a deformed pelvis.
- Malpresentation or position.
- Locked twins.
- Congenital abnormalities of the fetus.

Pelvic abnormalities and disproportion including shoulder dystocia

These can be caused by developmental anomalies of the pelvic bones, disease or injury of the bones (in the past rickets was more common) or abnormalities of the spine, hip joints or lower limbs.

Shoulder dystocia

Shoulder dystocia occurs when the shoulders remain impacted in the pelvis after delivery of the head. It is uncommon but serious and requires a high degree of skill on the obstetrician's part to manoeuvre the baby without causing problems.

Implications for bodywork

If there is a physical reason why labour is obstructed then bodywork is not usually going to be of much help and medical attention will be required.

Presentation and cord prolapse

Descent of the cord below the presenting part happens about once in 300 births. The risk is when the cord becomes compressed, which can create hypoxia to the baby. It may also create an obstruction to a progressing labour. Prolapse of the cord is not a medical issue for the woman but it is life-threatening for the baby. The usual response is immediate caesarean. If the therapist is with the mother when the cord prolapses and no primary care providers are present, contact for emergency care must be initiated immediately. The woman is advised to assume a knee to chest position to slow labour until the caesarean can be performed.

Fetal compromise (distress)

This term is used to describe oxygen deprivation and the following signs may be present:

- Fetal tachycardia.
- A pathological CTG and corresponding FBS result.
- Fetal bradycardia or severe changes in fetal heart rate or decelerations due to uterine contractions which do not recover between contractions or both.
- Passage of meconium-stained amniotic fluid.

(Fraser & Cooper 2003: 466).

If this happens in the first stage of labour, then a caesarean section may be indicated and in the second stage, forceps or ventouse may be used. A paediatrician will need to be present at the delivery to give any necessary treatment to the baby.

Implications for bodywork

Depending on the reason and severity, relaxation work may be beneficial. Sometimes it may feel appropriate to include direct work with the baby, through touching the abdomen, singing, talking or other energy work.

Rupture of the uterus

This is an uncommon complication and may be caused by:

- Obstructed labour.
- Intrauterine manipulations.
- Weak scar from previous caesarean section (1 in 2000). The classical vertical incision is more risky.
- Dilatation of the cervix.
- Oxytocic drugs.
- Many previous pregnancies.

It carries a high mortality rate but incidence in the UK has fallen from 5.7 per million in 1970 to 2.1 in 1981. *It is a medical emergency.*

Laceration of the perineum and vagina

These are classified as:

- First-degree tear – the tear occurs to the skin and a minor part of the perineal body and related posterior wall of the vagina.

- Second-degree tear – tear to the perineal body up to but not involving the anal sphincter with a corresponding tear in the vagina.
- Third-degree (complete) tear – includes the anal sphincter and usually extends for 2 cm or more into the anal canal. If it is not repaired there will be incontinence of flatus and stool.

Treatment of first- and second-degree tears is repair by suturing utilising local anaesthesia. Third-degree tears require repair by someone with expert knowledge and may need general or epidural anaesthesia.

Fistulae

This may occur due to pressure of the presenting part in labour or by injury during operative procedures. Pressure between the head and the pubic bone may cause local ischaemia and subsequent necrosis of the anterior vaginal wall and base of the bladder leading to the formation of a vesicovaginal fistula. If the rectum is involved this is called rectovaginal fistula.

This type of condition is not common in the UK and Canada but in countries with inadequate obstetrical services it is relatively common. It may cause urinary or faecal incontinence or both.

Haemorrhage

This is blood loss of more than 500 ml. Drugs are usually given to contract the uterus. With large blood loss a transfusion may be advised.

Shock

Can be caused by excessive blood loss.

Delayed placental delivery

Provided there are no indications of haemorrhage and the client is medically stable, as an alternative to surgical removal, energy work can be initiated. GB 21 is an especially effective point, or any of the labour focus points may help. If it is going to work then it will work fairly instantly, so it will not interfere with any medical procedures that may be deemed necessary.

Summary box for issues relating to the higher-risk client

- Always establish that the client is receiving care from her primary care provider for any health issue that arises. In most cases of higher-risk situations, close collaboration will be needed with the client's primary care provider.
- Bodywork is often beneficial for clients in a higher-risk category and may help decrease stress and physical discomforts related to the primary issue.
- Further training may be needed to ensure safe practice and increase knowledge about providing the best care possible to the client. If the therapist does not have sufficient training to deal with the condition of the client, referral to a more experienced practitioner is advisable.
- The therapist may be working in clinical, home or hospital settings depending on where the client is receiving her medical care. Creating professional relationships with a team-building approach is crucial in establishing the basis of sound therapeutic interaction.
- The goal of the therapist is always to ensure that the therapeutic interaction serves to benefit the client and does not increase risk of harm. As with medical treatment, bodywork should work from a model of reducing risk of mortality and morbidity in the client.

References and further reading

Agren, A., Berg, M., 2006. Tactile massage and severe nausea and vomiting during pregnancy – women's experiences. Scand. J. Caring Sci. 20 (2), 169–176.

Arafeh, J.M., 1997. Disseminated intravascular coagulation in pregnancy: an update. J. Perinat. Neonatal Nurs. 11 (3), 30–45.

Bennhagen, R., Holmberg, L., 1989. Protein C activity and antigen in premature and full term newborn infants. Acta Paediatr. Scand. 78 (1), 34–39.

Blackburn, S., 1985. Rho (D) isoimmunization: implications for the mother, fetus and newborn. In: NAAACOG Update Series (Vol. 3). Continuing Professional Education Centre, Princeton NJ.

Borg, W.P., Sherwin, R.S., 2000. Classification of diabetes mellitus. Adv. Intern. Med. 45, 279–295.

Buyon, J.P., 1998. The effects of pregnancy on autoimmune diseases. J. Leukoc. Biol. 63 (3), 281–287.

Center for Disease Control and Prevention, Achievements in public health, 1900–1999: healthier mothers and babies 1999. Morb. Mortal. Wkly. Rep. (MMWR) 48 (38), 849–858.

Chamberlain, G., 1991. ABC of antenatal care. Raised blood pressure in pregnancy. Br. Med. J. 302 (6790), 1454–1458.

Clayton, S.G., Lewis, T.L.T., Pinker, L.G., 1985. Obstetrics by Ten Teachers, fourteenth ed. Edward Arnold, London.

Crowley, P., 2000. Prophylactic corticosteroids for pre-term birth. Cochrane Database Syst. Rev. (2) CD000065.

Crowther, C.A., Middleton, P., 1999. Anti-D administration in pregnancy for preventing Rhesus alloimmunisation. Cochrane Database Syst. Rev. (2) CD000020. DOI: 10.1002/14651858.CD000020.

Cuckle, H.S., Densem, J.W., Wald, N.J., 1992. Detection of hydatidiform mole in maternal serum screening programmes for Down's syndrome. Br. J. Obstet. Gynaecol. 99 (6), 495–497.

De Boer, K., ten Cate, J.W., Sturk, A., et al., 1989. Enhanced thrombin generation in normal and hypertensive pregnancy. Am. J. Obstet. Gynecol. 160 (1), 95–100.

De Swiet, M., 1985. Thromboembolism. Clin. Haematol. 14 (3), 643–660.

De Swiet, M., 1995. Medical disorders in pregnancy (Chapter 22). In: Chamberlain, G. (Ed.), Turnbull's Obstetrics, second ed. Churchill Livingstone, Edinburgh.

Detels, R., McEwan, J., Beaglehole, R. (Eds.), et al., 2002. Oxford Textbook of Public Health. Vol 1: The Scope of Public Health, fourth ed. Oxford University Press, Oxford.

Dietl, J., 2000. The pathogenesis of pre-eclampsia: new aspects. J. Perinat. Med. 28 (6), 464–471.

Douglas, K.A., Redman, C.W., 1994. Eclampsia in the United Kingdom. Br. Med. J. 309 (6966), 1395–1400.

Formby, B., 1995. Immunologic response in pregnancy: its role in endocrine disorders of pregnancy and influence on the course of maternal autoimmune disease. Endocrinol. Metab. Clin. North Am. 24, 187–205.

Fraser, D.M., Cooper, M.A., 2003. Myles' Textbook for Midwives, fourteenth ed. Elsevier Churchill Livingstone, Edinburgh.

Gates, S., 2000. Thromboembolic disease in pregnancy. Curr. Opin. Obstet. Gynecol. 12 (2), 117–122.

Gilbert, E.S., Harmon, J.S., 1986. High Risk Pregnancy and Delivery. Mosby, St Louis, p. 269.

Gilbert, E., Harmon, J.S., 1993. Manual of High Risk Pregnancy and Delivery. Mosby, St Louis, p. 25.

Gilbert, E.S., Harmon, J.S., 2002. Manual of High Risk Pregnancy and Delivery, third ed. Mosby, St Louis.

Gillmer, M.D.G., Hurley, P.A., 1999. Diabetes and endocrine disorders in pregnancy. In: Edmonds, D.K. (Ed.), Dewhurst's Textbook of Obstetrics and Gynaecology for Postgraduates, sixth ed. Blackwell Science, Oxford, pp. 197–209.

Hathaway, W.E., Bonnar, J., 1987. Hemostatic Disorders of the Pregnant Woman and Newborn Infant. Elsevier, New York (Chapter 1).

Health Canada, 2004. Special Report on Maternal Mortality and Severe Morbidity in Canada. Enhanced Surveillance: The Path to Prevention. Minister of Public Works and Government Services, Ottawa.

Henderson, C., Macdonald, S., 2004. Mayes' Midwifery: A Textbook for Midwives, thirteenth ed. Baillère Tindall, Edinburgh.

Higgins, J.R., de Swiet, M., 2001. Blood pressure measurement and classification in pregnancy. Lancet 357 (9250), 131–135.

Howie, P.W., 1995. Coagulation and fibrinolytic systems and their disorders in obstetrics and gynaecology. In: Whitfield, C.R. (Ed.), Dewhurst's Textbook of Obstetrics and Gynaecology for Postgraduates, fifth ed. Blackwell Science, Oxford.

Johnson, A., Townshend, P., Yudkin, P., et al., 1993. Functional abilities at age 4 years of children born before 29 weeks gestation. Br. Med. J. 306 (6894), 1715–1718.

Jordan, J.A., 1994. Female genital mutilation (female circumcision). Br. J. Obstet. Gynaecol. 101 (2), 94–95.

Kadar, N., 1999. Ectopic and heterotopic pregnancies. In: Reece, E., Hobbins, J. (Eds.) Medicine of the Fetus and Mother. Lippincott, Philadelphia.

Kent, N., Leduc, L., Crane, J., et al., 2000. Prevention and treatment of venous thromboembolism (Vte) in obstetrics. J. SOGC 22, 736–749.

Kumar, V., Abbas, A.K., Fausto, N., 2004. Robbins and Cotran Pathologic Basis of Disease, seventh ed. Elsevier Saunders, Philadelphia, p. 470.

Landon, M.B., 1999. Diabetes mellitus and other endocrine disease (Chapter 31). In: Gabbe, S., Niebyl, J.R., Simpson, J.L. (Eds.) Obstetrics, Normal and Problem Pregnancies, fourth ed. Churchill Livingstone, New York.

Levero, F.G., Macdonald, P.C., Gant, N.F., et al., 1984. Obstet. Gynecol. 64: 608–610.

Lewis, T.G. (Ed.), 2001. Why Mothers Die 1997–99. Fifth Report of the Confidential Enquiries into Maternal Deaths in the United Kingdom. CEMD, NICE, RCOG, London.

Lewis, T.L.T., Chamberlain, G.V.P., 1990. Obstetrics by Ten Teachers, fifteenth ed. Edward Arnold, London.

Llewellyn-Jones, D., 1990. Fundamentals of Obstetrics and Gynaecology. Vol. 1: Obstetrics, fifth ed. Faber and Faber, London.

Lockwood, C.J., Kuczynski, E., 1999. Markers of risk for pre-term delivery. J. Perinat. Med. 27 (1), 5–20.

McGrath, M.M., Sullivan, M.C., Lester, B.M., et al., 2000. Longitudinal neurological follow-up in neonatal intensive care unit survivors with various neonatal morbidities. Pediatrics 106 (6), 1397–1405.

Magee, L.A., Helewa, M., Moulquin, J-M., et al., 2008. SOGC Clinical practice guideline; diagnosis, evaluation, and management of the hypertensive disorders of pregnancy. J. Obstet. Gynaecol. Can. 30 (3 Suppl. 1), S1–S49 Available at: <http://www.sogc.org/guidelines/documents/gui206CPG0803_001.pdf> (accessed 20.04.09).

Makhseed, M., Musini, V.M., Ahmed, M.A., et al., 1999. Influence of seasonal variation on pregnancy induced hypertension and/or pre-eclampsia. Aust. N. Z. J. Obstet. Gynaecol. 39 (2), 196–199.

Odent, M. McMillan, L., Kimmel, T., 1996. Prenatal Care and Sea Fish. Eur. J. Obstet. Gynecol. 68, 49–51.

Ontario Medical Association, 2005. Ontario antenatal record form. <https://www.oma.org/forms/ontarioantenatalrecord2005.pdf> (accessed 20.04.09).

Palanivelu, L.M., 2007. Chorea gravidarum. J. Obstet. Gynaecol. 27 (3), 310.

Parazzini, F., Mangili, G., La Vecchia, C., et al., 1991. Risk factors for gestational trophoblastic disease: a separate analysis of complete and partial hydatiform moles. Obstet. Gynecol. 78 (6), 1039–1045.

Parisi, V.N., 1988. Cervical incompetence and preterm labor. Clin. Obstet. Gynecol. 31(3), 585–598.

Pearson, J., 1997. Effective care. Pearson, J. 'High risk' coping with pregnancy complications. Great Expectations, Autumn 1997, p. 28.

Pharoah, P.O., Cooke, T., Cooke, R.W., et al., 1990. Birthweight specific trends in cerebral palsy. Arch. Dis. Child. 65 (6), 602–606.

Public Health Agency of Canada, 2006. Make Every Mother and Child Count: Report on Maternal and Child Health in Canada. Institute of Health Economics, Edmonton, p. 4.

Rabinerson, D., Neri, A., Yardena, O., 1992. Combined anomalies of the Mullerian and Wolffian systems. Acta Obstet. Gynecol. Scand. 71 (2), 156–157.

Sanderson, D.A., Milton, P.J.D., 1991. The effectiveness of ultrasound screening at 18–20 weeks gestational age for prediction of placenta previa. J. Obstet. Gynaecol. 11 (5), 320–323.

Scholl, T.O., Hediger, M.L., Fischer, R.L., et al., 1992. Anemia vs iron deficiency: increased risk of pre-term delivery in a prospective study. Am. J. Clin. Nutr. 55 (5), 985–988.

Sibai, B.M., Ramadan, M.K., 1993. Acute renal failure in pregnancies complicated by hemolysis, elevated liver enzymes, and low platelets (HELLP). Am. J. Obstet. Gynecol. 168 (6/1), 1682–1687.

Sibai, B.M., Ramadan, M.K., Usta, I., et al., 1993. Maternal morbidity and mortality in 442 pregnancies with hemolysis, elevated liver enzymes, and low platelets (HELLP syndrome). Am. J. Obstet. Gynecol. 169 (4), 1000–1006.

Silver, R.M., 1987. Lancet 2, 1297.

Silver, R.M., Branch, D.W., 1999. Sporadic and recurrent pregnancy loss. In: Reece, E.A., Hobbins, J.C. (Eds.) Medicine of the Fetus and the Mother, second ed. Lippincott Raven, Philadelphia, pp. 195–215.

Stabile, I., Grudzinskas, J.G., 1990. Ectopic pregnancy: a review of incidence, etiology and diagnostic aspects. Obstet. Gynecol. Surv. 45 (6), 335–347.

Symonds, E.M., 1992. Essential Obstetrics and Gynaecology, second ed. Churchill Livingstone, Edinburgh.

Thompson, J., 1989. Torture by tradition. Nurs. Times 85 (15), 16–17.

Tin Chiu, L., Bates, S., Pearce, M., 1999. Biochemical tests in complications in early pregnancy. In: O'Brien, P. (Ed.), The Yearbook of Obstetrics and Gynaecology, vol. 7. RCOG Press, London.

Tindall, V.R., 1987. Jeffcoate's Principles of Gynaecology. Butterworth-Heinemann, London.

Tseng, C.E., Buyon, J.P., 1997. Neonatal lupus syndromes. Rheum. Dis. Clin. North Am. 23 (1), 31–54.

Tsimoyiannis, E.C., Antoniou, N.C., Tsaboulas, C., et al., 1994. Cholelithiasis during pregnancy and lactation: prospective study. Eur. J. Surg. 160, 627–631.

United Nations, 1996. Report of the Fourth World Conference on Women: Beijing, 4–15 September 1995. United Nations, New York. Online: accessed 20 April 2009. A/CONF.177/20/Rev.1 of 1 January 1996.

Walker, J.J., 2000. Severe pre-eclampsia and eclampsia. Baillières Best Pract. Res. Clin. Obstet. Gynaecol. 14 (1), 57–71.

Williamson, C., Hems, L.M., Goulis, D.G., et al., 2004. Clinical outcome in a series of cases of obstetric cholestasis identified via a patient support group. Br. J. Obstet. Gynaecol. 111 (7), 676–681.

World Health Organization, 2004. Millennium development goals – indicators. WHO, Geneva. <http://www.who.int/mdg/goals/MDGsList_smartformat.pdf> (accessed 16.02.04.).

World Health Organization, 2005. Make every mother and child count: a toolkit for organizers of activities, World Health Day, 7 April 2005. WHO/RHR/04.10.

Zeitlin, J., Wildman, K., Breart, G., et al., 2003. PERISTAT: indicators for monitoring and evaluating perinatal health in Europe. Eur. J. Public Health 13 (3), 29–37.

Chapter contents

Learning outcomes

- Evaluate the relevant qualities needed to specialise in maternity work
- Identify relevant training issues
- Describe relevant practice considerations
- Describe aspects of the bodyworker's role

Introduction

While maternity bodywork is an exciting and expanding field in which to work, there are specific issues which need to be considered for the therapist. The potential role of the maternity bodyworker can cover more than simply one-to-one work with a client and the therapist needs to consider which aspects of it they wish to specialise in. Once they have undertaken a personal evaluation of the type of work they want to include in their practice, the next issue is to evaluate and access appropriate training and then begin to build one's practice. They need to identify the specific needs of the maternity client group and to take into account that this is one of the few times in life when healthy clients are under the care of a primary care provider.

15.1 Setting up a maternity-focused bodywork practice

Qualities needed to be a maternity bodyworker
Commonly asked questions
- Do I have to have had children to work with pregnancy and birth?
- Can a male practitioner successfully work in this area?
- What other qualities do I need?

Do I have to have had children to work with pregnancy?

Often one of the first questions that bodyworkers ponder is whether they have to have had children to work effectively with pregnant clients. Essentially the answer is 'no'. A bodyworker does not necessarily have to have had the experience of their clients. For example, it is possible to work with cancer patients without having had cancer. Furthermore, even if therapists have had children, the different range of experiences of pregnancy, birth and parenting vary enormously from woman to woman and from culture to culture. Furthermore:

Whether we ever choose pregnancy, every one of us has encoded in our cells the knowledge of what it is to conceive, gestate and give birth to something that grows out of our own substance. You don't have to have a baby to learn how to labour. Labour, whether physical or metaphorical, teaches us not to fight the process of giving birth, not matter what we're giving birth to, even when it hurts and we want to quit

(Northrup 1998: 416–417)

The most important aspect is for the therapist not to be carrying unresolved issues around pregnancy and birth which may impede their judgement and ability to support their client. Bodyworkers with children are sometimes drawn to specialise in the maternity field either because they have wonderful experiences which they want to share, or dreadful experiences which they want to 'save' other women from experiencing. For bodyworkers with no children, they may have issues with miscarriage and fertility or other issues and they need to be careful not to live out unfulfilled desires through their clients.

Suzanne (who has two children)

In some ways it has helped me to empathise with my clients through having experienced pregnancy first hand. It was this which motivated me to learn more about bodywork in pregnancy and certainly I felt more able to 'experiment' with different techniques on myself. During both my pregnancies I used bodywork as a major source of support. I had extremely positive experiences of pregnancy and birth and did not really suffer from any ailments; indeed I felt well and healthy throughout and they were positive times in my life. How much that was due to bodywork or from my hereditary patterning I do not know. However, I did support my health and I did trust my body. I have no experience of many of the ailments women suffer from, such as symphysis pubis problems, heartburn, carpal tunnel syndrome. I have never had a miscarriage or undergone a termination, so I cannot personally identify with those experiences, although I work a lot with women at those times in their lives. So while I feel that my own experiences gave me a foundation on which to build, it has been primarily through my work with women over the years that I have built up my knowledge of other conditions, situations and issues.

Cindy (who has no children)

I feel anyone interested in helping families have a positive birthing experience is an asset in the field. Many massage therapists I know attended their first birth as a result of being invited by their clients. That first experience whetted the appetite for attending more births and gaining additional training.

The key elements are passion for the work and an ability to work from a client-centred framework. I think professionals in the field should be mindful of their attitude towards practitioners who do not have children since I have heard unintentionally hurtful comments towards childless practitioners. For me, the bottom line is if you love this work then you have an important contribution to make.

Can the male practitioner work effectively with the maternity client?

Some people believe that pregnancy and birth is very much 'women's business' and it is not appropriate for men to be involved. It is true that in traditional cultures it was 'women's business' but male and female relationships were completely different and in many cultures men and women did not have much connection with each other. Modern culture has tended to value 'experts' who may often be male and many feminists see the rise of the male obstetrician in childbirth as a sign of male control over women. There is some truth in this. However, it is wise to remember that sometimes female obstetricians can be less sympathetic to women than male obstetricians.

Again, one of the main considerations is clarity, empathy and enthusiasm. Men have the experience of their own birth and many male practitioners are drawn to the field because of experiences they may have had with their partners during pregnancy and birth. The male practitioner does need to be sensitive to the fact that some women may not want to have a male practitioner, although some women may prefer a male practitioner. Working with the breasts and abdomen is likely to be more of an issue for the male therapist and they need to make sure that they provide a safe space and adequate draping for the client to feel comfortable.

What qualities do I need?

As pregnancy, birth and becoming a mother are such life-changing experiences, therapists need to be self-aware and not impose their own values and judgements on the client. Being able to support a client to learn to connect with her own knowledge and way of processing the experience is essential. It is vital to respect the choices that clients make, especially if they are different from the choices the therapist would make. Creating a safe space for the client to express herself and be heard is key. It is also important to recognise the limitations of one's role and know what other services and support the pregnant woman may need to access. The ability to reflect on one's work is fundamental.

Be knowledgeable about resources

It is important to be able to know about specific services pregnant women can access and to work to liaise with the relevant groups and individuals so that referrals can be made as necessary. The type of groups to be aware of are:

- Pre- and postnatal classes including yoga, pilates, Aquafit.
- Breastfeeding support groups such as La Leche League.

- Home birth support groups.
- Antenatal and postpartum support groups.
- Special interest support groups such as: twins and multiple birth support, parents of children with disabilities, SANDS (still birth and neonatal death support groups).
- Other therapists specialising in maternity work, e.g. counsellors, psychotherapists and so on.

Dealing with the more difficult aspects of pregnancy

Difficult issues can include loss, death, emotional or sexual trauma. Many therapists begin by wanting to work with pregnancy because they see it as a positive time in a woman's life. While this is true and it can be a very rewarding time to work, the maternity period is not always positive. Sexual issues often surface during pregnancy and birth, particularly if the mother has suffered from abuse. Birth and death are closely interlinked and the therapist needs to consider how they would feel if their client miscarried, or experienced stillbirth or loss in the early postnatal period. Birth itself may be a very traumatic experience for many women.

15.2 Reflective exercise

- Do you think you have the right qualities to work in the maternity period?
- Consider why you are drawn to working in the maternity field.
- What motivates you in your work?
- How would you feel if you are a big fan of home birth but your client wants to have an elective caesarean section?
- How you would you feel if your client had a miscarriage?

Appropriate training

It is important for the therapist to evaluate whether they have the relevant training and experience. Most bodywork training does not cover maternity care in sufficient depth for the therapist to be able to specialise without further training.

The quality of the maternity training required will depend on the context of the general training that the practitioner has received. This varies enormously from country to country and even between states in some countries. For example, massage therapists in Ontario receive 2200 hours of instruction over a period of 2 years. This has become the yardstick of

training in other Canadian provinces and is beginning to become accepted in other countries. In the USA and the UK programmes of 1 year's duration or less than 500–1000 hours are more common; however, most therapists will access further advanced training courses once the foundation training has been completed. Shiatsu therapist training in the UK is spread over 3 years with various residential and non-residential modules and home study and practice required. Osteopaths train for a minimum of 3 years full time.

The therapist needs to consider what specific maternity training was included as part of their course. They need to evaluate it in the context of number of hours, the content of the courses, the accuracy of the information, the experience of the trainers and the clinical practice which was offered.

In most cases, the therapist is likely to need to do a specialised course. They have to consider whether they want to specialise only in pregnancy or birth support work or postnatal work. In a way it makes sense to see the whole period as a continuum, but some therapists may prefer to work more with pregnant or postnatal women.

Length of course

It is hard to give a precise number of hours as it depends on the exact delivery of the course and how much pre- and post-course work is required as well as the therapist's initial level of bodywork training. As a guideline we would suggest that for pregnancy work a minimum of at least 20 contact hours would be required. For birth work an additional minimum of 20 contact hours would be needed. For postnatal work, if the therapist has already done some pregnancy/birth training, which is important as many of the themes of postnatal work may arise from the birth or pregnancy experience, then an additional minimum of 10 hours is likely to be sufficient. However, if the therapist is only doing a course in postnatal work then the contact hours would need to be more.

Course content

Consider what topics are covered on the course. This would need to include some coverage of the following topics:

1. Relevant anatomy and physiology.
2. Relevant eastern theory, if the therapist works with that model.
3. An overview of the medical care offered in the country in which the course is being taught and any issues this may raise.
4. Pre- and post-course reading and research.

5. Supervised practice working with pregnant women during the course.
6. Self-reflection exercises, including reflecting on things like qualities needed, how to evaluate the work and so on.

Some ideas/support on how to set up and run a maternity practice, including: creating appropriate intake forms and client information, promotion, marketing and networking.

Course reputation

- Is the course recognised by any relevant accrediting organisations?
- Is the course recognised in the community as providing accurate, client-centred content?
- What sort of feedback has there been from other participants?
- How many participants are currently working in the maternity field?

Credentials of the educators

It is important to consider who is teaching the course and ask:

- What is their training?
- How long have they been involved in maternity work?
- What is their philosophy of care?
- What is their educational experience and training?
- Are they recognised and well respected by their peers and others in the field?
- Are they affiliated to recognised institutions, governing bodies, primary care providers?
- What ongoing CPD and clinical activities are they currently engaged in?

Post-course consolidation

- What opportunities exist for post-course consolidation?
- Is course work or case study work required?
- What is the time frame?

Ongoing support and development: training, CPD

Once the course has been completed, what opportunities are there to continue learning? What kind of post-course support is offered in building, developing and maintaining the practice? Are there any student networks? Discussion groups? CPD possibilities?

As the issues and type of care are constantly changing and skills can always be refined and developed, it is important to see the initial maternity training as

only being a starting point. It is important to access continuing training, education and support in order to develop the work.

Practice management

Once the relevant training has been completed the therapist needs to consider how they are going to run their maternity practice.

Insurance cover

It is important to check that insurance cover is appropriate, as some companies will insure for all aspects of maternity work, while others may have certain exclusions such as no work in the first trimester, during labour, the first 6 weeks postnatally or with the newborn.

Appropriate cover can usually be arranged provided evidence of appropriate training for the intended activity can be provided.

Membership of professional bodies

In addition to having current membership of bodywork professional bodies, it may also be necessary, dependent on the country in which the therapist is working and the type of work being undertaken, to be a member of another organisation, e.g. doula or ante- and postnatal education organisations.

Research

As it is a developing field it is important to keep up to date with latest research and debates around research. This can be done by continuing to attend relevant workshops and lectures, peer support networks and by subscribing to journals such as *Birth*, *MIDIRS*.

Evaluating care

Record keeping, creating audits and adhering to quality assurance programmes, evaluating care are as important with maternity work as any aspect of work.

Analysing the intake form and having relevant information for the client

It is likely that the generic intake form for bodywork is inappropriate for maternity clients and will need to be modified. Further relevant information sheets specific to aspects of maternity care may need to be produced.

Promotion: brochures and websites, other media

This will define the kind of work that the therapist is offering and the potential benefits; backed up by research or testimonials where possible. It should give information about what to expect during a session, how long the session will last, how frequently the woman needs to come. It will also include information about whether home visits are offered and if the therapist is able to offer support in the hospital setting. The training and background of the therapist and their philosophy of care also need to be outlined. It is important to keep the information relevant and factual and not to make any false or misleading claims.

Handouts

These can be useful to have both as resources for individual clients and for teaching classes. They help to reinforce any learning which has occurred or information which has been given. The types of topics which can be useful to provide information on are:

- Exercises for pregnancy and the postpartum.
- Positions and movements for labour.
- Teaching the partner massage skills.
- Diet and nutrition.
- Emotional support.
- Other therapies.
- Support groups.

Distribution of informational leaflets and promotion

Many pregnant women are part of different groups. It can be useful to make contact with the other groups and sources of support in pregnancy, not only to access sources of support for the client but also as a means of promoting the practice. For example an aquanatal class may be a good place to distribute leaflets and then referrals can be made between the therapist and the aquanatal teacher to their mutual benefit.

Many therapists find that if they make a contact with a local childbirth educator or midwife or obstetrician, then they can offer free talks or put up posters. Private practices are often easier to connect with as in many areas there are lengthy bureaucratic procedures involved in making contact with state-run healthcare systems.

Remember that pregnant women often have other children and so family support networks and mother and toddler groups or schools can be good places to offer to give talks or distribute leaflets. Other options include:

- Websites designed for mums-to-be and new mums, e.g. Netmums.
- Radio presentations.
- Talks in local hospital.
- Links with National Childbirth Trust and other childbirth groups.
- Articles for local newspapers.

Charging

The therapist needs to decide how long they are going to have their session and what they are going to charge for the different types of session:

- Antenatal visits.
- Home visits.
- Postnatal home visits.
- Hospital visits.
- Mother and baby and partner work.
- Birth support work.
- Group work.

They may want to offer discounts or packages to encourage women to take advantage of the different types of work they may offer, and especially to encourage women to come for postnatal work.

Of course any charging and advertising needs to conform to the scope of practice of the therapist. If working in a hospital, there are several methods of payment:

- A fee for service basis with the client paying for the treatment.
- A contract with the hospital with fees paid directly by the hospital.
- Care provided within the context of a student-based or postgraduate training programme where the student does not receive a fee but is gaining increased knowledge and clinical experience under the supervision of an instructor who is working for either a recognised training college or for the hospital itself.

Birth support charging

The therapist needs to be clear what they are offering. If it is a commitment to attend the birth, it is important to understand what that involves. It means:

- Other clients may need to be cancelled.
- It is not possible to travel far from the client for 2 weeks before and after the due date.
- Refraining from alcohol.
- Being on call 24/7.

It is important to consider what would happen if the therapist became ill or there was a family crisis – what kind of back up can they offer to honour that commitment?

If this is what is being offered, then many therapists charge a fixed fee which reflects not only the time spent with the client and her family but the cost of cancelling other clients and the potential inconvenience and antisocial and challenging hours. Realistically with a busy bodywork practice this level of support is not likely to be practical to be offered very often. This type of service would also need to include at least one or two antenatal visits with the family and other birth support people plus at least one postnatal visit to debrief after the birth.

Some therapists prefer not to take on that guaranteed role but offer to be there for the client as a standby. They will do their best to attend the birth but will not guarantee a firm commitment. They may offer phone support or to be there for some but not all of the birth. It is important that the mother has considered the role of all her support people and is happy with this level of commitment from the therapist. In this situation, the therapist can offer to come for an initial callout fee which would cover the first couple of hours and then an hourly rate after that, depending to an extent on what is done. There is an element of trust in this kind of contract and it tends to work better when the client is a regular bodywork client.

15.3 Scope of practice: the bodyworker as maternity care provider

The role of the bodyworker

Specialising in maternity work opens up new options for working. The therapist can simply decide to focus on the provision of bodywork within an allotted appointment time, as with non-pregnant clients. However, the therapist may decide that they want to offer a more comprehensive package and, depending on their skills and training, offer additional options to support women at this crucial time of their lives.

In some respects the maternity bodywork specialist's role is potentially not unlike the traditional maternity caregiver. The TBA (traditional birth attendant) was often not medically trained and was respected as a 'wise' woman in the village who could give good support to other women. She would focus on the woman's social and emotional well-being. Pregnancy and birth was seen as a time when the mother would be encouraged to adapt to her new role in society. There would be an emphasis on lifestyle support and the 'normality' of the process. The wise woman would tend to give support at the birth and postnatally as well as during pregnancy.

Depending on the bodyworker's training, they may be offering a space where the client can explore some of the feelings which arise and be a person whom the client sees regularly. It is important to be aware of boundary issues and not offer 'counselling' as such, unless specifically trained to do so, but in the relaxed space offered by bodywork clients do often connect with their feelings about their pregnancy and how they are adapting to their role as a mother as well as physically how they are managing through the pregnancy. A vital part of the maternity therapist's role can be to listen, support and educate.

These days, the midwife is often a primary care provider who has a different relationship to the mother. It is important that the therapist recognise that, however beneficial the work they offer may be, they are not the primary care provider and must not assume those responsibilities. The client needs to be visiting a primary caregiver on a regular basis. The therapist needs to seek to support that relationship and not undermine it. It is important not to contradict information given by the care provider, even if the information appears to be misinformed regarding bodywork. It is vital to know when to refer to the primary care provider and how to work alongside them.

It is a time where the work is affecting not just the client and her baby but also her partner and immediate family. An important part of the maternity work, which is often expected by the client, is to be able to include the partner. Usually this is at the level of teaching simple massage skills but it could include supporting the family with resource material (e.g. written information on groups which can support them) or working with exercise or diet information. It could also involve work for birth preparation or involving the partner in postnatal massage of the mother and infant massage. It can include working directly with the partner with bodywork to reduce stress and support them in their changing role. In this respect, the therapist may be working more as a birth educator than simply a bodyworker and it is important to be clear about the role. Some bodyworkers extend their role in this field and run childbirth education classes based on bodywork therapy. Again it is vital to have appropriate skills and insurance in offering these types of classes.

In these days of increasingly medicalised maternity care, the bodyworker offers vital additional tools for pregnancy clients. Bodyworkers are independent professional practitioners who need to be accountable for the care they offer.

Bodywork has provided a pivotal foundation for women to continue to receive nurturing care amidst a worldwide culture which is insisting on moving maternity care in the direction of more and more technological intervention.

In what was once a powerful and mother/baby centred event, there has been a shift in recent years to care that is more focused on 'what is wrong' within the pregnancy/birth, and consequently a need to exercise 'control', with a resulting focus that moves the primary focus away from actual care for the family and towards a focus of reducing risk of lawsuit for the health care.

(Cindy)

The way forward can be to work alongside primary care givers to give women the best of both worlds: integrated care. Table 15.1 describes the bodyworker's role in relation to the primary maternity caregiver. These will vary to some extent dependent on the country and type of care offered.

Collaborating with the primary care provider

If the bodyworker is unsure about how to proceed with a particular condition and needs further medical information or diagnosis in order to be able to proceed safely, then they need to refer to the primary caregiver, either via the client or with her permission, for more diagnosis or information in order to proceed safely and effectively with the work.

In some countries therapists consider this 'asking for permission' from the primary caregiver in order to proceed with bodywork. There are some issues which arise with this approach.

1. The primary caregiver may not be well informed regarding bodywork and therefore not in a professional position to give advice regarding specific bodywork modifications. Indeed they may even be sceptical of or antagonistic to the benefits of bodywork. The bodyworker has the ultimate responsibility for any decisions he or she makes.

2. Often the primary caregiver simply does not have the time to respond to the bodyworker. It is worth making introductions to local primary care providers and explaining the nature of the work, but it is unrealistic to expect that busy primary care providers can dialogue with a bodyworker about every case. Ultimately this would be an ideal situation so that true integrated care can be an option and the most appropriate care for each client can be determined. This may happen if the bodyworker is working in a multidisciplinary way in the hospital situation.

We suggest, as a way of working towards integrated care, that the therapist write a letter to the client's

Table 15.1 The bodyworker's role in relation to primary maternity caregiver

Maternity body worker	Primary caregiver
Supports the woman's physical, emotional and (potentially) spiritual well-being	Has the ultimate responsibility for the woman's and baby's health and may have to make life or death decisions
Is the 'expert' in bodywork, including after care (breathing, exercises) if appropriately trained	Is the 'expert' in the medical assessment of the client, undertaking tests and risk assessment. May or may not know about bodywork
Is responsible for the decisions they make regarding the appropriateness of the bodywork	Is responsible for the overall health status of the client
Supports the client so that she can make appropriate decisions about her care: e.g. listening, giving emotional support and space, facilitating access to information and resources	Makes the medical care decisions in consultation with the client; informed choice
Places emphasis on lifestyle support choices	Places emphasis on medical care choices
Is open to dialogue with the primary care provider; seeks information which may inform the bodywork	Provides information about the medical condition of the client and the effects on the physiological and pathophysiological processes
Knows when to refer the client to the primary caregiver	Has the prime responsibility for dealing with emergency situations
Provides continuity of care with one person; this is often initiated prior to pregnancy and may include preconceptual support and continue for years into the postpartum and for other pregnancies	Usually involves care provided by a number of people, depending on the health status of the client: midwife, obstetrician, specialist, paediatrician
Listens, supports and educates	Educates, but this role has become less prominent. Listens and supports as much as possible, but often has limited time in which to do so.

Table 15.2 Identifying the role of the primary care provider and provision of maternity care

	United States	**United Kingdom**
Primary maternity care giver	Obstetricians (for 90% of women): midwives and family physicians for the remainder. In labour maternity nurses provide most of the care with the obstetrician managing complications	Mostly midwives with obstetricians caring for women with complications. Midwives provide all intrapartum care for most women, unless there are complications which are managed by the obstetrician
Autonomy of caregiver	Care varies depending on the individual physicians. However insurance providers and health maintenance organisations increasingly limit those practices which are not considered cost effective	NHS midwives have little individual autonomy and practice according to the policy of their institutions. This policy is established by local authorities, often using NICE guidelines, and the government. Independent midwives are more autonomous.
Participation by women in decision making	'Informed consent' is the law but most women expect the obstetrician to make decisions. Most midwives and family physicians share decision making.	'Informed choice' and 'woman-centred' care is a standard of care and the government and childbirth activists are making some efforts to ensure that women are able to make decisions.
Continuity of care giver	Not considered cost effective, feasible or desirable. Some women try to organise it through birth plans and employing doulas or independent midwives.	Considered important and some programmes are beginning to replace the system of seeing different midwives.
Influence of scientific evidence on practice	Varies considerably but customs, opinions and fear of litigation are more powerful influences.	Leaders in obstetrics, family medicine, nursing and midwifery are actively engaged in the scientific evaluation of numerous unproved clinical practices. There is a widespread acceptance of the need for evidence based practice.
Influence of fear of litigation on practice	The likelihood of doctors being sued is high and insurance expensive. Insurers advise on how to reduce the possibility of law suits. This advice is not based on science, safety or effectiveness but on risks of being sued.	There are similar trends although it has less impact on care than scientific findings, costs, customs and other factors.

primary care provider informing them that the client is receiving bodywork and inviting contact if there are any issues that the care provider has concerns about. This letter can be given to the client to give to her primary careprovider at her next visit.

Identifying the primary care provider

It is important to identify who provides primary care in the community and to find out more about them.

- What guidelines exist for the practice of these primary care providers?
- What services are included?
- Who pays for the services – e.g. government, extended healthcare plans, the client?
- Are there a variety of options for primary care provider and who makes that choice?

The answers to these questions vary from country to country. In the UK the main primary care provider for the low-risk client is often the midwife who is seen as 'the guardian of normal birth'. The woman tends to see the obstetrician more if there are complications as obstetricians specialise in the abnormal.

In the USA and Canada most women first go to see their obstetrician/gynaecologist and may not see a midwife at all. In many European countries there is a mixture of midwifery and obstetric care. Table 15.2 compares some of the main features of US and UK care.

Building positive relationships with primary care providers

In order to support a model of integrated care, the therapist can write to the clinics and hospitals in their area introducing themselves and their work. Free treatments or demonstrations, within the scope of practice, may be offered so that the primary care provider can experience at first hand the kind of work which is being offered by the therapist.

Some therapists offer to do a presentation at an antenatal class. This may be initially on a voluntary basis, for example offering to run a short session on the benefits of bodywork during labour with some practical demonstrations, but sometimes this can lead to paid work. Some therapists set up bodywork practices within hospital settings. Other therapists build relationships with primary caregivers where they can discuss cases, with the woman's consent, or ask for information on specific conditions.

Bodyworkers can put themselves forward to sit on medical boards or maternity committees in their local health authority. For example the principal author sat as the lay representative for 5 years on the maternity services liaison committee for Avon (1995–2000). This committee discussed issues relating to the maternity services. This offers a good opportunity to meet clinicians and be aware of local issues, as well as being able to represent the bodyworker's point of view and make oneself known within the community. From her contacts on this committee, she was then asked to sit on the labour ward committee in the local hospital.

Sometimes there are local campaigns which the therapist can get involved in, which link together not only primary caregivers but also all those in the area who are interested in maternity issues. For example in Bristol, in the UK, there is an on-going campaign for establishing midwifery-led birth centres.

Another way is to know the private care providers in the area and refer clients to those.

Developing practices within clinic and hospital settings

There are several options for working in the hospital setting:

- A clinic space can be established within the hospital; this can be on the basis of renting a room within the hospital and seeing clients there on a private basis.
- Work can be done with existing clients if they become hospitalised, either antenatally or postnatally.
- Clients can be supported during labour.
- Bodywork teachers can run bodywork programmes for their students in hospitals.
- Volunteer work can be offered with women from special needs groups.

- Sometimes the hospital will pay the therapist to offer specific services.

Hospital managers will want to check qualifications, insurance and experience. It can be a good idea to have a portfolio presenting a profile of the maternity work. Sometimes this forms part of course work required for maternity training.

Within the hospital setting it is important to be clear about:

- Roles/responsibilities.
- Working as part of a team.
- Identifying any specific considerations.
- Evaluating one's own work.
- Filling in hospital audit and evaluation.

Access to client/patient health information/ hospital charts

Some medical professionals and patients query the need for bodyworkers to have access to the medical charts but it can be an important adjunct to the information gathering of the therapist giving important insights into the client's background. Access to patient information/charts includes scrupulous attention to patient confidentiality which should be a basic standard of all bodywork professionals.

It is unlikely that the therapist who is hired externally by the patient on a fee for service basis would have access to the hospital data unless she has conferred with the primary care staff (with patient permission) directly.

If the therapist is working in the hospital they would possibly be required to fill out client records, fill in hospital charts, comply with hospital record keeping, evaluation and audit. These are usually quite brief and are likely to have limited space for detailed charting of bodywork. The therapist is likely to need to also complete their own longer client record form for bodywork to comply with their professional body standards.

Challenges to working in the postpartum unit

Patients can change their mind about having a treatment quite quickly depending on how long it takes to do the initial information gathering, whether the baby is fussing or not, the emotional state of the patient, her pain level, whether or not she has guests. PP treatments are often shorter.

Bodyworker as birth support person/doula

It is important to understand the role of the bodyworker at birth. They are secondary to the primary caregiver and must always defer to their expertise. Bodywork birth support is an addition to primary care. There are often legal requirements for specific primary caregivers to be present. For example in the UK it is illegal for a midwife not to be present at a home birth while in the USA it can be illegal in some states for the midwife to be present at birth. There are some specific issues which may arise in offering bodywork support.

Birth plans

Think about supporting the mother in writing a birth plan and its implications: does it encourage a flexible approach, or is it potentially setting the mother up for failure and disillusion? Wording and phraseology are important.

Working alongside the mother's partner

It is important not to take over the potential role of support that the woman's partner can offer. If the partner is engaged and involved, support and encourage them in their role and do not take over. The therapist needs to work alongside the partner as well as the primary caregiver.

Home birth or birth support at home prior to hospital admission

The therapist needs to consider what to do if the mother suddenly starts giving birth before the midwife has arrived. They would need to have basic knowledge of what to do and common scenarios which may arise as well as resuscitation skills, ideally including infant resuscitation.

How to decide when the mother is ready to go to hospital

This is a hard decision to make, simply because labour is so different for different women. The best advice is to at least make sure the contractions are regular in length and space and have been like this for at least an hour or more. They should be lasting at least 40 seconds and be 2–3 minutes apart. However, try to encourage the mother to wait till she feels she cannot cope any more.

It also depends on how far the woman is away from hospital. If it is not far, then it is usual to leave transfer as long as possible, to be sure the mother is in active labour. If the distance is greater, then the mother will have to go in earlier. The main thing is to encourage the mother to stay relaxed so that she can try to tune in to when she is ready. Bear in mind most women go to hospital too early, especially with a first baby, and this may have the effect of slowing labour down.

If the mother is in labour during the day, it is often possible to ask the primary caregiver to come and check her at home before she goes into hospital.

Knowing when to call the midwife if supporting a home birth

This is a little easier, as the midwife can always go away if the mother is in early labour. Again, usually women call the midwife out too early.

How to work with the midwife and other primary caregivers

The role of a midwife and other primary caregivers is to support normal birth. By working to support the mother's body the therapist is supporting that natural process. Most primary caregivers will be pleased that the mother has this additional support, especially as many mothers just want to lie down, have an epidural and not be actively involved in the process. Of course, if things are not going well and the mother needs to be monitored or have some kind of intervention, then it is important to cooperate with her medical carers. While not interfering with the tasks of primary carers in an emergency situation, if it is often possible to continue to support the mother to remain as in touch with her body as much as she can, in order to reduce stress. This is especially important if she wants to try to have as natural a birth as possible. For example primary caregivers may want the mother to lie on her back to be monitored, but if she wants to lie on her side or be on all fours then that is usually possible. If there really is no other option than to lie on her back and the birth becomes a medical emergency, then there will be no doubt that that is what needs to happen.

Bodyworker as childbirth educator

If the therapist starts to teach exercises or bodywork outside the one-to-one sessions with their clients they are getting into the realm of antenatal and postnatal education. It is important to be aware if there are any issues that entails, such as insurance cover and any particular training or affiliations to particular professional bodies.

Once the therapist has verified that they can apply bodywork skills to teaching classes, various options open up. There can be classes for example on massage that partners can do for the mother during pregnancy or in the postnatal period. Birth preparation classes can be run with a focus on using bodywork skills. The therapist might decide to team up with yoga teachers or midwives to offer a more complete package.

Collaborating with other complementary therapists

As always, it is important to recognise the limits to one's practice and know when the client might benefit from referral to another type of therapist. It can be useful to build up a referral list of local practitioners who specialise in working with pregnant and postpartum clients.

Testimonials

Diane

Great Expectations, Canada

After moving to the Windsor, Ontario, area, I was curious as to why there were not more RMTs in the area who focused principally on maternity work. If you peruse the yellow pages, most RMTs advertise pregnancy in their list of 'conditions' that they are willing to treat. But not one focused only on maternity work/support. After continuing my education and furthering my understanding in pregnancy, labour and delivery and the postpartum period through Trimesters Prenatal Education, I had a vision in my mind to instil these values into my every day practice. To lay my hands on a mom-to-be every so often just was not enough for me. I craved more practice, and more knowledge of the delicate balance between mom and baby's minds, bodies and souls; knowledge that would only come with time. I have a strong passion and desire to give moms the attention and reassurance that they deserve while growing, giving birth to and caring for their children.

I opened Great Expectations Family Massage Therapy in 2004 (Windsor area), a home-based business focusing on perinatal massage, labour support and shiatsu in maternity care. (I now also offer WATSU, a form of shiatsu performed in the water.) I advertised everywhere where I thought expectant women would be. Maternity clothing stores, yoga studios, daycares, the midwive's office, obstetrician's offices, fitness centres, and the list goes on. I developed a website that would direct women to learn more about the importance of massage therapy during pregnancy. I began to massage many expectant women, who told their expectant friends, who told their midwives and obstetricians about my services. I contacted the local midwives (who had just come to the Windsor area and gained hospital rights). Slowly but surely, 75% of new intakes were pregnant! My motto quickly became 'build it and they will come'.

I have built a good rapport with other healthcare providers by providing confident and individualised methods of massage. My dream is to one day be the first name that comes to mind when an expectant mother asks for help with a sore back, or swollen ankles, or stress relief.

I believe that my clients value the education that I have completed, the good working relationship I have built with other healthcare providers and most importantly the experience that I have gained in working with pregnancy and labour and delivery. Had I not focused my practice, the level of experience I have today might not have been gained until years down the road. I also believe that focusing my practice has opened my eyes to other avenues I will be able to explore once my career as an RMT is over. Entering midwifery, nursing, or continuing to attend deliveries as a doula are all sustainable ways to satisfy my passion for this field.

Catherine Tugnait

Birth Educator and Maternity Therapist, UK

My interest was aroused in becoming a maternity therapist in 2004 when I had been teaching National Childbirth Trust classes for 4 years. My clients often complained of normal pregnancy ailments and bemoaned the fact that they could not get a good massage as many therapist considered pregnancy to be a contraindication. I signed up for a general massage course and then completed Suzanne's massage and pregnancy diploma. Later I studied reflexology, specialising in maternity reflexology.

Now I work with pregnant women on a daily basis. In addition to my private work as a maternity therapist, I work as an NCT teacher and do outreach work in children's centres, with women who would not normally be able to access antenatal education and therapies. I also work at a local refuge for women who are victims of domestic violence and volunteer at a respite cafe for parents with children who have developmental and communication problems such as autism and Down syndrome. It feeds my soul to treat those parents with therapies to help them cope with the stress that life throws at them. I try to build therapies into all aspects of my work. I share lots of skills with birth partners, so that they can use therapies in labour and also with the women themselves to work their own shiatsu points for conditions such as morning sickness and carpal tunnel syndrome, and labour priming points when they are post dates. I am about to start running courses in the children's centre to teach women how to do some basic reflexology for friends and family including their children. I incorporate postnatal sessions into my NCT courses and children's centre workshops to teach the mums how to massage their babies and I use many shiatsu points in this, especially the stomach meridian for digestive issues.

Cindy

As bodyworkers, we need to be reminders – to the clients we serve and their families; to our professional colleagues in the field who may never have had the honour to attend to a 'normal' pregnancy or a 'healthy' home birth within an environment of both nurturance and empowerment which considers the 'CARE' of the family as the primary issue. We can encourage, support, celebrate and honour those who have babies at this time in our culture, as well as those who work in this field on every level. Whether working together or on our own, we can shift the milieu of pregnancy and birth back to a place of health and well-being. Our professional opportunity to do so makes our work an incredible gift.

Reference

Northrup, C., 1998. Women's Bodies, Women's Wisdom. Piatkus Books, London.

Useful contacts and resources

Initially this was intended to be a comprehensive list of all the useful contacts and information that therapists need to support their practice. The reality of compiling this for a worldwide audience, combined with the ever-changing details, meant that we decided to highlight areas of useful exploration with some ideas of starting points to guide the therapist, rather than a comprehensive list.

Physical resources

Cushions, bolsters, futons

As outlined in the chapter on equipment (Ch. 8), it is useful to have a wide range of cushions, beanbags and so on. There are many specialist massage suppliers but often cheaper and equally effective alternatives can be purchased from a futon or soft furnishing shop (for example IKEA sells relatively inexpensive cushions and futons). For plastic-covered wedges and cushions then it may be necessary to go direct to a massage suppliers. For large sausage or triangular pillows then specialist maternity shops which sell breastfeeding cushions can be an option.

Balls

These can be purchased from most sports shops as exercise balls. So-called 'maternity' balls are simply the same thing. Special ball cushions can also be brought from specialised places: these are like a plastic disc which can be placed on a chair to make it like a ball.

Beanbags

These can be brought from some soft-furnishing shops but there are some varieties on the market which have a 'hole' for the pregnant abdomen. One of the main ones is the 'belly bag', developed in Australia.

Thebellybag.co.uk
Bellybag.com.au

Charts and models

These can be useful tools for aiding explanations to clients. They include: model uterus with baby, model pelvis, chart of changes in uterus and fetal development.

Some suppliers

www.Physiomed.com – 01457 860444

A UK-based online company which sells massage and exercise equipment including plastic-covered wedges, balls, disc cushions.

www.limbsandthings.com

Health education models including model uterus www.healthedco.com and www.childbirthgraphics.com Are part of a company based in West Sussex, UK, which sell charts and models.

www.birthinternational.com

UK- and Australian-based company, incorporating ACE graphics which sell worldwide: books, charts, models and DVDS and books.

Icea.org

An American-based childbirth organisation which also sells books and charts.

Oil suppliers

Maternity clients benefit from the best-quality oils. There are many suppliers. Some of our favourites include:

Forest Essentials
www.forestessentialsindia.com
Ayurvedic oils including: neem oil, coconut, cocoa
  butter, and mother and baby blends.

Fragrant Earth
www.fragrantearth.com
Company founded by Jan Kismirek, author of Liquid Sunshine and consultant to Elemis. Based in Somerset, UK. Good-quality base oils.

Essential oil resource consultants
Bob and Rhiannon Harris. Providers of research, education and information in the field of essential oils.

www.essentialoil.com
essentialorc@club-internet.fr

The International Journal of Clinical Aromatherapy
www.ijca.net

The International Journal of Essential Oil Therapeutics
www.ijeot.com

Canadian oil and equipment suppliers:

Know Your Body Best
200 Queens Quay East #3-1
Toronto
Ontario M5A 4K9
Canada
tel: 416-367-3744
fax: 416-367-3364
1-800-881-1681
www.knowyourbodybest.com
info@knowyourbodybest.com

Canadian Massage Supplies

www.canadianmassagesupply.ca

Tui body balm; beeswax based wax.

Tui Bee Balme Co-operative Golden Bay New Zealand
tuibee@voyager.co.nz

Useful tools for mothers

It can be useful to have some local contacts for resources such as specialist nursing bras; Bravado is a good make.

www.bravadodesigns.com

It could also be useful to know local or web suppliers of things like:
Plastic disc to sit on
Belts for SPD
Or the bodyworker could have one or two of their own discs which they lend out to clients.

Books

There are some specialist pregnancy bookstores:
Parent Books

www.parentbooks.ca

Obstetric, physiotherapy and midwifery information

It is useful to access these organisations for information on current obstetric and midwifery guidelines as well as physiotherapist exercise and care guidelines.

Obstetricians

RCOG UK Royal College of Obstetricians and Gynaecologists
www.rcog.org.uk
AOCG American College of Obstetricians and Gynecologists
www.acog.org
SOGC Society of Obstetricians and Gynaecologists of Canada
www.sogc.org
sogc.org/guidelines
sogc.org/links
sogc.org/health/pregnancy
sogc.org/health/pregnancy-resources

Midwives

Canada:

Canadian Association of Midwives
www.canadianmidwives.org
www.canadianmidwives.org/links

UK:

Royal College of Midwives
www.rcm.org.uk

Australia:

www.midwives.org.au

USA:

amcbmidwife.org

Physiotherapists/physical therapists

UK:

www.csp.org.uk
Association of Chartered Physiotherapists in Obstetrics and Gynaecology
14 Bedford Row
London WC1R 4ED, UK

USA:

American Physical Therapists Association (APTA)
www.apta.org

Information sites
MIDIRS

www.midirs.org

Midwifery information and resource. Useful for leaflets, journal, digest and resources.
  NICE and NHS guidelines
www.nhs.uk
www.nice.org.uk

Cochrane Review; assesses research.

www.nelh.nhs.uk/cochrane.asp

Midwifery Today; US-based organisation, publishes newsletters and organises conferences.

www.midwiferytoday.com

General resource sites

Motherisk
www.motherisk.org

Childbirth Connection

www.childbirthconnection.org

March of Dimes

marchofdimes.com

MIDIRS Resources also on maternity organisations

Informed choice leaflets, MIDIRS digest

Support and special issues groups

There are support groups on most maternity issues from miscarriage to toxoplasmosis to specific genetic defects. MIDIRS in the UK has a directory of different groups and it is worth finding out what local contacts there are for these groups which are often national.
  To give some examples of some of the themes of the groups:

Sexual abuse
Prison women; Sheila Kitzinger:
  www.sheilakitzinger.com
TWINS and multiple birth groups.
Miscarriage
Pelvic girdle support groups:
  British Pelvic Girdle Support Group
  Pelvicpartnership.org.uk
  Pelvic instability network pelvicgirdlepaincom
    support (PINS)

Birth Crisis; this is an organisation that helps women who have had a difficult birth
Traumatic birth; www.sheilakitzinger.com/birthcrisis
NET mums; this is a UK web-based support and information resource for parents
Fathers to be: http://www.fatherstobe.org
Homebirth: http://www.homebirth.org.uk/
Spinning Babies is a step-by-step approach to optimal fetal positioning: http://spinningbabies.com/
AIMS: Association for Improvement in Maternity Services www.aims.org
Maternity Alliance: www.maternityalliance.co.uk

Breastfeeding
UK:
Association of Breastfeeding Mothers
www.abm.me.uk – 08444122949

National Childbirth Trust
www.nct.org.uk – 03003300771

La Leche League
www.laleche.org.uk – 08151202918

Breastfeeding Network
www.breastfeedingnetwork.org.uk – 08444124664

National breastfeeding helpline 08442090920 (run by the Association of Breastfeeding Mothers and the Breastfeeding Network).
Australia:
www.breastfeeding.asn.au

Exercise groups
There are some national organisations which regulate some of the main types of exercises which are useful in pregnancy such as: Yoga, Pilates, exercise. It is worth finding out the key maternity experts.

Childbirth education groups
Antenatal Alliance UK
NCT
www.nct.org

ICEA International Childbirth
www.icea.org

Birthing from Within:
http://www.birthingfromwithin.com/

Active Birth Centre:
http://www.activebirthcentre.com/

Other organisations:
Association for Pre and Perinatal Psychology and Health
APPAH www.birthpscyhology.com

Doula organisations

These are the most established in the USA where there are fewer midwives.
ALACE

www.alace.org

DONA

Doulas of North America
Doula UK

Bodywork professional organisations

It can be useful to know the main regulating bodywork organisations. This includes the main organisations which offer maternity education.

Index

Notes: Page numbers followed by "f" indicate figures, "t" indicate tables, and "b" indicate boxes.

Printed in the United States
By Bookmasters